Biostatistics for Nurses

Biostatistics for Nurses

BT Basavanthappa MN PhD
Ex-Professor and Principal
Government College of Nursing
Bengaluru, Karnataka, India
PhD Guide for Research Work

Member
Faculty of Nursing, Academic Council
Rajiv Gandhi University of Health Sciences
Bengaluru, Karnataka, India

Examiner
UG, PG and Doctoral Courses on Nursing, Various Universities

Ex-Program In-charge
Indira Gandhi National Open University
BSc Nursing Course, Karnataka and Goa, India

Life Member
Nursing Research Society of India
Trained Nurses Association of India
New Delhi, India

President
Nursing Teachers Association
Rajiv Gandhi University of Health Sciences
Bengaluru, Karnataka, India

Winner
Bharat Excellence Award and Gold Medal
Vikas Ratan Gold Award
United Writers Association (UWA) Lifetime Achievement Award
Shree Veeranjaneya "Shrujanashri" Award

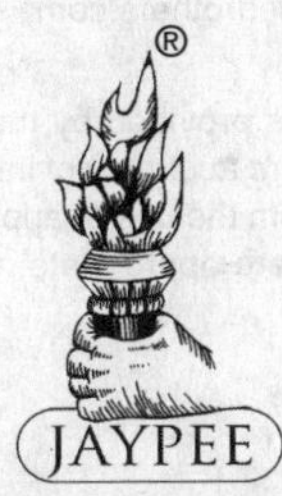

JAYPEE BROTHERS MEDICAL PUBLISHERS (P) LTD

New Delhi • London • Philadelphia • Panama

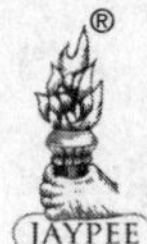

Jaypee Brothers Medical Publishers (P) Ltd

Headquarter

Jaypee Brothers Medical Publishers (P) Ltd
4838/24, Ansari Road, Daryaganj
New Delhi 110 002, India
Phone: +91-11-43574357
Fax: +91-11-43574314
Email: jaypee@jaypeebrothers.com

Overseas Offices

J.P. Medical Ltd.
83, Victoria Street, London
SW1H 0HW (UK)
Phone: +44-2031708910
Fax: +02-03-0086180
Email: info@jpmedpub.com

Jaypee-Highlights Medical Publishers Inc.
City of Knowledge, Bld. 237, Clayton
Panama City, Panama
Phone: + 507-301-0496
Fax: + 507-301-0499
Email: cservice@jphmedical.com

Jaypee Medical Inc.
The Bourse
111, South Independence Mall East
Suite 835, Philadelphia, PA 19106, USA
Phone: + 267-519-9789
Email: joe.rusko@jaypeebrothers.com

Jaypee Brothers Medical Publishers (P) Ltd
17/1-B Babar Road, Block-B, Shaymali
Mohammadpur, Dhaka-1207
Bangladesh
Mobile: +08801912003485
Email: jaypeedhaka@gmail.com

Jaypee Brothers Medical Publishers (P) Ltd
Shorakhute, Kathmandu
Nepal
Phone: +00977-9841528578
Email: jaypee.nepal@gmail.com

Website: www.jaypeebrothers.com
Website: www.jaypeedigital.com

Inquiries for bulk sales may be solicited at: jaypee@jaypeebrothers.com

Biostatistics for Nurses

First Edition: **2014**

ISBN 978-93-5025-372-4

Printed at Sanat Printers, Kundli

Dedicated to

My parents
Late Shri Thukkappa
&
Smt Hanumanthama
and also
My dear students of
Nursing Community

Preface

It gives me immense pleasure and satisfaction to present this book *Biostatistics for Nurses* to nursing community. In offering the title, I remain grateful to readers who have supported my all 22 titles on nursing and giving fruitful comments.

Nurses need Biostatistics in many ways. It helps nurses to calculate and know the biological values, laboratory values, vital statistics and calculate the dosage of drugs, infusion, transfusion and their duration and also helps to identify mistakes, abnormalities in values and others. All these help to plan the nursing care. Keeping these in view, I have designed the book to acquaint the nurses and nursing students with statistical techniques most commonly used and reported in the nursing literature. I have attempted to make the book user-friendly by keeping the things which are required for the nurses and nursing students. Without statistics, a research cannot be fulfilled one. Statistical analysis helps nurse researchers to make sense of quantitative information. Without statistics, quantitative data would be chaotic mass of numbers. Statistical procedure enables researchers to summarize, organize, evaluate, interpret, and communicate numeric information.

This book has been sequentially organized into 20 chapters and efforts have been made to keep contents that are prescribed by the regulatory bodies of nursing courses. Each chapter in the book is self-contained and serves the purpose of the course subject, and it has been made more concised and relevant to the needs of the students. This book is supposed to be valuable and serve the purpose.

I am aware that errors might be crept in and shall feel obliged if such errors are brought to my notice. I sincerely welcome any suggestions for further improvement of this title and that will be highly appreciated.

BT Basavanthappa

Acknowledgments

I owe a great deal of thanks to many who encouraged and supported me with their time and encouragement throughout.

- Shri G Basavannappa, Former Minister of Karnataka State, for having initiated and supported me to take up the "Noble Nursing Profession" as my career.
- Dr Manjula K Vasundhra, Former Professor and Head, Department of Community Medicine, Bangalore Medical College, Bengaluru, Karnataka, India, who continuously encouraged me to write texts in the field of Nursing because this is a major force in medical and health services.
- My father, Shri Thukkappa, who continued to grace for the progress of my career and all-round development of my personality for the welfare of the community.
- My mother, Smt Hanumanthama, who continues to be a bright spot in the lives of all who knew her and whose grace gave me strength to progress in my life.
- My wife, Smt Lalitha, who gives meaning to my life in so many ways. She is the one whose encouragement keeps me motivated, whose support gives me strength and whose gentleness gives me comfort.
- My lovely children, BB Mahesh and BB Ganashree, for all the joy they provided to me and all the hope that they instill in me and they bear with patience throughout my works of the nursing texts. They keep me young at heart.
- Finally, my warmest appreciation goes to M/s Jaypee Brothers Medical Publishers (P) Ltd, New Delhi, India, for sharing my vision for this book and giving me the chance to turn vision into reality.
- In addition, I am particularly indebted to the faculty, nursing students and nurses, who have put their faith in my titles to assist them on their path of excellence and also I appreciate the many who have shared their comments and suggestions in the previous editions of my titles.

Contents

CHAPTER 1 Concepts of Statistics

Introduction

The word 'Statistics' is very old and that similar words can be found in ancient languages such as 'Status' in Latin, 'Statista' in Italian and 'Statistik' in German. 'Status' means the position of affair at a particular time. The meaning of all these words is "Political State". In ancient times, the Government used to collect the information on the affairs of the state regarding population and property or wealth of the country, the former enabling the government to have an idea of the manpower of the country and the latter providing a basis for introducing new taxes and levies.

As stated earlier the word 'statistics' appears to have been derived from the word 'status' meaning a (political) state. In its origin, statistics was simply the collection of numerical datas by kings, on different aspects useful to the state. With the passage of time, however, its scope began to include collection of numerical data pertaining to almost every endeavor, calculations of percentages, etc. and presentation of data in tables and charts. Later on statistics of births, and deaths, marriages and divorces, of mental abilities of persons, of population, imports and exports and the like has been practiced. Now statistics is not only with the collection and presentation of data, but also with interpretation and drawing of inferences from the data.

Statistics is the practice or science of collecting and analyzing numerical data in large quantities, especially, for the purpose of inferring proportions in a whole, from those in a representational sample. For a layman it conveys an impression about numerical facts. Since health care, medical and nursing are considered scientific disciplines, statistics means the methodology of collection, compilation and interpretation of numerical facts.

The science of statistics is essentially a branch of mathematics and may be regarded as mathematics applied to observational data (RA Fisher).

Statistics is a branch of applied mathematics with roots in a part of mathematics called probability theory and it is fundamental to all observational sciences—physical science, biological science, social science, medical science and nursing science. Statistics is a main partner, wherever observations are made, recorded in numerical form and analyzed for the purpose of reaching scientific conclusions or judgments. The term 'statistics' has been used to indicate facts and figures of any kind: Health Statistics, Vital Statistics, Business Statistics, etc. Normally science with statistics bears good fruits. Statistics without scientific applications has no roots.

Definition of Statistics

Statistics are the classified facts representing the conditions of the people in a state especially those facts which can be stated in number or in a table of numbers or in any tabular or classified arrangements (Webster).

- Statistics is a numerical statement of facts in any department of enquiry placed in relation to each other (AL Bowley). According to him statistics is the science of counting, science of average and the science of measurement of social phenomena
- By statistics we mean the aggregate of facts affected to a marked extent by multiplicity of causes, numerically expressed, enumerated or estimated according to reasonable standards of accuracy, collected in a systematic manner for predetermined purpose and placed in relation to each other—(Horace Secrist)
- Statistics is the science of estimates and probabilities (AL Boddington)
- Statistics is the study of methods and procedures for collecting, classifying, summarizing and analyzing data and for making scientific inference from such data (PV Sukhatme)
- Statistics is a field of study concerned with the organization and summarization of data and the drawing of inferences about a body of data when only a part of the data are observed. (Wayne W Daniel)
- Statistics may be defined as the collection, organization, presentation, analysis and interpretation of numerical data (Croxton and Cowden). Accordingly, the terms used in this definition mean as given below:
  - ***Collection***: Collection of data constitutes first step in statistical investigation. Utmost care is required to collecting data because they form the foundation of Statistical Analysis. The conclusions drawn on faulty collection of data can never be reliable.
  - ***Organization***: Data collected from published sources has to be organized with the help of editing. The collected data must be edited very carefully so that the omission, inconsistencies, irrelevant answers and wrong computation may be corrected and adjusted. After the data has been edited, the next step is to classify them. The last step in organization is tabulation. The purpose of tabulation is to present data in row and column-wise, so that there is clarity in the data presented. So organization also includes classification and tabulation.
  - ***Presentation***: After the data have been collected and organized, they are ready for presentation in the form of diagrams and graphs.
  - ***Analysis***: The next step is analysis. The purpose of analyzing the data is to dig out information useful for decision-making using statistical analysis such as, measures of central tendency, measures of variation, correlation, regression, etc.
  - ***Interpretation***: The next stage in statistical investigation is interpretation, i.e., drawing conclusion from the data collected and analyzed. The interpretation of data is a difficult task and necessitates a high degree of skill and experience.
- Statistics is also defined as the "scientific study of numerical data based on natural phenomena". Terms used in this definition give more understanding. They are as follows:
  - ***Scientific study***: Statistics has criteria of validity of scientific evidence. Objectively in the presentation and evaluation of data in the general ethical code of scientific methodology must constantly be in evidence.
  - ***Data***: Statistics generally deals with populations and groups of individuals, hence it deals with quantities of information, not with single datum.
  - ***Numerical***: Unless the data of a study can be quantified in one way or the other, they would not be amenable to statistical analysis. Numerical data may be measurements, the length or width or width of a structure or the amount of a chemical in a body fluid—or counts—the number of bristles or teeth.
  - ***Natural Phenomena***: Which include all those events that happen in animate or inanimate nature not under the control of

man, plus those evoked by the scientists and partly under his control as in experiments.

Features of Statistics

According to the definitions stated above, the essential features of the statistics are as follows.

i. Principles and methods for the collection, presentation, analysis and interpretation of numerical data of different kinds include:
   - Observational data, quantitative data (measurement, survey data)
   - Data that has been obtained by repetitive operation (experimental data)
   - Data affected to a marked degree by a multiplicity of causes.

ii. The science of the art of dealing with variation in such a way as to obtain reliable results.

iii. Controlled, objective methods whereby group trends are abstracted from observations on many separate individuals.

iv. The science of experimentation, which may be regarded as mathematics applied to observational data.

Characteristics of Statistics

According to secrist the following are the characteristics of statistics:

- Statistics are the aggregate of facts.
- Statistics are numerically expressed.
- Statistics are affected to a marked extent by multiplicity of causes and not by a single cause.
- Statistics should be collected in a systematic manner.
- Statistics should be collected for a predetermined purpose.
- Statistics should be placed in relation to each other.
- The reasonable standard of accuracy should be maintained in statistics.

Merits of Statistics

- Statistics helps in presenting large quantity of data in a simple and classified form.
- It gives methods of comparison of data and it weighs and judges them in the right perspective.
- It enlarges the individual mind.
- It, when considered as the logic of figures, assists in arriving at correct views based on facts.
- It helps in finding the conditions of relationship between the variables.
- It tries to give material for the businessmen as well as the administrators so as to serve as a guide in planning and in shaping future policies and programs.
- It proves useful in a number of fields like Railways, Banks, Army, Health, including medical and nursing, etc.

Demerits of Statistics

1. *Statistical laws are held to be true on the average or in the long run.* They are not exact laws true in every case. Statistics deals with phenomena affected by a large number of causes. Many of these causes have to be neglected or studied jointly with other more important causes. As such the conclusions arrived under similar conditions at all times, are not identical though they are of the same nature.
2. *Statistics does not take cognizance of individual cases.* It deals with aggregates, though for purposes of analysis these aggregates are very often reduced to single figures. Thus, the average income of a group of persons in the group might have become poorer than what they were before.
3. *Statistical data must always be treated as approximations* or estimates and not as precise measurement. This is particularly so in business or economic studies where experiments cannot be carried out under controlled conditions.
4. *Statistical methods cannot be applied to facts, that cannot be measured quantitatively* such as, health, culture, intelligence, poverty, etc. These subjective concepts will have to be related in an indirect fashion to numerical data before they can be studied statistically.

5. *Statistical results are ascertained by samples.* If the selection of samples is biased, errors will accumulate and results will not be reliable.
6. The greatest limitation of statistics is that *only one who has an expert knowledge of statistical methods can efficiently handle statistical data. Statistic*s, like medicine in the hands of quacks are capable of being easily misused by the non-expert. Knowingly or unknowingly, such a person can draw faulty conclusions.
7. *Statistical results might lead to fallacious conclusions if they are quoted without their context.* Thus the average marks of two students for three examinations might be the same but one may be improving from bad preparation to good while the other may be deteriorating in his studies.

Statistical thinking and operations in research are very important from a variety of standpoints. The application of statistics pervades all subject matters. Its use has permeated almost every facet of our lives. It is a knot of all scieces, indispensable to search an intelligent judgment and has become a recognized discipline in its own right. It has been used in almost all fields including trade, industry, commerce, economics, biology, physics, chemistry, education, medicine, nursing and so on. For example, in nursing for assessment of conditions of the patient, nurse relies on actual data like temperature, pulse rate, respiration and blood pressure.

Generally, statistics permits the use of descriptive language which is more efficient and exact in communications. They disallow any vague conclusion and emphasize arriving at definite ones. These techniques enable us to present the results in a summarized, more meaningful and convenient form and thus bring order out of chaos. Further it enables us to draw generalizations and make predictions.

In addition, the study of statistics is gaining further impetus because of the facts as given below:

- Professional literature is replete with statistical symbols, concepts and ideas
- All advanced courses of study require a formal course work in statistics
- Professional training of a nurse scientists includes the requirements of the study of statistics
- Statistics are widely used in research in all fields of human knowledge

So, the main functions of statistics includes the following:

- It presents facts in a definite form
- It simplifies mass of figures
- It facilitates comparison
- It helps in formulating and testing hypothesis
- It helps in prediction
- It helps in formation of suitable policies.

Limitations of Statistics

1. The main limitation of statistics is that it cannot deal with a single observation or value.
2. Statistical methods are not applicable to studies which measure qualitative characters and cannot be coded in numerical value.
3. The statistical study does not take care of the changes occurring to the individuals. But it does reveal the changes occurring in a mass or group of individuals. For instance, per capita gross national product (GNP) at factor cost in 1980 is Rs. 673.80 and in 2000 it is Rs. 1690.30. On the basis of these figures it can definitely be concluded that per capita GNP has increased by more than Rs. 1000 but it must be kept in mind that it gives no information about an individual.
4. Statistical statements or conclusions are generally not true or applicable to individuals but are applicable to the majority of cases. For instance, the statistical information says that 90 per cent patients of a particular disease die during operation. If a doctor has performed nine operations so far and all the nine patients have died during operation, he still cannot assure the tenth patient will be cured after the operation.

There can be hundreds of situations which can be enunciated under the heading of limitations of statistics. These ideas are of common sense and can be thought of by individuals themselves.

Some people think that the inferences based on statistical data are very reliable as the numbers can not be false while others do not trust statistical results at all. According to the nonbelievers these numerals are the tissues of falsehood as Disraeli said "There are three degrees of lies—lies, damned lies and statistics." Darrell Huff said "A well wrapped statistics is better than Hitler's 'big lie', it misleads, yet it cannot be pinned on you. Another statement by Huff showing his distrust in statistics is "The secret language of statistics, so appealing in a fact minded culture, is employed to sensationalize, inflate, confuse and oversimplify." All this confusion has emerged due to the fact that it is not easy to differentiate between fictitious data and the data collected and tabulated in a well-planned manner.

Statistics is misused either deliberately or often due to the lack of knowledge. As defined earlier statistics is a tool, technique or an approach to deal with the data to arrive at correct conclusion or decision. If intelligibly used, it gives wonderfully good results and if misused, it can be disastrous. This can be very well supported by the statement, "Figures would not lie, but liars figure." Another statement in support of the misuse of statistics is "statistics is like clay, of which you can make a god or a devil."

Types of Statistics

There are many branches of applied statistics depending on the area of applications as given below:

- Biostatistics—Related to biological events
- Medical statistics—Data from clinical profession which usually tells us the proportion of change
- Vital Statistics—Data from all vital events, e.g. Birth, Deaths, Marriages, etc.
- Population Statistics—Data from demography, e.g. Age, Sex, Education, Income, etc.
- Hospital Statistics—Mortality, utility of, hospital service, utilization, etc.
- Health Statistics—Data of medical and health sciences. Most of the occasions it is quantitative data.

Meaning of Biostatistics

Biostatistics is the branch of statistics applied to biological science including medical science. It is also known as biometry, i.e. literally meaning "Biological measurement". In Greek 'Bio' means life and 'metro' means 'measured'. Hence biometry means measurement of life. It may be stated as the application of statistical methods to the solution of biological problems. Today 'Biostatistics' is the scientific study of handling quantitative information. Medical statistics or biostatistics can be called quantitative medicine. It embodies a methodology of collection, classification, description and interpretation of data obtained through the conduct of surveys and experiment. The main purpose is to draw and describe inferences about the numerical properties of populations. The population can be finite population that have enumerable elements or infinite population.

As stated earlier statistics is the study of methods and procedures for collection, organization, presentation, analysis and interpretation of numerical data. For a nurse or any health care provider, the statistics means the methodology of collection, compilation and interpretation of numerical facts. The numerical facts which one comes across in health sciences such as, pulse rate, hemoglobin percentage level, number of people suffering from various diseases, number of births and deaths taking place, etc. are all affected and controlled to a large extent by a number of factors —biological, environmental, social and so on. Hence, whenever the meaning of certain numerical figures is to be understood and their cause and effect in terms of different factors is to be elicited, certain procedures are to be followed. The methodology of such collection and meaningful interpretation of numerical facts is known as "Statistics".

Biostatistics which is an applied branch of statistics in very heavily utilized for health sciences including nursing science. Biostatistics is a applied scientific discipline rather than a basic or fundamental study. Its roots lie in mathematics, but its branches touch all areas of biology, medicine, nursing, and public health. When the data is being analyzed or derived from the biological sciences and health sciences, we use the term 'biostatistics' to distinguish the particular application of statistical tools and concepts as given below:

- Biostatistics is the science and art of collection, compilation presentation, analysis and interpretation of numerical data concerned with biological events which are affected by the multiple factors.
- Biostatistics is the science which applies the theory of probability to the making of estimates and inferences about the characteristics of population.
- Biostatistics is the branch of statistics which deals with the methodologies of collection, elucidation and interpretation of numerical facts relating to the biological sciences, particularly from the field of medicine, public health and nursing.
- Health statistics is the branch of biostatistics and particularly deals with the methodology of collection, compilation and interpretation of numerical facts concerned with the health and ill-health of the human population. Some of these are births, diseases, deaths and the different features related to them. However, when numerical facts dealing with only birth, death, marriages, divorces, etc. in the light of the then related facts are considered, the branch of statistics is known as "Vital Statistics".
- In plural form statistics denotes collection of numbers, facts, and figures. In singular form, it is science of figures.
- Health statistic is a science of collection, processing, analysis and transformation of data, which is required for organizing and implementing health services. As such, collected figure is 'data' which when analyzed, yield 'information'. By experience when information is put to practice it becomes intelligence.

There are several measures to help describe the characteristics of a population. Measurements of samples generate some numerical values like an arithmetical average. These values are termed as 'estimates or statistics'. Values which are descriptive of the population are called 'Parameters'. Parameters are generally estimated from sample statistics though the former description exists. These may, however, remain unknown for reasons of convenience. For example, generally, a preponderance of measurement occurs somewhere around the middle of the range of population of measurement. Thus, some indication of a population 'average' would express a useful bit of descriptive information. Such information is called a "measures of central tendency" and several such measures include the mean and the median. It is also important to describe how dispersed the measurements are around the 'average'. Such descriptive property is called 'measures of dispersion' and several such measures are the range and the standard deviation.

A quantity such as measures of central tendency or as measures of dispersion is called a parameter when it describes or characterizes a population. It is very difficult to calculate parameters but parameters can be estimated very well by random sampling of population. An estimate of a population parameter is called statistics. It is biostatistical convention to represent population parameters by Greek letter and sample statistics by Roman letters. For examples the symbols 'σ' and μ (Greek letter Sigma and Mu) may be used to represent population standard deviation and mean respectively. There are some variations in this usage and may be encountered in the literature related to statistics.

Categories of Statistics

Statistics is the study of methods and procedures for collecting, classifying, summarizing and analyzing data and for making scientific inferences from such data. Accordingly, the statistics breaks naturally into two reasonably distinct categories: descriptive statistics and inferential statistics.

Descriptive Statistics

Descriptive statistics refers to procedures for organizing, summarizing and describing quantitative data about the samples or about the population where complete population data is available. In other words, descriptive statistics serve as devices for organizing data and bringing into focus their essential characteristics for the purpose of reaching conclusions at a later stage.

Whenever our purpose is merely to describe a set of data, we are employing **descriptive statistics**. For example, one of the first things that we would want to do with our data is to graph them, to calculate means (averages) and other measures, and to look for extreme scores or oddly shaped distributions of scores. These procedures are called descriptive statistics because they are primarily aimed at describing the data. The field of descriptive statistics was once looked down on as a rather uninteresting field populated primarily by those who drew distorted-looking graphs for such publications as in magazines. In the last few years, however, the late John Tukey had developed what he calls exploratory statistics, or **exploratory data analysis (EDA)**. He has shown the necessity of paying close attention to the data and examining them in detail before invoking more technically involved procedures.

The area of descriptive statistics involves, through the use of graphic, tabular, or numerical devices, the abstraction of various properties of sets of observation. Such properties include the frequency with which various values occur, the notion of a typical or usual value, the amount of variability in a set of observation and measurement of relationship between two or more variables. So the statistical techniques, which are used in the descriptive statistics include, measures of central tendency (mean, median, mode) used measures of variability (standard deviation, average deviation and range).

Descriptive statistics does not involve the drawing of an inference from a sample to its population. It has been noticed that the field of descriptive statistics is not concerned with the implications or conclusions that can be drawn from sets of data. The primary function of descriptive statistics is to provide meaningful and convenient techniques for describing features of data that are of interest. The failure to choose appropriate descriptive statistics has often been responsible for faulty scientific inferences.

Inferential Statistics

Inferential statistics provides the procedures to draw an inference about conditions that exist in a large set of observations, from study of a part of that set. In other words, the statistical procedures used for drawing of inferences about the properties of populations from sample data are generally referred to as sampling or inferential techniques. So inferential statistics also known as sampling statistics.

After we have described our data in detail and are satisfied that we understand what the numbers have to say on a superficial level, we will be particularly interested in what is called **inferential statistics**. In fact, most of this book will deal with inferential statistics. In designing our experiment, we acknowledge that it was not possible to measure the entire population and therefore we draw samples from that population. Our basic questions, however, deal with the population itself. We might want to ask, for example, about the average self-esteem score for an entire population of students who could have taken our program, even though all that we really have is the average score for a sample of students who actually went through the program.

Inferences about population drawn from sample measures may involve some error or discrepancy, the magnitude of which can be estimated on the basis of probability theory. Hence, mere description of the numerical properties of samples is within the realm of descriptive statistics while making inferences from sample to larger groups of subjects or events on the basis of probability theory in the province of inferential statistics. Statistical inference is concerned with the procedures whereby such generalizations or inductions can be made.

This concern is most often limited to the quantitative aspects of the generalization, but more and more often in practice the statistician is asked to contribute to the process of reaching substantive conclusion as well. The ability to make generalized conclusions, inferring characteristics of the whole from characteristics of its parts, lies within the realm of inferential statistics.

Parameter Statistics

A measure, such as the average self-esteem score, that refers to an entire population is called a **parameter**. That same measure, when it is calculated from a sample of data that we have collected, is called a **statistic**. Parameters are the *real* entities of interest and the corresponding statistics are *guesses* at reality. Although, most of what we will do in this book deals with sample statistics (or guesses, if you prefer), keep in mind that the reality of interest is the corresponding population parameter. We want to *infer* something about the characteristics of the population (parameters) from what we know about the characteristics of the sample (statistics). In a similar vein, we are particularly interested in knowing whether the average self-esteem score of a population of students enrolled in our program is higher or lower, than the average self-esteem score of students not enrolled. Again we are dealing with the area of inferential statistics, since we are inferring characteristics of populations from characteristics of samples.

Variables and their Classification

The term variable refers to a property or characteristic on which the members of a group or set, differ from one another. A variable is measurable or a potentially measurable component of an object or event that may fluctuate in quantity or quality, from one individual object or event to another individual object or event of the same general class.

As stated earlier the variable is something which varies like the properties that differ from each other such as sex, age, religion, ethnicity, grade, height, weight, intelligence, attitudes, socioeconomic status and host of other such factors. So variable may be defined as 'changes or narrations that can be observed and measured'.

The term opposed to the term variable is 'constant' signifying the condition that the members of a group do not differ among themselves on this property. However, a particular property may be a variable in a specific situation and a constant in another situation. The property of sex, in a mixed group of boys and girls is a variable, while in a group of boys only, is a constant. The particular values of a variable are referred to as variable or variate values. There are two types of variations, i.e. variation between units and variation within variables can be Qualitative or Quantitative, as given below:

Qualitative Variables

A concept which can take on different quantitative values is called a variable. As stated earlier the concepts like weight, height, income are all examples of variables. Qualitative phenomena or the attributes are also quantified as the basis of the presence or absence of the concerning attributes. Variables can be on a scale consisting of values like red, white, black or white or presence or absence of a disease, etc.

Qualitative variables are also named as attributes. These variables are most capable of being described numerically. These refer to those variable which consist of categories that cannot be ordered in magnitude. For example, sex, race, religion, nationality, color of the eye or skin, etc. These characteristics are called "attributes" or attribute variate or descriptive characteristics. When classifications are to be made on the basis of attribute, groups are differentiated either by the presence and absence of the attributes (example presence or absence of a specific disease or color, etc.) or by its differing qualities. The qualities of an attribute can easily be differentiated by means of some natural or physical line of demarcation and their natural differences determine the group into which a particular item is to be placed. For example, if a specific particular is the basis of classification there will be a group of people with 'heart disease', 'diabetes', 'tuberculosis', 'diarrhea', 'cancer', 'hypertension', 'AIDS', 'malaria', etc.

Quantitative Variables

The quantitative variables refer to those variables which are composed of categories then can be ordered in magnitude. Magnitude is the quantum or quantity in which the attribute exists in various instances of the phenomena. Here the variables are those taking values on quantitative scale for which as comparison of magnitude is involved. For example height, weight, hemoglobin, calorie, natural content of food, blood count, etc.

The three categories of quantitative variables are as follows:

- **A continuous variable:** If a variable can take on any value between its minimum value and its maximum value, it is called a continuous variable. A combination variable is that which can assume any numerical value within a specific range. It may take an infinite number of values between any two points on the scale. So a continuous variable is one which is capable of being measured in any arbitrary degree of fitness or exactness. For example age, height, weight, intelligence, hemoglobin, etc.
- **A discrete variables:** The categorical variables are those variables which are not capable of being measured in any arbitrary degree of fitness/exactness because the variables contain a clear gap. A discrete variable can assume only a finite number of values between any two points on the scale. For example the size of the family—it may involve size as the variable taking the value of 0, 1, ...10 children for family or numbers cigarettes consumed per day or number of attacks of diarrhea in children during the given year.
- **An ordinal variable:** It takes the value like 'worse' 'unchanged' 'improved'. These values are often coded as 1, 2, 3,... this relative order is meaningful. The theoretical nature of the variable and not its operations of measurement makes a variable continuous or discrete.

Variables can be classified as dependent, independent and extraneous as given below:

Dependent and Independent Variables

In statistics, we also dichotomize the concept of a variable in an additional way. We speak of **independent variables** (those that are manipulated by the experimenter) and **dependent variables** (those that are not under the experimenter's control—the data). In our example, group membership is an independent variable, since we control it. We decide what the treatments will be and who will receive each treatment. The data—such as, self-esteem scores, age, personal control, and so on—are the dependent variables. Basically, the study is about the independent variables and the results of the study (the data) are the dependent variables. Independent variables may be either quantitative or qualitative, whereas dependent variables are generally, but certainly not always, quantitative.

Variables may be classified into independent and dependent categories, if their functional relationship is of interest. The expression $Y = f(x)$ signifies that the given value Y is the same unspecified function of another variable x. It stands that given a value of x and a knowledge of a functional relationship, Y can be predicted. For instance, if one variable depends upon or is a consequence of the other variable, it is termed as 'dependent variable' and the variable that is antecedent to the dependent variable is termed as independent variable. In experiments, the independent variable is the stimulus variable in whose effect the experiment is interested. The dependent variable or criterion variable appears, disappears, or varies as the independent variable is introduced, withdrawn or given in different quantities. Accordingly, dependent variable is referred to as one about which the experimenter makes a prediction.

The independent variable is referred as one which is manipulated, and selected by the experimenter for the purpose of producing observable changes in the behavioral measures. In other words, the independent variable is the one on the basis of which the prediction about the dependent variable is made. Independent variable is called the stimulus variable and dependent variable as response variable.

Independent variable may be classified into three categories depending upon the nature of the variable.

- Task variable refers to those characteristics which are associated with behavioral task presented to the subject. For example, Reaction time of experiment.
- Environmental variable refers to those characteristics of the environment which are not the physical parts of task and as such tend to produce changes in the behavioral measures. For example, Noise, temperature, illumination, etc.
- Subject variable refers to those characteristics of the subject which are likely to produce changes in the behavioral measures. For example, age, sex, weight, anxiety, intelligence, etc.

Extraneous variable: Independent variables those are not related to the purpose of the study, but may affect the dependent manipulates as 'extraneous variable'. In other words the experiment manipulates a variable only for the sake of controlling its unwanted effect upon the experimental results. Those variables are also called control variables or relevant variables. For example, if an investigator wants to study the relationship between the height and weight of the children, age will tend to affect the relationship. Because with advancement in age both height and weight of the children increase. So here it can be controlled. Whatever effect is noticed on dependent variable as a result of extraneous variable(s) is technically described as an 'experimental error'. A study must always be so designed than the effect upon the dependent variable attributes entirely to the independent variable(s) and not to some extraneous variable or variable(s).

A variable is any quantity or characteristic which may possess different numerical values or categories. Time, age, wages, prices, scores on intelligence tests, political party preference and sex are examples of variables. Some variables can be differentiated according to the number of units of some measure which they possess. Time and age are of this type since they are differentiated according to the number of years, days, months, or some other time units which are associated with them. Other variables can be differentiated only according to a described characteristic. Political preference is not divided into units of political preference, but is differentiated on the basis of Republican, Democrat, Socialist, and other political groupings. Sex is not variable in terms of numbers of units of sex, but in terms of the categories male and female. Variables which have a certain number of defined units, such as years, dollars, inches or pounds can be manipulated by the rules of mathematics and are called cardinally defined quantitative variables. Some variables do not have countable units associated with them, but can be differentiated according to some less precise definition of quantity. If each of several cakes at a country fair is judged to be best, second best, etc., down to poorest in the group, no number of units of "goodness" is indicated, but some loosely defined amount of "goodness" is implied in the differentiation. Variables which are ordered on a continuum according to some variable characteristic are said to be ordinary defined quantitative variables. Some variables cannot be differentiated according to either implied or explicity stated units. These are designated as qualitatively defined variables.

Variate values refer to the values indicated by a variable. When considered in the aggregate they constitute a series. Qualitatively defined variables are considered to have "all or nothing" variate values.

A distinction is usually made between quantitatively defined variables which are *continuous* and those which are *discrete*. A continuous variable has an unlimited number of possibilities ranging between the lowest and highest, with no gaps or breaks except at a limited number of specified values. It is said to be discontinuous at those points. A discrete variable is defined only for a series of specified values with no possibility of variate values between those points. A continuous variable is capable of indefinite refinement, but the discrete variable is distinct and separate, whereas the values of a continuous variable merge into one another by minute gradations. Age, weight, and temperature are examples of continuous variables; people, houses and automobiles are examples of discrete variables. In practice, all variables are treated as discrete units, the continuous type variables being refined to some specified discrete unit size according to the needs of the particular situation and the precision of the measuring instrument. Although length is subject to indefinite refinement in theory and can be considered to be continuous, in actual practice, length is described in discrete units of inches, hundredths of inches, milimicrons or some other specified length unit. The difference between discrete variables and the specified units used in describing a continuous variable becomes extremely important in connection with class boundaries and class limits in frequency distributions.

Measurement Scales

The aim of measurement is to provide accurate, objective, sensitive and communicable descriptions of characteristics of phenomena. The measurements are expressed in different units. Measurement refers to the process of assigning numerals to events, objects, etc. according to certain rules. The main properties of measurements include the following:

- In the process of measurement numbers are assigned according to some rules.
- Measurement is always concerned with certain attributes/features of the object.
- The measurement numerals are used to represent quantities of the attributes. Measurement can be defined as the assignment of numbers to objects and events according to logically accepted rules. The number system is highly logical and offers a multiplicity of possibilities for further logical manipulations. The measurement scale should possess the following attributes to allow for these logical manipulations.
- Magnitude is the quantum or quantity in which the attribute exists in various instances of phenomena. It allows us to tell whether one instance of attribute is greater than, less than, or equal to another instance of the attribute. For example, if Lalitha gets a score of 20 on aggressiveness scale and Mamatha, a score of 25, say Mamatha is more aggressive than Lalitha.
- *Equal intervals:* It denotes that the magnitude of the attribute represented by a unit of measurement on the scale is equal regardless of where on the scale the unit falls. For example, a difference in heights below 60 inches and 65 inches is equal to difference in height, between 67 inches and 72 inches. But it is not possible when working with psychological phenomena, for example a difference in IQ level.
- Absolute zero point indicates that a 'Zero' quantity of the attribute exists at that point or nothing. All the attributes being measured exist. For example, zero height indicates 'no height' at all. However, in the case of intelligence (IQ level) and aggressiveness one may assign zero score to a person but it does not mean a point of an absolute absence of all intelligence or aggressiveness in the person.

The comparison of observations on different individuals or villages is direct and valid. However, the problem of measurements is not so simple in cases like severity of illness, nutritional status of an individual and sanitary condition of a household. Measurement in these cases will have to be dependent on more than one factor simultaneously. A composite index giving weight, age to the different factors involved is formulated and used as a measure. In some situations instead of an index, the individuals or items are only ranked. These are examples of different levels of measurement. It is important to take into account the levels of measurement of the observations while selecting appropriate statistical tools for making comparison or for drawing conclusions.

Probably the foremost leader of those who see measurement scales as crucial to the choice of statistical procedures was SS Stevens. Basically, Stevens defined four types of scales: nominal, ordinal, interval, and ratio. These scales are distinguished on the basis of the relationships assumed to exist between items having different scale values.

Keeping in mind these above statistics three characteristics of measurements, the measurement scales can be divided into four different most widely used classification of measurement scales which include:

1. Nominal scale or classifying scale
2. Ordinal or ranking scale
3. Interval scale or equal interval scale
4. Ratio scale.

Nominal Scale or Classifying Scale

Nominal scale refers to the simple classification of objects or items into discrete groups which do not bear any magnitude relationships to another. In this scale the observations are placed into broad categories which may be denoted by symbol or labels or names. Generally numbering of houses, naming of streets, naming persons and cars is done for convenience and nor based on any of the three qualities mentioned about—magnitude, equal intervals and absolute zero point. For example classifying patients according to diagnostic groups or type of residence (rural, or urban or *kutcha* or *pucca* or *semipucca*) constitute a nominal scale. Another example, that a sample being studied may be classified as (a) Hindus (b) Muslims (c) Christians or same sample may be classified on the basis of sex, rural-urban variable, political party affiliation, etc. Here observations are placed into broad categories which may be denoted by symbol or labels or names. For example blood groups, diagnostic categories, gender, marital status, cause of death.

In a sense, **nominal scales** are not really scales at all; they do not scale items along any dimension, but rather label them. Variables such as gender and political-party affiliation are nominal variables. Such categorical data are usually measured on a nominal scale, since we merely assign category labels (e.g. male or female; Republican, Democrat, or Independent) to observations. A numerical example of a nominal scale is the set of numbers assigned to football players. Frequently, these numbers have no meaning other than that they are convenient labels to distinguish the players from one another. Letters or pictures of animals could just as easily be used.

In nominal measurement members of 2 groups are never equivalent, but all members of any one group are always equivalent. The relationship is reflexive, transitive and symmetrical. Statistical operations used are counting/frequency, percentage, proportion, mode, etc. Addition, division, subtractions and multiplication is not possible. Nominal scale is the least powerful level of measurement. Here there is restriction to use made as the measure of central tendency. There is no generally used measure of dispersion for nominal scales. Chi-square test is the most common test of statistical significance that can be utilized and for the measures of correlation, the contingency coefficient can be worked as it indicates no order or distance relationship and has no arithmetic origin. It simply describes difference between things by assigning them to categories. Nominal data are thus counted data. The scale wastes any information it may have about varying degrees of attitude, skills, understandings, etc. In spite of all, nominal scales are very useful and are widely used in survey research and export fact research. Nominal scale is elementary and simple.

Ordinal or Ranking Scale

After nominal scale, the next higher level scale is the ordinal scale. This consists of ranking all categories of a variable according to some criterion such as, grading of muscle strength or ranking of socioeconomic class. Here categories or observations are ranked or ordered. Each category is in unique position in relation to other categories but the distances between the categories are not known. For example severity of illness, socioeconomic status, ranking of students according to the marks obtained.

The simplest true scale is an **ordinal scale,** which orders people, objects, or events along some continuum. An excellent example of such a scale is the ranks in the Navy. A commander is lower in prestige than a captain, who in turn is lower than a rear admiral. However, there is no reason to think that the *difference* in prestige between a commander and a captain is the same as that between a captain and a rear admiral. An example from psychology would be the Holmes and Rahe (1967) scale of life stress. Using this scale, you count (sometimes with differential weightings) the number of changes (marriage, moving, new job, etc.) that have occurred during the past six months of a person's life. Someone who has a score of 20 is presumed to have experienced more stress than someone with a score of 15 and the latter in turn is presumed to have experienced more stress than someone with a score of 10. Thus, people are ordered, in terms of stress, by the number of changes in their recent lives. This is another example of an ordinal scale, because nothing is implied about the differences between points on the scale. We do not assume, for example, that the difference between 10 and 15 points represents the same difference in stress as the difference between 15 and 20 points. Distinctions of that sort must be left to interval scales.

Ordinal scale reflects only magnitude and does not possess the attributes of equal intervals or an absolute zero point. For example, instead of measuring height of students in a class with a tape, ask them to line up and decide their height. Here tallest receiving rank of '1' next tallest rank of '2'. The ordinal scale places events in order, but there is no attempt to make the intervals of scale equal in terms of some rule. Rank orders represent ordinal scales and are frequently used in research relating to qualitative phenomena. For example, students rank in degree class involve the use of ordinal scale. One has to be very careful in making statements about scores based on ordinal scale.

In ordinal scale, numbers denote the rank order of the objects or the individuals. Here numbers are arranged from highest to lowest or lowest to highest. Ordinal scales reflect which person or object is larger or smaller, harder or softer, heavier or lighter and brighter or duller, etc. A person may be grouped based on physical or psychological traits, to convey the relationship. Besides this relationship, equivalent relationship of greater than or lesser than, can be found out by the ordinal scale.

Here the statistical operations used are median, percentile, rank correlation, etc. since the numbers of this scale have only a rank measuring, the appropriate measures of central tendency is the median. A percentile or quartile measure is used for measures of depression. Correlations are restricted to various rank order methods. Measures of statistical significance are restricted to the non-parameter method. Ordinal scales are not absolute quantities nor do they convey that distance between the different rank value is equal.

Interval Scale or Equal Interval Scale

Interval scales include all the characteristics of ordinal or nominal scale. The interval scale possesses two out of three important requirements of a good measurement scale, i.e. magnitude and equal intervals but lacks the real or absolute zero point. The salient feature of this scale is that numerically equal distances in properties of the object are measured. Here the units of measurement are constant or equal, since they are at an equal interval, they are added and subtracted from each other, e.g. A = 20, B = 16, C = 8, D = 4. ∴ A – C = 20 – 8 = 12, B – D = 16 – 4 = 12.

With an **interval scale**, we have a measurement scale in which we can legitimately speak of differences between scale points. A common example is the Fahrenheit scale of temperature, where a 10-point difference has the same meaning anywhere along the scale. Thus, the difference in temperature between 10° F and 20° F is the same as the difference between 80° F and 90° F. Notice that this scale also satisfies the properties of the two preceding ones. What we do not have with an interval scale, however, is the ability to speak meaningfully about ratios. Thus, we cannot say, for example, that 40° F is half as hot as 80° F, or twice as hot as 20° F. We have to use ratio scales for that purpose. (In this regard, it is worth noting that when we perform perfectly legitimate conversions from one interval scale to another—for example, from the Fahrenheit to the Celsius scale of temperature—we do not even keep the same ratios. Thus, the ratio between 40° and 80° on a Fahrenheit scale is different from the ratio between 4.4° and 26.7° on a Celsius scale, although the temperatures are comparable. This highlights the arbitrary nature of ratios when dealing with interval scales.

In interval scale, the intervals are adjusted in terms of some rule that has been established as a basis for making the units equal. The units are equal only in so far as one accepts the assumptions on which the rule is based. Intervals scale have an arbitrary zero; it does not have the capacity to measure. The complete absence of a trait or characteristic and an important characteristic, namely distance between any two numbers (values of the variable) is fixed and equal. In this scale, the zero point and the unit of measurement are arbitrary. An excellent example of interval scale is measurement of temperature—centigrade or Fahrenheit. Interval scales provide more powerful measurement than ordinal scale, for internal scales also incorporate the concept of equality of interval. The statistical measure used for interval scale are arithmetic mean, standard deviation, product moment correlation technique (Pearson) and generally used tests for statistical significance are the 't' test and 'F' test. The only statistics, i.e. coefficient of variation is not used here because it is on the ratio.

Ratio Scale

The scale of measurement which has all the three attributes—magnitude, equal intervals and an absolute zero point is called 'ratio scale'. The interval scale does not have an absolute zero point at which a complete absence of particular property can be taken. Absolute zero point, which is an additional characteristic of ratio scales means, exactly the nothing of the quantity being measured, whether it is a physical or a psychological variable, that is concerned. Ratio scales are almost nonexistent in psychology and other social sciences, except in the area of psychological judgement. Ratio scaling allows for mathematical manipulations of multiplication, division and taking of square-roots, etc. and permit us to arrive at sensible results that can be verified. In statistical techniques we create meaningful zero points such as, at the mean of a distribution or at a difference of zero. Deviation from these statistically generative zero points can be treated as ratio scale measurement.

A ***ratio scale*** is one that has a *true* zero point. Notice that the zero point must be a true zero point and not an arbitrary one, such as 0° F or even 0° C. (A true zero point is the point corresponding to the absence of the thing being measured. Since 0° F and 0° C do not represent the absence of temperature or molecular motion, they are not true zero points). Examples of ratio scales are the common physical ones of length, volume, time, and so on. With these scales, we not only have the properties of the preceding scales but we also can speak about ratios. We can say that in physical terms 10 seconds is twice as long as 5 seconds, that 100 lbs is one-third as heavy as 300 lbs and so on.

You might think that the kind of scale with which we are working would be obvious. Unfortunately, especially with the kinds of measures we collect in the social sciences, this is rarely the case. Consider for a moment, the situation in which an anxiety questionnaire is administered to a group of high-school students. If you were foolish enough, you might think that this is a ratio scale of anxiety. You would maintain that a person who scored 0 had no anxiety at all and that a score of 80 reflected twice as much anxiety as did a score of 40. Although most people would find this position ridiculous, with certain questionnaires you might be able to build a reasonable case. Someone else might argue that it is an interval scale and that, although the zero point was somewhat arbitrary (the student receiving a 0 was somewhat anxious but your questions failed to detect it), equal differences in scores represent equal differences in anxiety. A more reasonable stance might be to say that the scores represent an ordinal scale: A 95 reflects more anxiety than an 85, which in turn reflects more than a 75, but equal differences in scores do not reflect equal differences in anxiety. For an excellent and readable discussion of measurement scales.

As an example of a form of measurement that has a scale that depends on its use, consider the temperature of a house. We generally speak of Fahrenheit temperature as an interval scale. We have just used it as an example of one and there is no doubt that, to a physicist, the difference between 62° F and 64° F is exactly the same as the difference between 72° F and 74° F. If we are measuring temperature as an index of *comfort,* rather than as an index of molecular activity however, the same numbers no longer form an interval scale. To a person sitting in a room at 62° F, a jump to 64° F would be distinctly noticeable (and welcome). The same cannot be said about the difference between room temperatures of 72° F and 74° F. This points up the important fact that *it is the underlying variable that we are measuring (e.g. comfort), not the numbers themselves, that is important in defining the scale.* As a scale of *comfort,* degrees Fahrenheit do not form an interval scale.

Since, there usually is no unanimous agreement concerning the measurement scale employed, it is up to the individual user of statistical procedures to decide which scale best fits the data. All that can be asked of the user is that he or she think about the problem carefully before coming to a decision and not simply assume that the standard answer is necessarily the best answer.

Ratio scale in the highest level of measurement and has properties of nominal, ordinal and interval scale, plus an absolute or true zero points. The salient feature of this scale is that ratio of any two members is independent of the unit of measurement and therefore can be meaningfully equated. For example 16:8 is equal to 4:7, here statistical operation like co-efficient of variation is also included. Measures of weight, height, length, loudness, etc are included in ratio scale. Ratio scale represents the actual amounts of variable.

Usually, all statistical techniques are usable with ratio scales and all manipulations that are carried out with real numbers can also be carried out with ratio-scale values. Multiplications and divisions can be used with this scale. Geometric and harmonic mean can be used as measures of central tendency and coefficient of variation may be calculated.

Thus, according to the nature of the variable permits, the investigator uses the scale that provides the most precise description. The investigator widely uses these above measurements for the following functions:

- Selection of personnel in industry/institutions
- Various types of classification effectively
- In order to compare two individuals
- It is a basic part of research
- Improving classroom instructions.

The Role of Measurement Scales

As stated earlier that writers disagree about the importance assigned to measurement scales. Some authors have ignored the problem totally, whereas others have organized whole textbooks around the different scales. A reasonable view is that, the central issue is the absolute necessity of separating in our minds, the numbers we collect from the objects or events to which they refer. Such an argument was made for the example of room temperature, where the scale (interval or ordinal) depended on whether we were interested in measuring some physical attribute of temperature or its effect on people (i.e., comfort). A difference of 2° F is the same, *physically,* anywhere on the scale, but a difference of 2° F when a room is already warm may not *feel* as large as does a difference of 2° F, when a room is relatively cool. In other words, we have an interval scale of the physical units but no more than an ordinal scale of comfort.

Because statistical tests use numbers without considering the objects or events to which those numbers refer, we may carry out any of the standard mathematical operations (addition, multiplication, etc.) regardless of the nature of the underlying scale. An excellent, entertaining and highly recommended paper on this point is one by Lord (1953), entitled, 'On the Statistical Treatment of Football Numbers', in which he argues that these numbers can be treated in any way you like because. "The numbers do not remember where they came from".

The problem arises when it is time to interpret the results of some form of statistical manipulation. At that point, we must ask whether the statistical results are related in any meaningful way to the objects or events in question. Here, we are no longer dealing with a statistical issue, but with a methodological one. No *statistical* procedure can tell us whether the fact that, one group received higher scores than another on an anxiety questionnaire, reveals anything about group differences in underlying anxiety levels. Moreover, to be satisfied because the questionnaire provides a ratio scale of anxiety *scores* (a score of 50 is twice as large as a score of 25) is to lose sight of the fact that we set out to measure anxiety, which may not increase in an orderly way with increases in scores. Our statistical tests can apply only to the numbers that we obtain and the validity of statements about the objects or events that we think we are measuring, hinges primarily on our knowledge of those objects or events, and not on the measurement scale. We do our best to ensure that our measures relate as closely as possible to what we want to measure, but our results are ultimately only the numbers we obtain and our faith in the relationship between those numbers and the underlying objects or events.

From the preceding discussion, the apparent conclusion—and the one accepted in this book—is that the underlying measurement scale is not crucial in our choice of statistical techniques. Obviously, a certain amount of common sense is required in interpreting the results of these statistical manipulations. Only a fool would conclude that a painting that was judged as excellent by one person and contemptible by another ought therefore to be classified as mediocre.

Regardless of the level of data used, the researcher must answer the question, "Are the differences I see caused by chance, or are other factors responsible, such as my treatment?" For example, when a researcher sees that two different groups have different means, the next task is to test the differences between the means to determine whether they are significantly different statistically. Based on the level of data, the researcher selects the statistical test that is the most appropriate to determine whether chance is the overriding factor.

The terms parametric statistics and nonparametric statistics are associated with level of measurement of the data to be analyzed. Each of these terms refers to a different group of inferential statistical techniques. Parametric statistical techniques are intended to be used with interval and ratio data; non-parametric statistical techniques are intended to be used with nominal and ordinal data. Details of the tests are explained chapters 16, 17, 18.

Table 1.1 summarizes selected statistical tests based on levels of data.

Table 1.1

Summary of selected statistical tests based on levels of data

Level of data	*Number of samples*	*Statistical test*	*Correlational statistics*
Nominal level	1 or more	Chi-squared	
Ordinal level	1 or more	Chi-squared	
	2	Mann-Whitney U	Spearman's rho
	3 or more	Kruskal-Wallace one-way analysis of variance by ranks	
		Friedman two-way analysis of variance by ranks	
Interval or ratio level	2	*t* test (must state if samples are independent or related)	Pearson's *r*
		Analysis of variance	
	3 or more	Analysis of variance	
		Analysis of covariance	
		Multiple analysis of variance	
		Multiple analysis of covariance	

Need for Statistics in Health Sciences including Nursing

As the result of an urgent need for more precise and objective methods, statistical techniques have been gaining increasingly, wide acceptance among health scientists including nursing. It will be found that the development of any science is marked by the extent to which exact quantitative data and techniques have superseded mere speculations and qualitative impressions. Sciences like physics, chemistry, astronomy and so on are frequently referred to as 'exact' or 'pure', sciences, largely because of their data and methodology, are relatively precise and quantitative. It seems, safe to say that, as the health sciences advance from the impressionistics and qualitative stages, statistical methods will become increasingly important. In fact, the researcher in nursing and any other field, should have a thorough knowledge of at least the fundamentals of statistics, is an indispensable part of equipping themselves.

As scientists, we all have beliefs and the purpose of the scientific experiment is to test those beliefs. Yet medical history is littered with untested beliefs acted upon for decades or even centuries until the application of scientific method had led to their being discarded, often with great reluctance. These might merely concern the theory of medicine or, more importantly, they might concern patients; for example, numerous futile operations were done to remove healthy organs of patients—tonsils, gall-bladders and colons—because of the untested and unproved hypothesis of focal sepsis. A scientific approach is more humane and careful clinical trials prevent useless and dangerous drugs being inflicted upon the public.

Earlier this century injections of gold were thought to benefit patients with tuberculosis. How did this belief arise? Perhaps somebody treated a patient suffering from tuberculosis with gold and they got better. Everytime a new patient treated with gold got better the belief was reinforced, and tended to lead to suppression of contrary data. Since the natural history of untreated tuberculosis leads to recovery in some patients and to death in others, chance results could easily lead to false conclusions about the efficacy of treatment. This is the problem with all therapies: real effects, whether beneficial or harmful, may be obscured and chance happenings may lead to false conclusions.

The purpose of a properly designed medical experiment is to eliminate the effect of belief (bias)

and the object of statistics is to disentangle the effects of chance from the true but unknown effects of treatment. The proper application of statistics to medicine is of relatively recent origin but this is not so in many other scientific disciplines. A statistician should be a member of, or available for consultation for, any scientific team, his function being to advise on the method of collecting, processing, analyzing and interpreting numerical data. However, statistical methods can never *prove* anything and the answer always comes out as a *probability;* the same applies to assessing results by intuition, except that the probability is not calculated but guessed.

A knowledge of basic statistical concepts and techniques is also necessary for an intelligent understanding of current writing in the nursing science literature. It is generally taken for granted by writers in the field of nursing and health sciences, that the reader knows the meaning of such basic terms as mean, median, mode, percentage, standard deviation, correlation and reliability. The profits which derive from reading professional/technical studies of this kind are largely in proportion to the understanding of statistical methods.

The advantages of statistics in the field of health care include the following:

- Helps in mapping health problems in the community
- Helps in deciding about health care used in hospitals, health centers and nursing homes
- Helps to ease comparison of related events, diseases and other things related to health and illness
- Helps to check the efficiency of health programs at National, Local and Global levels
- Helps to assess the health care utilization of government and private health organizations
- Helps in planning, implementing and evaluating health services at all levels

Now-a-days a number of professional journals show the extensive use of statistical methods in the collection, evaluation and presentation of biological data. This is a reflection of the need for precise quantitative assessments of different types of phenomena that are affected by sampling and biological variations and thus the need for making valid inferences. Now, nursing research is getting more importance in the field and research components are included in the nursing education to have orientation and to conduct research to improve the body of knowledge and its application in practice. Research workers, students and other professionals in their respective fields will need to study data presented by others and evaluate the evidence found in their data. Also, they have to plan and evaluate their own work. Knowledge of the logical basis of the statistical approach and the rationale of the commonly used statistical technique will be an essential prerequisite.

Much progress has been made in the theory of statistics in recent years in improving the techniques and methods of estimating and handling numerical data. Statistics as a science provides the investigator with powerful and sensitive tools to help him/her in determining the likelihood that a particular outcome of treating a group of patients in the result of treatment, the result of other factors, the result of chance whether a characteristic is truly associated with occurrence of disease or an artifact of observation. To ignore these fundamental questions and to scoff at the use of statistics in medicine, nursing and their research, as mere statistics is to ignore the systematic observation and measurement of the phenomena which are the very basis of science.

Statistics finds its place wherever numerical facts enter into the picture. Health Sciences including nursing sciences deal with various numerical measurements and as such statistics is an essential part of health sciences and its varied uses are as follows:

i. As health sciences deal with measurements and comparisons, effective comparisons are possible only through the principles of statistics.
ii. Inherent features of all biological observations is their variability. A health science

being part and parcel of biological sciences is not exceptional for this variability. Each individual varies from one another with respect to different medical phenomenon. Similarly, each group of individuals is different from other groups. As an example, the pulse rate, the hemoglobin level or the total number of white blood cells in a given volume of blood, etc. vary from person to person even amongst healthy ones. Though, a single fixed value for any of the above measurements cannot be called as a standard value for a healthy individual, a range can always be expressed as a standard or normal value. Again these ranges may vary from one group to the other due to various factors. As an example, the pulse rate per minute varies from the infant age group to the older age group. Similarly, the normal hemoglobin level varies from one part of the country to the other. As such, in order to obtain these normal values and also to compare them from one group to another, statistical methodology plays an important part.

iii. Statistical quantities serve as indices for the measurement of health of a community in terms of rates and ratios of fatalities, morbidities, mortalities, health facilities, their availability or usage and so on. These indicators are useful in comparing the health status of a community or group in one place with the other or from one season or period to the other. They are also of help in studying in detail the influence of environmental, social, economical, seasonal and other numerous factors on health of a community. As an illustration the typhoid prevalence in a community may be associated with numerous factors. The prevalence may be higher with poor socioeconomic standard. The prevalence may be common in unhygienic areas of the community such as, those with unsafe water supply or with unhygienic eating places, etc. The disease may also be highly prevalent during certain seasons. The disease may be more prevalent with those people who were not protected. By a systematic statistical analysis of the factors related to a disease, a health worker can define the problems in terms of contrasts.

iv. There may be a number of factors responsible for the variations in the health of a community. For example, the higher prevalence of typhoid amongst lower socioeconomic group of the community may be due to drinking of unsafe water or consumption of unprotected food or lack of resistance due to under nourishment or insufficient protection against disease because of nonacceptance of immunization. As such by analyzing the causes for the contrasts, with the help of statistical methodologies, effective control measures can be taken.

v. Preventive and control measures undertaken in a community can be assessed only through statistical evaluation of the data, as apparent change in any of the factors may not be otherwise significant.

vi. Records of morbidities, births, deaths and other health activities maintained and analyzed statistically will help in understanding the health of the community.

vii. Periodical investigations or surveys are to be undertaken in the community to define the problems and to elucidate the reasons for the contrasts. These investigations are to be planned and analyzed with the help of statistical methodologies.

viii. The statistical methodologies are useful in defining the epidemiological aspects of diseases.

ix. Continuous research is going on in health sciences and all research investigation should be properly planned and the results of the investigations are to be scientifically analyzed. These aspects of planning and analysis form the core of statistical methodology.

In brief, in the words of an eminent health statistician, it is said that "statistics are the eyes and ears of a health worker". The statistician's job is to extract all available information from the given data to make the figures tell their own story and reveal what is concealed in them. Depending on his/her experience and knowledge of the area of enquiry and varying degrees of collaboration with experts in the field, statisticians make deeper probes into data to understand the underlying phenomena. Those who work with statistics might fall in following categories:

- Those who need to know statistics in order to appreciate reports of findings in their professional field
- Those who must select and apply statistical treatment in the course of their own inquiry

For interest of these categories in their own subject matter, statistics is an aid in organizing and making meaningful the evidence that bears on questions that have been raised. Medical researcher, nurse researcher, engineers, psychologists, counselors, and many more regularly find that statistical procedures can be of assistance.

In addition, there are other two categories of statistics which include the professional statistician and the mathematical statistician.

- Professional statisticians are those who have been trained in the university (Department of Mathematics or Statistics) undergone extensive training in statistical theory and relevant mathematics. The advantage that they have is that of expert knowledge of statistical theory and of its general applicability. The practicing statistician is the one who assists those with substantive questions in finding and applying statistical models, with which to examine, evidence relative to their enquiry. Their primary interest is applied statistics and that too, applicable.
- The mathematical statistician is the one who trained in the university like a professional, but his/her primary interest is in pure statistics and probability theory and that too theoretical.

The active participation and involvement of statisticians is extremely essential for the formulation of research programs, not only in the field, but also in the clinic, the laboratory and the hospital and for interpretation of data. It is also important that research scientists, health scientists and nursing scientists get adequate training at least in elements of biostatistics. In the same way, it is also important that biostatisticians who are involved in health, including medical and nursing research acquire basic knowledge with respect to health and nursing science. Since we have included statistics and biostatistics in the nursing curriculum, nursing students should not depend on a statistician for statistical applications in nursing. For professional interpretations of their research results, he/she should learn application of the method, regarding, which does not require knowledge of mathematics, higher than what she/he had acquired in school. However, he/she should take guidance of a qualified statistician right from the beginning of any scientific study till drawing conclusion.

Evolution of Biostatistics in Nursing

Biostatistics is defined as the application of the statistical methods to the problems of biology, including human biology, medicine, public health and nursing.

Perhaps the earliest important figure in biostatistics is thought to be Adolphe Quetelet (1796-1874), a Belgian astronomer and mathematician, who in his work combined the theory and practical methods of statistics and applied them to the problems of biology, medicine and sociology. Francis Galton (1822-1911), a cousin of Charles Darwin, has been called the **Father of Biostatistics and Eugenics**, the two subjects that he studied interrelatedly. The inadequacy of Darwin's genetic theories stimulated Galton to try to solve the problems of heredity. Gallon's major contribution to biology is his application of statistical methodology to the analysis of variability and the study of regression and correlation in biological measurements. His hope of unravelling the laws of genetics through these procedures was in vain. He started with the most difficult material and with the wrong assumptions. However, his methodology has become the foundation for the application of statistics to biology. Karl Pearson (1857-1936) at the University College, London, became interested in the application of statistical methods to biology, particularly in the demonstration of natural selection, through the influence of WFR Weldon (1860-1906), a zoologist at the same institution. Weldon, incidentally, is credited with coining the term biometry for the type of studies pursued by him. Pearson continued in the tradition of Galton and laid the foundation for much of the descriptive and correlational statistics. The dominant figure in statistics and biometry in this century has been Ronald A Fisher (1890-1962). His many contributions to statistical theory will become obvious.

Florence Nightingale as Statistician

Florence Nightingale may well be assigned a position in the history of social statistics next to those occupied by Quetelet and Farr. Her ardent, genuine sympathy for the sick and distressed was greatly augmented by a positive genius for marshalling definite knowledge of the forces which make for disease and suffering. The same intellect which sharply separated the formulae, procedures, and practical methods of nursing from its abiding principles as one of the humanities, also discerned the statistical facts of sickness and other forms of disharmony between the individual and his environment. In hospital care of the sick, as an instance, Miss Nightingale replaced the astigmatic case viewpoint with one embodying a grasp of total situations. This is one function of statistics.

Her earnest perception of this truth—an essential in the equipment of the statistician—was firmly supported by her control over laborious detail and by her scrupulous care in testing the statistical foundations of her premises. The interpretations she placed upon the facts developed in her researches show a careful regard for the competent counsel which she so often consulted. In all these respects Nightingale exhibited the prime qualities of one thoroughly versed in the art of preparing and reflectively analyzing social data.

The ever-increasing importance and application of statistics to biological data is evident even on cursory inspection of almost any medical and nursing journal. There has been such a marked increase in the use of statistics in nursing. It has apparently come with the realization that, in nursing the interplay of casual and response variables obey laws that are not in the classic mold of the 19th century.

Thus, many nurse scientists even to this day have retained the tradition of strictly mechanistic and deterministic concepts of thinking, while physicists, as their science became more refined and came to deal with ever more "elementary" particles, began to resort to statistical approaches. *In nursing, most phenomena are affected by many casual factors, uncontrollable in their variation and often unidentifiable. Statistics is needed to measure such variable phenomena with a predictable error and to ascertain the reality of minute, but important differences.*

Florence Nightingale's contribution to statistics is given below:

Health statistics comprise of an important tool for public health practice. From statistics, we learn about a community's morbidity and mortality rates, accident patterns, demographics and use of systems and resources. Statistics provide the facts from which positive changes in health care can be launched. They form the basis for designing community nursing interventions, for planning and evaluating community health programs and for analyzing and developing health policy and legislation. Florence Nightingale, the Pioneer of modern nursing long ago recognized the value of statistics and used them, described as a basis of major reforms in the health care of her day.

The somewhat legendary accounts of this remarkable woman contain but a few references to that part of life and work which should appeal to the students of the history of modern social statistics. More or less is understood of her radical innovations in the nursing care of the sick in institutions and especially in military hospitals, a definite idea exists of her capacities as reformer, administrator and nurse. Comparatively little is known of her, however, as a constructive compiler and interpreter of descriptive social statistics. One biographer alone, Sir Edward T Cook, speaks with sympathy and understanding of her as a statistician. He calls her a "passionate statistician".

The activities of Nightingale in statistics may be classed under several broad categories. We may think of her in terms of her forty years of thought and achievement in the Indian context; in safeguarding the health of the British soldier; in recognizing civil and military hospital administration at home and abroad; and in this later regard, of her pioneer services to the profession of nursing. Her keen intellect, applied to these major projects of her career, comprehended the utility of the statistical method as a means of developing a basis of established fact for social reform.

In early life, Nightingale showed peculiar aptitude for collecting and methodically recording current historical facts. Her observations during the travels of the Nightingales in Europe over the period 1837–1839 are a curious mixture of comment and criticism on the then existing laws, land systems, social conditions and benevolent institutions. Throughout her life she collected an immense number of pamphlets, reports, and returns which she skillfully analyzed with telling effect in her campaigns for hospital and sanitary reform. Following her nursing apprenticeship with the Fliedners at Kaiserswerth, she undertook further training at the *Maison de la Providence* in Paris; here she proceeded to collect hospital reports, returns, statistical forms and general information on hospital construction and sanitation. Among her papers then, were elaborately tabulated analyzes of hospital organizations, nursing systems and their end results. These inquires extended to both France and Germany. She seems also to have addressed circulars of inquiry on the same subjects to representative hospitals in the United Kingdom.

Nightingale was profoundly influenced by the works of Adolphe Quetelet, the Belgian astromoner, meteorologist, and statistician. Perhaps her practice of methodically recording the facts of her botanical researches led her to one of Quetelet's laws of flowering plants. The common lilac flowers, he averred, were the sum of the squares of the mean of daily temperatures, counted from the end of the forests, equals 4,264° centigrade. While the "law" delighted her, she regarded it as a lesser example of Quetelet's researches and statistical conclusions. She was fascinated most by Quetelet's "*Sur l'Homme et le Development de ses Facultes*", published in the year 1835, in which he outlined his conception of statistical method as applied to the life of man. From Quetelet, Nightingale learned much of the science and art which describes human society in terms of numbers. From him she learned the methods, general aims, and results of qualified inquiry into social facts and forces.

Influence on Military and Sanitary Statistics

The discipline of Quetelet's new science of social inquiry was to have its first influence upon the military and sanitary statistics of the Crimean War. Nightingale found the medical records of the Scutari hospitals in lamentable condition. Even the number of deaths was not accurately recorded. The three separate registers then maintained gave each a totally different account of the deaths among the military forces. None of the statistical records was kept in an uniform manner. She was able to introduce an orderly plan of recording the principal sickness and mortality data of the military hospital establishments which came within the sphere of her influence.

Nightingale's experience in Crimea filled her with an ardent desire to remedy the scandalous neglect of sanitary precautions in the Army; her study of the available data convinced her that the greater number of deaths in hospitals need not have occurred at all. During the first seven months of the Crimean campaign, a mortality of 60 percent per annum from disease alone occurred, a rate of mortality which exceeded even that of the Great Plague in London and a higher ratio than in the case of mortality of cholera. Nightingale's vigorous use of these facts resulted in a series of reforms, which in turn reduced this terrible rate of mortality. She observed, also, that if sanitary neglect prevailed in the Army on field, it probably affected the Army at home in considerable degree likewise. She compared the mortality in civil life with the mortality among soldiers and found out that it was nearly double that of civil life. In her writing to Sir John McNeil she said: "It is as criminal to have mortality of 17, 19, and 20 per thousand in the Line, Artillery and Guards, when that in civil life is only 11 per 1,000, as it would be to take 1,100 men out upon Salisbury Plain and shoot them".

Her further observations on the Chatham military hospitals were: "This disgraceful state of our Chatham Hospitals is only one more symptom of a system, which, in the Crimea, put to death 16,000 men—the finest experiment modern history has seen upon a large scale, viz., as to what given number may be put to death at will by the sole agency of bad food and bad air". Among her private notes of 1856, her biographer found this: "I stand at the altar of the murdered men and while I live, I fight their cause". The one weapon upon which she placed most dependence was her collection of sanitary statistics.

Influence on Hospital Administration

The results of her personal studies of army medical statistics were embodied in a report, from the beginning intended as a confidential communication to the War Office and the Army Medical Department. There had been considerable delay in the formation of the Royal Commission on the Health of the Army which she had requested in her November, 1856, interview with Lord Panmure. The Royal Warrant establishing the Commission was not issued until May 5, 1857. During the exasperating period of delay Nightingale held in reserve her array of statistics, until, having begun her agitation with the sovereign rulers and continuing through the politicians, she was almost ready to plead her cause with the people. In three months from the day the Royal Warrant was issued, the Commission presented its report. In the meantime, Lord Panmure had asked Nightingale for her "Notes Affecting the Health, Efficiency, and Hospital Administration of the British Army". These notes are the least known of her works, because they were never officially published. It has never become known how much of the final report of the Royal Commission was actually the work of Nightingale. Printed at her private expense and circulated among influential people, her "Notes" made a profound impression. They have been termed "a treasury of authentic fact … affording a complete elucidation of the causes which had brought about failure and showing the means by which the country could best hope to safeguard the truly sacred task of providing for the health of its troops in future wars". Another of her friends who read the proof said: "It has so much the character of good, sincere, enlightened conversation on a subject which is thoroughly understood and appreciated and so little the appearance of having been 'got up' or of pretension of any kind, literacy or artistic". Another reader said: "I regard it as a gift to the Army, and to the country altogether priceless".

The preface to the Notes gave the keynote. Hospitals were shown to be, but part of wider programs involving the general health and efficiency of the Army. This was emphasized by the fact that those who fell before Sevastopol by disease were above seven times the number who fell by the enemy. The introductory chapter gave the history of the health of the British armies in previous campaigns. Six of the twenty sections of the 'Notes' dealt with the medical history of the Crimean War. Two other sections discussed the mortality of armies in peace and war and the necessity for a statistical department of the army. There were also numerous appendices, supplementary notes, graphic illustrations and diagrams.

Pioneer in Graphic Illustration

It must be remembered that these notes were written by Nightingale in the short space of six months and while in delicate health. In the preparation of her report she had but little assistance; the gathering of the data was facilitated, however, by the friendly cooperation of many broadminded men in the public service. Dr Farr, for instance, aided materially in the preparation of the comparisons between the mortality of civil and army life and in editing the graphical illustrations which he especially commended. These graphical diagrams were at that time somewhat of an innovation in statistics and had not significant precedent, save in the statistical works of AM Guerry, a contemporary of Quetelet. The report of the commission, containing some thirty-three written answers by Nightingale to leading questions by the Commission, together with her original tabulation of the appalling morbidity and mortality statistics of the British Army, was issued to the public in January, 1858. The graphical illustrations in her own Notes portrayed, by means of shaded or colored squares, circles and wedges, (1) the deaths due to preventable causes in the hospitals during the Crimean War and (2) the rate of mortality in the British Army at home. "Our soldiers enlist," as she put it, "to death in the barracks". She reprinted this graphic section and distributed it, with a brief memorandum, to leading members of Parliament and to medical and commanding officers throughout the country, in India, and in the Colonies. "It is our flank march upon the enemy", she said.

The chief product of the commission's work of interest from the statistical standpoint was the report of the subcommittee on Army Medical Statistics. This committee, consisting of Mr Sidney Herbert, Sir A Tulloch, and Dr Farr, reported in June, 1858, and published its "First Annual Report on the Health of the Army" in March, 1861. The compilations were directed by Dr Thomas Graham Balfour, under whose leadership British army statistics became the best and most useful obtainables in Europe.

The facts published in the "Notes" did not go unchallenged. A pamphlet appeared anonymously calling them in question. Nightingale immediately prepared a reply. This second note was entitled "A Contribution to the Sanitary History of the British Army during the late War with Russia", and constituted a scathing and eloquent account of the preventable mortality which she had witnessed in the East. The graphic charts of the "Notes" were reproduced.

Management of Civil Hospitals

The opposition to the recommendations of the subcommission on Army Barracks stimulated Nightingale to prepare a more extended discussion of hospital construction, organization and management. From her extensive experience in and study of hospital systems in Germany, France, and Ireland and in the Crimea, she prepared two addresses on hospital construction and sanitation for the Liverpool meeting of the National Association for the Promotion of Social Science. These papers were reprinted as "Notes on Hospitals". These "Notes" in three editions, the last in 1863, revolutionized ideas of hospital construction.

It was pointed out that the hospital statistics then available gave little information of real value on the proportion of recoveries, of deaths and the average duration of hospital treatment for different diseases, duly qualified by sex and age. A common agreement on the number and nature of statistical data to be tabulated was recommended. A unique feature of this Liverpool address was a mortality table for hospital nurses and attendants showing the greatly increased prevalence of communicable diseases among this class of hospital nurses and attendants showing the greatly increased prevalence of communicable diseases among this class of hospital employees, as compared with the mortality from the same causes in civil life. The deplorable existence of "hospital gangrene" and "hospital septicemia" in that day of defective hospital sanitation and construction was effectively portrayed by these mortality statistics.

A brief inquiry into the precedent circumstances will be of interest. When Nightingale returned from the Crimea she directed much thought and attention to hospital statistics as an adjunct to administration of institutions for the care of the sick. She found a complete lack of scientific coordination. The statistics were not kept along uniform lines. Each hospital followed its own nomenclature and classification of diseases. The available data had never been tabulated upon forms which would render the statistics of one hospital comparable with those of another. The data had little value for advancing medical knowledge or as an adjunct to hospital management. With the assistance of Dr Farr and of other friendly physicians, she drew up a standard list of diseases (largely a selection from the Espine-Farr system) and a set of model hospital statistical forms. She had her model forms printed in 1859 and persuaded some of the London hospitals to adopt them experimentally. She and Dr Farr studied the tabulated results, which had sufficient value to show how large a field of qualified statistical inquiry had been opened by the introduction of her forms.

Miss Nightingale's skill in so effectively employing the statistical method in army sanitary reform had led to her election, in 1858, to Fellowship in the Royal Statistical Society. On October 16, 1874, the American Statistical Association elected her an honorary member.

International Statistical Congress of 1860

This growing association with the leaders of thought in the statistical world of her time enabled her to take an active part in drawing up the program of the second section of the International Statistical Congress, held at London in 1860. This section dealt with sanitary statistics. Nightingale and Dr Farr incorporated the forms for uniform hospital statistics, which had been experimentally introduced into a group of London hospitals in 1859, in a paper read for her before the section by Dr McMillian. Additions and recommendations, chiefly by Dr Berg of Sweden and Dr Neumann of Berlin, were concurred in a letter to the Earl of Shaftesbury, President of the Section.

This paper on uniform classifications and forms for hospital statistics was afterward widely circulated among physicians and hospital officials. Large quantities of the forms were supplied to hospitals in various parts of the country. The Paris hospitals took up the plan. Guy's Hospital, London, prepared a statistical analysis of its experience for the years 1854 to 1861; St Thomas for the years 1857 to 1860; and St Bartholomew's for 1860. At a meeting held on registration it was decided that each hospital should publish its own statistics annually and that the forms devised by Miss Nightingale should be used so far as practicable.

Elements of Hospital Medical Statistics

Nightingale then prepared a detailed paper on "Hospital Statistics and Hospital Plans" for the Dublin meeting of the National Association for the Promotion of Social Science in 1861. In this paper she emphasized the seven primary tabulation elements of hospital sickness statistics, which were:

1. Number of patients remaining in hospital on first day of the year
2. Patients admitted during the year
3. Patients recovered or relieved during the year
4. Patients discharged as incurable, unrelieved, for irregularities or at own request
5. Patients dead during the year
6. Patients remaining at the end of the year
7. Mean duration of cases in days and fractions of a day.

These tabulation "elements" were to be compiled as seven separate tables, each showing diseases classified there under sex and age (by single years under five and by five years periods thereafter). The additional consideration of diseases contracted in hospital while under treatment was also provided for. These extensions of the original paper were suggested by Drs Berg and Neumann. Nightingale held that these supplementary tables would bring out the fact of the then scandalous prevalence of "hospital diseases" such as gangrene and septicemia.

The statistics of the various hospitals adopting her forms were published in the *Journal* of the Royal Statistical Society for September, 1862. Nightingale's system of uniform hospital statistics was never generally successful over any considerable period of time. The plan, but partly realized, in the requirements of the King's Hospital Fund, demands for its complete and effective operation a more intelligent appreciation of and a finer enthusiasm for statistical facts than is afforded even by present day voluntary and competitive hospital systems in metropolitan districts.

A further example of Nightingale's use of the statistical method in hospital economy was her study of the questions relating to the possible removal of St Thomas Hospital at the instance of the Southeastern Railway. The railway company proposed the removal of the hospital to provide for an extension of the right-of-way from London Bridge to Charing Cross. She analyzed the origins of cases served by the hospital, tabulated the proportions of cases within certain radial distances, and showed the probable effect upon patients of the removal of the hospital to the several possible sites suggested. This method of fitting hospital accommodation to the needs of populations has only recently been revived. It represents a legitimate application of demographic principles to the study of the relief of dire human needs.

The statistics of surgical operations from the standpoint of hospital cost and practical end results were next considered by Nightingale. In a commentary on St Bartholomew's statistical report, Nightingale outlined the minimum requirements of a report form for the nature and result of surgical operations. The subject was further developed in a paper read for her before the Berlin meeting of the International Statistical Congress in 1863.

Before the close of the London meeting of the International Statistical Congress, 1860, Nightingale addressed a letter a Lord Shaftesbury. The letter was read to the whole Congress and adopted by it as a resolution. The resolution impressed upon governments, the prime necessity for publishing more extensive and numerous abstracts of the statistical information in their possession.

Nightingale and the Census of England 1861

Nightingale made a determined effort to extend the scope and application of the Census of 1861, largely in the direction of collecting statistics which would serve as a foundation for sanitary reform. Her aim was twofold: one was to enumerate the sick and infirm on Census Day. To those who denied that it could be accomplished, she pointed out that it had been done elsewhere, notably in Ireland. Her second ambition was to obtain complete data on the housing of the population; this, too, had been practicable in Ireland, she urged. In pressing her point with the Census officials she said: "The connection between the *health* and the *dwellings* of the population is one of the most important that exists. The 'diseases' can be approximated also. In all the more important – all those which affect the national health, there will be very little error. Where there is error in these things, the error is uniform … and corrects itself….." These few remarks still serve as prolegomena to any future census plans for England or any other country.

The Census Bill came up late in the session and not much comment can be found on the foregoing suggestion for a development of Census inquiry. The only critical comment made in the debate proceeded from Lord Ellenborough, who, far from considering the innovations of sickness and housing statistics, proposed to exclude most of the inquires already suggested. Nightingale, in her conception of census methods and results, was far ahead of her day and generation. Subsequent censuses, chiefly in the United States, in Tasmania, and in one or two countries, have included sickness and housing inquiries.

Scope and Use of Statistics

Nightingale's activities in furthering statistical progress were the outgrowth of her deep conviction, variously expressed in her several papers, that the social and moral sciences are in method and substance statistical sciences. In her several papers on metaphysical topics, she asserts that statistics were to her almost a religious exercise. Her conception of theology was that, its true function was to ascertain the "character of God". Statistics, she mused, discovered and codified law in the social sphere and thereby revealed certain aspects of "the character of God". Doubtless, in these speculations she was profoundly influenced by the studies of Quetelet in moral statistics, as typified in his "*Recerches statistiques sur le Royaume de Pays-Bas*".

Statistics as an element in political education also appealed with peculiar force to Miss Nightingale. In a letter to Benjamin Jowett she said: "The Cabinet Ministers, the army of their subordinates ... have for the most part received a university education, but no education in statistical method. We legislate without knowing what we are doing. The War Office has some of the finest statistics in the world. What comes of them? Little or nothing. Why? Because the Heads do not know how to make anything of them. Our Indian Statistics are really better than those of England. Of these no use is made in administration. What we want is not so much (or at least not at present) an accumulation of facts, as to teach men who are to govern the country, the use of statistical facts".

She proposed a number of leading questions which she desired to see investigated by the statistical method: What had been the result of twenty years of compulsory education? What is the effect of town life on offspring in number and in health? What are the contributions of the several social classes to the population of the next generation? In proposing these inquiries she anticipated by more than a generation, the work of the eugenists and biometricians of the Galton-Pearson school. Her friend, Adolphe Quetelet, had inaugurated studies of this character. In conversation with Benjamin Jowett she proposed to found at Oxford a Professorship or Lectureship in Applied Statistics. Jowett seems to have discussed the matter with Arthur Balfour and Professor Alfred Marshall. Nightingale, on her part, consulted Francis Galton, who responded earnestly and worked out a detailed plan. There was more or less discussion over the matter, but in the press of other affairs, the proposition was discarded. It is certainly of very great interest in this connection to observe that many years afterward such an enterprise was undertaken by the University College in London; probably, however, not directly issuing from Miss Nightingale's suggestion.

Vitality of Aboriginal Races

Following her disciplines on army, medical, and civil hospital statistics, came her statistical investigations into colonial questions: the first into the vitality of native or aboriginal races in the colonies; the second into the sanitary condition and material welfare of the population and military establishment of India, In a paper before the National Association for the Promotion of Social Science, meeting at Edinburgh in 1863, she discussed the gradual disappearance of the native races when brought into contact with the influences of civilization. The paper was suggested by Sir George Grey, who, at that time, was deeply engaged with questions of Colonial policy. The preliminary inquiry related to the probable effect of European school usages and school education generally, upon the health of children, of parents and of races which had not heretofore been brought under any system of education. With the assistance of the Duke of Newcastle, she prepared a form which was sent by the Colonial Office, to the governors of the various colonies. From the returns of 143 schools she deduced the mortality of school children by age period and by sex and further classified the data gave important information on the causes of high institutional mortality among the native races. The numbers involved were small and the results were considerably in error; but, in the main, the conclusions as to the neglect of sanitary precautions and the change in the living habits of native race were sound.

A further paper on the aboriginal races in Australia was read before the same Association at York, England, in 1864. This essay contained copious quotations from correspondence with colonial governors over points raised by the first paper. The Colonial Office circulated the reprint of the Edinburgh paper widely. Nightingale has been considered a pioneer in work for arresting the decline of native races, so far as such work had been possible.

British Army in India

After the death of Sidney Herbert, Nightingale devoted the larger portion of her time and attention to the Indian question. Her earlier years of service to the British Army at home were not significant than her later years of endeavor for the army and the people in India. The greater proportion of the lives of soldiers lost in India was not chargeable to battle, but to disease caused by insanitation and general ignorance of military tropical hygiene. In 1859, it was found out that the average annual death rate of the British armies in India had been 69 per 1,000 since the year 1817. In recent times the figure has been 5 per 1,000. The changes in living and working accommodations which brought about this reduction in army mortality are directly traceable to the recommendations of the Royal Commission, appointed in 1859, which reported in 1863. An unrecorded fact, however, is that Nightingale's suggestion led directly to the appointment of the Commission and that the greater part of the Report was her handiwork. The suggestions upon which permanent reforms in army sanitation in India were based were also her work.

For eight months, during the latter part of 1858 and the earlier part of 1859, Nightingale importuned Lord Stanley for the appointment of a Royal Sanitary Commission which would do for the armies in India what had been done for the armies at home. She had contemplated for two years before the appointment of a Commission to investigate the entire question of the armies in British India. The mutiny of almost the whole of the Bengal native army and the contingents in northern India in 1857, which had filled the minds of the British population with thoughts of vengeance and repression against the native army, had only served to fix her attention upon sanitary and other administrative reform on behalf of the soldiers. Her analysis of the statistics of army mortality in India convinced her that there was murder committed not by the Sepoys alone. To their mind, it was murder to doom British soldiers to death by neglect of the most elementary sanitary precautions.

Anticipating the appointment of the Commission, she began collecting, tabulating, and interpreting data she had derived from circulars of inquiry which she had drafted and sent to all the stations in India. The inquiry form lacked little in requisite completeness and precision of detail. In the meantime, Nightingale and Dr Farr searched the sickness and mortality records of the India Office.

The report of the Indian Sanitary Commission when issued in 1863 comprised in all 2,028 pages, mostly in small print. The greater part of the statistical work in the report bore clear evidence of Nightingale's influence. Her inquiry blank, in the first instance, provided the vehicle for the transmission of much of the evidence. The replies to her question occupy the whole of the second volume of the report. In October, 1861, the commission requested her to submit her interpretation of these stational reports. Her observations upon these reports occupied 23 pages and are the most remarkable of all of her published works. Her unusual treatment of the subject by the addition of illustrative wood-cuts describing Indian hospitals and barracks, made the treasury demur, however, at the cost, but Nightingale was permitted to pay for the printing, out of her private purse. Copies of these observations were sent to the Queen and to influential members of the government. Sir John McNeill wrote: "The picture is terrible, but it is all true. There is no one statement from beginning to the end, that I feel disposed to question and there are many which my own observation and experience enable me to confirm". In detail, her notes related to the camp diseases which follow the selection of poor sites, defective disposal of human waste, over-crowding in barracks, lack of suitable occupation and exercise, dietaries and defective hospital arrangements. The sources of statistical data for the armies in India were also criticized. In addition to her observations, Nightingale prepared with Dr Sutherland an abstract of the returns upon which her "observations" were founded.

Moreover, when the report was published she moved with her characteristic decision to secure for it the newspaper and periodical publicity which it deserved. She contributed a popular resume of the Royal Commissions Report to the National Association for the Promotion of Social Science, meeting at Edinburgh in 1863, entitled "How People may Live and not Die in India". The paper was republished in 1864, with a preface and an account of what the Commission had actually achieved in sanitary works and measures. In 1868, the Secretary of State printed her resume of the Indian Sanitary Question from 1859 to 1867 and her memorandum of advice and suggestions on the entire situation as it then stood. The dispatch from Sir Stafford North core under date of April 23, 1863 (drafted by Nightingale), was printed at the same time. This dispatch resulted in the first of the annual series of Indian Sanitary Reports. In the reports for 1868 and 1869 appear two of Nightingale's contributions: in the first an introduction of eight pages and in the second her paper on "Sanitary Progress in India".

Her statistical enterprises of this period are well summarized in a few phrases which are here quoted from one of her letters: "I am all in the arithmetical line now… I find that every year . . . there are in the Home Army, 729 men alive every year who would have been dead but for Sidney Herbert's measures, and 5,184 men always on active duty who would have been constantly sick in bed. In India the differences is still more striking. Taken on the last two years, the death rate of Bombay is lower than that of London, the healthiest city in Europe. And the death rate of Calcutta is lower than that of Liverpool and Manchester. But this is not the greatest victory. The Municipal Commissioner of Bombay writes that the huddled native masses clamorously invoke the aid of the Health Department if but one death from cholera occurs; whereas formerly half of them might be swept away and the other half think it all right".

In 1873, the National Association for the Promotion of Social Science invited her to contribute a paper on the ten years of progress in India since her "How People May Live and Not Die in India". The India Office reprinted the paper in its 1874 bluebook. The salient fact developed in this report was that the death rate in the Indian Army had been reduced from 69 per 1,000 to 18 per 1,000. This summary of ten years of sanitary progress in India she was qualified to prepare in consequence of her editorial work on the annals issued by the sanitary department of the India Office.

In 1877, Nightingale published two letters on famine in India and followed these by an article in the *Nineteenth Century* magazine. This article, "The People in India", gave the principal facts about the Indian famines and proceeded further to describe in considerable detail the evils of usury in the Bombay Deccan. Beginning with 1874, Nightingale collected statistics of irrigation in India, and of the effect of irrigation on the life and health of the people. These data, the appendix of the second part of an unpublished work on the Indian Land Question and Irrigation Systems, were afterward partially used in several isolated papers. She thought much on education in India. There had been a neglect of elementary education. The exception was found in the system of village schools established by Lieutenant-Governor James Thomason, of what was then the Agra Province. The report of the Indian Education Commission of 1883 directed attention to the essential difficulties residing in the language, creedal, race, and traditional differences of the populations of the several provinces. The two chief difficulties in the way of a diffusion of education among the masses in India are the large agricultural population, among whom it is in all countries difficult to advance any system of education, and the existence of a hereditary class, whose object has been to maintain their monopoly of learning as the chief buttress of their social supremacy. Questions such as these occupied Nightingale's attention in the years 1881 and 1882.

The succeeding years were taken up in turn by Army Hospital Service reform, district nursing organization, nursing education and Indian finance problems.

In 1891, Nightingale finally laid aside her ambition to found at Oxford a Professorship in Applied Statistics. This relinquishment of active interest in the progress of statistics was indicative only of her physical powers. The gradual failure of sight, memory, and mental apprehension proceeded during the last fifteen years of her life. Her death occurred on August 13, 1910.

EXERCISES

1. State three definitions of statistics. Explain which one you consider the most appropriate.
2. Define statistics and explain the features of statistics.
3. Define statistics and list the characteristics of statistics.
4. Give an account of merits and demerits of statistics.
5. State the meaning of biostatistics and explain the need for statistics in nursing and health sciences.
6. Discuss Florence Nightingale's contribution to statistics.
7. Write short notes on the following:
   a. Descriptive statistics.
   b. Inferential statistics.
8. Define variable and explain the quantitative variables.
9. Write the notes on the following:
   a. Dependent variable and independent variable.
   b. Extraneous variable.
10. What are measurement scales? Explain them with proper illustration.

CHAPTER 2 Evidence-based Nursing Practice and Use of Computer in Nursing and Research

EVIDENCE-BASED NURSING PRACTICE

Introduction

Evidence-based practice refers to a practice that involves making clinical decisions on the best available evidence, with an emphasis on evidence from disciplined research. Since three decades, nursing research has experienced remarkable growth, providing nurses with an increasingly sound base knowledge from which to practice.

Nursing practices are generally based on nurses' past experiences; however there is little scientific evidence to support nurses' clinical decision making and expected outcome. While, nursing practices based on research evidences contribute to achieving client outcome and making nursing practices credible. Therefore, nurses need to base their practices on empirical evidences to optimize client outcomes, to provide cost effective safe practices and to enhance the credibility of nursing care.

Roots of evidence-based nursing can be traced in Florence Nightingale's era of nursing practices. Her concepts of promoting health, prevention of disease, and care of the sick were central ideas of her system. It involves identifying solid research findings and implementing them in nursing practices, in order to increase the quality of patient care. Sometimes, the term *research utilization* and *evidence-based practices* are used interchangeably. However, in real sense, the term *research utilization* is a narrow term, which is used for the use of empirically generated knowledge for nursing practices. In addition, research utilization has been defined as the use of research findings in any or all aspects of one's work as a registered nurse or at its simplest, the use of research.

Nurses are managing their clinical responsibilities at a time, when the nursing profession and the large health-care system require an extraordinary range of skills and talents from them. Nurses are expected to deliver the highest possible quality of care in a compassionate manner, while also being mindful of the cost. To accomplish these, evaluate extensive clinical information and incorporate it into clinical decision-making. Nurses increasingly are expected to adopt an evidence-based practice (EBP), which is broadly defined as the use of the best clinical evidence in making patient-care decisions.

The term evidence-based practice may be defined as the conscientious, explicit and judicious use of current best evidence in making decisions about the care of individual clients. The meanings used in this definition are as follows:

- *Conscientious* means carefully and with diligence
- *Explicit* means precisely and clearly
- *Judicious* means sensibly and with good judgment

Thus evidence–based nursing is the use of best evidence carefully, diligently, precisely and with good judgment in making decision about the care of an individual patient.

Evidence-based nursing (EBN), is a term that has been coined to mean the use of firm data rather than anecdotes, traditions, intuition or belief in making decisions about nursing practice. Evidence-based nursing practice needs to integrate individual clinical expertise with the best available clinical evidence from systematic research.

- Individual clinical expertise means the skill and judgements which nurses have acquired through clinical experience and clinical practice.
- Best available clinical evidence means, clinically relevant research, both basic system medical sciences including nursing and from client-centered clinical research into the safety and efficiency of therapeutic nursing interventions.

Evidence-based practice (EBP) in nursing is a process of locating, appraising, and applying the best evidence from the nursing and medical literature to improve the quality of clinical nursing practices.

More recently, the term *evidence-based nursing* (EBN) has emerged. This term has evolved from the initial work done in 'evidence-based medicine' defined as: the conscientious, explicit, and judicious use of current best evidences in making decisions about the care of individual patients. The practice of evidence-based medicine means integrating individual clinical expertise with the best available external clinical evidence from systematic research. If we use this same definition for 'evidence-based nursing', its meaning is broader than that of 'research utilization'. The practice of evidence-based nursing involves the following steps: formulation of an answerable question to address a specific patient problem or situation; systematic searching for the research evidence that could be used to answer the question; appraisal of the validity, relevance and applicability of the research evidence; integration of the research evidence with other information that might influence the management of the patient's problems: clinical expertise, patient preference for alternative forms of care, and available resources; implementation of the evidence-based practice decisions; and finally, evaluation of the outcome of the decision.

Evidence-based nursing (EBN) is a type of evidence-based practice in nursing. It involves identifying solid research findings and implementing them in nursing practices, in order to increase the qualtiy of patient care.

Evidence-based nursing (EBN) is a process founded on the collection, interpretation, and integration of valid, important, and applicable research. Some define EBN tightly, considering only the application of the findings of randomized clinical trials, while others are include the use of case reports and expert opinions.

Thus, evidence-based nursing is a term that has been coined to mean the use of firm data rather than anecdotes, traditions, institutions or belief in making decisions about nursing practice in field of health.

- The goal of evidence-based practice is to identify the most effective and cost-efficient treatments for a particular disease or conditions.
- A number of health-care organizations and groups are devoted to compiling study results that provide evidence to use in formulating guidelines for medical and nursing practice.
- We can find such compiled information in
  - Clinical practice guidelines
  - Evidence reports
  - Local health-care agency tools (e.g. clinical pathways and protocols).

Clinical Practice Guidelines are systematically developed statements to assist practitioners and patients in making decisions about appropriate health-care for a particular disease or procedure. Clinical practice guidelines are usually developed by clinicians, patients and advocacy groups and are published by specialty organizations, universities and government agencies.

Evidence Reports: Evidence reports are state-of-the-art, systematic reviews on clinical topics for the purpose of providing evidence for guidelines, quality improvement, quality measures and insurance coverage decisions. Evidence reports are usually developed by scientists, rather than clinicians, patients and advocacy groups, in the form of theory or phenomenon, i.e. competent in theory as given below:

- A theory is an organized set of related ideas and concepts that help us find meaning in our experiences (such as nursing), organize our thinking around an idea (such as caring) and develop new ideas and insights into the work we do.
- Phenomena are aspects of reality that you can observe and experience. They are the subject matter of a discipline often called phenomena of concern. Ex. Pharmacist—drugs, nurses – concerns of human being.

Purposes

- Evidence-based practices is an approach which tries to specify the way in which professionals or other decision-makers should make decisions by identifying such evidence that there may be for a practice and rating it according to how scientifically sound it may be.
- Its goal is to eliminate unsound or excessively risky practices in favor of those that have better outcomes.
- Evidence-based practice has contributed a lot towards better patient outcome. Heater and colleagues reported that patients who receive research-based nursing care make 'sizeable gains' in behavioral knowledge, and physiological and psychosocial outcomes compared with those receiving routine nursing over.
- The ultimate goal of evidence-based nursing is to provide the highest quality and most cost-efficient nursing care possible.
- The purpose or utility of evidence-based practice in nursing is mainly to improve the quality of nursing care.

Significance of Research

Research is a careful investigation or inquiry, especially through scientific methods, aimed at searching new facts or verification of established facts under various situations, in any branch of knowledge. Scientific research is a systematic and objective attempt to provide answers to certain questions. The purpose of research is to discover and develop an organized body of knowledge through application of scientific procedures.

Numerous definitions are available of the term "Research". The appropriate definition would be, "an honest, exhaustive, intelligent searching for facts and their implications with reference to a given problem, which may lead to development of theories, concepts, generalizations and principles". The ultimate outcome of any research should be to define authentic and verifiable knowledge leading to definite contributions in the field studied.

Nurses increasingly are expected to adopt an evidence-based practice, which is broadly defined as the use of the best clinical evidence in making patient care decisions.

Although there is no consensus about what types of 'evidence' are appropriate for evidence-based practice, there is general agreement that research finding from rigorous studies constitute the best type of evidence for informing nurses about 'decisions', actions and interactions with patients. Nurses are accepting the need to base specific nursing actions and decisions on evidence indicating that the actions are clinically appropriate, cost effective, and result in positive outcomes for clients. Nurses who incorporate high-quality research evidence into their patient decisions and advice are being professionally accountable to their patients. They are also reinforcing the identity of nursing as a profession.

Another reason for nurses to engage in and use research involves the spiraling costs of health-care and the cost containment practices being instituted in health-care facilities. Now, more than ever, nurses need to document the social relevance and effectiveness of their practice, not only to the profession but to nursing care consumers, health care administration, third-party payers (ex. Insurance companies) and government agencies. Some research findings will help to eliminate nursing actions that do not achieve desired outcomes. Other findings will help nurses identify practices that improve health-care outcomes and contain costs as well.

Nursing research is essential if nurses are to understand the varied dimension of their profession. Research enables nurses to describe the characteristics of a particular nursing situation about which little is known; to explain the phenomenon that must be considered in planning nursing care; to predict the probable outcomes of certain nursing decisions; to control the occurrence of undesired outcomes and to initiate activities to promote desired client behavior.

Research is systematic inquiry that uses disciplined methods to answer questions or solve problems. The ultimate goal of research is to develop, refine and expand the body of knowledge. Nurses are increasingly engaged in disciplined studies that benefit the profession and its patients and that contributes to improvement in the entire health-care system.

Nursing research is the systematic, objective process of analyzing phenomena of importance to nursing. Research in nursing encompass all clinical practice arenas, nursing education and nursing administration.

Thus, nursing research is systemic inquiry, designed to develop knowledge about issues of importance to the nursing profession, including nursing practice, education, administration and information.

Nurse researchers currently are making important contributions to the evidence-based practice necessary for professional nursing. Nurses participate in research by:

- Identifying ideas that should be examined through the research process
- Assisting in designing and/or performing research
- Using research as a basis for their practice.

There is a need at each level of educational preparation. Nurses function in different roles in the research process as given below:

i. Diploma in Nursing
   - Be aware of the importance of research to evidence-based practice
   - Help to identify problem areas in nursing
   - Help to collect data with a more experienced nurse researcher.

ii. Bachelor Degree in Nursing
   - Critique research for application to clinical practice
   - Identify nursing research problems and help to implement research studies
   - Apply research findings to establish sound, evidence based clinical practice.

iii. Master Degree in Nursing
   - Analyze problems so that appropriately designed research can be used to solve problems
   - Through clinical expertise, apply research-based practice to nursing care situations
   - Provide support to on-going research projects
   - Conduct research for the purpose of assuring quality nursing care.

iv. Doctoral Degree in Nursing
   - Conduct nursing research
   - Serve as leaders in applying research results to the clinical arena
   - Develop ways to monitor the quality of nursing care being administered by nurses.

Scientific Method

"Scientific inquiry is the process in which the researcher, through use of the senses, systematically collects observable, verifiable data to describe, explain or predict events".

- The goals of scientific enquiry are to find solutions to problems and to develop explanations of the Universe (Theories)
- The scientific method has two unique characteristics that the other ways of knowing do not:

– Objectivity or self-correction—this means that the researcher uses techniques to keep her personal beliefs, values and attitudes separate from the research process
– Use of empirical data—it consists of information gathered through sight, hearing, task, touch or smell. Conclusions based on reality and not on beliefs or hunches.

In brief characteristics of scientific method include the following:

- It begins with an identified problem or need to be studied.
- It uses theories, models and conceptual themes that have been empirically tested.
- It uses systematic, orderly methods to acquire empirical evidence to test theories.
- It uses methods of control for ruling out other variables that might affect the relationships between the variables they are studying.
- It avoids explanations that cannot be empirically tested.
- It prefers to generalize the findings (knowledge) so that it can be applied in cases other than those in the study.
- It uses built in mechanism for self-correction.

The scientific method makes use of a variety of procedures and study designs aimed to increase the chances that the data collected will be reliable, relevant and unbiased. There are two major categories of research design, i.e. quantitative and qualitative. Each category has within its several specific types of research methodology.

Quantitative Research: The main purpose of this research is to gather data from enough subjects (People being studied) to be able to generalize results to a similar population.

Generalized results mean that you say, "What I found to be so, for this group of people will probably be the same for all people, who are similar".

- In quantitative research, researcher carefully controls data collection and are careful to maintain the objectivity of the process. Data are reported as numbers. Numerical data, ex. Questionnaires, number of incidents, or reactions to a medication.
- Persons studied are large numbers of subjects, so it can be generalized to other similar population.
- It has hypothesis.
- *Environment:* It can be in a laboratory setting: needs to be a controlled environment.

Qualitative Research: Focuses on the lived experience of people. The purpose is not to generalize the data, but to share the experience of the person or persons in the study.

- Data—Non-numerical data: Data may consist of words from interviews, observations, written documents and even art or photos.
- Persons studied are small number of participants; is not designed to be generalized.
- It has no hypothesis, because it is the research of the "lived experience" of the person or person being studied.
- *Environment:* It is done in the "natural settings", i.e. the person's home or work setting.

Researchers usually work within a paradigm that is consistent with their world view and that gives rise to the types of question that excite their curiosity. The maturity of the concept of interest also may lead to one or the other paradigm: when little is known about a topic, a qualitative approach is often more fruitful than a quantitative one.

Quantitative Research includes Experimental and Non-experimental Studies: A basic distinction in quantitative studies is the difference between experimental and nonexperimental research. In experimental research, researchers actively introduce an intervention of treatment. In non-experimental research, on the other hand, researchers collect data without making changes or introducing treatments. For example, if a researcher gave bran flakes to one group of subjects and prune juice to another to evaluate which method facilitated elimination more effectively, the study would be experimental because the researcher intervened in the normal course of things. In this example, the researcher created an "active variable" involving a dietary intervention. If, on the other hand, a researcher compared elimination patterns of two groups of people whose regular eating patterns differed – for example, some normally took foods that stimulated bowel elimination and others did not—there is no existing attributes and is non-experimental.

Experimental studies are explicity designed to test causal relationships. Sometimes non-experimental studies also seek to elucidate or detect causal relationships, but doing so is tricky and usually is less conclusive. Experimental studies offer the possibility of greater control over extraneous variables than nonexperimental studies.

Qualitative studies are often rooted in research traditions that originate in the disciplines of anthropology, sociology, and psychology. Three such traditions have had especially strong influences on qualitative nursing research and are briefly described here.

- **The grounded theory** tradition, which has its roots in sociology, seeks to describe and understand the key social psychological and structural processes that occur in a social setting. Grounded theory was developed in the 1960s by two sociologists, Glaser and Strauss (1967). The focus of most grounded theory studies is on a developing social experience – the social and psychological stages and phases that characterize a particular event or episode. A major component of grounded theory is the discovery of a core variable that is central in explaining what is going on in that social scene. Grounded theory researchers strive to generate comprehensive explanations of phenomena that are grounded in reality.
- **Phenomenology**, which has its disciplinary roots in both philosophy and psychology and is rooted in a philosophical tradition developed by Husserl and Heidegger, is concerned with the lived experiences of humans. Phenomenology is an approach to thinking about what life experiences of people are like and what they mean. The phenomenological researcher asks the questions: What is the essence of this phenomenon as experienced by these people? Or, What is the meaning of the phenomena to those who experience it?
- **Ethnography** is the primary research tradition within anthropology, and provides a framework for studying the meanings, patterns, and experiences of a defined cultural group in a holistic fashion. Ethnographers typically engage in extensive fieldwork, often participating to the extent possible in the life of the culture under study. Ethnographic research is in some cases concerned with broadly defined cultures (e.g. Haitian in refugee communities), but sometimes focuses on more narrowly defined cultural (e.g. the culture of emergency departments). The aim of ethnographers is to learn from (rather than to study) members of a cultural group, to understand their world view as they perceive and live it.

Steps of Quantitative Research

In quantitative studies, researchers move from the beginning point of a study (the posing of a question) to the end point (the obtaining of an answer) in a fairly linear sequence of steps that is broadly similar across studies. In some studies, the steps overlap, whereas in others, certain steps are unnecessary. Still, there is general flow of activities that is typical of a quantitative study.

The early steps in a quantitative research project typically involve activities with a strong conceptual or intellectual element. These activities include reading, conceptualizing, theorizing, reconceptualizing and reviewing ideas with colleagues or advisers. During this phase, researchers call on such skills as creativity, deductive reasoning, insight, and a firm grounding in previous research on the topic of interest. The early steps include the following:

Step 1: Formulating and Delimiting the Problem

One of the first things a researcher must do is develop a research problem and research questions. Good research depends to a great degree on good questions. Without a significant, interesting problem, the most carefully and skillfully designed research project is of little value.

It is important that individuals work *closely together* to reach the optimum outcome for the chosen topic. Some things that would ensure *collaboration* are working in groups to review performance improvement data, *brainstorming* about ideas, and achieving consenus about the final selection. When selecting a question, nurses should formulate questions that are likely to gain support from people within the organization. An interdisciplinary medical team should work together to come up with an agreement about the topic selection. The priority of the question should be considered as well as the severity of the problem. Nurses should consider whether the topic would apply to many or few clinical areas. Also, the availability of solid evidence should be considered because providing proof of the research. This will increase staffs' willingness to implement into nursing practice.

One of the most challenging issues in using EBP in the clinical setting is learning how to adequately frame a clinical question so that an appropriate literature review can be performed. When forming a clinical question, the following should be included: the disorder or disease of the patient, the intervention or finding being reviewed, possibly a comparison intervention, and the outcome.

Quantitative researchers usually proceed from the selection of a broad problem area to the development of specific questions that are amenable to empirical inquiry. In developing a research question to be studied, nurse researchers must pay close attention to substantive issues (Is the research question significant, given the existing base of knowledge?); clinical issues (Could findings from this research be useful in clinical practice?); and methodologic issues (How can this question best be studied to yield high-quality evidence?). The identification of research questions must also take into consideration practical and ethical concerns.

Step 2: Reviewing the Related Literature

Quantitative research is typically conducted within the context of previous knowledge. To build on existing theory or research, quantitative researchers strive to understand what is already known about a research problem. A thorough literature review provides a foundation on which to base new knowledge and usually is conducted well before any data is collected in quantitative studies. For clinical problems, it would also be necessary to learn as much as possible about the "status quo" of current procedures relating to the topic and to review existing practice guidelines or protocols.

A familiarization with previous studies can also be useful in suggesting research topics or in identifying aspects of a problem about which more research is needed. Thus, a literature review sometimes precedes the delineation of the research problem.

Literature review to search for the best available evidence: Once the topic is selected, the research relevant to the topic must be reviewed, in addition to other relevant literature. It is important that clinical studies, integrative literature reviews, meta-analyses, and well-known and reliable existing EBP guidelines are accessed in the literature retrieval process. With the Internet at one's fingertips, a plethora of research is just a few clicks away. However, just because you found it in a respectable journal does not signify high quality research. When reviewing any article for evidence retrieval, read it very closely. Articles can appear to be precise and factual on the surface but with further and much closer examination, flaws can be found. The article can be loaded with opinionated and/or biased statements that would clearly taint the findings, thus lowering the creditability and quality of the article. Time management is crucial to information retrieval. Nurses making their way through the vast amount of research available may find it helpful to read research articles or critical reviews instead of clinical journals. To maintain high standards for EBP implementation, education in research review is necessary to distinguish good research from poorly conducted research. Equally important is to consider if the materials being reviewed are current. Once the literature is located, it is helpful to classify the articles as either conceptual (theory and clinical articles) or data-based (systematic research reviews). Before reading and critiquing the research, it is useful to read theoretical and clinical articles to have a broad view of the nature of the topic and related concepts, and then to review exiting EBP guidelines.

Step 3: Undertaking Clinical Fieldwork

In addition to refreshing or updating clinical knowledge based on written work, researchers embarking on a clinical nursing study benefit from spending time in clinical settings, discussing the topic with clinicians and health-care administrators and observing current practices. Sterling (2001) notes that such clinical fieldwork can provide perspectives on recent clinical trends, current diagnostic procedures and relevant health-care delivery models; it can also help researchers better understand affected clients and the settings in which care is provided. In addition to expanding the researchers' clinical and conceptual knowledge, such fieldwork can be valuable in developing methodologic tolls for strengthening the study. For example, in the course of clinical fieldwork researchers might learn what extraneous variables need to be controlled or might discover the need for Spanish-speaking research assistants.

As with literature reviews, clinical fieldwork may serve as a stimulus for developing research questions and may be the first step in the process for some researchers.

Step 4: Defining the Framework and Developing Conceptual Definitions

Theory is the ultimate aim of science in that it transcends the specifics of a particular time, place and group of people and aims to identify regularities in the relationships among variables. When quantitative research is performed within the context of a theoretical framework—that is, when previous theory is used as a basis for generating predictions that can be tested through empirical research—the findings may have broader significance and utility.

Even when the research question is not embedded in a theory, researchers must have a clear sense of the concepts under study. Thus, an important task in the initial phase of a project is the development of conceptual definitions.

Step 5: Formulating Hypotheses

A hypothesis is a statement of the researchers' expectations about relationships between the variables under investigation. Hypothesis, in other words, is predictions of expected outcomes. They state the relationships researchers expect to find as a result of the study.

The research question identifies the concepts under investigation and asks how the concepts might be related; a hypothesis is the predicted answer. For example, the initial research question might be phrased as follows: Is preeclamptic toxemia in pregnant women associated with stress factors present during pregnancy? This might be translated into the following hypothesis: Pregnant women with a higher incidence of stressful events during pregnancy will be more likely to have preeclamptic toxemia than women with a lower incidence of stress. The experience of the patients is designed to test hypotheses through statistical analysis.

In the next phase of a quantitative research project, researchers make decisions about the methods and procedures to be used to address the research question and plan for the actual collection of data. Sometimes the nature of the question dictates the methods to be used, but more often than not, researchers have considerable flexibility to be creative and make many decisions. These methodologic decisions usually have crucial implications for the validity and reliability of the study findings. If the methods used to collect and analyze research data are seriously flawed, then the evidence from the study may be of little value. For which following steps should be followed.

Step 6: Selecting a Research Design

The research design is the overall plan for obtaining answers to the questions being studied and for handling some of the difficulties encountered during the research process. A wide variety of research designs are available for quantitative studies, including numerous experimental and non-experimental designs.

In designing the study, the researchers specify which specific designs will be adopted and what controls will be used to minimize bias and enhance the interpretability of results. In quantitative studies, research designs tend to be highly structured, with tight controls over extraneous variables. Research designs also indicate other aspects of the research – for example, how often subjects will be measured or observed, what types of comparisons will be made and where will the study take place. The research design is essentially the architectural backbone of the study.

Study designs may be:

- Observational – where one or more groups of patients are "observed" by the researcher and certain characteristics of the observed group or groups that are of relevance to the research question are recorded.
- Experimental – an intervention or "experiment" is performed (e.g. giving a drug) on one or more groups of patients, and the effects of the intervention are recorded by the researcher.

There are different types of observational studies.

a. **Case control studies (Fig. 2.1)**

The study begins with the absence or presence of an outcome and the investigators then look backwards in time to try and detect possible causes or risk factors.

For example, you could study a group of babies, some of whom are of low birth-weight and others are normally grown and compare the smoking habits of the parents in the two groups. The outcome here is low birth-weight and the possible risk factor is parental smoking habits.

b. **Cross-sectional studies**

The investigators analyze data collected on a group of subjects at one time rather than over a period of time. Cross-sectional studies are designed to determine "What is happening?" right now.

For example, you could study hemoglobin levels at the first antenatal visit to study the prevalence of anemia in early pregnancy.

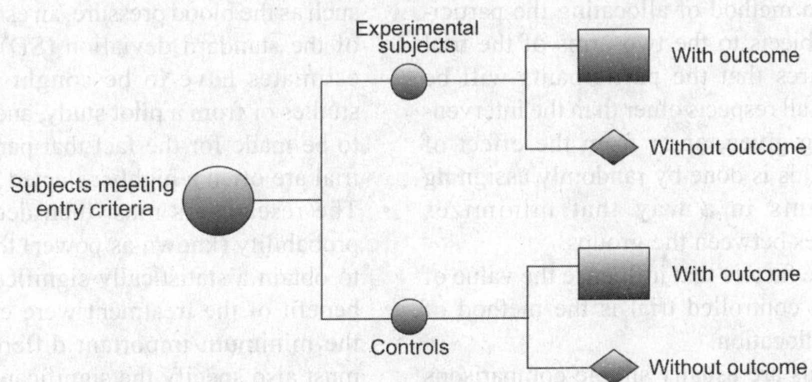

Fig. 2.1: Observation Study Designs

c. **Case control studies**

A cohort is a group of people who have something in common and who remain part of a group over an extended period of time. Investigators record outcomes after observing the group over a period of time.

For example, you could study a group of women after menopause over several years to study the effects of menopause on women's health.

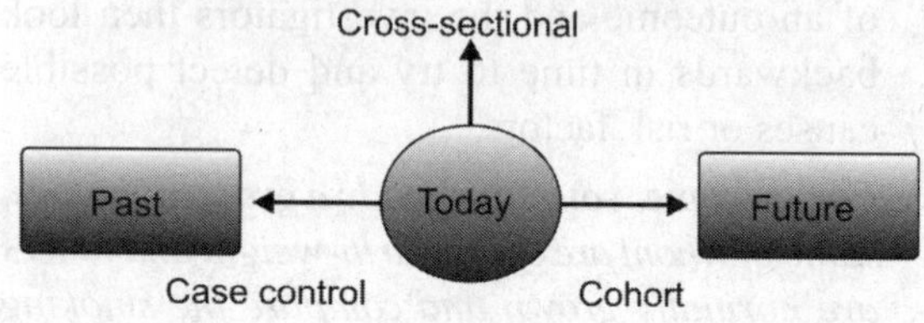

Among experimental studies, the different types of trials include:

a. **Non-randomized controlled trials**

A control trial compares an intervention group with a control group, the two arms of the trial. In a non-randomized trial, participants are not always allocated to the different arms of the trial in a random manner. This can lead to imbalances between the groups being compared and would have a negative influence on the results of the trial.

b. **Randomized controlled trial**

i. This is the principal research design in the evaluation of medical interventions. The aim is to use a method of allocating the participating subjects to the two arms of the trial that ensures that the participants will be similar in all respects other than the intervention being given, apart from the effect of chance. This is done by randomly assigning participants in a way that minimizes imbalances between the groups.

ii. One of the factors that influence the value of a random controlled trial is the method of random allocation.

Clinical trials are usually simple comparisons between two randomised groups, and the number of patients entered into a trial is nearly always determined in advance—and clinical objectives are seldom taken into account when the size of the sample is chosen. Hence, the numbers are usually estimated by the length of time or amount of money available, or even by choosing some arbitrarily "round" number. Altman (1983) pointed out that recent reviews of general medical publications and of clinical trials in particular have shown that many studies are too small to have any reasonable chance of detecting clinical benefit of the treatment under investigation and he gives guidelines for getting the numbers right:

- The usual method by which the size of the sample is determined is closely related to significance testing. The object of this is to reduce to an acceptable level the risk of obtaining a misleading result by making statistical significance and clinical importance coincide as nearly as possible.
- The physician should specify either the smallest benefit of the new treatment that would be considered to be of clinical importance or the smallest benefit that it would be important not to miss.
- For trials where the measure is qualitative (or categorical)—improved or not improved, survived or died—an estimate is needed of the proportion with that outcome (such as the death rate) that may be expected in one group, usually the control.
- If the measured outcome is a continuous variable such as the blood pressure, an estimate is needed of the standard deviation (SD) of this. These estimates have to be sought from previous studies or from a pilot study, and allowance has to be made for the fact that participants in the trial are often a highly selected group.
- The researchers must then decide with what probability (known as power) they would wish to obtain a statistically significant result if the benefit of the treatment were exactly equal to the minimum important difference, and they must also specify the significance level, which is usually set at 5 percent (see later).

If too few patients are used, important therapeutic benefits may not be detected or false-positive findings may be reported, a possibility enhanced by the likely publication being biased in favor of a "significant" result. Unfortunately, the continuing uncertainty about various forms of therapy is usually due to the size of the original clinical trials being too small. Large number of patients are needed when small differences in response to a drug are expected or when the natural history of the disease varies greatly; an example of this is the use of penicillamine in rheumatoid arthritis, and this type of trial usually has to be done on a multicenter basis. The best way to ensure that numbers in any clinical trial are satisfactory is, of course, to get the expert advice of a statistician.

c. **Methods of randomization include:**

i. *Quasi-random allocation:* A method of allocating participants that is not truly random, for example, allocation by date, of birth, day of the week, medical record number, day of the year or the order in which participants are included in the study (e.g. allotting participants alternately to two arms of a trial).

ii. *True random allocation:* A method of allocation that uses the play to assign participants to comparison groups in a trial, e.g. by using a random numbers table or a computer-generated random sequence. Random allocation implies that each individual being entered into a trial has the same chance of receiving each of the possible interventions. It also implies that the probability an individual will receive a particular intervention is independent of the probability that any other individual will receive the same intervention.

Step 7: Developing Protocols for the Intervention

In experimental research, researchers actively intervene and create the independent variable, which means that people in the sample will be exposed to different treatments or conditions. For example, if we were interested in testing the effect of biofeedback in treating hypertension, the independent variable would be biofeedback compared with either an alternative treatment (e.g. relaxation therapy), or with no treatment. The intervention protocol for the study would need to be developed, specifying exactly what the biofeedback treatment would entail (e.g. who would administer it, how frequently and over how long a period the treatment would last, what specific equipment would be used, and so on) and what the alternative condition would be. The goal of well-articulated protocols is to have all subjects in each group treated in the same way. (In non-experimental research, of course, this step would not be necessary).

Step 8: Identifying the Population to be Studied

Before selecting subjects, quantitative researchers need to know what characteristics participants should possess. Researchers and others using the findings also need to know, to whom study results can be generalized. Thus, during the planning phase of quantitative studies, researchers must identify the population to be studied. The term population refers to the aggregate or totality of those confirming to a set of specifications. For example, we might specify nurses (RNs) and residence in India as attributes of interest; the study population would then consist of all licensed RNs who reside in India.

Step 9: Designing the Sampling Plan

The word 'population' or 'universe' means an aggregate of all "elementary units", each unit may be animate or inanimate, about which an information is required.

Universe or whole population may be "finitie" (e.g. 100 kgs of rice in a sac (Bag) or all the inhabitants of a city) or it may be "infinite" (e.g. stars in the sky etc.). Universe may be "homogeneous" i.e. made up of uniform class (e.g. Polished rice in a sack; all Hindu

Table 2.1

Difference between census and sampling enumeration

Census enumeration	Sampling enumeration
1. Investigation is carried out for the entire population (all units).	Investigation is carried out only for a sample.
2. Useful when detailed information is required.	Useful when overall information is required.
3. Organization is costly and consumes more time.	Organization is cheap and consumes less time.
4. Greater attention cannot be paid for each unit because of the vastness of the population.	Greater attention can be paid for each unit because of relative smallness of the sample.
5. Difficult to achieve a complete and accurate study.	Easy to achieve a complete and accurate study.
6. Requires more personnel for study.	Requires less personnel for study.

women of reproductive age in the city etc.) or it may be heterogeneous, made of dissimilar classes of persons or animals or objects.

It is not possible for any scientific study to cover the whole population because of the cost, time and practicability. So a representative portion of the universe is taken for the study. It is called a "Sample". For example, a handful of rice from a sac (Bag) of 100 kgs rice, a group of people attending a public meeting etc. The observations made out of a representative sample is then applied to the universe at large, but generalization is valid, only if the sample is sufficiently large and representative.

Sampling is a procedure, adopted for selection of a representative units of the universe units. The sampling procedure can be adopted with the help of "Sampling frame", which consists of a list of "enumeration units".

When the investigation is carried out for the entire population it is called the "Census Enumeration" and when it is carried out for the sample, it is called "Sample Enumeration". The difference between these two are described in Table 2.1.

Research studies almost, always rely on a sample of subjects, who are a subset of the population. It is clearly more practical and less costly to collect data from a sample, than from an entire population. The risk, however, is that the sample might not adequately reflect the populations behavior, traits, symptoms or beliefs.

In most research projects it is impossible or impractical to study the effect of treatment on all patients available who might be suffering from a given condition. The total number is referred to statistically as the "population" and the group chosen for study "the sample". It follows that the more representative the sample is of the total population, the more applicable will be the results to that population.

The study of a sample will save time, money and effort; also, since the number of people making the observations will be less, it will be easier to find good specialists and to train them adequately, and the methodology can be more tightly controlled as fewer research instruments will be needed—so their performance can be constantly verified. The disadvantage is the problem of sampling errors, so that the sample may not represent the population itself. This can be reduced by simply increasing the size of the sample and it can be quantified by means of a statistical constant called the standard error.

Suppose a sample is selected by selecting only those units of the population, so that it suits a specific purpose as per the desire of the investigator, it is called as "Purposive Sampling". This method serves only a limited purpose. Suppose a sample is selected in such a way that the characteristic of the population is represented, it is called as "Representative Sampling". The characteristics of a representative sample includes:

- It is selected by a sampling technique from the universe or population it represents.
- Usually it does not differ from the universe in compostion. If it differs, it is solely by chance.

- Each member of the universe from which it is taken has an equal opportunity of being selected.
- Bias has been ruled out and the sample will give an estimate of the attribute under study, almost equal to the population value called "true value".
- It is chosen according to a rule that is independent of the observations to be made on the sample.
- Sample should be sufficiently large in size to represent population from which it is drawn.

When a sample is not representative of its population, it is known as a "selected sample". By definition a selected sample cannot be used to draw conclusions about a population, unless it is known fairly precisely in what way the sample differs. There are three ways in which samples may become selected:

1. Instances where the sample is taken from a sector of a population with the erroneous belief that this sector forms the whole population.
2. Cases where individuals are chosen by a method other than random sampling, for choosing individuals by a random procedure is the only advisable method for providing samples.
3. Cases where the sample is chosen correctly but circumstances make it impossible to obtain information from the individuals under study. This happens, for example, when doing surveys by post, where only the people interested in the subject being researched with answer. These people usually have characteristics that are quite different from the rest of the population, and omission of those not replying to any questionnaire will produce wrong conclusions.

Various methods of obtaining samples are available. These methods vary in cost, effort and skills required, but their adequacy is assessed by the same criterion: the representativeness of the selected sample. That is, the quality of the sample for quantitative studies depends on how typical or representative, the sample is of the population with respect to the variables of concern in the study. Sophisticated sampling procedures can produce samples that have a high likelihood of being representative. The most sophisticated methods are **probability sampling** methods, which use random procedures for selecting subjects. In a probability sample, every member of the population has an equal probability of being included in the sample. With **non-probability sampling**, by contrast, there is no way of ensuring that each member of the population could be selected; consequently, the risk of a biased (unrepresentative) sample is greater. The design of a **sampling plan** includes the selection of a sampling method, the specification of the sample size (i.e. number of subjects) and the development of procedures for recruiting subjects.

Step 10: Specifying Methods to Measure the Research Variables

Quantitative researchers must develop methods to observe or measure the research variables as accurately as possible. Based on the conceptual definitions, the researcher selects or designs appropriate methods of operationalizing the variables and collecting data. A variety of quantitative data collection approaches exist. **Biophysiologic measurements** often play an important role in clinical nursing research. Through self-reports, another popular method of data collection, subjects are asked directly about their feelings, behaviors, attitudes and personal traits (for example, in an interview with research personnel). Another technique is observation, wherein researchers collect data by observing and recording aspects of peoples' behavior.

Data collection methods vary in the degree of structure imposed on subjects. Quantitative approaches tend to be fairly structured, involving the use of a formal instrument that elicits the same information from every subject. Sometimes researchers need to develop their own instruments, but more often they use or adapt measuring instruments that have been developed by others. The task of measuring research variables and developing a data collection plan is a complex and challenging process that permits a great deal of creativity and choice. Before finalizing the data collection plan, researchers must carefully evaluate whether the chosen methods capture key concepts accurately.

Step 11: Developing Methods for Safeguarding Human/Animal Rights

Most nursing research involves human subjects, although some studies involve animals. In either case, procedures need to be developed to ensure that the study adheres to ethical principles. For example, forms often need to be developed to document that the subjects' participation in the study plan needs to be reviewed to determine whether the rights of the subjects have been adequately protected. Often that review involves a formal presentation to an external committee.

Step 12: Finalizing and Reviewing the Research Plan

Before actually collecting research data, researchers often perform a number of "tests" to ensure that plans will work smoothly. For example, they may evaluate the readability of any written material to determine if people with below-average reading skills can comprehend them, or they may need to test whether technical equipment is functioning properly. If questionnaires are used, it is important to know whether respondents understand questions or find certain ones objectionable; this is usually referred to as pre-testing the questionnaire. During final study preparations, researchers also have to determine the type of training that is to be provided to those responsible for collecting data. If researchers have concerns about their study plans, they may undertake a pilot study, which is a small-scale version or trial run of the major study.

Normally, researchers have their research plan critiqued by peers, consultants, or other reviewers to obtain substantive, clinical or methodologic feedback before implementing the plan. When researchers seek financial support for the study, a proposal typically is submitted to a funding source and reviewers of the proposed plan usually suggest improvements. Students conducting a study as part of a course or degree requirement have their plans reviewed by faculty advisers. Even under other circumstances, however, researchers are well advised to ask individuals external to the project to assess preliminary plans.

Experienced researchers with fresh perspective can often be invaluable in identifying pitfalls and shortcomings that otherwise night not have been recognized.

After finalizing and reviewing research plan the empirical portion of quantitative studies involves collecting research data and preparing that data for analysis. In many studies, the empirical phase is one of the most time-consuming parts of the investigation, although the amount of time spent collecting data varies considerably from one study to the next. If data are collected by distributing a written questionnaire to intact groups, this task may be accomplished in a matter of days. More often, however, data collection requires several weeks, or even months, of work for which following steps are to be followed.

Step 13: Collecting the Data

The actual collection of data in a quantitative study often proceeds according to a pre-established plan. The researcher's plan typically specifies procedures for the actual collection of data (e.g. where and when the data will be gathered); for describing the study to participants and for recording information. Technological advances in the past few decades have expanded possibilities for automating data collection.

A considerable amount of both clerical and administrative work is required during data collection. Researchers typically must be sure, for example, that enough material is available to complete the study; that participants are informed of the time and place that their presence may be required; that research personnel (such as interviewers) are conscientious in keeping their appointments; that schedules do not conflict; and that a suitable system of maintaining confidentiality of information has been implemented.

Step 14: Preparing the Data for Analysis

After data is collected, a few preliminary activities must be performed before data analysis begins. For instance, it is normally necessary to look through the questionnaire to determine if they are usable. Sometimes forms are left almost entirely blank or contain other indications of misinterpretation or noncompliance. Another step is to assign identification numbers to the responses or observation of different subjects, if this was not done previously.

Coding of the data is typically needed at this point. Coding involves the transition of verbal data into numeric form, according to a specified plan. This might mean assigning numeric codes to categorical variables such as gender (e.g. 1 for females and 2 for males). Coding might also be needed to categorize narrative responses to certain questions. For example, patients' verbatim responses to a question about the quality of nursing care they received during hospitalization might be coded into: (1) positive reactions (2) negative reactions, (3) neutral reactions, (4) or mixed reactions, another preliminary step involves transferring the data from written documents onto computer files for subsequent analysis.

After preparing the data for the next move is analysis of the data. Here quantitative data gathered in the empirical phase are not reported in raw form. They are subjected to analysis and interpretation, which occurs in the fourth major phase of a project for which the following steps should be followed.

Step 15: Analyzing the Data

The data themselves do not provide answers to research questions. Ordinarily, the amount of data collected in a study is rather extensive; research questions cannot be answered by a simple perusal of numeric information. Data need to be processed and analyzed in an orderly, coherent fashion. Quantitative information is usually analyzed through statistical procedures. Statistical analyses cover a broad range of techniques, from simple procedures that we all use regularly (e.g. computing an average) to complex and sophisticated methods. Although some methods are computationally formidable, the underlying logic of statistical tests is relatively easy to grasp, and computers have eliminated the need to get bogged down with detailed mathematic operations.

Step 16: Interpreting the Results

Before the results of a study can be communicated effectively, they must be systematically interpreted. **Interpretation** is the process of making sense of the results and of examining their implications. The process of interpretation begins with an attempt to explain the findings within the context of the theoretical framework, prior empirical knowledge, and clinical experience.

If research hypotheses have been supported, an explanation of the results may be straightforward because the findings fit into a previously conceived argument. If hypotheses are not supported, researchers must explain why this might be so. Is the underlying conceptualization wrong, or was it inappropriate for the research problem? Or do the findings reflect problems with the research methods rather than the framework (e.g. was the measuring tool inappropriate)? To provide sound explanations, researchers not only must be familiar with clinical issues, prior research and conceptual underspinning, but must be able to understand methodologic limitations of the study. In other words, the interpretation of the findings must take into account all available evidence about the study's reliability and validity. Researchers need to evaluate critically the decision they made in designing the study and to recommend alternatives to others interested in the same research problem.

Actually the analytic phase brings researchers full circle: it provides answers to the questions posed in the first phase of the project. However, researcher's responsibilities are not complete until the study results are disseminated.

Step 17: Communicating the Findings

A study cannot contribute evidence to nursing practice if the results are not communicated. The most compelling hypothesis, the most rigorous study, the most dramatic results are of no value to the nursing community, if they are unknown. Another – and often final – task of a research project, therefore, is the preparation of a **research report** that can be shared with others.

Research reports can take various forms: term papers, dissertations, journal articles, presentations at professional conferences and so on. **Journal articles** – reports appearing in such professional journals as *Nursing Research* – usually are the most useful because they are available to a broad, international audience. There is also a growing number of outlets for research dissemination on the internet.

Step 18: Utilizing the Findings in Practice

Many interesting studies have been conducted by nurses without having any effect on nursing practice or nursing education. Ideally, the concluding step of a high-quality study is to plan for its' utilization in practice settings. Although, nurse researchers may not themselves be in a position to implement a plan for utilizing research findings, they can contribute to the process by including in their research reports recommendations regarding how the evidence from the study could be incorporated into the practice of nursing and by vigorously pursuing opportunities to disseminate the findings to practicing nurses.

- ***Evaluating and analyzing the strengths and weaknesses of that evidence in terms of validity and generalisability:*** Use of rating systems to determine the quality of the research is crucial to the development of EBP. There are several rating systems available online.
- ***Implementing useful findings in clinical practice based on valid evidence; evidence is used alongside clinical expertise and the patients' perspective to plan care:*** After determining the internal and external validity of the study, a decision is arrived at whether the information gathered does apply to your initial question. It is important to address questions related to diagnosis, therapy, harm, and prognosis. The information gathered should be interpreted according to many criteria and should always be shared with other nurses and/ or fellow researchers.
- ***Evaluating efficacy and performance of evidences through a process of self reflection, audit, or peer assessment:*** Finally after the implementation of the useful findings for the clinical practices; efficacy and performance is evaluated through processes of self reflection, internal or external audit or peer assessment.

Quantitative Research Process—An Illustration

The steps described in the preceding section represent an idealized conception of what researchers do. The research process rarely follows a neatly prescribed pattern of sequential procedures. Developments in one step, for example, may require alterations in a previously completed activity. Nevertheless, for the quantitative researcher, careful organization is very important.

Almost all research projects are conducted under time pressure. Students in research courses have end-of-term deadlines; government sponsored research involves funds granted for a specified time. Those who may not have such formal time constraints (e.g. graduate students working on these or dissertations) normally have their own goals for completion. Setting up a timetable in advance may be an important means of meeting such goals. Having deadlines for tasks—even tentative ones—helps to impose order and delimits tasks that might otherwise continue indefinitely, such as problem selection and literature reviews.

It is not possible to give even approximate figures for the relative percentage of time that should be spent on each task in quantitative studies. Some projects require many months to develop and pretest the measuring instruments, whereas other studies use previously existing ones, for example; the write-up of the study may take many months or only a few days. Clearly, not all steps are equally time-consuming. It would make little sense simply to divide the available time by the number of tasks.

Let us suppose a researcher was studying the following problem: Is a woman's decision to have an annual mammogram related to her perceived susceptibility to breast cancer? Using the organization of steps outlined earlier, here are some of the tasks that might be undertaken:

1. The researcher, who lost her mother to breast cancer, is concerned that many older women do not get a mammogram regularly. Her specific research question is whether mammogram practices are different for women who have different views about their susceptibility to breast cancer.
2. The researcher reviews the research literature on mammograms, factors affecting mammography decisions and interventions designed to promote it.
3. The researcher does clinical fieldwork by discussing the problem with nurses and other health-care professionals in various clinical settings (health clinics, private obstetrics and gynecology practices) and by informally discussing the problem with women in a support group for breast cancer victims.
4. The researcher examines frameworks for conceptualizing the problem. She finds that the Health Belief Model is relevant and this helps her to develop a conceptual definition of susceptibility to breast cancer.
5. Based on what the researcher has learned, the following hypothesis is developed: Women who perceive themselves as not susceptible to breast cancer are less likely than other women to get an annual mammogram.
6. The researcher adopts a non-experimental research design that involves collecting data from subjects at a single point in time. She designs the study to control the extraneous variables of age, marital status and general health status.
7. There is no intervention in this study (the design is non-experimental) and so this step does not need to be undertaken.
8. The researcher designates that the population of interest is women between the ages of 50 and 65 years living in Karnataka who have not been previously diagnosed as having any form of cancer.
9. The researcher decides to recruit for research a sample of 200 women living in Bangalore; they are identified at random using a telephone procedure known as random-digit dialing.
10. The research variables will be measured through self-report; that is, the independent variable (perceived susceptibility), dependent variable (mammogram history) and extraneous variable will be measured by asking the subjects a series of questions. The researcher decides to use existing measures of key variables, rather than developing new ones.
11. A human subjects committee at the researchers' institution is asked to review the research plans to determine whether the study adheres to ethical standards.
12. Plans for the study are finalized: the methods are reviewed and refined by colleagues with clinical and methodologic expertise; the data collection instruments are pretested; and interviewers who will collect the data are trained.
13. *Data are collected* by conducting telephone interviews with the research sample.
14. *Data are prepared for analysis* by coding them and entering them onto a computer file.
15. *Data are analyzed* using a statistical software package.
16. The results indicate that the hypothesis is supported; however, the researchers *interpretation* must take into consideration that many women who were asked to

participate in the study declined to do so. Moreover, the analysis revealed that the mammogram used in the sample was substantially higher than had been reported in earlier studies.

17. The researcher presents an early report on the findings and interpretations at a conference of National Nurses Association. She subsequently publishes the report in The *Nursing Journal of India* or any registered journal of nurses.
18. The researcher seeks out clinicians to discuss how the study findings can be *utilized in practice.*

The researcher in this study wants to conduct the study over a 2-year period. Figure 2.2 presents a hypothetical schedule for the research tasks to be completed (The selection of the problem is not included because the research topic has already been identified). Note that many steps overlap or are undertaken concurrently. Some steps are projected to involve little time, whereas others require months of work.

In developing a time schedule of this sort, a number of considerations should be kept in mind, including researchers level of knowledge and methodologic competence. Resources available to researchers, in terms of research funds and personnel, greatly influence time estimates. In the present example, the researcher almost certainly would have required funding from a sponsor to help pay for the cost of hiring interviewers, unless the researchers were able to depend on colleagues or students.

It is also important to consider the practical aspects of performing the study, which were not all enumerated in the preceding section. Obtaining supplies, securing permissions, getting approval for using forms and instruments, hiring staff and holding meetings are all time-consuming, but necessary activities.

Individuals differ in the kinds of tasks that appeal to them. Some people enjoy the preliminary phase, which has a strong intellectual component, whereas, others are more eager to collect the data, a task that is more interpersonal. Researchers

0	2	4	6	8	10	12	14	16	18	20	22	24
Conceptual phase												
Step 2												
Step 3												
Step 4												
Step 5												
Planning phase												
Step 6												
Step 7												
Step 8												
Step 9												
Step 10												
Step 11												
Step 12												
Empirical phase												
Step 13												
Step 14												
Analytic phase												
Step 15												
Step 16												
Dissemination phase												
Step 17												
Step 18												
0	2	4	6	8	10	12	14	16	18	20	22	24

Fig. 2.2: Hypothetical schedule for research task to be completed

should, however, allocate a reasonable amount of time to do justice to each activity.

Qualitative Research Process

As we have just seen, quantitative research involves a fairly linear progression of tasks—researchers plan in advance the steps to be taken to maximize study integrity and then follow those steps as faithfully as possible. In qualitative studies, by contrast, the progression is closer to a circle than to a straight line—qualitative researchers are continually examining and interpreting data and making decisions about how to proceed, based on what has already been discovered.

Because qualitative researchers have a flexible approach to the collection and analysis of data, it is impossible to define the flow of activities precisely—the flow varies from one study to another and researchers themselves do not know ahead of time exactly how the study will proceed. The following sections provide a sense of how qualitative studies are conducted by describing some major activities and indicating how and when they might be performed are as given below:

Identifying the Research Problem

Like quantitative researchers, qualitative researchers usually begin with a broad topic area to be studied. However, qualitative researchers usually focus on an aspect of a topic that is poorly understood and about which little is known. Therefore, they do not develop hypotheses or pose highly refined research questions before going into the field. The general topic area may be narrowed and clarified on the basis of self reflection and discussion with colleagues (or clients), but researchers may proceed with a fairly broad research question that allows the focus to be sharpened and delineated more clearly once the study is underway. (Qualitative researchers may also decide to focus on a topic that has been extensively researched quantitatively, but has had little qualitative attention).

Performing Literature Reviews

There are conflicting opinions among qualitative researchers about doing a literature review at the outset of a study. At one extreme are those who believe that researchers should not consult the literature before collecting data. Their concern is that prior studies or clinical writings might influence researchers conceptualization of the phenomena under study. According to this view, the phenomena should be elucidated based on participants viewpoints rather than on any prior information. Those sharing this viewpoint often do a literature review at the end of the study rather than at the beginning. Others feel that researchers should conduct at least a preliminary up-front literature review to obtain some possible guidance (including guidance in identifying the kinds of biases that have emerged in studying the topic). Still others believe that a full up-front literature review is appropriate. In any case, qualitative researchers typically find a relatively small body of relevant previous work because of the types of question they ask.

Selecting and Gaining Entry into Research Sites

During the planning phase, qualitative researchers must also select a site that is consistent with the topic under study. For example, if the topic is the health beliefs of the urban poor, an inner-city neighborhood with a high percentage of low-income residents must be identified. In making such a decision, researchers may need to engage in anticipatory fieldwork (and perhaps some clinical fieldwork) to identify the most suitable and information-rich environment for the conduct of the study. For a qualitative researcher, an ideal site is one in which (1) entry is possible; (2) a rich mix of people, interactions and situations relating to the research question is present; and (3) the researcher can adopt – and maintain – an appropriate role vis-à-vis study participants. It is critical to appraise the suitability of the site (and the settings within the site where data will be collected) before entering the field.

In some cases, researchers may have access to the site selected for the study. In others, however, researchers need to gain entry into the site or settings within it. A site may be well suited to the needs of the research, but if researchers cannot "get in", the study cannot proceed. Gaining entry typically involves negotiations with gatekeepers who have the authority to permit entry into their world. Gaining entry requires strong interpersonal skills, as well as familiarity with the customs and language of the site. In addition, certain strategies are more likely to succeed than others. For example, gatekeepers might be persuaded to be cooperative if it can be demonstrated that there will be direct benefits to them or their constituents – or if a great humanitarian purpose will be served. Researchers also need to gain the gatekeepers trust, and that can only occur if researchers are congenial, persuasive, forthright about research requirements (e.g. how much time the fieldwork will require), (and – perhaps most important – express genuine interest in and concern for the situation of the people in the site. In qualitative research, gaining entry is likely to be an ongoing process of establishing relationships and rapport with gatekeepers and others at the site, including prospective informants.

Research Design in Qualitative Studies

As we have seen, quantitative researchers do not collect data until the research design has been finalized. In a qualitative study, by contrast, the research design is often referred to, as an emergent design—a design that emerges during the course of data collection. Certain design features are guided by the qualitative research tradition within which the researcher is working, but nevertheless few qualitative studies have rigidly structured designs that prohibit changes while in the field. As previously noted, qualitative designs are not concerned with the control of extraneous variables. The full context of the phenomenon is considered an important factor in understanding, how it plays out in, the lives of people experiencing it.

Although qualitative researchers do not always know in advance exactly how the study will progress in the field, they nevertheless must have some sense of how much time is available for field work and must also arrange for and test the needed equipment; such as tape recorders or videotaping equipment. Other planning activities include such tasks as hiring and training interviewers to assist in the collection of data; securing interpreters if the informants speak a different language; and hiring appropriate consultants, transcribers and support staff.

Addressing Ethical Issues

Qualitative researchers, like quantitative researchers, must also develop plans for addressing ethical issues—and, indeed, there are special concerns in qualitative studies because of the more intimate nature of the relationship that typically develops between researchers and study participants.

Conducting the Qualitative Study

In qualitative studies, the tasks of sampling, data collection, data analysis and interpretation typically take place iteratively. Qualitative researchers begin by talking with or observing a few people who have first-hand experience with the phenomenon under study. The discussions and observations are loosely structured, allowing for the expression of a full range of beliefs, feelings, and behaviors. Analysis and interpretation are ongoing, Concurrent activities guide choices about the kind of people to sample next and the types of questions to ask or observations to make. The actual process of data analysis involves clustering together related types of narrative information into a coherent scheme. The analysis of qualitative data is an intensive, time-consuming activity.

As analysis and interpretation progress, researchers begin to identify themes and categories, which are used to build a rich description or theory of the phenomenon. The kinds of data obtained and the people selected as participants tend to become increasingly focused and purposeful as the conceptualization is developed and refined. Concept development and verification shape the sampling process – as a conceptualization or theory develops, the researcher seeks participants who can confirm and enrich the theoretical understandings, as well as participants who can potentially challenge them and lead to further theoretical development.

Quantitative researchers decide in advance how many subjects to include in the study, but qualitative researchers sampling decision, are guided by the data themselves. Many qualitative researchers use the principle of data saturation, which occurs when themes and categories in the data become repetitive and redundant, such that no information can be gleaned by further data collection.

In quantitative studies, researchers seek to collect high-quality data by using measuring instruments that have been demonstrated to be accurate and valid. Qualitative researchers, by contrast, must take steps to demonstrate the trust worthiness of the data while in the field. The central feature of these efforts is to confirm that the findings accurately reflect the experiences and viewpoints of participants, rather than perceptions of the researchers. One confirmatory activity, for example, involves going back to the participants and sharing preliminary interpretations with them, so that they can evaluate whether the researchers thematic analysis is consistent with their experiences. Another strategy is to use triangulation to converge on a thorough depiction of the target phenomena.

An issue that qualitative researchers sometimes need to address is the development of appropriate strategies for leaving the field. Because qualitative researchers may develop strong relationships with study participants and entire communities. They need to be sensitive to the act that their departure from the field might seem like a form of rejection or abandonment. Graceful departure and methods of achieving closure are important.

Disseminating Qualitative Findings

Qualitative nursing researchers also strive to share their findings with others at conferences and in journal articles. Qualitative findings, because of their depth and richness, also lend themselves more readily to book-length manuscripts than do quantitative findings. Regardless of researcher's position about when a literature review should be conducted, they usually include a summary of prior research in their reports, as a means of providing context for the study.

Quantitative reports almost never present raw data – that is, data in the form they were collected, which are numeric values. Qualitative reports, by contrast, are usually filled with rich verbatim passages directly from participants. The excerpts are used in an evidentiary fashion to support or illustrate researcher's interpretations and theoretical formulations.

Utilization of Research Findings

The research utilization/innovation diffusion process begins with an empirically based innovation or new idea that gets scrutinized for possible adoption in practice settings. The Evidence-based practice (EBP), by contrast, begins with a search for information about how best to solve specific practice problems. Findings from rigorous research are considered the best possible source of information, but EBP also draws on other sources. A basic feature of EBP is that it de-emphasizes decision making based on custom, authority opinion, or ritual. Rather, the emphasis is on identifying the best available research evidence and *integrating* it with clinical expertise, patient input, and existing resources.

The EBP movement has given rise to considerable debate, with both staunch, zealous advocates and skeptics who urge caution and a balanced approach to health-care practice. Supporters argue that EBP offers a solution to sustaining high health-care quality in our current cost-constrained environment. Their position is that rational approach is needed to provide the best possible care to most of the people, with the most cost-effective use of resources. Critics worry that the advantages of EBP are exaggerated and that individual clinical judgments and patient inputs are being devalued. Although there is a need for close scrutiny on how the EBP journey unfolds, it seems likely that the EBP path is the one that health-care professions will follow in the early 21st century.

There are many barriers to promoting evidence-based practice; some of the significant ones are discussed below:

- Lack of professional ability to critically appraise research. This includes having a considerable amount of research evaluation skills, access to journals, and clinic/hospital support to spend time on EPN are limited for the nurses.
- Lack of time, workload pressures, and competing priorities of patient care can impede use of Evidence-Based Practices.
- Lack of knowledge of research methods is also one of the significant barriers in promotion of Evidence-Based Practices.
- Lack of support from professional colleagues and organizations, and lack of confidence and authority in the research arena.
- Practice environment can be resistant to changing trend and true conventional methods of practice. This can be caused because of reluctance to believe results of research study over safe, traditional practices, cost of adopting new practices, or gaining momentum to rewrite existing protocols. It is important to show nurses who may be resistant to changes in nursing practice the benefits that nurses, their patients, and their institutions can reap from the implementation of evidence-based nursing practice, which is to provide better nursing care.
- Values, resources and evidence are the three factors that influence decision-making with regard to health care. All registered nurses and health-care professionals should be taught to read and critically interpret research and know where to find articles which relate to their field of care. In addition, nurses need to be more aware of how to assess the information and determine its applicability to their practice.
- Lack of continuing education programs. Practices do not have the means to provide workshops to teach new skills due to lack of funding, staff, and time; therefore, the research may be tossed dismissed. If this occurs, valuable treatments may never be utilized in patient care. Not only will the patients suffer but the staff will not have the opportunity to learn a new skill. Also, the practitioners may not be willing to implement change regardless of the benefits to patient care.
- Introducing newly learned methods for improving treatments or patients' health is the fear of 'stepping on one's toes'. New nurses might feel it is not their place to suggest or even tell a superior nurse that newer, more efficient methods and/or practices are available.
- The perceived threat to clinical freedom offered by evidence-based practice is neither logical nor surprising. Resistance to change and to authority is part of human nature. When we make decisions based upon good quality information we are inconsistent and biased. Human nature offers many challenges to evidence-based practice.

USE OF COMPUTER IN NURSING AND RESEARCH

Introduction

A computer is an electronic device that accepts data, manipulates the data and produces the output in a fast and efficient way. Computers are able to process large volumes of data or information in a fraction of second. Using computer, people can communicate information across globe. It is easy to process large amount of data. Results obtained from the computer will be an accurate one. Data computer storage and retrieval is in a fast manner. A powerful could form as many as three million calculations in a second. Being a machine it does not suffer from the human trials of tiredness and lack of concentration. Computers are essential parts of our day-to-day life. They are useful for people of all ages in every occupation. As the computer increases the accuracy, productivity and work efficiency, so these are considered inevitable in medical profession which includes nursing profession.

Now the uses of computers virtually in every environment even the areas that are unconnected with number manipulation. From the executive in any office to the house-wife and her washing machine to the teenage recording his/her favorite television program. Computers have entered into practically every sphere of human activity. With the development of technology in computers such as internet and various softwares, the work can be easily done. The nurses sitting at their own work place can get information related to health with the facts by using internet and can apply the latest evidence based knowledge for the care of patients. Not only this, the softwares developed in statistics helped the nurses to analyze the data collected with a short span of time for research work.

Main Uses of Computer

a. **Data storage:** A person can feed the data into the system through the input device and that can be stored. At any time that can retrieve the stored data. Data means Text, Numbers, Object, Images, Pictures and Sounds, etc.
b. **Communication:** A person can communicate to others through computers via E-mail, Video Conferencing, Voice Chatting, Video Chatting, etc.
c. **Entertainment:** People can use the computers to watch movies, listen to music and playing games. Computers have been used extensively in the creative arts as well. Sound, Still Pictures, and Video are now routinely created (through synthesizers, computer graphics and computer animation), universally edited by computer. Computers have also been used for entertainment, with the video game becoming a huge industry.
d. **Education:** In education, computers play a vital role. The e-Learning, materials in the retrieval media, presentations enhance the literacy among the people and help in research also. The role of computers in education has become important in recent times. Education through internet and computer aided learning has simplified education in schools. Most of the relevant information (both recent and past) and subject material is available online from where students can easily download and refer as and when required. Due to the benefits of computers in education, internet and computer based learning has become commonplace in schools and colleges.

Uses of Computers in Nursing

a. **Nursing practice:** In hospital admission, discharge and transfers system allows nurses to obtain basic biographical information about the clients before they arrive to the ward/unit. When a discharge or transfer is entered in the computer, all the appropriate departments will be notified, e.g. Pharmacy, dietary and also help nurses in following aspects:
   i. To keep the records of patient's health status during hospital stay and also as OPD patient.
   ii. Hospital management information system helps to have an access of patient's treatment chart, operation list or anesthetic record, etc. This is possible after the knowledge of computers.
   iii. Helps nurses in managing the routine documents on computers in a fraction of time, which otherwise take up a lot of time manually.
   iv. Increases the productivity of nurses.
   v. Knowledge of computers with hospital management information package, nurse

generally generates a prescription, fixes an appointment for next visit, once the diagnosis is entered. Due to which the time spent on routine matters is generally cut down.

vi. Other functions in hospitals with appropriate software is automatic generation of reminder letters, determination of milestones, etc., is achieved.

vii. Computer typing is very legible. Nursing process, care of pain, implementation of activities, nursing notes and discharge plans can be computerized. It can be stored in a format determined by the institution.

b. Nursing education: Computer assisted instruction programs are very useful in self-placed learning. Online presentations (preparing course material using presentation packages) make teaching effective. Without spending a lot of time in the class room the E-learning facilitates the students to do their higher education. In nursing education use of computer helps as mentioned below:

i. Knowledge of computers can be applied to prepare the slides on MS–Power Point on the topics to be taught to students.

ii. Knowledge of multimedia helps the nursing teachers and nursing students to make teaching effective.

iii. Education through internet and computer aided learning has simplified education in nursing schools.

c. Nursing administration: In nursing administration computer helps the nurses:

i. For preparation of records of nursing students by the nursing teachers and nursing superintendent.

ii. For preparing and keeping records of assessment and results of nursing students.

iii. In preparing the rules, letters, etc.

iv. Knowledge of computers helps in preparing the duty rosters and saves the time.

v. For preparing drafts of plan—annual or monthly or weekly such as rotational plans, time-tables, etc.

vi. Computerized patients classification system can be used to assign nursing staff based on how severely-ill the clients are.

vii. Computerized inventory system keeps track of supplies received and disbursed client billing system, diagnosis or reports, budget planning, maintenance of personal records.

d. Nursing research: Statistical methodology girds its place whenever numerical facts enter into picture. Statistics is an intergral part of nursing research since of deals with numerical aspect. So computer helps in many ways for example.

Examples for statistical packages: SPSS is the package, which provides the complete solution for the statistician as well as the researcher. For research in nursing, following are some of the useful functions in statistics which are supported by SPSS. Probability and survival modeling techniques are suitable for the use of complex nursing research situations. These methods may help to connect the qualitative-quantitative gap. The complex calculations can be solved easily by using such software. The use of statistical packages for windows in a variety of areas, including:

- Survey and research
- Administrative research, human resources, and resource planning
- Medical, scientific, clinical, and social science research
- Planning and forecasting
- Quality improvement
- Analytic application development

In addition, during research works computer helps nursing resource as follows:

- Computers are used to get informations on the researches carried out through internet. For examples: websites like pubmed, medlar, indmd provide a lot of information for the health care professionals (via Internet), data collection tool, dissemination of findings and results, tabulations, preparation of research reports and project report.

- Knowledge of computers helps the nurses in preparing class teachings and health education interesting and effective. However, it reduces the dependency of nurses for their work on others and helps them to become self-reliant in operating computers, creates awareness among the nurses to make the use of various monitors used to analyze the condition of patients. The basic knowledge of computers improves the work efficiency of nurses as these reduce the time spent on the written work and provide sufficient time to be spent with the patients. Even they are able to access the data related to patients without leaving their station and patients alone. So the computer's knowledge helps nurses to increase their productivity and to provide best patient centered care. Knowledge of computers reduces the time taken to do the documentation, which usually takes time if done manually.

EXERCISES

1. What is evidence-based practice?
2. Define research and discuss the significance of research in nursing.
3. Define research and explain the steps of scientific research.
4. Define qualitative research and explain the steps to be followed in qualitative research.

CHAPTER

3 Collection of Data

Introduction

Statistics generally deals with population and groups of individuals, hence it deals with quantities of information and not with a single datum. The plural form of datum is data. It is necessary to understand the meaning of data and various types of data before discussing details of data collection. The collection of data constitutes the first step in a statistical investigation. Utmost care is required in collecting data because they form the foundation of statistical analysis. If data are faulty, the conclusion drawn can never be reliable. Any group of measurement which provide information is referred as data.

Data are the observable and measurable facts that provide information about phenomenon under study. *For example*, when physical growth of infant is the phenomenon under study, the data to measure about physical growth would be the body weight, height, chest, and head circumferences. In other words, using the data and information, indicators are developed which are the reflection of indirect or partial measures of a real situation. The aim of gathering and summarizing data is to transform this into meaningful information in order to identify and measure variables, describe behavior, and compute empirical evidences that are objective, reliable, and valid.

Once it is decided what type of study is to be made, it becomes necessary to collect information about the concerned study, mostly in the form of data. For this, information has to be collected from certain individuals directly or indirectly. Such a technique is known as survey method. These are commonly used in social sciences, i.e. the problems relating to sociology, political science, psychology and various economic studies. In surveys, the required information is supplied by the individual under study or is based on measurements of certain units. Generally, the respondents or units are selected from a population using some standard sampling techniques. Another way of collecting data is by experimentation, i.e. an actual experiment is conducted on certain individuals or units about which the inference is to be drawn. Such experimental studies are common in agriculture, biology, medical science, nursing, etc.

Classification of Data

Data can be classified on the basis of characteristic, source, field and contents.

Data Based on Characteristics

It includes qualitative and quantitative. Here qualitative relates to attributes and quantitative relates to discrete variates and continuous variates. Whenever an observation is made, it will be recorded and a collective recording of these observations either numerical or otherwise is called as data. These observations may be collected in a simple way like recording the sex of a person in a group or noting down the number of cases of disease in a community or may be done through an experiment such as, finding vital capacity of an individual or total white blood cell count in a given volume of blood, etc. In each of the above cases a certain observation is made of a characteristic which varies from one observation to other is called variable. Depending upon the nature of the variable, data may be termed as qualitative or quantitative. For example, Qualitative data – sex, type of disease, causes of death, etc. quantitative data – vital capacity of lungs, total WBC count in given volume.

Qualitative data are non-numeric features or experimental units, where as quantitative data are with numerical properties.

Quantitative data can be classified into two kinds, namely discrete and continuous when the variable under observation can take only fixed values in a given range like whole numbers or in other words the variable jumps from one number to another without taking the in-between values, the data is called as 'discrete data'. Instead, if the variable can take any value in the given range, then the data is called 'continuous data'. For example, the number of white blood cells in a given volume of blood is a discrete data as it can be expressed only in whole numbers. And the hemoglobin percentage level of a person is a continuous data as it can be measured to any decimal value depending on the precision of the measuring instruments.

Data Based on the Source

There are two categories of data namely, (i) primary data and (ii) secondary data.

Primary data: The data, which are collected from the units or individual respondents directly for the purpose of certain study or information, are known as primary data. For instance, an enquiry is made from each tax payer in a city to obtain their opinion about the tax collecting machinery. The data obtained in a study by the investigator are termed as primary data. If an experiment is conducted to know the effect of certain fertilizer doses on the yield or the effect of a drug on the patients, the observations taken on each plot or patient constitute the primary data. Hundreds of such examples can be cited.

Secondary data: The data, which had been collected by certain people or agency, and statistically treated. Now the information contained in it is used again from records, processed and statistically analysed to extract some information for other purpose, is termed as secondary data. For instance, if the data given in different census years is again processed to obtain trends of population growth, professional changes, changes in sex ratio, mortality rate, etc. it is termed as secondary data. Usually, secondary data is obtained from year books, census reports, survey reports, official records or reported experimental findings. Different organisations and government agencies publish information (data) in the form of reports, periodicals, journals, etc. Names of organisations and their publications with relevant details are given in the chapter on Statistical Organisation in India.

The sources that the student should tap, vary with his/her interests and the type of his/her study. Generally, sources are divided into documentary and field sources. The later includes living persons who have a fund of knowledge about or have been in intimate contact with, social conditions and changes over a considerable period of time. These people are in a position to describe not only the existing state of affairs but also the observable trends and significant change in a social process. These persons regarded as personal sources or direct sources. If discretion is in their selection, various professional and business persons, old residents and community leaders may be utilized as a sources of information. Each person supplying information may often serve as a check on the other until the account is reliably constructed. The documentary sources of information are those which are contained in the published and unpublished documents, reports, statistical accounts, manuscript, letters, diaries, etc. These sources are generally divided into '*primary sources*' which provide data gathered at first hand, the responsibility for their compilation and promulgation remaining under the same authority that originally gathered them; and '*secondary sources*' which provide data that have been transcribed or compiled from original sources and of which the promulgating authority is different from that which controlled the collection of the data at first hand, for example, census. In other words, if the data is derived from the direct measurements/observations on the population units, it is 'primary data'. For example, observations based on the actual measurement of height, weight, Hb%, etc. of individuals by the investigator/or his team – when the data is not derived from the primary source, but is derived from sources like search, it is secondary data.

There are two systems of sources of data which include regular or routine and non-routine or ad-hoc data collect system:

- Regular or Routine system: examples: Census Birth and Death registration, notification of disease, cancer registers, reporting under surveillance of diseases
- Ad-hoc or non-routine system: example: National sample survey, investigation of an epidemic, Knowledge Attitude Perception (KAP) on healthy habits, etc.

i. *Regular system includes the following*

- Census: It is a population estimate and is a process of complete enumeration of all individuals in a country on a fixed date. It contains aspects like general, economic, social, cultural, migration, establishment, fertility and special information if any.
- Vital registration: Includes births, deaths, marriages, divorces, adoptions, legitimations, legal separations, recognitions and annulments. These are vital events that need recording and are helpful in day-to-day civilian affair regulations.
- Notification of disease: It is regulation and policy as a part of prevention and control of diseases. Notifiable disease are cholera, plague, yellow fever, polio, influenza, malaria, typhoid, hepatitis and locally epidemics.
- Disease registry: Permanent record of specific diseases like cancer, shock, blindness, birth defects, tuberculosis and leprosy.
- Medical records: Cumulative health record in educational institutions and working places.
- Hospital records.
- Environmental health information.

ii. *Ad-hoc system includes the following*

- Sample registration system – to get quick required data for policy making and planning
- Disease surveillance – AIDS surveillance, malaria surveillance, etc.
- Manpower statistics
- Surveys – population based surveys, National health survey
- Additional ad-hoc demographic data – situational analysis of population movement, natural calamities, major epidermis
- Economic and Fiscal data
- Security scheme and serial schemes – Medical insurance, sickness, absenteeism, disability benefits and other benefits and welfare scheme.

Data Based on Field

In computer data base management software, data is arranged in tabular form. The columns are called fields and rows are records. Each field can hold record of its' type which needs to be described at the time of creation of data base. The common types of fields are character type, numeric type, date type, and logical type.

- ***Character type***, e.g. Name, address
- ***Numeric type***, e.g. Age, height, weight, blood sugar level, systolic/diastolic BP, serial numbers, etc.

- ***Date type***, e.g. Date of birth, date of admission, date of discharge, etc.
  - The data can be expressed dd/mm/yyyy (British format)
  - The data can be expressed mm/dd/yyy (American format)
  - The data can be expressed yyyy/mm/dd (ANSE format)
- ***Logical type***: This refers to dichotomous data for example, sex (male/female), result of drug trial (cured/not cured, residence (urban/rural).

Data Based on Content

The data can be classified, depending on the contents which include, nominal, ordinal, interval and ratio data, according to scales of measurements

- ***Nominal data:*** It is another name for qualitative data. Here, the data is presented as frequency distribution of some characteristics such as sex, religion, etc. The groups do not have any logical order. There is no implication of order or ratio of the adjacent categories. When there are only two possible categories, the data is named dichotomous for example
  - Smoking—smokers/non-smoking
  - Sex—male/female
  - Outcome of MI—death/survival
  - Goals of NAMP—achieved/not achieved
  - Cause of illness—heredity/environment
- ***Ordinal data:*** In this type, the data is presented according to rank or order. There is thus, a logical order, for example:
  - Frequency, distribution, of student according to the rank in examinations
  - Degree of malnutrition—severe, moderate, mild
  - Socioeconomic status—upper, middle, lower

  Here there no implication of class-interval. The groups are thus not equidistant, since it relates to, true zero does not exist. Ordinal data are with implicit order of inter-relationship.
- ***Interval data:*** In this type, the data is placed in meaningful intervals and order. Here, the number between characters. For example:
  - Body temperature – Degree of Fahrenheit or Celsius
  - Heart rate – per second

  To quote frequency distributions of patients according to temperature groups, like below 37°C and above 37°C. Here the groups are meaningful because, the difference in the temperature of 37°C and 36°C and 38°C and 37°C is equal, i.e. 1°C. however there is no implication of ratio in the sense that 30°C is not twice as hot as 15°C.
- ***Ratio data***: Here there is relative magnitude. In this type, the data is presented in frequency distribution in logical order and meaningful groups. In addition a meaningful ratio exists. For example, frequency distribution of pulse rate, height, weight, etc. Thus, pulse rate of 120/minute is twice as fast as that of 60 per minute. Similarly, a person with weight 80 kgs is twice heavy as the one with weight of 40 kg. Further, in this data type, a true zero exists. For example, pulse rate of zero means no pulse at all.

Thus, identification of the type of data is essential in any statistical exercise for reasons given below:

- It helps in further analysis
- It helps selection of data presentation method
- It helps selection of test of significance.

Methods of Data Collection

The objective of a study, the population under study, the units or individuals from whom the information is to be collected is ascertained first. Then keeping in view the purpose and importance of the investigation and types of respondents, the statistician has to choose one of the three methods of enquiry given below.

1. Personal enquiry method.
2. Correspondence, i.e. mailed questionnaire method.
3. Direct observational method.

Personal Enquiry Method

Before starting the investigation, a question sheet is prepared which is called *schedule*. The schedule contains all the questions which would extract a complete information from a respondent. Often, the schedule contains the likely answers also. As a precaution in any method a few schedules are tested by filling them before the commencement of the survey. This pre-testing of schedules removes certain discrepancies like ambiguity of the questions and irrelevant questions in the schedule. Such pre-testing is known as a *pilot survey*.

In this type of enquiry, the investigator contacts the respondent personally and asks him questions given in the schedule one by one and notes down his replies on the schedule. If the unit is a household, the investigator contacts the head of the family to fill up the schedule. Such a practice is called a *direct personal interview method*.

The interview is a process of communication or interaction in which the subjects or interviewee gives the needed information verbally in a face-to-face situation. Although the interview is generally associated with counseling or psychotherapy, it is used effectively to collect useful information about individual in many research situations.

Interviewing is a popular way of gathering information in qualitative research. Interview provides a wide range of data. It provides information about person's feelings, perceptions, and opinions. Interviewers should not make preassumptions about the respondents. Interview requires high-level questioning skills and active participation.

Interviewing requires face-to-face contact or contact over telephone and calls for interviewing skills. Interview may be used either as a main method or as a supplementary one in collection of research-related data.

These are most often used to gather detailed, qualitative data. Interviews are conducted one-on-one, while focus group interviews are conducted in small groups. Both are usually conducted with targeted samples of staff, administrators, youth, families, community members, and so on. These can be conducted in person or by phone. Questions are generally open-ended, and responses are documented.

Sometimes, the information is not collected directly from the respondent, but from a third person who is expected to know him well. Such an approach is useful in case where the respondent is expected to conceal information about himself. For instance, a person who is addicted to alcoholic drinks or suffering from some infectious disease may hide correct information about certain things. Hence, an indirect enquiry will give better information. Such a method of enquiry is known as *indirect personal enquiry method*. The main advantage of this method is that the information is likely to be complete, more correct and some additional information can be retrieved. The person may be persuaded to reply to some of the more personal questions too.

Mailed Questionnaire Method

Questionnaires are one of the most popular methods of conducting research. They provide a convenient way of gathering information from a target population. They are cost-effective and easy to construct and analyse. A questionnaire is a planned self-reported form designed to elicit information though written or verbal responses of the subjects. In other words, a questionnaire is a research instrument used for data collection. It is a set of questions that may or may not provide with response alternatives which are to be answered by subject.

When a survey is spread over a vast area and the respondents are educated, a mailed questionnaire method is preferred in comparison to the personal interview method. In this method, a questionnaire is mailed to each and every respondent. They are requested to fill up the questionnaire and send it back. This method is less costly and less time consuming. The difficulty in this method is that a large number of respondents do not return the duly filled in questionnaires.

Direct Observational Method

Observation is a way of gathering data by watching behavior, events, or noting physical characteristics in their natural setting. Observation is a method of data collection that can be used to gather such information as characteristics and conditions of individual, verbal and nonverbal communication, etc. Observation method of data collection is particularly well suited to nursing research. There are several situations that require nurses to use the observation method for data collection such as behavior and attributes of the patients, their families, and hospital staff, and so on.

In this approach an investigator stays at the place of survey. He does not make enquiries, but notes down the observations himself. For instance, to understand the migratory habits of a variety of birds, the investigator stays at the birds sanctuary and notes down the movements to and fro every day. This method of survey is not used frequently.

Observation may be defined as systematic viewing, coupled with consideration of the seen phenomena. That is, consideration minor be given to the larger unit of activity in which the specific observed phenomena occur. Overall phenomena of course are open to observations, not all those open to observation find a ready observer at hand. Not all occurrence lend themselves to study by observational techniques.

Research observation involves the systematic selection, observation and recording of behaviors, events and settings relevant to a problem under study. When nurse researchers observe an event – such as nurse interacting with a patient – they have to know at least broadly what to observe. Nurse researchers make observations of human behavior or the characteristics of individuals, events, environments or objects. The common observable phenomena involved in nursing research are:

1. *Characteristics and conditions of individual:* By direct observation investigator can get lots of information about person's attributes and states, which include both enduring traits such as, physical appearance and more temporary conditions such as rashes. Physiologic conditions can be observed either directly through the senses or with the help of observational apparatus such as, radiograph, MRI, ECG, etc.
2. *Activities and behavior:* Number of actions are amenable to observation and constitute valuable data for nurse researchers. Activities and behavior that indicate health status physical status and emotional functioning are particularly important. For example, activities or behaviors that lend themselves to observational study, include patient's eating habits, length and number of visits by friends and relatives and aggressive actions among children in the hospital play room.
3. *Skill attainment and performance:* Nurses are routinely called on to develop skills among clients. Skill attainment is often demonstrated behaviorally and is therefore amenable to observation. For example, diabetic patients skill in testing their urine for sugar and acetone or infants ability to suck when positioned for breast feeding and also nurses on-the-job performance and decision-making behaviors.
4. *Verbal communication:* The content and structure of people's conversation are readily observable, easy to record. A nurse researcher may be interested in observing information given by nurses to patients, exchange of information among nurses at change-of-shift reports, conversation among patients about health-care services of hospitals.
5. *Non-verbal communication:* Individuals communicate their attitudes and emotions in many ways, other than just with words. The kind of non-verbal behavior amenable to observational methods include, facial expressions, touch, posture, gestures and other body movements, crying or laughing and extra linguistic behavior, i.e. the manner in which people speak aside from the content, such as the intonation, loudness and continuity of speech.
6. *Environmental characteristics:* Individuals surrounding can be affect their behavior. For example, observable environmental attributes includes hospital noise levels, nursing homes' decor, safety hazards in schools or the cleanliness of the households in a community.

In selecting behaviors, attribute or situations to be observed the researcher must decide what constitute a unit. There are two apparatus as given below. The choice of approach depends mostly on the nature of the probe.

- The most approved entails, observing large units of behavior and treating then as a whole. For example, Psychiatric nurse researcher might study patients' mood swings. An entire constellation of verbal and non-verbal behavior might be construed as signaling aggressive behavior
- The molecular approach uses small, highly specific behavior, as observational units. Each movement, action, gesture or phrase is treated as a separate entity.

The types of observation used are unstructured and structured observation

In case the observation is characterized by careful definition of the units to be observed, the style of recording the observed information, standardized condition of observation and the selection of pertinent data of observation, then the observation is called as "structured observation". But when the observation is to take place without these characteristics to be thought in advance, the same is termed as 'unstructured observation'. Descriptive studies use "structured observation". Exploration studies use mostly "unstructured observation".

Unstructured Observation

Unstructured observational data are most often gathered in field setting, through a process known as "Participant observation". Participant observes and participates in the functioning of the social group under investigation and strive to observe, ask questions and record information within the contexts, structures and symbols that are relevant to group members. Most of the qualitative studies use this approach. When the observer observes by making himself, more or less, a member of the group he is observing so that he can experience what the members of the group experience, thus the observation is called as the participant observation. But when the observer observes as a detached emissary without any attempt on his part to experience through participation what others feel, the observation of this type is often termed as "non participant observation". When the observer is observing in such a manner that his presence may be unknown to people he is observing, such observation is described as "disguised observation".

The most common form of record keeping participant observations are logs and field notes, but photographs and videotapes may about be used

- A log book or field book daily records events and conversation in the field
- Field notes are much broader, more analytic and more interpretive than a simple listing of occurrences. Field notes are both descriptive and reflective
  - Descriptive or observational notes are objective descriptions of observed events, conversations; information about actions, dialogue contexts which are recorded as completely and objectively as possible
  - Reflective notes which document the researcher, personal experience, reflections and progress while in the field, can serve a number of different purposes; which include methodological notes, theoretical notes and personal notes.

Structured Observation

Researchers using structure/observational methods specify in advance the behavior or events to be observed and use record-keeping forms that yield numeric information. Observers using structured observation are still required to make some inferences and exercise judgement; but they are restrained with regard to the kinds of phenomena than will be watched and recorded.

In structured observation investigator uses category, checklists and rating scale.

- A category system represents an attempt to designate in a systematic or quantitative fashion, the qualitative behaviors or events transpiring in observational setting. It requires the careful and explicit definitions of behavior and characteristics to be observed. Each category must be explained in detail with an operational definition, so the observers have a relatively clear-cut criteria for determining the occurrence of specified phenomena. For example, interaction between mother and infants during periods of feeding and sleeping. Here for the observer categorized sleep – wakeful states are made into mutually exclusive categories: Sleep, Drowse/Transition, Alert and active waking. Here the 'alert' category is defined as "the infant's eyes are open and scanning, motor activity is typically low, etc.

- Checklist referred to an instrument that the observer uses to record observed phenomena, which is constructed on the basis of the category system. In an exhausting checklist usually formatted with a list of behaviors or events from the category system on the left and space for tallying, the frequency or duration of occurrence of behaviors is placed on the right. The observer's task, with an exhaustive checklist, is to place behavior in only one category for each element. The element refers to either a unit of behavior, such as a sentence in a conversation, to a time interval, checklist for non-exhaustive systems is referred to as a sign system, begins with a list of behaviors (or symptoms) that subjects may manifest or may not manifest. The observers task is to watch for instances of behavior on the list.
- Rating scales – an alternative to checklist for recording structure observations is a rating scale. This requires the observers to rate a phenomena along a descriptive continuum, that is typically bipolar. The ratings are quantified for subsequent statistical analysis. A seven-point scale or a five- point scale can be used:

1 2 3 4 5 6 7

Extremely relaxed (R) |—|—|—|—|—|—|—| Extremely tensed (T)

Neither R and T

Self-Report

The self-report is a method of collecting data that involves a direct report of information by the person who is being studied. This method is used by the nurse researcher in both quantitative and qualitative research. The self-report data usually are collected by an oral interview or written questionnaire.

Qualitative Self-report Tools

Methods of collecting qualitative self-report data include the following:

1. Unstructured interviews are conversational discussions on the topic of interest. They are the mode of choice when researchers do not have a clear idea of what it is that they do not know. In conducting unstructured intervals, it is critical to let participants tell their stories, with little interruptions. Phenomenological, grounded theory and ethnographic studies usually rely heavily on unstructural interviews. These interviews are characteristics by a flexibility of approach to questioning.
2. Semi-structural interviews are in which interviewers are guided by a topic guide of questions to be asked. Here the researchers know what they want to ask, but cannot predict what the answers will be. Their role in the process is somewhat structured, where as, the participant is not. The interviewers function is to encourage the participant to talk freely about all the topics on the list and tell the stories in their own words. In preparing the list of questions, care needs to be taken to order questions in a logical sequence, perhaps chronologically or perhaps from the general to the specific.
3. Focus group interviews are which involve discussions with small, homogeneous groups about topics covered in a topic guide. These types of interviews are becoming increasingly popular in the study of health problems. In this group four or more persons are assembled for a discussion. People selected for a group

usually through purposive or snowball sampling are a fairly homogenous group. The interviewer (moderator) guides the discussion according to a written set of questions or topic, to be covered, as in a semi-structural interview...FCG sessions are carefully planned discussions that take advantage of group dynamics for accessing rich information in an efficient manner.

4. Joint interviews, which involve simultaneously talking with members of a family, e.g. a couple. Nurse researchers are sometimes interested in phenomena that involves a relationship between two or three people or that require understanding the perspective of more than one person, e.g. the experiences of cancer patients and their caretaker.
5. Life histories are narrative self-disclosures about individual life experiences. The life-history encourage respondents to narrate in chronological sequence, their experiences. Ethnographers frequently use individual life histories to learn about cultural patterns. Comparative life stories are especially valuable for the study of the patterns, meanings of health and health-care particulars among elderly persons.
6. Oral histories, are used to gather personal recollections of events and their perceived causes and consequences. These are very important methods for the historical researcher. When the topic under study and scrutiny is not too distant past and people who experienced that event can still be asked to narrate those experiences.
7. Critical incidents interviews, involve probes about the circumstances surrounding a behavior or incident that is critical to an outcome of interest. For example, understanding humor in clinical practice of sample of nurses about an incident that took place in the hospital.
8. Diaries and journals, are in which respondents are asked to maintain daily records about some aspects of their lives.
9. Think aloud method, involves having people use audio-recording devices to talk about decisions as and when they are making them. This method has been used in both natural and simulated settings.
10. Photo-elicitation interviews, involve, interviews stimulated and guided by photographic images. It is often used in ethnographics.
11. Self-report narratives on the internet – it is available through the internet.

When preparing for in-depth interviews researchers learn about the language and customs of participants, formulate broad questions, make decisions about how to present themselves, develop ideas about interview settings, and take stock of equipment needs. When conducting in-depth interviews researchers require considerable interviewer skill in putting people at ease, developing trust, listening intently and managing possible crises in the field.

Quantitative Self-report Tools

To obtain self-report data for quantitative study usually formal, written instruments are used. The instrument is an interview schedule. When questions are asked orally either face-to-face, as telephone interviews. It is called a questionnaire or an SAQ (Self-administered Questionnaire) when respondents complete the instrument themselves, usually in a paper-and-pencil format and occasionally directly onto a computer.

Structured instrument consists of a set of questions (also known as items) in which the wording of both questions and in most cases, response alternative is predetermined. When structured interviews or questionnaires are used, subjects are asked to responds to the same questions, in the same order and with the same set of response options. In developing structured instruments, much effort is usually devoted to the content, form and wording of questions. Structured self-report instruments may include open or closed-ended questions.

- Open-ended questions permit respondents to reply in narrative fashion, which allow respondents to respond in their own words. For example, what was the main problem you face in your nursing college.

- Closed-ended questions or fixed alternatives questions offer respondents alternative replies, from which subjects must choose the one that most closely matches the appropriate answer. Types of close-ended questions include:
  i. Dichotomous questions, which require a choice between two options. For example, have you ever been hospitalized. (a) yes (b) No. These types of questions are considered most appropriate for gathering factual information.
  ii. Multiple-choice questions, are which offer a range of alternatives. MCQ's usually offer three to seven alternatives. For example, How important is it to you to avoid a pregnancy this time?
     a. Extremely important
     b. Very important
     c. Somewhat important
     d. Not important?
  iii. Cafeteria questions, in which respondents are asked to select a statement best representing their view. For example, people have different opinions about the use of chemotherapy in cancer which of the following statements best represents your point of view?
     a. Chemotherapy is dangerous
     b. Chemotherapy has undesirable side-effects that suggest need for caution in its use
     c. I am undecided about my views on chemotherapy
     d. Chemotherapy has many beneficial effects that merit its use
     e. Chemotherapy is a wonder treatment that should be administered routinely to all cancer victims
  iv. Rank order questions, in which respondents are asked to rank a list of alternatives along a continuum. For example: students want to select some course for their career in life. Below is a list of things that many students want. Please indicate their order of importance to you by placing a "1" beside most important '2' beside the second most important are so on:
     a. Medical
     b. Dental
     c. Nursing
     d. Engineering
     e. Management
     f. Law
  v. Forced choice questions, which require respondents to choose between two competing questions used in personality tests. For example: which statement closely represents your point of view?
     a. I feel very bored in my dealings
     b. Sometimes I feel I do not have control over my dealings
  vi. Rating questions which ask respondents to make judgments along an order, bipolar dimension. For example, on a scale from 0 to 10, where '0' means "extremely dissatisfied and '10' means "extremely satisfied", how satisfied were your with the nursing care you received during your hospitalization.

  Checklist or matrix questions, in which several questions requiring the same response format are listed. For example, Table 3.1.
  viii. Calendar questions, which ask the stop and start dates of various events, recorded on a calendar of grid (Fig. 3.2). Page 68.
  viiii. Visual analog scales (VAS), are continuously used to measure subjective experience such as pain.

  No pain 0_________10 Severe pain.

Composite Scales

A scale is a device designed to assign a numeric score to people to place them on a continuum with respect to attributes being measured, like a scale for measuring attitude or weight or so on.

Table 3.1

Response data of a checklist or matrix questions regarding some of the aspects of a person's career

	Yes within a year	*Yes 2 years*	*Yes more than 2 years*	*No never*
a. Has any one harassed you in your career	1	2	3	4
b. Has some one helped you in your career	1	2	3	4
c. Has any one threatened you in your career	1	2	3	4
d. Has any one counselled you in your career	1	2	3	4

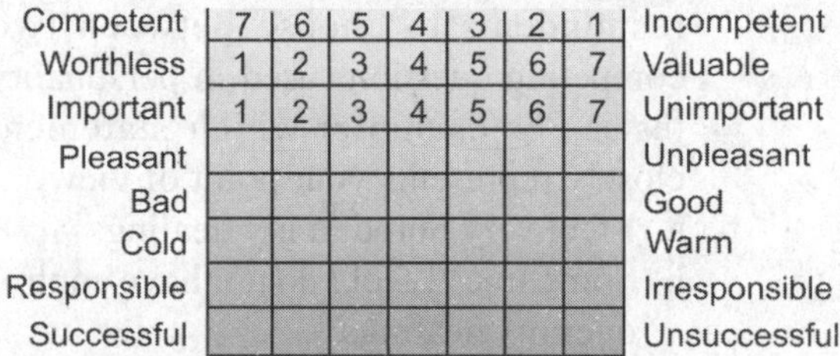

Fig. 3.1: An example of semantic differential

Note: This is an example, but when administering actual subjects, the score values should not be printed

These rating scales can also be used to assess the attitudes or feelings of self-concept. The expressions of the any point of view are accounted as measurements towards any item, object, or concept; they show the person's positive or negative attitude towards any concept. Measuring the score between two opposite concepts tells us about the attitude, feeling, and perception of a person or study subject towards the directions of positive or negative attitude in a scale. Visual scales illustrate visual depiction of any culture; photographs are given to get the feelings, beliefs, opinions about contrast, texture, color, and elements.

'Composite scales are socio-psychological measurements, which are directed towards quantifying the qualitative attributes such as feelings, attitude, self-concept, perceptions, and beliefs etc.'

'Composite scales are socio-psychological rating scale, which are generally used for qualitative measures and discriminate people with different attribute, perception, fears, motives, personality traits and needs those are often incorporated into interviews or questionnaires.'

A scale provides a numeric score to place respondents on a continuum with respect to attributes being measured, like a scale for measuring peoples' weight. Many studies that collect data through self-report use a psychological scale, which is used to discriminate quantitatively among people with different attitudes, fears, motives, perceptions, personality traits and needs. Scales are usually created by several close-ended items into a single composite score.

1. Likert scale—named after the psychologist Rensis Likert. It is also called summated rating scale. It consists of several declarative items that express a view point on a topic. Respondents are asked to indicate the degree to which they agree or disagree with the opinion expressed by the statement (e.g. Table 3.2).
2. Semantic differential scales—consists of a series of bipolar rating scales on which respondents indicate their reaction toward some phenomenon; scales can measure an evaluative (e.g. good/bad) activity (e.g. active/passive), potency (e.g. strong/weak) dimension (Fig. 3.1).

Biophysiologic Measurement Data

'Biophysiological method involves the collection of biophysiological data from subjects by using the specialized equipments to determine physical and biological status of subjects.' *For example*, blood pressure measurement by using special equipments such as sphygmomanometer and stethoscope.

Table 3.2

Example of a Likert scale to measure attitudes toward condoms

Direction of item scoring		*Responses*						*Score*
		SA	A	?	D	SD	Person 1 (√)	Person 2 (**X**)
+	1. Using a condom shows you care about your partner.		√			**X**	4	1
–	2. My partner would be angry if I talked about condoms			**X**		√	5	3
–	3. I would not enjoy sex as much if my partner and I used condoms		**X**		√		4	2
+	4. Condoms are a good protection against AIDS and other sexually transmitted diseases			√	**X**		3	2
+	5. My partner would respect me if I insisted on using condoms	√				**X**	5	1
–	6. I would be too embarrassed to ask my partner about using a condom		**X**			√	5	2
	Total Score						**26**	**11**

SA = Strongly agree, A = Agree, ? = Not decided, D = Disagree, SD = Strongly disagree

This trend is an expanded use of measures to assess the physiological status of a person. Specific technical instruments and equipments are used to measure the physiological and physical variables, and specialized training is needed for the interpretation of results. Data on physiological activity or dysfunction can often be gathered through direct observation. *For example*, phenomenon such vomiting, cyanosis, postcardiotomy delirium, edema, and wound status can be observed for presence or absence and intensity. Other biophysiological data can be gathered by asking people directly. The biophysiological phenomenon requires the use of specialized technical apparatus that yield quantitative measures.

The research community views biophysiological measures as objective data. Researchers may use the biophysiological data collection process either alone or in combination with other methods. In order to identify the measurement collection methods best for the project, the investigator should first list the variables of interest in the study and include them within the hypotheses or research questions. Once the methods of data collection are identified, the researcher should become aware of the limitations of the particular method of data collection chosen and implement procedures to limit the difficulties whenever possible.

The trend in nursing research is increasing the use of measures to assess the physiologic status of study participants and to evaluate clinical outcomes. Clinical nursing studies may involve specialized equipment and instruments, both for creating independent variable and for measuring dependent variable. Most nursing studies in which biophysiologic measures have been used fall into one of the six classes:

	January	February	March	April	May	June	July	August	September	October	November	December	January	February	March	April	May	June	July	August	September	October	November	December	January	February	March	April	May	June	July	August	September	October	November	December
Pregnancy (code no. is pregnancy no.)							1								1														2							2
Employment 1=Employed (write in name of each employer)	1			GCN Blore					1													1				RRCN Blore				1						
Child care																																				
1 = Kindergarten/elementary school																						6			6											
2 = After/before school program																																				
3 = Summer program/ day camp																									7					7						
4 = Head start																																				
5 = Day care center/nursery school/preschool																																				
6 = Family day care/baby sitter																																				
7 = Grandparent																																				
8 = Other relative																																				
9 = Boyfriend/husband																																				

Fig. 3.2: Example of a calendar grid (completed)
(For each period, enter code in beginning month and end month and connect with solid line)

1. *Basic physiologic processes:* Some studies investigate basic physiologic processes that are relevant to nursing care. Such studies often involve subjects which are healthy and normal or animal species one of the studies can be the plasma and nipple aspirate level in lactating women.
2. *Physiologic outcomes of nursing care:* Nurse researchers are increasingly interested in exploring and documenting ways in which nursing actions affect patient's bio-physiologic outcomes, e.g. effect of tepid sponge on fever patients (beneficial): This is used to update standard procedure.
3. *Evaluations of nursing intervention:* This is used for testing a new procedure invented in the field of nursing. Typically these studies involve a hypothesis stating that innovative nursing procedure will result in improved bio-physiologic outcomes among patients. For example: Assess anxiety means BP and respiratory rate used.
4. *Product assessments:* A number of studies are designed to evaluate alternative products desired to enhance patterns of health or comfort rather than to evaluate nursing interventions. Example: Recording temperature on prescribed intervals.
5. *Measurement and diagnoses improvement:* Nurse researchers sometime undertake studies to improve the measurement and recording of bio-physiologic information regularly gathered by nurses. Similarly, some researchers investigate methods to improve clinical diagnoses. Example: Urodynamic testing.
6. *Studies of physiologic correlates:* Nurse researchers have also studied biophysiologic outcomes in relation to social and psychological characteristics, e.g. Physiological problem and psychological states of the people with different physiologic condition, e.g. functional tests of lungs in COPD.

Types of Biophysiologic Measures

Biophysiologic measurements can be classified into *in vivo* and *in vitro* measurements.

1. *In vivo* measurements are those performed directly in or on living organism. For example: Oxygen saturation, blood pressure and body temperature. *In vivo* measures involve the use of instrumentation system, i.e. the apparatus and equipment used to measure one or more attributes of a subject and the presentation of the measurement data in a manner that humans can interpret. Now-a-days *in vivo* instruments have been developed to measure all bodily functions and technologic improvements continue to advance our ability to measure biophysiologic functions more accurately, more conveniently and more rapidly than ever before. For example, electronic monitors.
2. *In vitro* measures, are those performed outside the organism's body as in the case of measuring serum potassium concentrates in the blood. Nurse researchers may or may not be involved in the extraction of the material; however the analysis is normally done by specialized laboratory technicians. Usually each laboratories establish a range of normal values for interpreting results. The common laboratory analysis to be used in studies by nurse researchers are as given below:
   - Chemical measurements, such as, the measure of hormone levels, sugar levels or potassium levels
   - Microbial measures such as, bacterial count and identifiable blood count
   - Cytologic or histologic measures, such as tissue biopsies.

Biophysiologic measures have the advantage of being objective, accurate and precise, but care must be taken in using such measures with regard to practical, technical and ethical considerations.

Records, Documents and Available Data

Existing records and documents provide an economical source of research data. The places where nurse researchers can find useful records and documents are too numerous to list. A few suggestions may be helpful. In hospitals and other health-care settings, excellent records are kept routinely. For example: patient charts, doctors and nurse orders, care plan statements and shift reports. In addition there are financial records, personal records, nutrition records and so on.

'Q' Methodology

The history of the use of Q-sorts in research is relatively new. It was developed in 1930s by a British physicist-psychologist William Stephenson. The idea behind the development of this method was to inquire into the *subjectivity of human mind*. The examples of such subjectivity are limitless and include aesthetic judgement, appreciation of art, preferences for music, experiences of family after tragic events, and attitudes towards political groups. These were difficult, if not impossible, areas that could not measured and reported scientifically by the conventional quantitative methods available at that time.

Q-sorts are the powerful tools in which the participants are presented with card arrangement. In this technique, participants are provided prewritten cards with words, phrases, or statements, and asked to arrange these cards in an order along with a specific bipolar dimension. There are approximately 60 to 100 such cards that can be sorted out in 9 to 11 piles with few numbers of cards placed in each pile.

- Q-sorts can be used in a variety of ways, depending on the interest of the researchers. As one of the major variables in health science research is often the subjective viewpoint of individuals, Q-sorts can be a perfect tool in a variety of settings. With appropriate modifications, the scope of the research can be expanded to answer many difficult issues. *For example*, to analyse the nurse–patient relationship in greater depth, data derived from the Q-sort can be used to categorize major models of nurse–patient relationship, to determine the physicians' qualities that are important for the patients, and to identify the nurses' attributes that are associated with poor evaluation from patients.
- The Q-sorts can also be applied before and after an intervention to evaluate the effectiveness of intervention. *For example*, we can utilize the Q method to evaluate whether attitudes or perceptions of nurses change following implementation of a course on nurse–patient relationship. Thus, the Q method has the potential to be used in diverse situations depending upon the interest of the researchers and the area of study.

Q Methodology refers to a constellation of substantive, statistical and psychometric concepts for research on individuals. It uses a Q-sort procedure, in which people sort a set of card statements into piles according to specified criteria, which can be used to measure attitudes, personality and other psychological traits. One limitation of Q sorts is that, they yield ipsative measures; the average across cards is irrelevant basis of comparison because the forced-choice approach produces the same average for all subjects. This differs from other techniques that produce normative measures, e.g. Likert scale, because each choice is independent of others.

Projective Techniques

These are methods for measuring psychological attributes (value, attitudes, and personality) by providing respondents with unstructured stimuli to which they respond.

A wide range of tasks and games in which respondents can be asked to participate during an interview or group, designed to facilitate, extend, or enhance the nature of the discussion. Some are known as 'projective' techniques, being loosely based on approaches originally taken in a psychotherapeutic setting. These rely on the idea that someone will 'project' their own feelings or beliefs onto an imaginary other person or situation. It enable the participants to say more about the research subject than they can say spontaneously, accessing thoughts, feelings, or meanings which are not immediately available.

These are data collection methods that rely on people's projection of psychological traits in response to vaguely structured stimuli. They present participants with a stimulus of low structure, permitting them to 'read-in' their own interpretations and in this way provide researchers with information about their way of thinking. Here, the manner in which people react to unstructured stimuli is a reflection of their needs, motives, values or personality traits. There are different methods.

- Pictorial methods present pictures or cartoon and ask participants for their reaction. Rorschach inkblot test and thematic appreciation test (TAT) are other methods.
- Verbal methods present people with an ambiguous verbal stimulus rather than a picture. There were two types of verbal methods word association and sentence completion. Word association, which presents participant with a series of words, to which they respond with the first thing that comes to mind. This method helps study creativity, interests and attitudes. Sentence completion test, is one in which a person is given a set of incomplete sentences and asked to complete them in any desired manner.

  Ex. When I think of a nurse, I feel__________

  A good nurse always________________
- Expressive methods take the form of play, drawing or role playing. These techniques encourage self-expression, in most cases, through the construction of some product out of raw materials.

Vignettes

These are benefit descriptions of an event or situation to which respondents are asked to react. They are used to assess respondents' hypothetical behavior, opinions and percepts, e.g. naxal activity.

Cognitive and Neuropsychologic Test

Various aspects of cognitive functioning can be measured by cognitive tests including intelligence or aptitude, neuropsychological functioning and achievement.

Collection of Secondary Data

Secondary data means data that are already available, i.e. they refer to the data which have already been collected and analyzed by someone else. When the researcher utilizes secondary data, then, he has to look into various sources from where he can obtain them. In this case he is certainly not confronted with the problems that are usually associated with the collection of original data. Secondary data may either be published data or unpublished data. Usually published data are available in: (a) various publications of the central, state and local governments; (b) various publications of foreign governments or of international bodies and their subsidiary organizations; (c) technical and trade journals; (d) books, magazines and newspapers; (e) reports and publications of various associations connected with business and industry, banks, stock exchanges, etc.; (f) reports prepared by research scholars, universities, economists, etc. in different fields, and (g) public records and statistics, historical documents, and other sources of published information. The sources of unpublished data are many; they may be found in diaries, letters, unpublished biographies and autobiographies and also may be available with scholars and research workers, trade associations, labor bureaus and other public/private individuals and organizations.

The researcher must be very careful in using secondary data. He must make a minute scrutiny because, it is just possible that the secondary data may be unsuitable or may be inadequate in the context of the problem, which the researcher wants to study. In this connection, Dr AL Bowley very aptly observes that, it is never safe to take published statistics at their face value without knowing their meaning and limitations and it is always necessary to criticize arguments that can be based on them.

By way of caution, the researcher, before using secondary data, must see that they possess following characteristics:

1. **Reliability of data:** The reliability can be tested by finding out such things about the said data: (a) Who collected the data? (b) What were the sources of data? (c) Were they collected by using proper methods? (d) At what time were they collected? (e) Was there any bias on part of the compiler? (f) What level of accuracy was desired? Was it achieved?
2. **Suitability of data:** The data that are suitable for one enquiry may not necessarily be found suitable in another enquiry. Hence, if the available data are found to be unsuitable, they should not be used by the researcher. In this context, the researcher must very carefully scrutinize the definition of various terms and units of collection used at the time of collecting the data from the primary source originally. Similarly, the object, scope and nature of the original enquiry must also be studied. If the researcher finds differences in these, the data will remain unsuitable for the present enquiry and should not be used.
3. **Adequacy of data:** If the level of accuracy achieved in data is found inadequate for the purpose of the present enquiry, they will be considered as inadequate and should not be used by the researcher. The data will also be considered inadequate, if they are related to an area which may be either narrower or wider than the area of the present enquiry.

From all of this we can say that it is very risky to use the already available data. The already available data should be used by the researcher only when he finds them reliable, suitable and adequate. But he should not blindly discard the use of such data if they are readily available from authentic sources and are also suitable and adequate. For in that case, it will not be economical to spend time and energy in field surveys for collecting information. At times, there may be wealth of usable information in the already available data which must be used by an intelligent researcher, but with due precaution.

Selection of Appropriate Method for Data Collection

There are various of methods of data collection. Complete and appropriate answer of a research question largely depends on the selection of appropriate methods of data collection, which generally begin at the time of selection of a research design. A research question or hypotheses may be answered by using one or more number of methods of data collection. However, selection of appropriate method of data collection is influenced by several factors as discussed below:

- **The nature of phenomenon under study:** The nature of the phenomenon under study largely influences the choice of the method of the data collection. Each research phenomenon has its particular characteristics and, therefore, needs different approaches and methods of data collection. *For example,* some of the phenomenon only can be studied appropriately through observation such as clinical practices or processes in particular nursing procedures. Similarly, knowledge of a group of nurses only can be assessed through questioning or interviews. Therefore, the nature of the phenomenon under study significantly affects the selection of particular method of data collection.
- **Type of research subjects:** Data collection methods are also influenced by the type of subjects under study. *For example*, data collection from physically or psychologically disabled subjects can be done either by interviews or through observation, where data collection through questionnaires is not feasible. On the other hand, if data has to be collected from objects or institutions, questionnaries or interviews may not be possible at all, and researchers will have to depend mostly on observation to collect relevant data.
- **The type of research study:** Quantitative and qualitative research studies need different methods of data collection. *For example*, in

qualitative research, more in-depth information is required, therefore, focused group interviews or unstructured participatory interviews are feasible for data collection, while for quantitative research studies more structured interviews, questioning or observation is used for data collection.

- **The purpose of the research study:** The purpose of the study also influences the choice of the methods of data collection, such as in a study conducted with the purpose of the exploration of phenomenon, in-depth interviews may be needed for data collection, while studies conducted with purpose of description or correlation of study variables may need more structured methods of data collection.
- **Size of the study sample:** When a study is conducted on a small sample, interviews or direct observation may be possible, while these methods can be tedious for large samples. For larger samples, questionnaires can be better and more preferable methods for data collection. Interviews and observation methods will also be cost-effective and easy for smaller groups, while questionnaires will be convenient, easier, and cost-effective methods of data collection for larger samples.
- **Distribution of the target population:** If target population is spread in a large geographical area, it will not be possible to carry out interviews or observation, and therefore mailed questionnaires may be a better option, which will be more convenient and cost-effective in such conditions.
- **Time frame of the study:** If a research is conducted for the long time, it may permit the researcher to use the less-structured methods of data collection to gain in-depth information, while short time-frame studies may not allow the researcher to use the unstructured methods of data collection, where he or she gets very little time for data collection and analysis. Therefore, structured methods of data collection are used more for short-term research designs.
- **Literacy level of the subjects:** Illiterate subjects put constrains on the use of self-responding methods of data collection such as questionnaires. For illiterate subjects, interviews conducted in native language is one of the few possible methods of data collection used, while more varied and numerous options in methods of data collection are available for literate subjects.
- **Availability of recourses and manpower:** Some of the methods of data collection require more quantities of resources and manpower, such as conducting interviews and observation compared to the use of questionnaires. Therefore, availability of resources and manpower also affects the selection of methods of data collection.
- **Researcher's knowledge level and competence:** The researcher's knowledge and competence also affects the selection of methods of data collection, *for example* conducting an interview observation may require special social and psychological knowledge, skills, and competence, while the use of questionnaires may not demand these skills, however for the development and construction of a good questionnaire, good writing skills may be required.

As such the researcher must judiciously select the method/methods for his own study, keeping in view the following factors:

1. **Nature, scope and object of enquiry:** This constitutes the most important factor affecting the choice of a particular method. The method selected should be such that it suits the type of enquiry that is to be conducted by the researcher. This factor is also important in deciding whether the data already available (secondary data) are to be used or the data not yet available (primary data) are to be collected.
2. **Availability of funds:** Availability of funds for the research project determines to a large extent the method to be used for the collection of data. When funds at the disposal of the researcher are very limited, he will have to select a comparatively cheaper method, which may not be as

efficient and effective as some other costly method. Finance, in fact, is a big constraint in practice and the researcher has to act within this limitation.

3. **Time factor:** Availability of time has also to be taken into account in deciding a particular method of data collection. Some methods take relatively more time, whereas with others the data can be collected in a comparatively shorter duration. The time at the disposal of the researcher, thus, affects the selection of the method by which the data are to be collected.
4. **Precision required:** Precision required is yet another important factor to be considered at the time of selecting the method of collection of data.

But one must always remember that each method of data collection has its' uses and none is superior in all situations. For instance, telephone interview method may be considered appropriate (assuming telephone population) if funds are restricted, time is also restricted and the data is to be collected in respect of few items with or without a certain degree of precision. In case funds permit and more information is desired, personal interview method may be said to be relatively better. In case time is ample, funds are limited and much information is to be gathered with no precision, then mail-questionnaire method can be regarded more reasonable. When funds are ample, time is also ample and much information with no precision is to be collected, then either personal interview or the mail-questionnaire or the joint use of these two methods may be taken as an appropriate method of collecting data. Where a wide geographic area is to be covered, the use of mail-questionnaires supplemented by personal interviews will yield more reliable results per rupee spent than, either method alone. The secondary data may be used in case the researcher finds them reliable, adequate and appropriate for his research. While studying motivating influences in market researches or studying people's attitudes in psychological/social surveys, we can resort to the use of one or more of the projective techniques stated earlier. Such techniques are of immense value in case the reason is obtainable from the respondent who knows the reason, but does not want to admit it or the reason relates to some underlying psychological attitude and the respondent is not aware of it. But when the respondent knows the reason and can tell the same if asked, than a non-projective questionnaire, using direct questions, may yield satisfactory results even in case of attitude surveys. Since projective techniques are as yet in an early stage of development and with the validity of many of them remaining an open question, it is usually considered better to rely on the straight-forward statistical methods with only supplementary use of projective techniques. Nevertheless, in pre-testing and in searching for hypotheses, they can be highly valuable.

Thus, the most desirable approach with regard to the selection of the method depends on the nature of the particular problem and on the time and resources (money and personnel) available along with the desired degree of accuracy. But, over and above all this, much depends upon the ability and experience of the researcher. Dr AL Bowley's remark in this context is very appropriate when he says that "in collection of statistical data commonsense is the chief requisite and experience the chief teacher".

Before results can be analyzed, the data must be collected and this means making measurements of one sort or another. This poses several subsidiary questions:

1. What are measurements?
2. Are the measurements valid?
3. Has bias been eliminated?
4. Have the observations been recorded and transcribed correctly?

The description of these questions as given below:

1. As stated earlier, there are essentially three types of measurements:
   i. *Interval (numerical):* This records quantitative data and represents the highest level of measurement. Examples

are weighing an object on a balance, using a ruler or blood pressure machine, and levels of biochemical substances in blood or urine.

ii. *Ordinal (ranked):* This term is used for the recording of semi-quantitative data or when reponses are ranked in order—best result … worst result.

iii. *Nominal (classified):* Each category or class must be well-defined, exclusive (no observation may belong to more than one category) and exhaustive, meaning that all observations must belong to one of the categories. This is often difficult in clinical medicine but a simple example is where an outcome is recorded such as "alive" or "dead", "asleep" or "awake".

It is important to define the type of measurement since different statistical methods have to be applied to each of the above. There is, however, often overlap in the forms of measurement. For example, at necropsy the spleens of 100 patients may be weighed in grams and the interval scale used; but later the ordinal one may be preferred where spleens are specified as very large, large, average or small. Similarly, nominal data may be partially ordered since categories of response can in themselves have a rank order—excellent, good, fair, poor, very poor—although it may be difficult to say that the step from poor to fair is the same interval as the step from fair to good.

2. A ruler is a valid measure of height and an accurate pair of scales a valid measurement of weight. But does a cheese grater strapped to the arm under a blood pressure cuff give a valid measurement of pain intensity as the mercury column rises, and would it be right to describe it as a hundred millimeters of pain if that is when the subject begs you to stop doing it? Some measuring instruments are like this and it must be considered whether such measurements can be extrapolated to headache, or abdominal pain after operation, as some people might wish to do when they perfom a clinical trial of an analgesic drug. In medicine, there is often no clear dividing line.
3. It is easier to round up or round down blood pressure recordings and if a drug that you favor is being given, you might be tempted to round down rather than round up. This type of bias is eliminated in two ways: first by ensuring that at least the observer is unaware which treatment the patient is receiving and secondly by using instruments which do not disclose the true reading until after it has been made. In research on blood pressure, this can be done by the use of a Hawksley Random Zero machine or the more sophisticated though less portable London School of Hygiene machine.
4. Figures are often recorded incorrectly and different observers can disagree substantially about measurements. It is therefore important to have some knowledge of both inter- and intra-observer error. Most data from record cards or sheets are nowadays transcribed to punch cards or computers and their floppy disk storage facilities. Data must be transcribed correctly and the more transcribing is done, the greater the number of possible errors.

EXERCISES

1. State the meaning of data with example.
2. Discuss the classification of data on the basis of characteristics.
3. Explain the classification of data on the basis of its sources, field and content.
4. Explain in detail the sources of data collection in nursing research.
5. Describe briefly the factors influence in selection of appropriate method of data collection.

CHAPTER 4 Processing Statistical Data

Introduction

In the earlier chapter various methods of gathering statistical and other kind of data were discussed at some length. Where a mass of data has been assembled, it is necessary to arrange the material in some kind of concise and logical order. This procedure is referred to as tabulation.

Before tabulation of primary data, it should be scrutinized for (i) completeness, (ii) consistency, (iii) accuracy and (iv) editing.

Completeness: If the answer to some important question in a schedule or questionnaire is missing, it becomes necessary to contact the informant again and complete the missing information in the report. In case, such an information cannot be completed, the schedule or questionnaire should be discarded or revised.

Consistency: Some information given by the respondent may not be compatible in the sense that an information furnished by the individual either does not justify some other information or is contradictory or earlier one. For example, the total expenditure exceeds the income reported by the respondent, the number of children mentioned is less than total number of sons and daughters, then the respondent should again be contacted to rectify the mistake.

Accuracy: It is of vital importance. If the data are inaccurate, the conclusions drawn from it have no relevance or reliability. By checking the schedules or questionnaire only a little improvement can be made, e.g. if the sum of certain figures is wrong, it can be corrected. But if the investigator has either made a false report or the respondent has deliberately supplied wrong information about his income, age or assets, etc. editing will be of no use. In recent times, checks have been evolved to attain accuracy, e.g. by sending supervisors to check the work of investigators or reinvestigating a few respondents after a certain gap of time.

As already stated in the field of health, the data collected from various sources such as census, survey conducted by health institution and Government, medical records in the hospitals, registration of vital events and diseases, sample registration system and epidemiological surveillance of certain diseases like tuberculosis, leprosy, malaria, filaria, etc. Technically speaking, the processing of data implies, editing, coding, classification and tabulation of collected data, so that they are amenable to analysis. The term 'analysis' refers to the computation of certain measures along with searching for patterns of relationships that exist among data group. The process of analysis, relationships or differences supporting or conflicting with original or new hypothesis should be subjected to statistical significance to determine with what validity data can be said to indicate any conclusion.

Editing

Editing of data is a process of examining the collected raw data to detect errors and omissions and to correct these when possible. If is a fact that editing involves a careful scrutiny of the completed questionnaires/or schedules. Editing is done to assure that the data are accurate, consistent with other facts gathered, uniformly entered, as complete as possible and have been well arranged to facilitate cooling and tabulation. Researchers using the editing style act as interpreters who read through the data in search of meaningful segment and units. Once segments are identified and reviewed, they develop a categorization scheme and corresponding codes that can be used to sort and organize data. The researchers then search for the patterns and structures that connect the thematic categories.

To maintain homogeneity, the information sheets are checked to see whether the unit of information or measurement is the same in all the schedules. For instance, some people might have reported income per month and some annual income. In such a situation, it has to be converted to the same unit during editing. It should also be checked whether or not the same information has been supplied for a particular question in all the information sheets. The ambiguity arises due to various interpretations of the same question and should be removed.

Once the primary data have undergone the above four processes it is fit for further analysis.

Large scale data cannot be collected repeatedly because of the paucity of time, money and personnel. Hence the use of secondary data for certain studies is inevitable. While making use of the secondary data, one should always take care of the following points:

a. One should see whether the data are suitable for study.
b. The source of data should also be viewed, keeping in mind whether at any time, it is reliable or not. If there is any doubt about the reliability of data, it should not be used.
c. It should be noted that the data is not obsolete.
d. In case the data are based on a sample, one should see whether the sample is a proper representative of the population.
e. The primary data has been handled carefully by skilled persons only.

Once the above points are observed in the secondary data, it is ready to be used for further analysis.

Coding

Coding is the process of transforming raw data into standardized form of data processing and analysis; in quantitative research, the process of attaching numbers to categories. In qualitative research, the process of identifying recurring words, threads, or concepts within the data. In other words coding refers to the process of assigning numerals or other symbols to answers, so that the response can be put into a limited number of categories or classes. Such classes should be appropriate to the research problem under consideration. They must also possess the characteristic of exhaustiveness, i.e. there must be a class for every data item and also mutual exhaustivity, which means that a specific answer can be placed in one and only one cell in a given category set. Another rule to be observed is that of unidimensionality, by which it means that every class is defined in terms of only one concept.

Coding is necessary for efficient analysis and through it several replies may be reduced to a smaller number of classes which contain critical information required for analysis. Coding decisions should usually be taken up at the designing stage of the questionnaire. This makes it possible to precode the questionnaire choices and which in turn is helpful for computer tabulation, as one can straight forward key punch from the original questionnaire. Precoding the questionnaire has some obvious advantage such as, making it possible to eliminate all or major portions of an office coding operation.

The other method can be to transcribe data from questionnaire to a coding sheet or a transcription sheet. Transcription sheets are also useful for:

i. Combing information that has been reported on an individual basis into units representing several persons, such as household or family units and
ii. Drawing together related items of information about an individual reported in different sections of a questionnaire. One example of this integrating process is in fertility studies, where a variety of personal characteristics of the individual is analyzed in conjunction with other pertinent data such as, size of family, number of children born and similar information.

Accuracy of a measurement: Depends on the precision required, the tools available for the measurement and the skill of the person undertaking the task. Though absolute accuracy is neither possible nor desired in statistics, a reasonable degree of accuracy is a must. For instance, the monthly income of a person should be rounded to the nearest of ten of rupees, height is measured up to one-tenth of a cm and calculation of age in years and months is fairly accurate.

Sometimes the figures (values) are rounded by reducing one or more decimal places to the unit place or nearest to the ten or hundredth of a number. The universal rules of rounding are, if the decimal place value to be rounded is less than 5, it should be deleted straightway, and if greater than 5, the preceding number is increased by 1. In case the decimal place value to be rounded off is 5, the rule is to delete it if the preceding number is even and increase the preceding number by one if it is odd.

For instance, 9.74 will be rounded to one decimal place as 9.7 and 9.78 will be rounded as 9.8. Moreover, 9.75 will be rounded as 9.8 and 9.85 will also be rounded as 9.8 according to the rule. The rule is applicable in general for any numerical value.

Before giving absolute and relative error it is worth pointing out that in statistics an error is different from a mistake. The mistakes in counting, weighing, measuring or reporting are not errors in statistical sense and should be regarded as mistakes only. Error in statistical sense means the difference between the actual value and the value under consideration, generally an estimated value. An absolute error (AE) is the absolute difference between the actual value (X) and its estimated value (x).

$$AE = |X - x| \quad \text{...(4.1)}$$

The relative error (RE) is the ratio of the absolute error to the actual value, i.e.

$$RE = \frac{|X - x|}{X} \quad \text{...(4.2)}$$

Very often the relative error is given in percent, i.e.

$$RE = \frac{|X - x|}{X} \times 100 \quad \text{...(4.2.1)}$$

The smaller the relative error, the better is the result.

Classification

According to LR Connor, classification is the process of arranging things (either actually or notionally) in groups or classes according to their resemblance and affinities and gives expression to the unity of attributes that may subsist amongst the diversity of individuals. Professor AR Illersic has stated that the statistician's first task is to reduce and simplify the details into a form so that the salient features may be brought out, while still facilitating the interpretation of the assembled data. This procedure is known as classifying and tabulating the data.

In short, a table is a systematic arrangement of data in rows and/or columns. As a matter of fact, the kind of classification or tabulation mostly depends on the type of information required for study and the type of further statistical treatment to be undertaken. Though, there are no hard and fast rules, still some norms can be given for an ideal classification and tabulation of data. Norms for an ideal classification are:

1. The classes should be complete and there should be no-overlapping. It means that each

observation or unit must belong to an unique class. For instance, if we classify people according to their marital status, generally, we classify them as married and unmarried. But, there are many who do not belong to either of these groups namely, divorcees, widows or widowers. Since the number of such people is very small as compared to the number of married and unmarried people, they can be classified as 'others'.

2. Clarity of classes is another important property. It means that classes should be such that one can place a unit or an observation in a class without confusion.
3. One should use standardized classes, so that the comparison of results can be possible from time to time. For example, to know educational development, we should use classification like, illiterate, literate, primary, secondary, graduate, postgraduate and technical. Further, the unit of each class should be the same. The classification of data is generally done on geographical, chronological, qualitative or quantitative basis, on the following lines:
   i. *In geographical classification*, data are arranged according to places, areas or region.
   ii. *In chronological classification*, data are arranged according to time, i.e. weekly, monthly, quarterly, halfyearly, annually, etc.
   iii. *In qualitative classification*, the data are arranged according to attributes like sex, marital status, educational standards, state or intensity of disease, etc. It is not essential that a table should have only one attribute. The data can be classified according to any number of attributes. If the data can be classified into two classes only, it is said to be classified according to dichotomy. If the number of classes is more than two, it is said to be *a manifold classification*. The readers will come across many examples for these situations in the discussion later.
   iv. *Quantitative classification* means arranging data according to a certain characteristic that has been measured, e.g. according to height, weight or income of persons, vitamin content in a substance, etc. In this type of classification, certain classes are formed and the units belonging to these classes are attached to them. One problem that arises is of determining the class intervals. This class interval will depend upon the number of classes which will be arbitrarily decided keeping in view the quantum of data, measurement of characteristic and type of information required. A numerical formula as suggested by HA Sturges may be used for determining approximately the class interval and number of classes. The formula is,

$$i = \frac{L - S}{1 + 3.322 \log_{10} n} \qquad ...(4.3)$$

where $1 + 3.322 \log_{10} n = k$, the number of classes

i = Class interval

L = Largest observation

S = Smallest observation

n = Total number of observations

   v. *Time Series:* Another type of classification is the time series in which data or the derived values from data for each time period are arranged chronologically. A extensive example of the time series data is given in the chapter on Time Series Analysis.

After collection and editing of data the first step towards further processing is classification. Classification is the grouping of related facts into classes. Raw data as recorded in the Proforma or cards is not helpful in understanding their meaning or underlying trends. As such the data should be rearranged and classified in a suitable manner. Most of the research studies result in a large volume of raw data which must be reduced into a homogeneous group to get meaningful relationships. This fact necessitates classification of data, which happens to be the process of arranging data in groups or classes on the basis of common characteristics. Data having common characteristics are placed in one class and in this way the entire data gets divided into a number of groups or classes.

Classification is fundamental to any kind of scientific analysis. The general scheme of classification is commonly determined before the data are gathered but seldom actually completed until all the data have been collected. The basis of any statistical classification is determined by the problem at hand as well as by the characteristic features of the data.

The major objectives of classification of data include the following:

- To condense the mass of data in such a manner that similarities and dissimilarities can be apprehended
- To facilitate comparison
- To highlight the most significant feature of the data
- To enable a statistical treatment of the material collected.

In actual practice it will be found that one or more of the following criteria are almost invariably used in statistical classifications:

- Geographical
- Chronological or temporal
- Qualitative or attributive and
- Quantitative.

i. *Geographical:* In this type of classification data are classified on the basis of geographical or vocational differences between the various items like states, cities, regions, zones, area, etc. Geographical classifications are usually listed in alphabetical order for easy reference and are also based on size.

ii. *Chronological:* It is a type of classification on the basis of time. Here some units of time such as a day, week, month or year may serve as the basis of classification for certain kinds of statistical data. So when data are observed over a period of time, the type of classification is known as chronological classification. For example: The population of India as follows in each year (Census) (Table 4.1).

iii. *Qualitative:* Certain qualities or attributes of the individuals or groups are the basis of this classification. In this type of classification, data are classified on the basis of some attributes or quality such as sex, color, nativity, occupation, marital status, color of hair, literacy, religion, etc. Here the attributes cannot be measured, one can only find out whether it is present or absent in the units of population under study. For example, by the attributes under study in a given population one can find out how many persons are living in urban areas and how many persons are living in rural areas:

iv. *Quantitative:* A quantitative criterion as expressed by size or magnitude is particularly a common basis of classification in statistical work. Quantitative classification refers to the

Table 4.1

Population trends in India

Year	*Population (millions)*
1901	238
1911	252
1921	251
1931	279
1941	318
1951	361
1961	439
1971	548
1981	683
1991	839
2001	1027

classification of data according to some characteristics then can be measured, such as height, weight, income, sales, production, etc. Frequency distribution is an excellent illustration of this type of classifications (Table 4.2), i.e. income groups of Bedavatti Village of Sorab Taluk Shimoga Dist. in Karnataka, India.

Tabulation

Tabulation is the first step before the data is used for analysis and inter pretation by tabulation, the data becomes simple from a lot of collection of statistical data. Compilation of data involves two important steps, i.e. data editing and data reduction. Data editing is correction for incompleteness, inaccuracies, illegal entries and inconsistencies in data. Use of standard/pretested formats, inclusion of detailed instruction with data entry schedule, training of person involved, supervision, sample checking, checks introduced in data schedules, computerization of data entry are some of the data editing technology. Data reduction is the reduction of voluminous raw data in manageable amount for the purpose of presentation and analysis. In epidemiological studies people are interested in person, place and time distributions. Obviously this requires grouping of raw data in various person, place and time units. It needs tabulation.

This clear that tabulation is the most common method of data reduction. When a mass of data has been assembled, it becomes necessary for the researcher to arrange the same in some kind of concise and logical order. This procedure is called a 'tabulation'. So tabulation is the process of summarizing raw data and displaying the same in compact form for further analysis. In other words tabulation is an orderly arrangement of data, in columns and rows. Tabulation is essential, because:

- It conserves space and reduces explanatory and descriptive statement to a minimum
- It facilitates the process of comparison
- It facilitates the summation of items and the detection of errors and omissions
- It provides a basis for various statistical computations.

Tabulations can be done by manual, mechanical or electronic devices. The choice depends on the size and type of study, cost consideration, time pressures and the availability of tabulating machines or computers. If the objectives of the study are clear and preset, dummy tables are created in the profiles itself. Conversion of raw data into tables and groups with the help of various computer applications software like MS-Excel, Lotus, SPSS, EPI-Info is also possible. Data reduction involves a compromise between loss of details and compactness achieved.

In relatively large inquiries, we may use mechanical or computer tabulation if other factors are favorable and necessary facilities are available. Hand tabulation is usually preferred in case of small inquiries where the number of questionnaires is small and they are of relatively short length. Hand tabulation may be done using the direct tally, tally or the card sort and count methods. When there are simple codes, it is feasible to tally directly from the questionnaire. Under this method, the codes are written on a sheet of paper, called tally sheet and for each response a stroke is marked against the code in which it falls. Usually after every four strokes against a particular code, the fifth response is indicated by drawing a diagonal or horizontal line through the strokes. These groups of five are easy to count and the data are sorted against each code conveniently. In the listing method, the code responses may be transcribed onto a large work-

Table 4.2

Income groups of Bedavatti Village consisting of 70 families

Income groups (Rupees)	*Number of families (or Class frequency)*
Below 1000	13
1001 – 2000	20
2001 – 3000	12
3001 – 4000	18
4001 and above	7
Total	**70**

sheet, allowing a line for each questionnaire. This way a large number of questionnaires can be listed on one work sheet. Tallies are then made for each question. The card sorting method is the most flexible hand tabulation. In this method the data are recorded on special cards of convenient size and shape with a series of holes. Each hole stands for a code and when cards are stacked, a needle passes through particular hole representing a particular code. These cards are then separated and counted. In this way frequencies of various codes can be found out by the repetition of this technique. We can as well use the mechanical devices or the computer facility for tabulation purpose in case we want quick results, our budget permits their use and we have a large volume of straight forward tabulation involving a number of cross-breaks.

Tabulation may also be classified as simple and complex tabulation. The former type of tabulation gives information about one or more groups of independent questions, whereas the latter type of tabulation shows the division of data in two or more categories and as such, is designed to give information concerning one or more sets of inter-related questions. Simple tabulation generally results in one-way tables which supply answers to questions about one characteristic of data only. As against this, complex tabulation usually results in two-way tables (which give information about two inter-related characteristic of data), three-way tables (give information about three interrelated characteristics of data), or still higher order tables, also known as manifold tables, which supply information about several interrelated characteristics of data. Two-way tables, three-way tables or manifold tables are all examples of what is sometimes described as cross tabulation.

Formation of Statistical Series

In the series of organizing the data pertaining to a quantitative phenomenon, the following four series are considered:

a. Individual series
b. Discrete series
c. Grouped series
d. Continuous series

We shall explain the various stages of presenting the data by means of numerical illustration. The following are the marks of 100 students in an examination, arranged in order or roll numbers.

Raw Data or Unorganized Data

5	14	10	16	8	15	1	14	9	6
11	3	8	12	6	4	11	17	7	10
18	10	15	9	8	14	8	5	15	4
10	13	4	18	2	6	10	7	13	8
16	7	14	11	9	4	11	9	3	7
1	8	10	5	13	7	15	8	19	16
6	17	11	15	6	3	18	12	9	4
14	11	9	4	14	11	8	7	19	10
15	8	19	11	7	16	10	3	6	14
10	19	3	20	8	11	20	14	9	19

The data recorded as above are called the 'raw or unorganized' data. The marks are so unwieldy and scattered. Even after a careful reading, the various details contained in them are not clear. The marks are recorded as they are collected. They are not organized. However, they can be organized and presented in a better way in an array form.

Array

The raw data can be arranged in an ascending or descending order of values. This arrangement is called "arraying" the format of arraying the data is called as an "array".

The marks of 100 students in the examination are now presented in an organized form as under: Marks of 100 students (out of 20) organized and arrayed.

In arraying the raw data, serial numbers are used instead of roll numbers to maintain the order of the values of variables. By arraying, the data is not condensed. The size of the observation remains the same. However, the presentation of data looks better than the raw data. Such a type of data is essential for statistical analysis.

Though the arraying method gives a better picture, it is very difficult to grasp the significance of the data at a glance. So, the data is presented in

Sl.No	Marks	Sl.No	Marks	Sl.No	Marks	Sl.No	Marks
1	1	26	7	51	10	76	14
2	1	27	7	52	10	77	14
3	2	28	7	53	10	78	14
4	3	29	7	54	10	79	15
5	3	30	7	55	10	80	15
6	3	31	8	56	10	81	15
7	3	32	8	57	11	82	15
8	3	33	8	58	11	83	15
9	4	34	8	59	11	84	15
10	4	35	8	60	11	85	16
11	4	36	8	61	11	86	16
12	4	37	8	62	11	87	16
13	4	38	8	63	11	88	16
14	4	39	8	64	11	89	17
15	5	40	8	65	12	90	17
16	5	41	9	66	12	91	17
17	5	42	9	67	12	92	18
18	6	43	9	68	13	93	18
19	6	44	9	69	13	94	18
20	6	45	9	70	13	95	19
21	6	46	9	71	14	96	19
22	6	47	9	72	14	97	19
23	6	48	10	73	14	98	19
24	7	49	10	74	14	99	20
25	7	50	10	75	14	100	20

a still more attractive and condensed manner with the help of frequency distributions.

Variables that are classified according to the magnitude or size are very often arranged in the form of a frequency distribution. Figure 4.1 is a simple illustration of a frequency distribution. It will be observed that the class-intervals expressed are indicated on the left and the number of cases or frequencies in each interval are shown on the right.

In constructing a frequency distribution, it is necessary at the very beginning to determine

1. The number of class-intervals to be used,
2. The size of the class-intervals, and
3. The designation of the class-intervals.

1. Ordinarily there should be not less than eight or ten and not more than 18 or 20 class-intervals, depending on nature of the data and on the number of cases being studied. In order to obtain a clear understanding of the original data, the individual items are frequently arranged in either ascending or descending order of magnitude. Such a classification is known as an array. After noting the highest and lowest values as well as

Weight	Tabulation	Frequency
90-99	I	1
100-109	I	1
110-119	卌 IIII	9
120-129	卌 卌 卌 卌 卌 卌	30
130-139	卌 卌 卌 卌 卌 卌 卌 卌 II	42
140-149	卌 卌 卌 卌 卌 卌 卌 卌 卌 卌 卌 卌 卌 I	66
150-159	卌 卌 卌 卌 卌 卌 卌 卌 卌 II	47
160-169	卌 卌 卌 卌 卌 卌 卌 IIII	39
170-179	卌 卌 卌	15
180-189	卌 卌 I	11
190-199	I	1
200-209	III	3
Total number of cases		**265**

Fig. 4.1: Tabular work sheet for a frequency distribution. Data represents weights of 265 students at the Rajarajeswari College of Nursing, Bengaluru, Karnataka, India

characteristic features of the data, the number of intervals can be determined more easily.

2. For many types of data it is extremely important to have intervals of uniform size. The intervals should not be so small as to lose the advantages of summarization or so large as to conceal the more important characteristics of the distribution. Moreover, if the class-intervals are too small, vacant or blank intervals might occur. If comparisons are to be made between similar data, it is advisable to select class-intervals of the same size for all distribution. Whenever, possible the class-intervals should represent common and convenient numerical divisions such as five or ten, rather than odd divisions such as three or seven.
3. After the size of the class-intervals has been determined, it is important that they be clearly designated in the frequency table. Each interval must have definite lower and upper limits and must be expressed in such a way as to obviate any possibility of misinterpretation or confusion. The class-intervals are generally indicated by the first and last numbers of the interval. Thus, for example, 20 to 24 represents an interval of five; 10 to 19, an interval of ten; 2 to 3, an interval of two; and 9 to 11, an interval of three. A distinction should be made between the expressed limits and the actual limits of a class-interval. The actual separation between the intervals depends upon the precision of measurement in the original data. If the measures are carried to two decimal places then the actual upper limits, say of an interval of ten, would be 0 to 9.99. As will be observed from (Fig. 4.2). It is a commonly accepted practice in statistics to express the upper limits of class-intervals as integral numbers. In a discrete series the class-intervals are self-evident numbers. In a discrete series the class-intervals are self-evident since, a single unit determines the limits of the class-intervals.

Every class-interval has a midpoint which is midway between the upper and lower limits. Figure 4.2 illustrates the midpoints of an even of an odd interval. It will be observed that the midpoint of the interval 10 to 19 is 15 and that of the interval 10 to 14 is 12.5. After the class-intervals have been determined, it is a relatively simple matter to count the number of cases that fall in each interval.

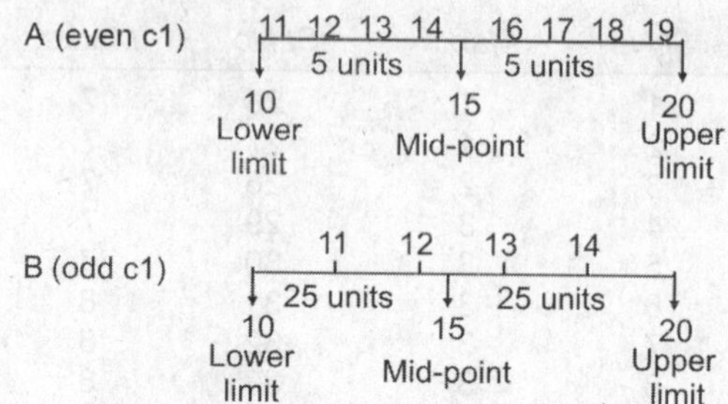

Fig. 4.2: Class-intervals and mid-point

Frequency Distribution

It is defined as the number of times each value of variable occurs in the series. It refers to the number of repetitions of a particular value of variables. It is shown with the help of counting against the particular value of class.

It is a summary presentation of values of variables arranged according to their magnitude either individually or in groups or classes. It depicts the different values of variable in one column and their respective frequencies in another. It is also called as "Frequency table", "Frequency chart" and "Frequency series".

There are three types of frequency distribution:
1. Discrete (discontinuous) frequency distribution
2. Grouped frequency distribution
3. Continuous frequency distribution.

Discrete Frequency Distribution

The variables which can take only definite or particular integers are called discrete frequency distribution, while constructing the discrete frequency distribution we count the number of times each value of variable occurs in the series. This is facilitated through the technique of "Tally bars" or "Tally Marks" method.

Tally Marks method: Tally bars are small vertical lines or bars scored parallel to each other. They are put opposite to a particular value or class to facilitate the counting of the frequencies. Usually a block of five bars is used in the counting process as ~~||||~~. This procedure makes the counting process more easy in the form of a unit of five frequencies.

Marks of 100 students (out of 20 marks) has been plotted in the form of discrete frequency distribution method (Refer Raw Data Table).

Marks	*Tally bars*	*Frequencies*	*Marks*	*Tally bars*	*Frequencies*
1	II	2	11	~~IIII~~ IIII	9
2	I	1	12	II	2
3	IIII	5	13	III	3
4	~~IIII~~ I	6	14	~~IIII~~ III	8
5	III	3	15	~~IIII~~ I	6
6	~~IIII~~ I	6	16	IIII	4
7	~~IIII~~ II	7	17	II	2
8	~~IIII~~ ~~IIII~~	10	18	III	3
9	~~IIII~~ II	7	19	~~IIII~~	5
10	~~IIII~~ IIII	9	20	II	2

The entire data is condensed and shown in which we count the number of times each value of variable occurs. The phenomenon of marks is called a **variable.** The marks themselves are called **values of variable.** The number of students scoring marks is called frequency. This type of distribution is suitable when the values of variable are less and the number of observations are more.

Grouped Frequency Distribution

When both the number of observations and the number of values of variable are large in size, the discrete frequency distribution is not suitable.

The entire range of the values of variable is to be condensed by dividing it into suitable groups or classes. Each class has two limits: Upper limit and lower limit (As the values of variable are integers or whole numbers (not fractional) "inclusive method" of classes are prepared). Both the limits are included while counting the number of observations against the particular class. However, there is a gap of one between the upper limit of the proceeding class interval and the lower limit of the succeeding class interval.

With reference to the previous table, though the values of variable are 20 in number and assured that they are large in size, we can divide them into different classes suitably, as 1-3, 4-6, 7-9.., and so on. The next step is to count the number of observations with the use of "tally bars" to form the frequency distribution. The "tally bars" are scored against the respective classes to which the values are referred.

Class-interval	*Tally marks*	*Frequency (f)*
1-3	~~IIII~~ III	8
4-6	~~IIII~~ ~~IIII~~ ~~IIII~~	15
7-9	~~IIII~~ ~~IIII~~ ~~IIII~~ ~~IIII~~ IIII	24
10-12	~~IIII~~ ~~IIII~~ ~~IIII~~ ~~IIII~~	20
13-15	~~IIII~~ ~~IIII~~ ~~IIII~~ II	17
16-18	~~IIII~~ IIII	9
19-21	~~IIII~~ II	7

The inclusive method is not in general use. So, inclusive method is converted into exclusive method for all the purposes. There will be a gap of one between the upper limit of the proceeding class and lower limit of the succeeding class. The gap is adjusted by correction factor. The correction factor is generally 0.5 which is adjusted. Correction factor of 0.5 is deducted from all the lower limit and added to all the upper limit.

For example, inclusive method of classes converted into exclusive method of classes.

Inclusive method	*Exclusive method*
1-3	0.5-3.5
4-6	3.5-6.5
7-9	6.5-9.5
10-12	9.5-12.5
13-15	12.5-15.5
16-18	15.5-18.5
19-21	18.5-21.5

The magnitudes of the class interval is two before the adjustment, but it is three after the adjustment. However, the mid-value remains the same in both the cases.

Continuous Frequency Distribution

When both the number of observations and the number of values of variable are large in size and the values of variable are both integers and fractional, the grouped frequency distribution is not suitable. The entire range of values is to be condensed by dividing it into suitable groups or classes. Each class has 2 limits – upper limit and lower limit. As the values of the variable are integers and fractional "Exclusive method" of classes are prepared. There will not be a gap of 1 between the upper limit of the proceeding class and the lower limit of the succeeding class. Because both the limits are the same.

For example:

Height in cm	Tally marks	No. of persons
150-160	𝍸 𝍸 𝍸 𝍸 IIII	24
160-170	𝍸 𝍸 𝍸 𝍸 𝍸 𝍸 IIII	34
170-180	𝍸 𝍸 𝍸 𝍸 𝍸	25
180-190	𝍸 𝍸 𝍸 𝍸 𝍸 𝍸 𝍸 𝍸 II	42
190-200	𝍸 𝍸 𝍸 𝍸 𝍸 𝍸 𝍸	35
		Total = 160

The class intervals are formed without any gaps in between them.

Class interval is defined as the size of each group of the data beginning with the lower limit and ending with the upper limit. So, it is a group constituted by two limits.

For example:

Inclusive method	Exclusive method
10-19	10-20
20-29	20-30
30-39	30-40

Principles of Tabulation

The collected and classified data can be presented in a tabular form. Tabulation stands for the systematic and scientific presentation of quantitative data in such a form as to elucidate the problem under consideration. Thus, tabulation is an orderly arrangement of data in columns and rows systematically in a tabular form. In fact tabulation is the first step before the data is used for analysis or interpretation. By tabulation, the data becomes simple, for collection of a lot of statistical data.

Basic principles for tabulation of data are as given below:

1. The tables should be numbered like table :1, table 2 and so on
2. Title of the table must be brief and self-explanatory
3. The heading of the columns and rows should be clear and concise, e.g.: - Height in cm, weight in kg, Age in years, etc.
4. The data must be presented according to size or importance
5. If percentage or averages are to be compared they should be placed as close as possible to the actual numbers in the data
6. The table should not be too large or too small. 10–20 rows are allowed in a table. Ideal is 20 rows
7. The class-interval should be the same throughout the table except in case of age
8. Groups should be tabulated in ascending or descending order from the lowest value in the range to the highest value
9. If certain data is omitted or extended, details should be given.

Objectives of tabulation include the following:

1. To summarize the data systematically
2. To classify the data in a simple form
3. To facilitate the data for a comparative study
4. To present the data in a minimum space.

Guidelines for Constructing a Statistical Table

After the data have been tabulated, the next step is to arrange at least part of them in statistical tables. Statistical tables have been referred to as the "shorthand of statistics". No matter what type of statistical problem one is investigating, there will almost invariably be a need for tables. It is therefore of extreme importance for the student of social research to have a thorough understanding of table construction. The advantages of presenting statistical data in tabular form are so obvious as to make extended comment unnecessary. It might, however, be pointed out that:

1. Statistical tables conserve space and reduce explanatory and descriptive statements to a minimum;
2. The visualization of relations and the process of comparison is greatly facilitated by tables;
3. Tabulated data can be more easily remembered than data which are not tabulated;
4. A tabular arrangement facilitates the summation of items and the detection of errors and omissions; and
5. Statistical tables provide a basis for computations.

In any discussion of the rules and practices which should be followed in the construction of statistical tables, it is important to make a distinction between the general purpose table and the special purpose table. The first type of table is also known as an original, primary or reference table and the latter type has been variously referred to as an analytical, summary, interpretative, derivative, or secondary table. The general purpose table is designed to include large amounts of source data in convenient and accessible form, whereas the special purpose table aims to illustrate or demonstrate certain points in a statistical analysis or to emphasize significant relationships in the data. The difference between the general purpose and the special purpose tables is well illustrated by the many published reports of the National Bureau of the Census. Virtually all of the tables in the reports on population, vital statistics, agriculture, manufacturing and other subjects are of the general purpose type. They represent extensive repositories of statistical information. Examples of the special purpose table are to be found in monographs and articles in which the table is fundamentally an instrument of analysis. The purpose of such tables is to reveal significant relations among the data or to emphasize certain facts. In the present discussion our main interest is in the special purpose table. The rules and procedures in constructing statistical tables are not entirely standardized, but there are certain generally accepted principles and usages which should be adhered to closely.

1. Every table should have a title. The title should represent a succinct description of the contents of the table and should make the table intelligible without reference to the text. The title should be clear, concise and adequate and should answer the questions *what? where? and when?* The title should always be placed above the body of the table.
2. Every table should be identified by a number to facilitate easy reference. The number may be either Arabic or Roman and it can be centered above the title or placed on the first line of the title.
3. The captions or column headings and the stubs or row headings of the table should be clear and brief.
4. Any explanatory footnotes such as reference symbols as the asterisk (*), dagger, double dagger and section mark ($) should be used.
5. If the data in a series of tables have been obtained from different sources, it is ordinarily advisable to indicate the specific sources in an inconspicuous place just below the table.
6. In order to emphasize the relative significance of certain categories, different kinds of type, spacing and indentation can be used.
7. Letters are generally used to guide the eye from the stubs to the first column, except where the column is set so closely that no guide is required.
8. It is important that all column figures be properly aligned. Decimal points and plus-minus signs also should be in perfect alignment.
9. Usually the columns are separated from one another by lines. Lines of this kind bring out the relations of the data more clearly and make the table more readable and attractive.

Lines are always drawn at the top and bottom of the table and below the captions. It is not at all necessary to draw lines along the sides of the table.

10. Sometimes the columns are numbered to facilitate reference.
11. Miscellaneous and exceptional items are generally placed in the last row of the table.
12. Since it may be found very confusing to read a long table when all the rows or lines are spaced, it is a common practice to group the stubs, as these side-heads are called. Generally, grouping of stubs by fives or fours is very satisfactory.
13. Abbreviations should be avoided whenever, possible and ditto marks should not be used in a statistical table.
14. The actual arrangement of the major classes in the table depends on the facts and relationships that are to be emphasized. It should always be kept in mind, however, that a statistical table should be made as logical, clear, accurate and simple as possible.
15. Columns and rows which are to be compared with one another should be brought close together.
16. Totals can be placed either at the top or at the bottom. It might be pointed out in this connection that the most conspicuous part of a table is the upper left-hand corner.

The arrangement of the categories in a table may be chronological, geographical, alphabetical, or according to magnitude. Chronological series may read to the left, depending on the emphasis or importance of the data in the series. With the exception of time series, categories as a rule should be arranged according to magnitude. If the order of importance has no particular significance, geographical order may be employed. Alphabetical arrangement is used much more frequently in general purpose than in special purpose tables.

EXERCISES

1. Define and discuss classifications.
2. Give reasons for tabulation.
3. Discuss the guidelines for constructing table with an illustration.
4. Discuss the following terms with an illustration:
   a. Frequency distribution
   b. Cumulative frequency distribution
   c. Random variable
5. What are the objectives and principles of tabulation? Also mention the different parts of standard table.

CHAPTER 5 Presentation of Data

Introduction

As stated in earlier, data collected as such do not give out any meaning. Raw data should be presented in a correct manner. So that, it gives meaning and it helps in many ways as given below:

- It arouses interest among the readers
- It reduces the data without compromising details
- It makes the data sufficiently concise without loosing important ones
- It enables readers to quickly grasp and draw quick impressions and arrive at some meaningful conclusion directly or indirectly
- It facilitates further statistical analysis
- It facilitates good communication

Generally, the presentation of data is done by tabular and graphical presentation.

The information collected through an enquiry or experiment may be presented in the form of tables or graphs. These tables enable us to come to some conclusion and make certain comparisons. Besides this, they set a stage fit for analysing the data. A table is a systematic arrangement of data in rows and columns, which is easy to understand and makes data fit for further analysis and drawing conclusions. On the other hand, a diagram, a chart or a graph is the visual form for presentation of data. Such a presentation makes it easy for a common man to understand the fluctuations, variations and the existing state of affairs of a phenomenon. The diagrams, charts or graphs may be two or three dimensional. The charts containing pictures with captions are called pictograms.

Regarding the discussion on tabulation of data, a table in general consists of the following parts:

Title: It gives information about the contents of the table. In a two-way table *captioning* levels the data to be presented in the columns whereas *stub* levels the data to be presented in the row.

Body of the table: It contains the numerical information pertaining to the various factors or characters.

Footnote: It is a statement which gives some specific information about the contents given in the body of the table.

Source note: It gives information about the source of data given in the table if it has not been collected by the person presenting them.

Keeping in view the above mentioned features of a table, a number of tables having varied classification can be constructed. Some tables with their methods of construction are discussed later.

Tabular Presentation of Data

Tabular presentation is the most common method of data reduction and of consolidation of data. The collected and classified data can be presented in a tabular form. Tabulation stands for the systematic and scientific presentation of quantitative data in such it involves an orderly arrangement of raw data in columns and rows systematically in a tabular form.

As stated earlier, the tabulation is helpful to:

- Summarize the data systematically
- Classify the data in a simple form
- Facilitate the data for comparative study and
- Present the data in a minimum space.

Formation of Frequency Table

Frequency distribution table is the method by which data of a long series of observation are systematically organized and recorded. Each one of the observations should fall into one and only one of the categories and there should be at least one category for each observation, i.e. categories should be medially exclusive. It is also called, frequency table, frequency chart and frequency series. Frequency table helps in grouping the data from master table. Consolidation of data into a table provides information at a glance. This throws light on how frequently a characteristic occurs in an individual or individuals of the same group.

The data obtained from the conduct of experiments or surveys are frequently a collection of numbers or scores. *A frequency distribution, shows a tallying of the number of times each score value (or interval of score values) occurs in a group of scores.* Classification and description of scores in the form of a frequency distribution have merits. The task of communication becomes easier and briefer and is better understood; and the important features of the data may become clearer. Frequency distribution make manual calculations of statistics easier. However, the main *flaw* is that the individual scores lose their identity and take over the central value of their respective class interval. It may lead to some error. Frequency distributions may be unnecessary when computer or calculating machines are to be used. Following Table 5.1 is an example of formations of frequency distribution:

Suppose a statistics test was given to 10 student nurses and their scores noted. How can we arrange these scores into a frequency distribution? Table 5.1 shows the procedure for the same. In part A, the scores obtained by the students have been given. For a better understanding of the scores, they have been listed in descending order (decreasing order). In Part B. it is evident that there are two values of 14, two of 13, three of 12, two of 11, and one of 10. We designate score value as "X" and the tally marks are made next to the X for each occurrence of the value and the tallies counted and written as frequency, *f*, against each score. The result is the frequency distribution as presented in Part C of Table 5.1. This frequency distribution indicates the frequency for any given value of the variable X. Note that the sum of the frequencies is equal to N, the total number of values of X, is 10. In the final form, the tally marks are deleted and only X and *f* values retained.

A distribution that indicates the percentage of the total number of cases which were observed at each score value (or interval of values) is called a

Table 5.1

The formation of a frequency distribution

Part A. Scores on a statistics test			
Given 12	12		
	14		14
	13		10
	11		12
	13		11
Part B. Scores presented in decreasing order (Preparation of an Array)			
Step I	14		12
	14		12
	13		11
	13		11
	12		10
Part C. Putting tally marks and frequencies			
Step II	Score X	Tally	Frequency
	14	II	2
	13	II	2
	12	III	3
	11	II	2
	10	I	1
			N = 10

relative frequency distribution. The frequency distribution given in Table 5.1 is reproduced in Table 5.2 to facilitate the calculation of relative frequency for each score and explain the procedure.

Frequency for each score (or class interval of scores) is divided by N and the proportions thus obtained are entered as relative frequency in column (3) of Table 5.2. The relative frequencies thus sum up to 1.00. Percentages instead of proportions may also be used. The advantages of a relative frequency distribution is that it expresses the pattern of scores in a manner which is not so convenient in the case of simple frequency distributions. Of course, it is always informative to know the total number of persons or N, in each case. The above example illustrating the concept of a frequency distribution had very small number of cases and a narrow range of scores. It was used to demonstrate through a simple case, the various aspect of this technique. An example of formation of frequency distributors for large number.

Table 5.2

Relative frequency distribution based on data of Table 5.1 (Part C)

Score' X (1)	*f (2)*	*Relative frequency (3)*
14	2	0.2
13	2	0.2
12	3	0.3
11	2	0.2
10	1	0.1
	N = 10	1.00

Frequency distribution is used to its great advantage where there are a large number of scores and a wide range of score values. In the formation of a frequency distribution, a decision regarding the size and number of class intervals is to be taken. It is to be based on some general principles and widely accepted distribution is illustrated on a set of 100 hypothetical scores given in Table 5.3.

The frequency distribution obtained from the above scores is given in Table 5.4.

Steps

Determine the Range

Range means the highest score minus the lowest score. In Table 5.3, the highest score is 192 and the lowest is 101. The range therefore is equal to 192 – 101 = 91.

Decide about the Number and Size of Class Intervals

A class interval (CI) is a band of scores. As a convention, the number of class intervals is generally kept between 10 and 20. However, depending upon the size of N, this number can vary beyond the two limits. In fact, the smaller number of class intervals leads to a coarser grouping and may introduce small errors into calculations of various statistics. The larger number of class

Table 5.3

One hundred hypothetical scores obtained by nursing students

101	107	152	153	159	153	182	191	192	180
153	156	162	172	175	176	133	134	135	138
157	158	172	140	141	145	147	110	111	131
134	150	150	120	122	183	172	161	163	165
167	164	172	151	157	158	160	159	160	172
181	172	171	149	152	154	155	157	158	160
161	171	151	154	152	155	157	154	156	153
102	101	106	171	109	117	116	119	118	110
142	146	132	171	145	155	157	158	150	154
105	171	172	162	152	175	153	157	153	152

intervals provides for a greater accuracy but may involve complications of calculations especially when N is not very large.

The sizes of class intervals generally recommended are 1, 2, 3, 5, 10 and 20. These six sizes fit into all types of data generally used by the social scientists. In our case, we preferred to have a class interval size of 10 for our data. The number of class intervals thus would be: Range ÷ class interval size, i.e. 91 ÷ 10 = 10 (raised to the next higher number). Had we decided to have a class interval size of 5, the number of class intervals would have been 21; and with a size of three, thirty one.

Determine the Starting Point

As a good rule, start the intervals with their lowest scores at multiples of the size of interval. In our case, having CI size equal to 10, we started with 10, 20, 30, 40, etc; for a size of 3, start with 3, 9, 12, 15, etc. and for a size of 5, start with 5, 10, 15, 20, 25, etc. Starting with an odd number when the CI size is also odd, gives an additional advantage that the midpoints of the class intervals will also be multiples of the CI size. In our case, we decided to start with 100, the lower limit of the lowest class interval. It is the first multiple of 10, below the smallest score in our data, i.e. 101. The class intervals thus formed are shown in Table 5.4. Instead of writing all the scores like 100, 101, 102, 103, 104, 105, 106, 107, 108 and 109, we have written only the lowest and the highest limits, i.e. 100-109. This is to save space and to avoid unnecessary lengthening of the table of frequency distribution. Moreover, the brief version, 100-109, means that all the ten scores between 100 and 109 are included. The class intervals as a convention, are written in a descending order, keeping the highest CI at the top and the lowest CI at the bottom. They should also form a continuous series and not broken ones.

Tally the Frequencies

In Table 5.4, Col. (2), the tally marks have been shown. Taking each score from Table 5.3, we locate it within the proper interval and write a tally mark "/", against the interval. Complete the tallying so as to cover all the scores. As a general convention based on convenience in counting, after four tallies have been placed before a CI, the fifth tally is marked from right to left across the first four so as to make clearly distinguishable groups of five tallies each. Tallies for each CI are then counted and noted as frequency for that CI (see Col. 3 of Table 5.4).

Table 5.4

Frequency distribution of 100 hypothetical scores obtained by nursing students with class interval (CI) size = 10

Class Interval (1)	*Tally (2)*	*f (3)*
190-199	II	2
180-189	IIII	4
170-179	~~IIII~~ ~~IIII~~ ~~IIII~~	15
160-169	~~IIII~~ ~~IIII~~ I	11
150-159	~~IIII~~ ~~IIII~~ ~~IIII~~ ~~IIII~~ ~~IIII~~ ~~IIII~~ ~~IIII~~ III	38
140-149	~~IIII~~ III	8
130-139	~~IIII~~ I	6
120-129	II	2
110-119	~~IIII~~ II	7
100-109	~~IIII~~ II	7
		N = 100

The sum of frequencies should be equal to the total number of scores or N. In case any score has been omitted or duplicated. In tallying, the total number of frequencies will not equal the total number of scores, or N. In case a tally has been placed in a wrong interval, there is no way of checking this error. However, in case of an error or doubt, the whole process of tallying should be done over again.

The sum of frequencies is written as $\sum f$ in which $\sum$ (capital Greek letter Sigma) stands for "the sum of *f*", and *f* for frequencies. The total number of scores of an individual is symbolized by the capital letter N which stands for number.

General Rules and Conventions

1. Select a class interval size that leads to the formation of 10 to 20 class intervals covering the whole range of scores
2. As far as possible, select class intervals of size 1, 2, 3, 4, 5, 10, or 20 points. These are likely to meet the requirements of most sets of data
3. Start the class interval at a score which is multiple of the size of that interval
4. Place the class interval containing the largest observations at the top; and that containing the smallest observations, at the bottom. All other class intervals should be arranged in descending order in between.
5. Make class intervals of uniform size and without any break in the series.

Exact Limits and Mid-points of the Class Intervals

In the case of continuous variables, recording of observations or scores as discrete values like, 10, 11, 12, 13, etc is based on the assumption that the value recorded represents a value falling within certain limits. These limits are usually taken as one-half or 0.5 unit above and below the value reported. A score of 51 on a test of general intelligence would imply that if a more accurate form of measurement has been used, this value would fall within the limits 50.5 and 51.5. In more precise terms, these limits are 50.5 to 51.499, in which the latter value has a recurring decimal, but for convenience, we write the limits as 50.5 to 51.5. If the measuring process allows for a higher level of accuracy like measurement to the nearer thousandth of a second, an observation of say, 0.285 seconds would fall within the limits of 0.2,845 and 0.2,855 seconds. These limits are often known as *exact limits* of the class interval. The terms, *real limits, class boundaries* or *end values* are also used for the purpose.

In the case of discrete variables, the class intervals themselves as given, represent the exact limits and no subtraction and addition of one-half unit is required to arrive at the exact limits. In Table 5.5, the exact limits of class intervals based on the data of Table 5.4 have been shown. For instance, the lowest class interval of 100–109 has the exact limits of 99.5–109.5.

For this purpose, 99.5 the lowest exact limit of the score 100 has become the lower exact limit of the class interval. Similarly, 109.5, the upper exact limit of the score 109, has become the upper exact limit of the same class interval.

The *mid-point* of class intervals are required in the calculation of further statistics like mean, median and standard deviation, etc. for which the frequency distributions are generally constructed. Moreover, all the individual scores in a class interval lose their identity and take over the value of the mid-point of the class interval to which they belong.

It is not difficult to determine the mid-points of the class intervals. The mid-point of any class interval can be obtained by adding one-half of the range of the class interval to the lower exact limit of that interval. To illustrate the point, we may refer to the two lowest class intervals of the frequency distribution in Table 5.5. The CI has a size of 10 units.

The important point is to take the lower exact limit and not the stated limit.

Generally, the midpoint of a class interval can also be obtained by using the formula.

Table 5.5

Exact limits and mid-point of class intervals

Class interval	*Exact limits (Lower-Upper)*	*Mid-points of Intervals (X)*	*Frequency (f)*
190-199	189.5-199.5	194.5	2
180-189	179.5-189.5	184.5	4
170-179	169.5-179.5	174.5	15
160-169	159.5-169.5	164.5	11
150-159	149.5-159.5	154.5	38
140-149	139.5-149.5	144.5	8
130-139	129.5-139.5	134.5	6
120-129	119.5-129.5	124.5	2
110-119	109.5-119.5	114.5	7
100-109	99.5-109.5	104.5	7
			$\Sigma f = 100$

Class interval	*Lower exact limit*		*One-half of range*	*Mid-point*
110-119	109.5	+	5	114.5
100-109	99.5	+	5	104.5

Mid-point = (Lower limit + Upper limit)/2 ...(5.1)

This applies to both the stated as well as the exact limits. In our case,

Mid-point of class interval 110-119 = (110+119)/2 = 114.5

Mid-point of class interval 100-109 = (100+109)/2 = 104.5

Using the exact limits also, we obtain the same values:

Mid-point of Class interval 110-119 = (109.5+119.5)/2 = 114.5

Mid-point of Class interval 100-109 = (99.5 + 109.5)/2 = 104.5

The concepts of size, exact limits and mid-points of a class interval are illustrated in Figure 5.1.

It may seem a bit baffling that the size of the class interval 100–109 is 10 as it might initially appear. But if all the scores contained in the class interval 100–109 are listed (100, 101, 102, 103, 104, 105, 106, 107, 108 and 109), these are clearly 10 and not 9 of them. Moreover, it may be kept in mind that both the scores of 100 and 109 are included in the interval. Hence, it is advisable that we do not calculate the size of the class interval simply by subtracting the stated lower limit from the stated upper limit of the interval. It would mean a size deficient by one unit. However, if the lower and upper exact limits are used for the purpose, the answer will be correct as in the case of the class interval 100–109.

Size of class interval = 109.5 – 99.5 = 10.

Assumptions Regarding Values within the Intervals

The grouping of data in class intervals leads to a loss of information about individual scores. Moreover, class intervals having identical lower and upper limits may be based on entirely different values as shown below. Let us take the class interval 5–9 for illustration:

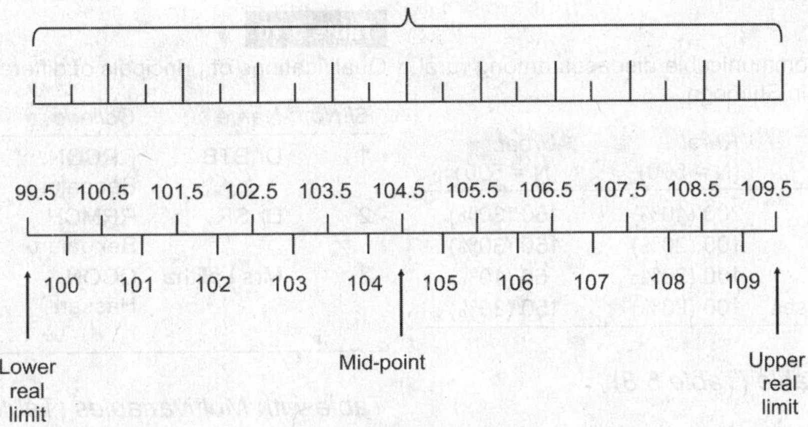

Fig. 5.1: Illustration of size, lower and upper exact limits and mid-point of the interval 100–109

Individual scores	*Class interval*
1. 5,5,5,5,5	5-9
2. 5,6,7,8,9	5-9
3. 9,9,9,9,9	5-9

In case 1, all the scores are concentrated at the lower limit, while in case 3, at the upper limit of the class interval. In case 2, the scores are evenly spread over the entire range of the class interval. Many other combinations of these scores are possible which can lead to the formation of this class interval.

Hence, in the calculation of various statistics, two important assumptions about values within the intervals are made.

- The first assumption which is generally used in the calculation of statistics like, median, quartiles, percentiles, etc, is that *the observations or scores are uniformly distributed over the entire range of the interval.*
- In the calculation of means, standard deviations and in drawing frequency polygons, another assumption is made that *all the values or scores in the class interval are the same and equal to the value corresponding to the mid-point of the interval.*

Types of Tables

Master Table

It is also known as reference table in which table shows all variables that can be cross classified. In fact it contains all the result of data reduction. It is the key score from where data are taken for tabulation. Each individual or each unit will have characteristics noted against them.

Table 5.6

Taluk-wise Malaria cases in Shimoga district in July 2007

Sl.No.	*Taluk*	*Number*
1	Bhadravathi	24
2	Hosanagar	20
3	Sagar	23
4	Shikaripur	23
5	Shimoga	20
6	Sorab	25
7	Thirthahalli	25
	Total	**160**

Simple Table (Table 5.6)

Above taken is simple shows talukwise positive cases of malaria during July 2007.

Correlation Table (Table 5.7)

It is also known as cross table, when two or more variables are recorded simultaneously, the data are recorded in row and column according to the corresponding frequency in each category.

Table 5.7

Distribution of communicable diseases among rural and urban area in Shimoga

Communicable diseases	*Rural (N = 500)*	*Urban (N = 500)*
Malaria	200 (40%)	150 (30%)
Tuberculosis	100 (20%)	150 (30%)
Leprosy	100 (20%)	50 (10%)
Diarrheal diseases	100 (20%)	150 (30%)

Association Table (Table 5.8)

This table, reveals the association between two qualitative variables, it is also required for calculating sensitivity and specificity of screening test.

Table 5.8

Association between tuberculosis and Lepromen test

	Tuberculosis Test	*Lepromen test*	*Total*
Positive	100	10	110
Negative	05	85	90
Total	105	95	200

Two by Two Table (Table 5.9)

This table shows, frequency distribution of two variables or two classes.

Table 5.9

Sex distribution of student in two colleges

College	*Male*	*Female*	*Total*
Govt Medical College	60	40	100
Govt Nursing College	20	80	100
Total	80	120	200

Text Table (Table 5.10)

It is descriptive table. It does not contain any numerical data.

Table 5.10

Qualifications of principals of different colleges

Sl.No.	*Name*	*College*	*Qualifications*
1	Dr BTB	RRCON, Bengaluru	MN PhD
2	Dr SR	RRMCH, Bengaluru	MBBS MD
3	Mrs Lalitha	CCON, Hassan	MSc Nursing (Ped)

Table with Multivariables (Table 5.11)

More than two variables or attributes are put to analysis for a set of character and is presented as multi-table.

Table 5.11

Distribution of antenatal case by gravida and health checking

Gravida I	12th Week	16th Week	20th Week	30th Week

Graphical Presentation of Data

A graph is the geometrical image of a frequency distribution. It is a mathematical picture. Frequency distributions are converted into visual models to facilitate understanding. It is easier, more convenient and quicker to draw inferences from graphs than from frequency distributions. Comparison of data also becomes easier. Graphical representation in the form of histograms, frequency polygons, cumulative frequency curves, pie-graphs, etc. appear almost daily in the newspapers, magazines, trade publications, business reports, and scientific periodicals. However, we shall discuss only the first three types of graphical representation because of their wider use and greater popularity.

Graphs and diagrams are very useful in presentation of statistical data. They provide a visual method of examining quantitative and qualitative data. They give better grasp of the information at a glance. Graphs are not substitutes for the table. However, they help to have an overall picture rather than detail. It is important to note the scale while interpreting a graph (particularly a line graph) for comparison of graphs because change in the scale will show a different pattern. Graphs must have clear and fully defined headings so that the contents could be grasped without referring to the text.

Graphs and charges are especially valuable in rendering large masses of statistical data clear and comprehensible. The meaning of series of figures in termed or tabular form may be difficult for the mind to grasp or retain. Properly constructed graphs and charts reliever the mind for burden some details be portraying facts concisely, logically, and simply. Graphs and charts, by emphasizing new and significant relationship, also may be immense service in discovering new facts and in developing hypothesis. Poorly constructed charts not only may seriously cheaper an otherwise good report, but they may actual misrepresent or distort the facts. So graphic techniques must be used with much care and discrimination. Besides possessing a thorough mastery of technique of graphic presentation, it is also important to be extremely thorough and meticulous in the actual construction of drawings.

Diagrams and charts prove nothing but they bring outstanding features to the eye. In tabulation find the columns and rows in a table may makes eye strain and there are chances of poor visual impression of data presented in a tabular form. In such circumstances data can be presented in the form of pictures, charts, diagram, or figures which will help in good comparison through good visual impression.

Merits and Demerits of Graphical Representation

The representation of quantitative data is done suitably through charts and diagrams. After tabulation the frequencies of a characteristic can be presented by two kinds of drawings, i.e. graphs and diagrams. They may be shown either by lines and dots or by figures. The drawings are meant for non-statistical minded people who want to study the relative values of frequencies of persons or events. For statistical minded persons they are for quick eye reading. As stated earlier a graphical representation is the geometrical image of a set of data. It is a mathematical picture. It enables us to think statistical problem in visual terms, i.e. it is a visual presentation of data. A picture is said to be more effective than words for describing a particular thing or phenomenon. Consequently, the graphical representation of data proves quite an effective and economic device for presentation, understanding and interpretation of the collected statistical data. It makes data interesting and makes its understanding easy even for lay persons. A meaningful impression can be attained even before one starts analyzing the data in depth.

The merits and demerits of graphical representation are as follows:

Merits

- It is easily understood by all.
- The data can be presented in a more attractive form appealing to the eye
- Observations in Change can be noticed with respect to time
- It shows the trends and tendency of values of the variables
- It helps interpolation of the values of the variables
- Valuable statistics like median, mode, percentile, quartiles, may be easily observed and can be calculated
- It helps for easy comparison
- Comparative analysis and interpretation may be made effectively
- Real value of graphical representation lies in its' economy and effectiveness
- It carries a lot of communication power
- It may help in the proper estimation, evaluation and interpretation of the characteristics of items and individuals

- It helps in forecasting as it indicates the trend and movements of the data in the past.

The semi log or double graphs need when a lot of fluctuations are seen for smoothening the irregularities (that are seen in arithmetic scale).

Demerits

1. It consumes a lot of time to construct a graph
2. A graph does not show all the facts or data in detail
3. It depicts only appropriate values.

Techniques of Constructing Graphs

To understand the mechanics of constructing graphs, it would be helpful to learn the basic terminology, principles and conventions as illustrated in Figure 5.2 and discussed below:

- *Coordinate Axes*. The two lines XOX′ and YOY' which intersect each other at right angles and at point O. Both the axes should be appropriately labeled.

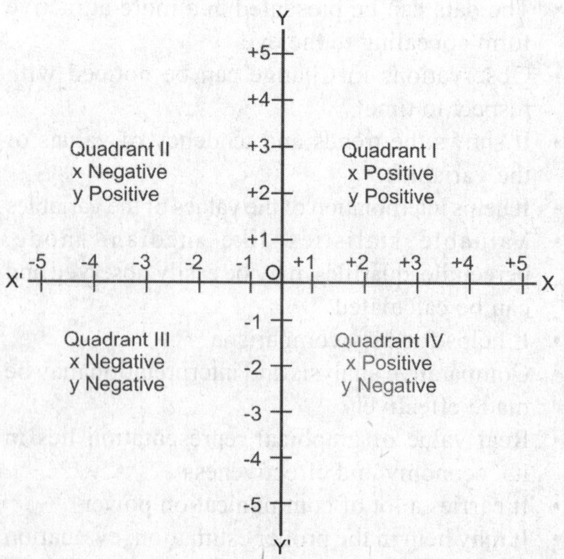

Fig. 5.2: The coordinate system

- *Abscissa* is the X-axis or XOX′ line along which the X values are located. It is the horizontal line in Figure 5.2.
- *Ordinate* is the vertical line or YOY′ line or Y-axis along which Y values are located.
- *Origin,* the point of origin or the zero point is the point of intersections of XOX′ and YOY′.
- *Quadrants.* The whole area of the plane is divided into four quadrants showing the signs of the values of X and Y as below:
  - Quadrant I: X positive and Y positive
  - Quadrant II: X negative and Y positive
  - Quadrant III: X negative and Y negative
  - Quadrant IV: X positive and Y negative
- *Signs of values:*

  On ordinate : signs above O, positive; and signs below O, negative

  On abscissa : signs to the right of O, positive; and to the left of O, negative
- By convention, the scores are laid off on horizontal or X axis and the frequencies on the vertical or Y axis.
- It is customary to assign a self-explanatory title to every graph.
- The distance along either axis selected to serve as a unit should be such that ratio of height to length is roughly 3:5. It adds to the aesthetic appearance of the graph.

Rectangular Coordinate Graphs

One of the most useful forms of graphic presentation used in nursing research is the well-known line graph. Figure 5.3 is an illustration of this type of graph. In statistical work it is called a *rectangular, rectilinear or Cartesian coordinate graph*. The basic form of this type of graph is derived by plotting figures in relation to two lines or axes.

As in Figure 5.3, these lines are drawn at right angles, the horizontal being called the *abscissal* or X-axis and the vertical, the *ordinal* or Y-axis. These two lines divide the region of the plane into four compartments called *quadrants* which are numbered counter-clockwise. The point of intersection (O) of the two axes is referred to as the origin of coordinates. Measurements to the right and above O are positive (plus) and measurements to the left and below O are negative (minus). To locate any point

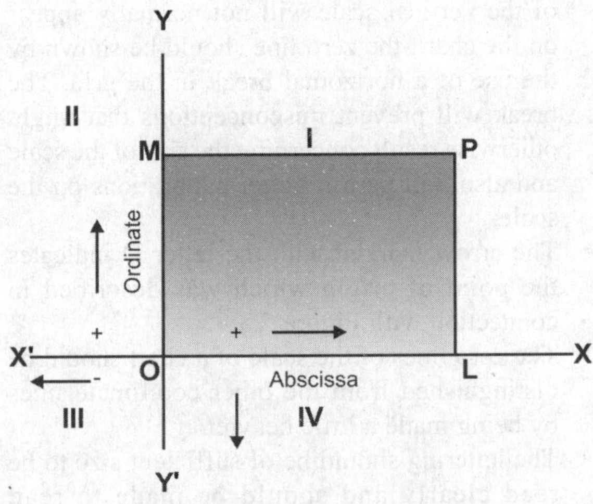

Fig. 5.3: Rectangular coordinates

in the plane of the two axes, measurements are made in terms of the two axes. The point P in Figure 5.3 has been located by taking a certain distance from the axis of ordinates and the axis of abscissae. The two axes can be marked off according to any desired unit beginning with the point of origin O as zero. In ordinary graphic presentation, quadrant I is the only one used. Sometimes, however, quadrant IV may be used to show such facts as immigration and emigration, profits and losses and imports and exports.

Figure 5.4 shows the characteristic features of the rectangular coordinate graph as well as certain general rules for graphic presentation. It can be observed that time is represented by the X-axis, or axis of abscissae and the other variable by the Y-axis, or axis of ordinates. The distance chosen to represent the units on the scales of the two axes is largely a matter of experimentation and judgment, but such factors as the following are always taken into consideration:

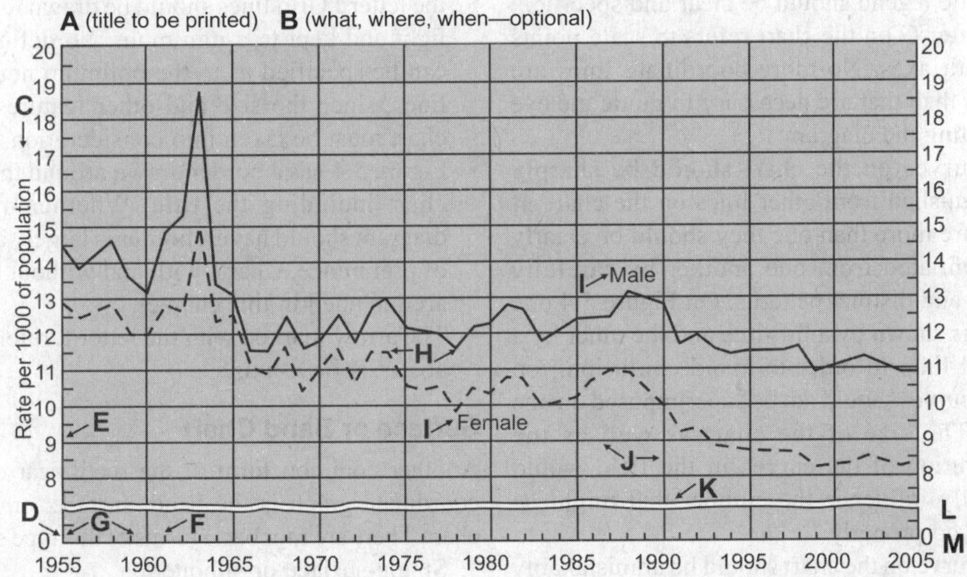

Fig. 5.4: Sample chart showing essential characteristics and rules for graphic presentation. A: Title at top. B: Optional. C: Scale legend for Y-axis. D: Origin. E: Axis of ordinates or Y-axis. F: X-axis or axis of abscissae. G: Scale points. H: Curves differentiated—solid and dashed. I: Contiguous legend for curves. J: Grid or coordinates lines—no more should be shown than are necessary to guide the eye in reading the diagram. K: Broken line—scale not complete. L: Zero line heavier than other coordinate lines. M: Lettering reads horizontally whenever possible

- Characteristics of the data
- Purpose of the chart
- Pleasing proportions
- Accuracy of presentation.

It will be observed further from Figure 5.4 that: Mortality Trends by sex 1955 to 2005.

The chart has a title, which has been placed directly above the grid.

- The title of the chart should be clear, concise, and simple and it should generally answer the questions *what? Where?* and *When?* The title may be drawn as part of the chart or set in type by the printer.
- The Y- or ordinal axis is designated by the arrow marked with the letter E. The scale reads from bottom to top.
- The arrow marked with the letter C refers to the scale legend. The scale legend for the ordinal axis can be placed to the left or at the top of the scale. If the chart is relatively wide, the scale legend may be placed on the right side as well, but this is not absolutely essential. Of course, the scale legend should be clear and specific.
- The letter G on the chart refers to scale points for both axes. No more coordinate lines are shown than that are necessary to guide the eye in reading the diagram.
- The curves on the chart should be sharply distinguished from other lines on the chart. If there are more than one they should be clearly differentiated from one another by carefully drawn and distinct patterns. On Figure 5.4 one curve is shown by a full-line and the other by a dashed line. In order to avoid confusion, too many curves should not be superimposed on one grid. The size of the chart as well as the distribution of the curves in the field would naturally influence the number that might be portrayed properly.
- Each curve on the chart should be unmistakably labeled. Generally, the most satisfactory method is to place the designation or legend contiguous to the curve. Sometimes the legend may be boxed off in one corner of the grid.
- It is frequently to indicate the plotting points on which the curves are based.
- In every rectangular coordinate chart it is essential for the vertical zero to be placed in the field of the chart. If, however, the zero line of the vertical scale will not normally appear on the chart, the zero line should be shown by the use of a horizontal break in the grid. The break will prevent misconceptions that might otherwise result concerning the size of the scale and also will permit larger calibrations on the scale.
- The arrow marked with the letter D indicates the point of origin which was described in connection with Figure 5.3.
- The zero lines of the scale of a chart should be distinguished from the other coordinate lines by being made a little heavier.
- The lettering should be of sufficient size to be read clearly and should be made to read horizontally whenever possible.
- The grid or coordinate lines are indicated by the letter J Grid lines should be drawn relatively light and kept to a minimum. No definite rule can be specified as to the optimum number of lines, since the size and other features of the chart must be taken into consideration.
- Figure 5.4 has a border drawn around the entire chart including the title. Whether or not a diagram should have a border is largely a matter of preference. Charts with and without borders are included in this chapter.
- The arrow marked with the letter L refers to the abscissal or X-axis.

Surface or Band Chart

Another common form of the rectilinear close to coordinate graph is the band, surface, or stratum chart. There are four basic forms of this type of chart:

1. Single-surface or silhouette
2. Staircase
3. Multiple-surface or band showing numerical values
4. One hundred percent multiple-surface or band.

General Principles of Constructing Graphs

- Every graph or diagram should have a suitable title. The position of the title for a graph is one of personal choice. In a published graph, however, the title is commonly placed below the graph. The title should convey meaning in as few words as possible and the main idea that the diagrams intend to portray
- Every graph or diagram should be completely self-explanatory. Therefore, it should be correctly labeled as to title, source scales and explanatory keys or legends
- A proper proportion between the height and width of a diagram/graph should be maintained. If the height and width is too short or too long in proportion, it will give an ugly look
- When more than a variable is shown on a graph, each should be clearly differentiated by means of legends or keys
- Scale division should be clearly indicated as well as the units into which scale is divided. On an arithmetic scale equal increments on the scale must represent equal numerical units
- On the scale reproducing frequency, the numerical scale should start with zero. If this is not possible the position of zero line should be shown with a break in the vertical scale clearly indicating that a break has been made
- Frequency is generally represented on the vertical scales, method of classifications on the horizontal. Horizontal axis (X-axis) is ordinate. The scales for both the axis should start from zero. The scales should be so selected that there is an optimal utilization of paper. The scale should be indicated, with an unit of measurement, at an appropriate place in the presentation. If there is break in continuity it should be shown with a broken line. The scale showing the values should be in even number or in multiples of five or ten, e.g. 25, 50, 75 or 20, 40, 60, odd values should be avoided, e.g. 1, 3, 5, 7, etc
- The graph or diagram generally precedes from left to right and from bottom to top. All writings should be placed therefore, so as to be read from the bottom right-hand side of the page
- In order to clarify certain points about the diagram, foot notes may be given at the bottom of the diagram/graph
- For an index illustrating different types of lines or different shades, colors should be given so that the reader can easily make meaning of the graph/diagram
- Graphs/diagrams should be absolutely neat and clean
- Graphs/diagrams should be as simple as possible so that the reader can understand their meaning clearly and easily
- Frequency is generally represented on the vertical scale, while the method of classification is on the horizontal scale
- Scale divisions should be clearly indicated as well as the units into which the scale is divided
- On an arithmetic scale equal increments on the scale must represent equal numerical units
- On the scale representing frequency, the numerical scale should start with zero. If this is not possible, the position of the zero line should be shown with a break in the vertical scale clearly indicating that a break has been made.

Modes of Graphical Presentation of Data

It has been known that the data in the form of raw scores is known as ungrouped data and when it is organized distribution, it is referred to as grouped data. Separate modes and methods are used to represent these two types of data—ungrouped and grouped. Let us discuss them under separate heads.

Graphical Presentation of Ungrouped Data

For the ungrouped data (data not grouped into a frequency distribution) we usually make use of the following graphical representation:

1. Line graphs
2. Bar graph or Bar diagrams
3. Circle graph or Pie diagrams
4. Pictograms.

Line Graph (Fig. 5.5)

Line graphs are simple mathematical graphs that are drawn on the graph paper by plotting the data concerning one variable on the horizontal X-axis and the other variable of data on the vertical Y-axis. With the help of such graphs the effect of one variable upon another variable during an experimental or normative study may be clearly demonstrated. The construction of these graphs can be understood through the following example:

A test was administered on a First year student of BSc Nursing to demonstrate the effect of practice of monitoring vital signs. The data so obtained may be studied from the following table.

Trial No.	1	2	3	4	5	6	7	8	9	10	11	12
Score	4	5	8	8	10	13	12	12	14	16	16	16

Draw a line graph for the representation and interpretation of the above data.

Plot the point (1,4), (2,5), (3,8), (4,8), (5,10), (6,13), (7,12), (8,10), (9,14) and (10,16).

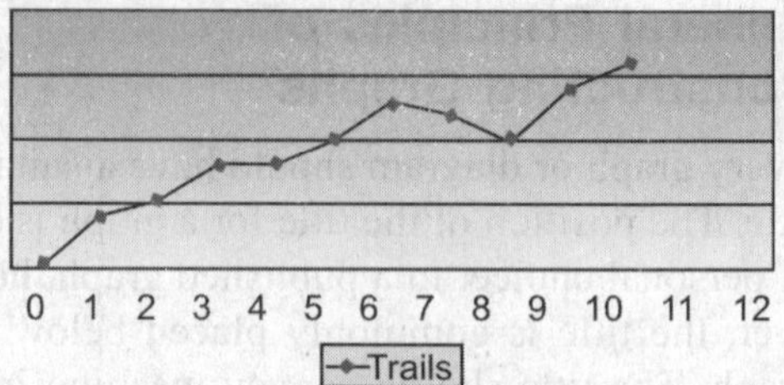

Fig. 5.5. Line Graph—the effect of practice on monitor vital signs

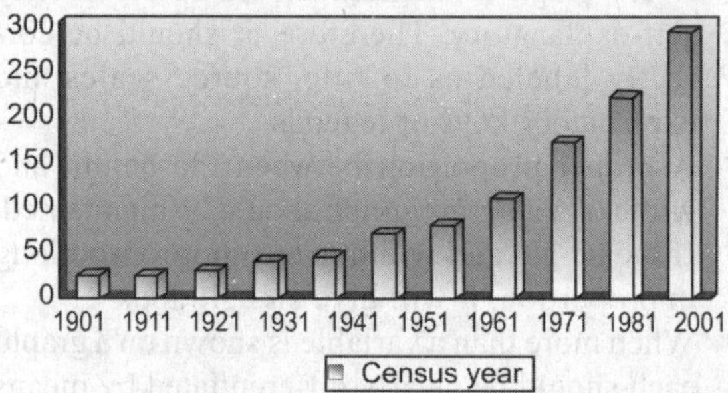

Fig. 5.6: India—growth of urban population 1901–2001

Bar and Column Charts

Bar and column charts are simple, flexible and effective techniques for computing the size of coordinate values or of parts of a total. The basis of comparison is linear or one-dimensional. This means that the length of each bar or column is proportional to the value portrayed. Fundamentally, the bar and column are very much alike. In a bar chart the bars are arranged horizontally and in a column chart, vertically. Another distinguishing feature is that, the bar chart is seldom used for depicting time series, whereas the column chart is used mainly for that purpose.

In graphic presentation, three different geometrical forms can be utilized for purposes of comparing magnitudes of coordinate items:

1. Linear or one-dimensional
2. A real or two-dimensional
3. Or three-dimensional.

In graphic presentation, the simplest and most exact comparisons can be made on a linear basis. This fact represents the real advantage of bar and column charts. Comparison of the relative sizes of areas is more difficult and of volumes, most difficult. Accordingly, where possible the use of a real and cubic forms should be avoided in graphic presentation.

There are several kinds of bar and column charts, including simple, subdivided, bilateral, step, area, as well as special variations of these types. All have one thing in common, namely, the length of the bar or column is proportional to the size or magnitude portrayed. The most widely used bar and column chart is the simple type. The simple bar chart is illustrated by Figure 5.6 and the grouped bar chart, by Figures 5.7A and B.

Urban Population in Millions

Subdivided bar and column charts not only show variations in total values but also components of the respective totals. This breakdown is accomplished by subdividing the bars and columns and

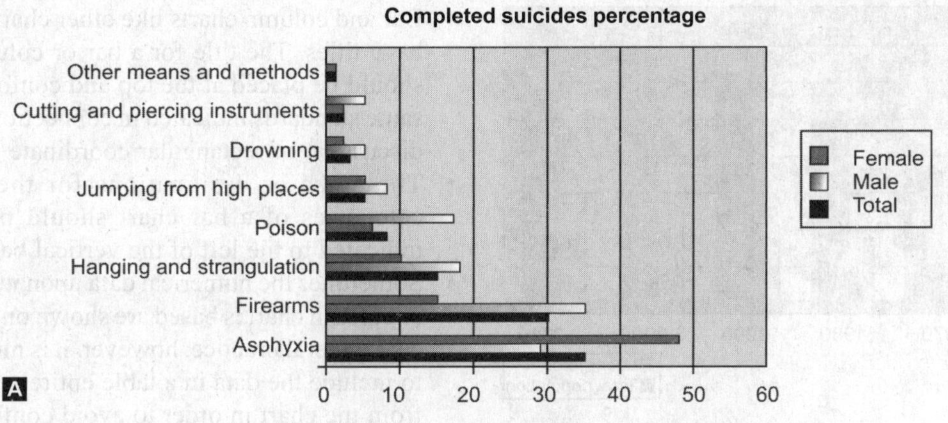

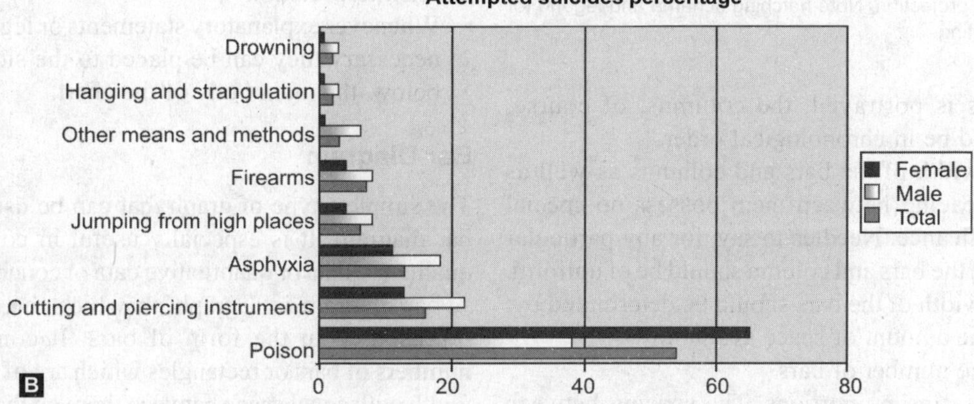

Figs 5.7A and B: An example of the grouped bar chart

differentiating the component parts by cross-hatching patterns (Figure 5.8). Another type is the bilateral or two-way bar or column chart. Bars or columns extend in two directions from a zero or base line. They may show positive and negative values or the comparison of two related categories (Figure 5.9). Limitation of space precludes a more detailed discussion of other more specialized types of bar and column charts.

In constructing bar and column charts, careful consideration should be given to the following standards and principles of design.

- The bars should be arranged in some systematic order usually according to magnitude, starting with the largest. In a column chart, where a time

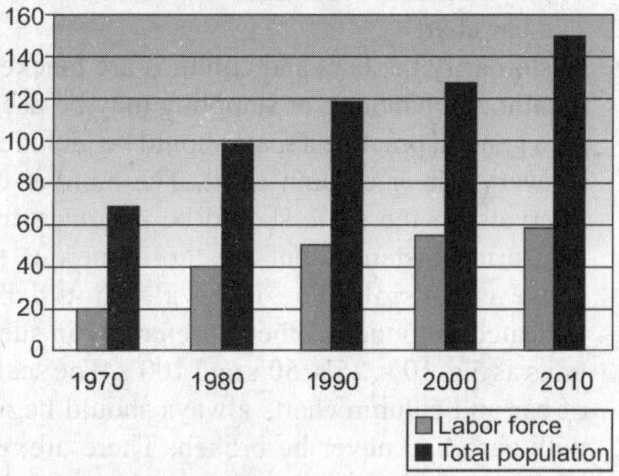

Fig. 5.8: Illustration of a grouped column chart

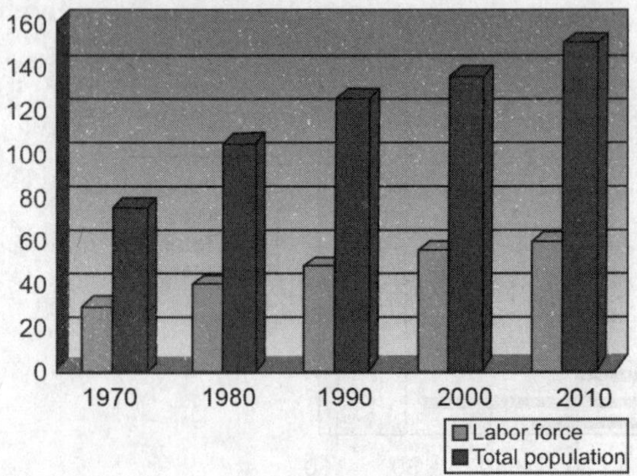

Fig. 5.9: Another illustration of a grouped column chart drawn in oblique projection. Note hatching scheme and legend for differentiating

series is portrayed, the columns, of course, should be in chronological order.

- The width of the bars and columns as well as the spacing between them possess no special significance. Needles to say, for any particular chart, the bars and column should be of uniform. The width of the bars should be determined by:
  - The amount of space available
  - The number of bars
  - Pleasing proportions. The spacing between the bars should be from one-half to three-fourth of the width of a bar. Frequently, in a column chart the spacing between columns may be much wider than between the bars in a bar chart
- Customarily the bars and columns are blacked in although hatching or stappling may be used
- As a general practice a scale should be included in every bar or column chart. The number of intervals on the scale should be adequate for measuring distances but not too numerous to cause confusion. The intervals should be indicated in round numbers, preferably in such units as 5's, 10's, 25's, 50's and 100's. The scale of bar and column charts always should begin with zero and never be broken. There are, of course, scale lines, scale points, scale numerals, and a scale legend.
- Bar and column charts like other charts, should have titles. The title for a bar or column chart should be placed at the top and conform to the same standards indicated in connection with the discussion of rectangular coordinate charts.
- The stubs or designations for the various categories of a bar chart should be clearly indicated to the left of the vertical base line
- Sometimes the numerical data upon which a bar or column chart is based are shown on the chart. As a general practice, however, it is much better to include the data in a table entirely separated from the chart in order to avoid confusion and misinterpretation
- Whenever explanatory statements or legends are necessary they can be placed to the side of, or below, the main body of the chart.

Bar Diagram

The simplest type of graph that can be used is the bar diagram. It is especially useful in comparing qualitative data or quantitative data of concrete type. A bar diagram is a graph on which the data are represented in the form of bars. It consists of numbers of bars or rectangles which are of uniform width with equal space between them on the X-axis. The length of the bar is proportional to the value it represents. It should be seen that the bars are neither too short nor too long. The scale should be clearly indicated and the base line be clearly shown.

In this diagram the bars representing births to White and Black women are drawn of equal width and with lengths equal to the respective number of births. Their area, therefore, is proportional to their length. Hence, comparison of the lengths of the two bars gives a visual picture of the births at this hospital by race, showing that there were about ten times as many babies born to Black mothers as to White mothers.

Bars may be drawn either horizontally or vertically. A good rule to use in determining the direction is that, if the legend describing the bar can be written under the bars when drawn vertically, vertical bars should be used; when it cannot be, horizontal ones must be used. In this way the legends can be read without turning the graph. The descriptive legend should not be written at the ends of the bars or within the bars, since such writing may distort the comparison. Usually the diagram will be more attractive if the bars are wider than the spaces between them.

The width of bars is not governed by any set rules. It is an arbitrary factor. Regarding the space between two bars, it is conventional to have a space about one half of the width of a bar (Fig. 5.10).

The data capable of representation through bar diagrams, may be in the form of raw scores, total scores or frequencies, computed statistics and summarized figures like percentages and averages, etc.

The bar diagram is generally used for comparison of quantitative data. It is also used in presenting data involving time factor. When two or more sets of data over a certain period of time are to be compared, a group bar diagram is prepared by placing the related data side by side in the shape of bars. The bars may be vertical or horizontal in a bar diagram. If the bars are placed horizontally, it is called a **Horizontal Bar Diagram.** When the bars are placed vertically, it is called a **Vertical Bar Diagram.** There are four types of Bar diagram: **(i) Simple Bar diagram, (ii) Multiple or Grouped Bar diagram. (iii) Subdivided or Component Bar diagram. (iv) Percentage Subdivided Bar diagram.**

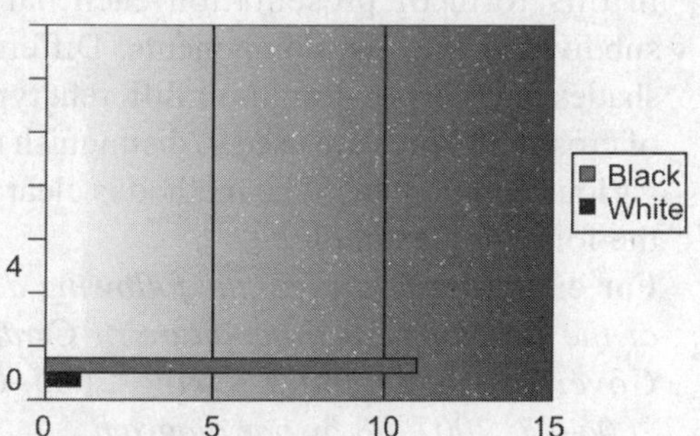

Fig. 5.10: Number of livebirths to white and black women

i. **Simple bar diagram:** It is used to compare two or more items related to a variable. In this case the data are presented with the help of bars. These bars are usually arranged according to relative magnitude of bars. The length of a bar is determined by the value or the amount of the variables. A limitation of **Simple bar diagram** is that only one variable can be represented on it. The method is illustrated by the following example (Fig. 5.11):

For example: *Draw a Bar Chart of the procurement of rice (in tons) in Karnataka state:*

Year	2003	2004	2005	2006	2007	2008
Rice (in tons)	4500	5700	6100	6500	4300	7800

Solution. The given data is represented by the **Simple Bar Diagram** as only one variable is to be represented.

Here we represent years on the X-axis and procurement of rice on the Y-axis.

ii. **Multiple or grouped bar diagram:** A multiple or grouped bar diagram is used when a number of items are to be compared in respect of two, three or more values. In this case, the numerical values of major categories are arranged in ascending or descending order so that the categories can be readily distinguished. Different shades or

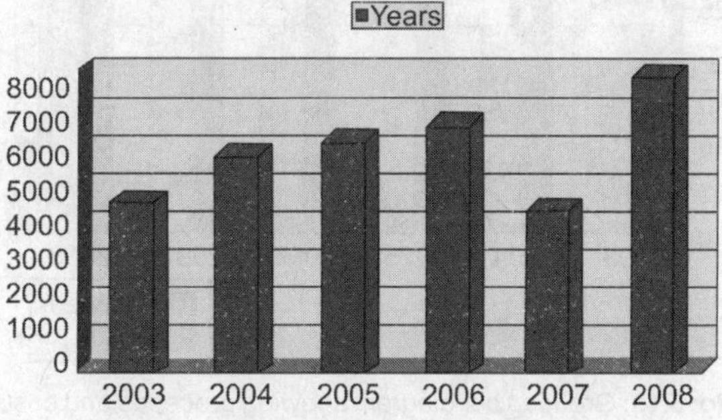

Fig. 5.11: Procurement of rice in Karnataka

colors are used for each category. Sub-classification of qualitative data may be shown by the use of multiple bars (Fig. 5.12). When using multiple bars there are two alternatives: either the bars representing the sub-classification may be drawn contiguous to one another as in Figure 5.13 or they may be separated by a small space. If the latter method is used, the space between the bars in a single group should be narrower than the space between the group of bars. In all cases when multiple bars are used, a key is necessary for differentiating the various sub-classifications.

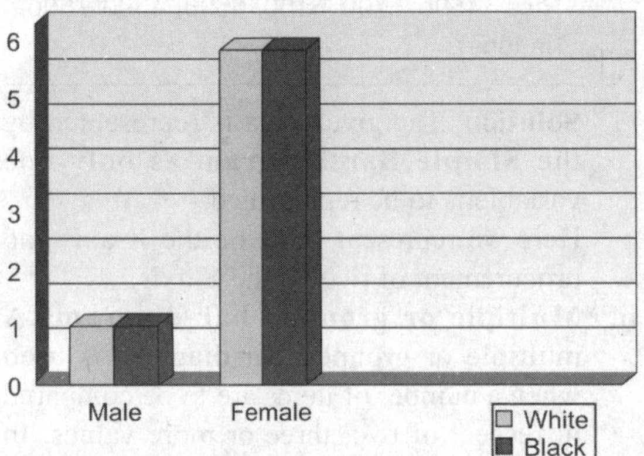

Fig. 5.12: Number of livebirths by sex to white and black women

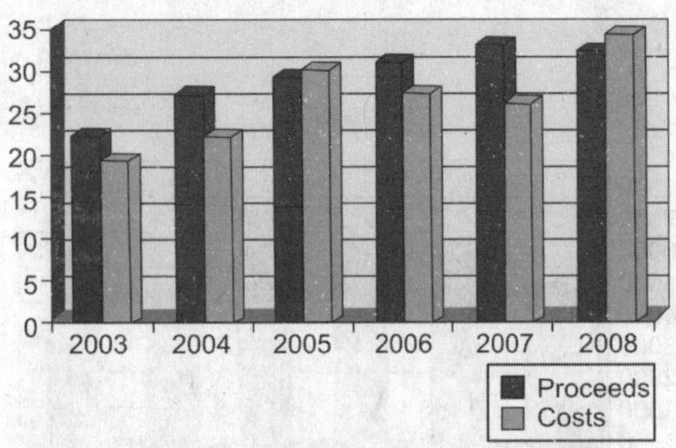

Fig. 5.13: Grouped bar diagram showing proceeds and costs

For example: *Represent the following data by a suitable diagram showing the difference between proceeds and costs:*

Proceeds and costs of a firm (in thousands of rupees)

Year	*Total proceeds*	*Total costs*
2003	22.0	19.5
2004	27.3	21.7
2005	28.2	30.0
2006	30.3	25.6
2007	32.7	26.1
2008	33.3	34.2

In this case the two types of information, i.e. proceeds and costs are shown on a diagram indicating the difference between them. The two types of information for each year are placed in such a way that a comparison may be made between them. So a grouped bar diagram is drawn in order to represent the given data.

iii. **Subdivided or component bar diagram:** A component bar diagram is one which is formed by dividing a single bar into several component parts. A single bar represents the aggregate value whereas, the component parts represent the component values of the aggregate value. It shows the relationship among the different parts and also between the different parts and the main bar. The design and procedure of constructing it, is similar to simple bar diagrams except, that in this form of presentation each bar is subdivided into its' components. Different shades or colors or designs or different types of cross hatchings are used to distinguish the various components. The method is clear by the following example.

For example: *Represent the following data of the development expenditure of Central Governments in India during 2005–06, 2006–07, 2007–08 by bar diagram.*

Year	*Loans and Advances*	*Capital*	*Revenue*	*Total*
2005-06	8,601	3,787	3,477	15,865
2006-07	10,535	4,456	4,036	18,827
2007-08	11,549	4,803	3,709	20,061

In this case we use subdivided bar diagram. Here the data for different years is represented by various parts of the single bar for the year (Fig. 5.14). Different parts are indicating loans and advances capital and revenues for each year. Different parts are indicating loans and advances capital and revenues for each year as shown in the figure.

i. Percentage subdivided Bar Diagram: It consists of one or more than one bar where each bar totals 100 percent. Its construction is similar to the subdivided bar diagram with the only difference that in the subdivided bar diagram segments are used in absolute quantities, in the percentage bar diagram the quantities are transformed into percentages. Its' construction is based on the following steps:

Step I Convert the quantities in each case into percentage of the whole

Step II Take the cumulative percentages

Step III Represent each category of items in different shades or colors or different types of cross-hatchings.

Step IV In case two diagrams showing different periods are given, then show each category of item with the same shade or color or cross-hatching.

For example: *Following are the heads of income of Railways during 2007 and 2008.*

	2007 (in crores of rupees)	*2008 (in crores of rupees)*
Coaching	26	31
Goods	40	39
Others	4.50	3.50

Represent the above data by a bar chart (Fig. 5.15)

We are given three types of information – coaching, goods and others are two years. In order to facilitate comparison among them and also between the two years, a component bar chart is drawn to represent the given data. The graph has been drawn on percentage figures. Percentage of each item has been expressed on the total income of respective years by the formula.

$$\text{Percentage} = \frac{\text{Income of the item}}{\text{Total income of respective year}} \times 100$$

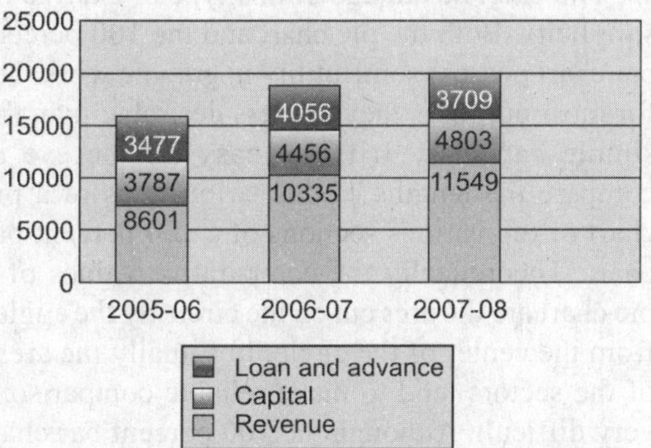

Fig. 5.14: Development expenditure of central and state Government in India

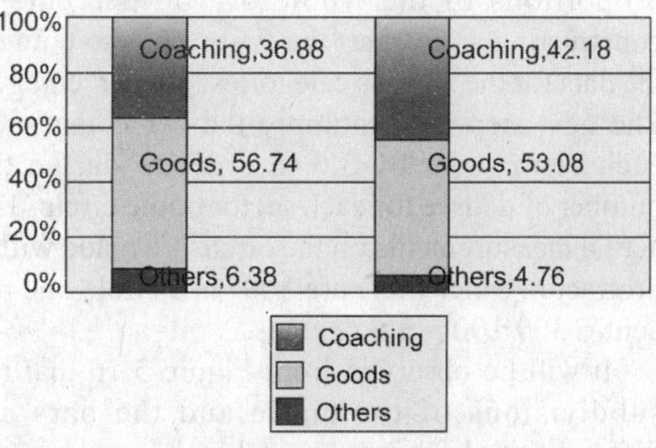

Fig. 5.15: Percentage subdivided bar chart showing incomes of Railways

Calculation of Percentage

Items	2007		2008	
	Income	Percentage	Income	Percentage
Coaching	26	36.88	31	42.18
Goods	40	56.74	39	53.06
Other	4.50	6.38	3.50	4.76
	70.50	100.00	73.50	100.00

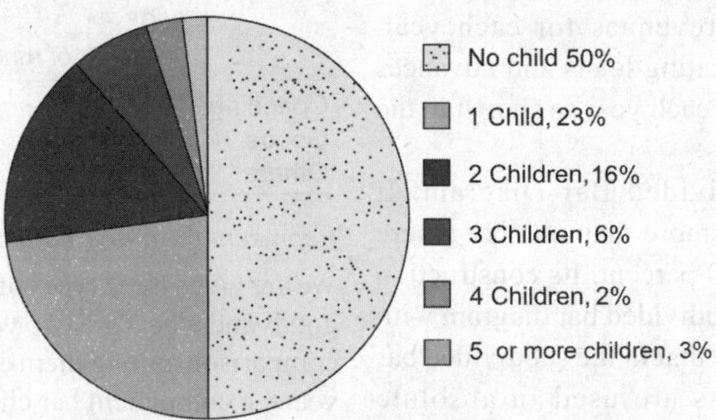

Fig. 5.16: Pie-chart drawn in axonometric projection

Pie chart and component bar chart: In both the pie and component bar charts, the emphasis is centered on the subdivision of a geometric form in relation to the whole. The pie chart is a circle divided into sectors representing various parts of the whole. Similarly, the component bar chart is subdivided into two or more parts to show proportions of the whole or 100 percent. In constructing a pie chart the first step is to convert the data for the various categories into percentages. The next step is to multiply the percentages for each component by 3.6 in order to derive the number of degree for each sector of the circle. The actual measurements on the circle are made with a protractor. Since there are 360° in a circle one per cent = 360/100 = 3.6 degrees.

It will be observed from Figure 5.16 that the subdivisions of the circle and the bars are differentiated by means of hatching schemes. Sometimes the various subdivisions are left blank, but in order to avoid optical illusions as well as confusion in interpretation, it is more satisfactory to cross-hatch or shade the diagrams. It will also be observed that the diagrams are specifically described by means of explanatory labels or legends.

The chief advantage of this type of chart is its simplicity. Both the pie chart and the 100 percent bar chart possess some utility in graphic work, but for most purposes they are less desirable than the simple bar chart. It is not easy for the eye to compare the lengths of the various arcs of a pie chart or the various sections of a 100 percent bar chart. Theoretically the comparative values of a pie chart are the arcs cut on the circle by the angles from the center of the circle. In actually the areas of the sectors tend to make reliable comparisons very difficult. Although the 100 percent bar chart has a scale, it may be difficult to relate the various component parts to the scale for precise

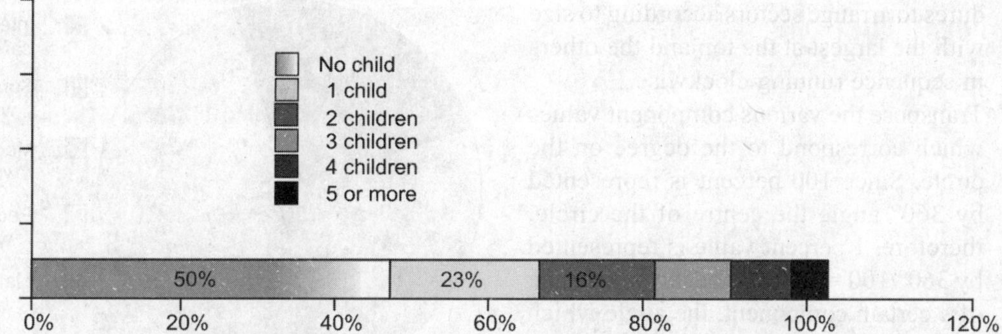

Fig. 5.17: The age and sex composition of the population of the state of Washington for 1991 and 2001. Increases in population between 1991 and 2001 for the various age groups are represented by a shading scheme

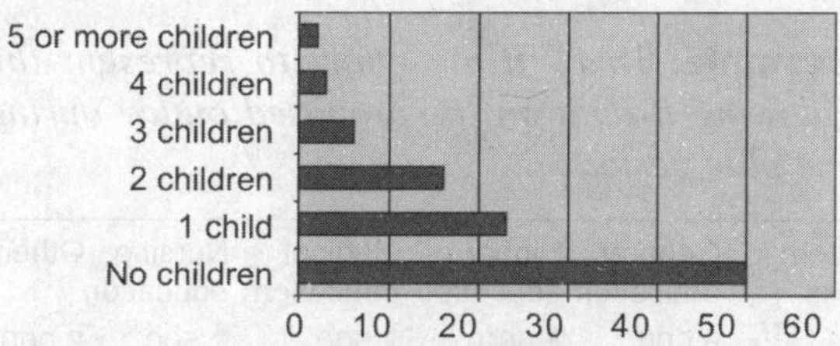

Fig. 5.18: Simple bar chart

interpretation, such as can be done with a simple bar chart where the separate bars extend from a common base line.

It also will be observed from Figure 5.17 that the simple bar chart can be used to depict component relations. In fact, because of its' emphasis on one-dimensional comparisons and because of its' common base line, it is superior for many purposes to either the pie chart or the one hundred percent bar chart (Fig. 5.18).

Pie Chart or Circle Chart or Sector Chart

A pie chart is a circular graph which represents the total value with its' components. The area of a circle represents the total value and the different sectors of the circle represent the different parts. The circle is divided into sectors by radii and the areas of the sectors are proportional to the angles at the centre. It is generally used for comparing the relation between various components of a value and between components and the total value. In pie chart, the data is expressed as percentage. Each component is expressed as percentage of the total value. A pie chart is also known as **circular chart** or **sector chart.**

The name pie diagram is given to a circle diagram because in determining the circumstances of a circle we have to take into consideration a quantity known as 'pie' (written as p).

Method of construction: The surface area of a circle is known to cover 2p radius or 360 degrees. The data to be represented through a circle diagram may therefore be presented through 360 degrees, parts or sections of a circle. The total frequencies or value is equated to 360° and then the angles corresponding to component parts are calculated (or the component parts are expressed as percentages of the total and then multiplied by 360/100 or 3.6). After determining these angles, the required sectors in the circle are drawn. The Steps of Construction Pie chart are as follows:

Step I Plot a circle of appropriate size with protractor, pencil and compass. The angles of a circle total 360°.

Step II Convert the given value of the components of an item in percentage of the total value of the item.

Step III In laying out the sector for a pie chart it is logical to adopt the common procedures to arrange sectors according to size with the largest at the top and the others in sequence running clockwise.

Step IV Transpose the various component values which correspond to the degree on the circle. Since 100 percent is represented by 360° angle the centre of the circle, therefore, 1 percent value is represented by 360°/100 = 3.6°. If 8 be the percentage of a certain component, the angle which represents the percentage of such component is (3.6 × 8) degrees.

Step V Measure with protector the points on a circle representing the size of each sector.

Step VI Label each sector for identification. The method is illustrated by the following example.

The calculation for Pie chart is shown in tabular form of following:

Example: *120 BSc Nursing students of a college were asked to opt for different ward experiences. The details of these options are as under.*

Areas of work experience	*No. of students*
Intensive care unit	6
Surgical ward	30
Medical ward	48
Pediatric ward	12
Maternity	24

Represent the above data through a pie chart.

The numerical data may be converted into the angles of the circle as given below (Pie-chart Fig. 5.19):

Areas of work experience	*No. of students*	*Angle of the circle*
Intensive care unit	6	6/120 × 360 = 18°
Surgical ward	30	30/120 × 360 = 90°
Medical ward	48	48/120 × 360 = 144°
Pediatric ward	12	12/120 × 360 = 36°
Maternity	24	24/120 × 360 = 72°
Total	120	360°

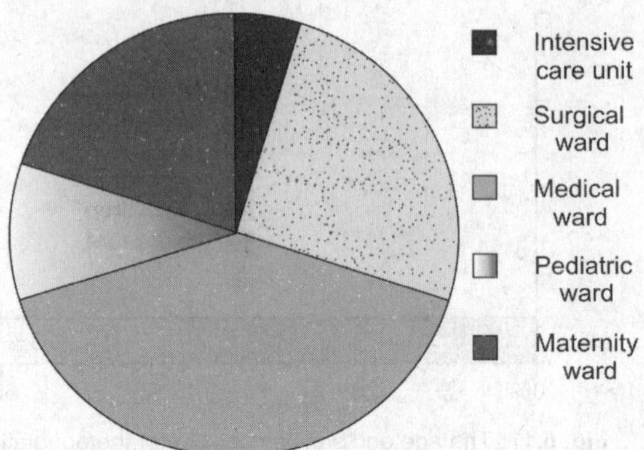

Fig. 5.19: Pie diagram area of work experience opted for students of BSc Nursing

Example: *Draw a pie chart to represent the following if data on the proposed outlay during one plan period.*

Item Rs.	General education	Higher education	Medical education	Nursing education	Other
(in Crs)	6,000	4,000	2,500	4,500	3,000

Solution. In constructing a pie chart, it is necessary to convert the percentages into angles of different degrees as given in Table 5.12.

Age and sex pyramid: Another type of chart similar to the bar chart is the age and sex pyramid or triangle. The age and sex pyramid is actually a double histogram with the bars arranged horizontally instead of vertically. A common base line extends vertically through the center of the chart for both sets of bars. The vertical axis always represents age. Wherever possible, equal intervals should be used. The horizontal axis represents the number or percentage of the total population in each age interval according to sex. The male sex is usually placed on the left and the female sex on the right of the center line. The figures on the horizontal axis may indicate percentages or absolute numbers (Fig. 5.20).

Area and Volume Charts

As a rule, diagrams involving real and cubic comparisons should be avoided, because instead

Table 5.12

Calculation for pie chart

Items	*Amount (Rs in Crores)*	*Percentage on Total (%)*	*Angle for each percentage (360°/100)*	*Angle for each item at the center of the pie chart*
General education	6,000	$\frac{6{,}000 \times 100}{20{,}000} = 30$	3.6	30 × 3.6 = 108
Higher education	4,000	$\frac{4{,}000 \times 100}{20{,}000} = 20$	3.6	20 × 3.6 = 72
Medical education	2,500	$\frac{2{,}500 \times 100}{20{,}000} = 12.5$	3.6	12.5 × 3.6 = 45
Nursing education	4,500	$\frac{4{,}500 \times 100}{20{,}000} = 22.5$	3.6	22.5 × 3.6 = 81
Others	3,000	$\frac{3{,}000 \times 100}{20{,}000} = 15$	3.6	15 × 3.6 = 54
Total	20,000	100		360

of simplifying the comparison desired, they are likely to confuse. It is extremely difficult to differentiate with any degree of accuracy the sizes of areas or cubes.

The lines or bars vary in one dimension only (length) areas in two dimensions (length and breadth) and volumes in three dimensions (length, breadth and thickness). In each form the smaller figure is one-half of the larger. From this simple illustration it is apparent that the relative numerical values of lines or bars can be more reliably estimated than those of either a surface or a solid.

Sometimes comparisons of areas and solids are further complicated when the forms are irregular in shape. Such is the case of certain types of pictorial charts. Charts of this type are frequently used in popular articles on social and economic questions and for propagandistic purposes. In comparing the sizes of two standing armies, for example, pictures of soldiers have been used.

Pictorial Unit Charts

On the other hand, pictorial charts of the one-dimensional type, is used with care and discrimination. They are effective and acceptable for social science reports, especially where popular appeal is to be made. Pictorial charts of this type have had wide acceptance and deserve an important place in the field of graphic presentation. Beginning in the early 1920's in Vienna, Dr Otto Neurath has been largely responsible for the development of this newer type of pictorial statistics. During the latter 1920's and early 1930,s Dr Neurath was Director of the Gesellschafts and Wirtschaftsmuseum in Vienna where he developed many pictographic techniques as well as the ideas of a universal "visual language".

The basic type of pictorial charts developed by Neurath and others is very much like the simple bar graph already discussed, but the units are represented by pictorial symbols instead of points on a scale. Each pictorial unit represents a certain value in the same way that a division on the scale of a bar chart represents a given value. Comparisons in both instances are in terms of one dimension only—length. Of course, there are many variations of this basic type of chart as well as combinations with other geometric forms (Fig. 5.21).

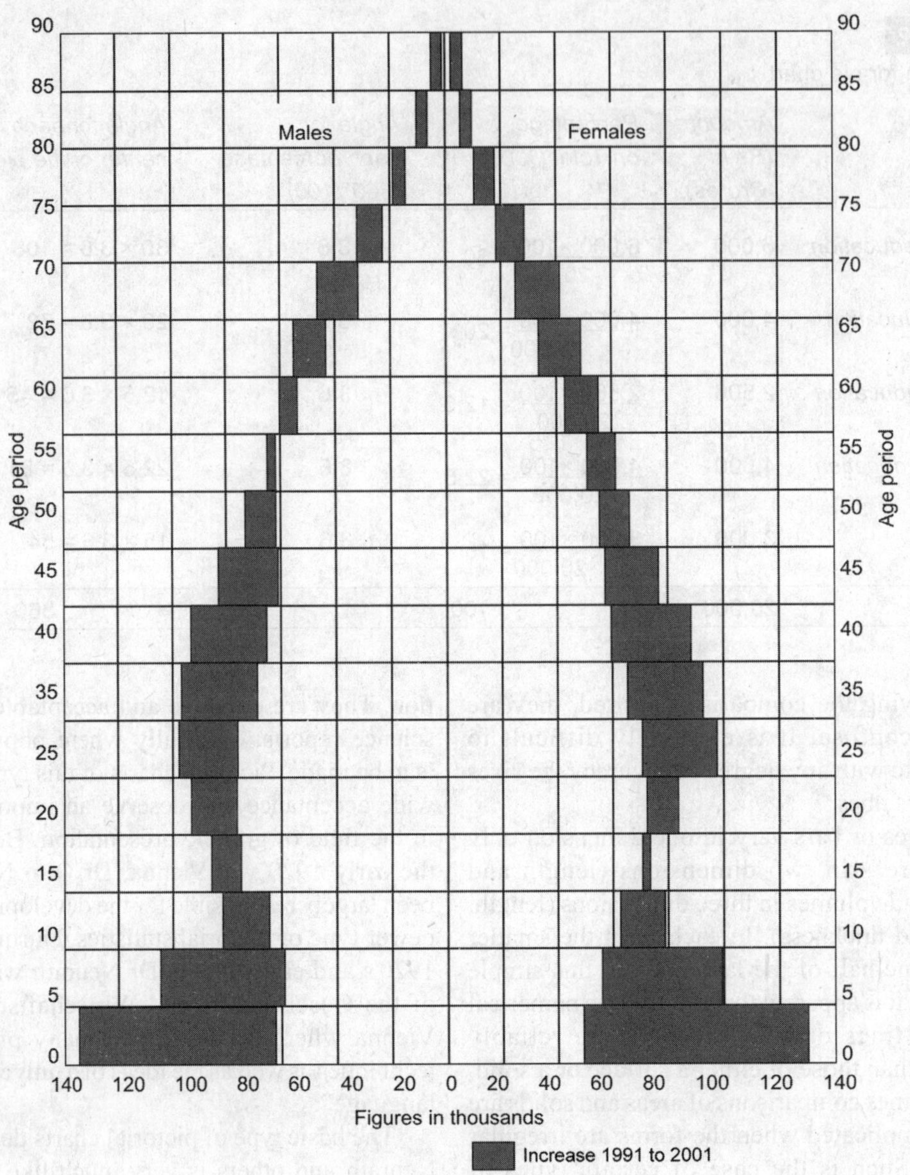

Fig. 5.20: Age and sex pyramid

In developing a pictorial unit chart, the following basic rules should be observed:

1. The symbols should be self-explanatory. If the chart is concerned with ships, the symbol should be an outline of a ship
2. All the symbols on the chart should represent a definite unit of value. Each symbol usually represents a convenient sum of individuals
3. The chart should be made as simple and clear as possible. The number of facts presented should be kept at a minimum
4. Pictographs should give only an overall picture; they should not show minute details

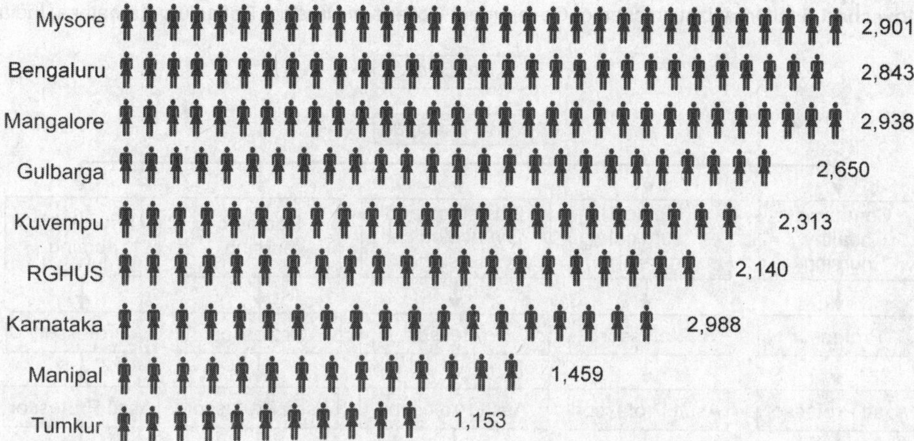

Fig. 5.21: An illustration of pictorial unit chart. Each symbol indicates one hundred graduates in different universities in Karnataka, India

5. Only comparisons should be charted. Isolated facts in themselves cannot be effectively presented by this method
6. There are many facts that by their very nature cannot be shown pictorially. This is true of large bodies of data that require more refined and elaborate techniques of analysis.

Organization and Flow Charts

Unlike the other forms of graphic presentation discussed in this chapter, the typical organization chart is not used to analyze or interpret statistical facts. Nevertheless, this type of chart possess definite utility for certain kinds of research and administrative problems. Characteristically the organization chart issued to present structural forms and relationships. An example of the organization chart is shown in Flow chart 5.1. This chart presents in simple graphic form a considerable body of information relating to *Government College of Nursing*, Bangalore an institution of Karnataka State Government as well as their organizational relationships.

The flow chart emphasizes process or movement rather than mere structure or organization. Flow charts are used to present both statistical and nonstatistical data.

Ranking Charts

The purpose of ranking charts is to portray the position of certain items or categories, usually on the basis of magnitude or frequency. Emphasis is placed on rank-order or rating of various items, rather than on their values. Figure 5.22 shows the ranking of the ten major causes of death in the year 2005 and in 2010.

Pictograph or Pictogram

It is a device of representing statistical data in pictures. In pictograph, a number of pictures of same size and equal in value are drawn. Each picture represents a number of units. Pictures are generally drawn side by side horizontally or vertically. It is widely used by government organizations as well as by private institutions. The chief advantage of this method is its' attraction. In this method of representation each picture is assigned some numerical value which can be expressed either by denoting it or writing it on the edge of each picture. While drawing pictograph, it should be borne in mind that the pictures drawn are simple, clear, easy to understand and the number of units which each picture represents should be clearly stated.

Flow chart 5.1: Organization chart of Government College of Nursing, Bengaluru Karnataka, India

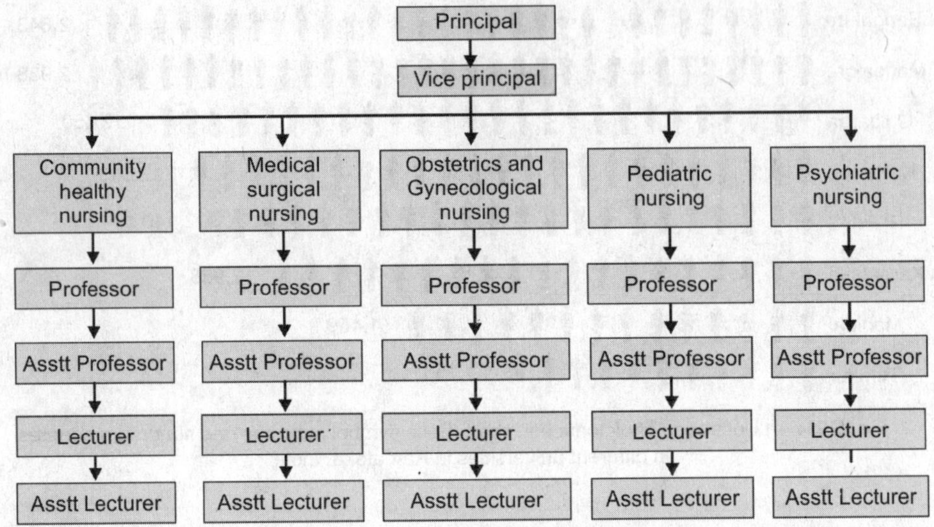

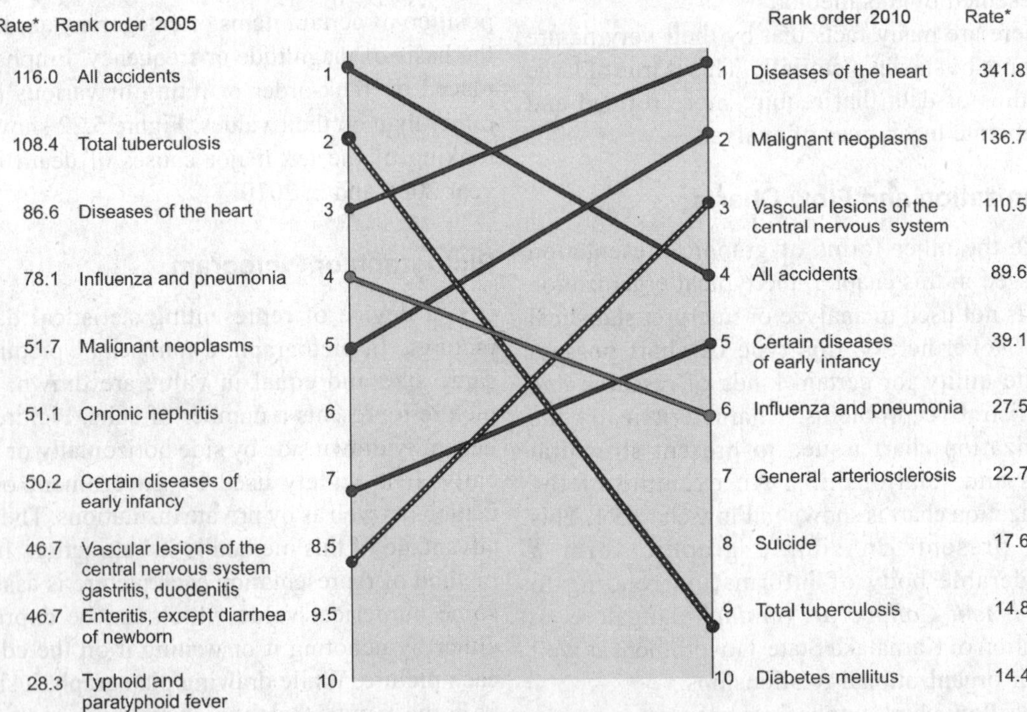

Fig. 5.22: A ranking chart

Graphical Representation of Grouped Data (Frequency Distribution)

There are five methods of representing a frequency distribution graphically:

1. Histogram
2. Frequency polygon
3. Cumulative frequency curve or ogive
4. Proportional change diagram
5. Ratio diagram or Arithlog.

Histogram

A histogram is a graph containing a set of rectangles, each being constructed to represent the size of the class interval by its' width and the frequency in each class-interval by its' height. The area of each rectangle is proportional to the frequency in the respective class-interval and the total area of the histogram is proportional to the total frequency. A histogram is used to depict a frequency distribution.

In constructing a histogram, the class-boundaries are considered to be very important; and they are located on the horizontal axis of the graph. The vertical rectangles are erected side by side on the basis of the frequencies over the class-interval which are extended to their class-boundaries.

When the class-intervals are unequal, difficulty arises, because the rectangles so formed will also be of unequal width. So in order to remove this difficulty, the heights of rectangles are made proportional not to the class frequencies, but to the frequency densities.

This type of diagram is used exclusively for showing frequency distributions of quantitative data that are continuous in nature. It is essentially an area diagram composed of a series of adjacent rectangles. Hence, the area used to represent the frequency in groups or class intervals when added together will give the composite area for the entire group.

A histogram is a set of vertical bars with equal base but different heights. Therefore, it is also known as bar-graph. It is known as frequency histogram also. The mechanics of its' construction will be explained with reference to the data of Table 5.13. Plotted as a histogram in Figure 5.23.

In Figure 5.23, the baseline is labeled with the score intervals rather than with the exact limits. Thus, the first interval in the histogram actually begins at 4.5, the exact lower limit of the interval, and ends at 9.5, the exact upper limit of the interval. The one score or frequency in the interval 5–9 is represented by a rectangle, the base of which is the length of the interval and the height of which is one unit up on the Y-axis. The two scores of frequencies on the next interval, 10–14, are represented by a rectangle with a length of one interval and height of 3Y units. The highest rectangle is on interval 25–29, which has a frequency of 13. The numbers written at the top of each rectangle will in the initial stage facilitate reading of the frequencies.

However, these are not always necessary. In selecting scales for the X axis and Y axis, the consideration of an approximate ratio of 3:5 between the height and length should be kept in view.

The histogram is composed of rectangles with different heights. It is not necessary to project the sides of the rectangles down to the base as is done in Figure 5.23. Still it will bring out the important fact of the rise and fall of the frequencies from interval to interval.

Construction of Histogram

A histogram or column diagram is essentially a bar graph of a frequency distribution. The following points are to be kept in mind while constructing the histogram for a frequency distribution.

Table 5.13

Cumulative frequency and cumulative percentage frequency in a frequency distribution

Class interval (1)	*Exact limits (2)*	*Frequency (3)*	*Cumulative frequency (4)*	*Cumulative percentage (5)*
45-49	44.5-49.5	2	50	100.00
40-44	39.5-44.5	3	48	96.00
35-39	34.5-39.5	6	45	90.00
30-34	29.5-34.5	9	39	78.00
25-29	24.5-29.5	13	30	60.00
20-24	19.5-24.5	8	17	34.00
15-19	14.5-19.5	6	9	18.00
10-14	9.5-14.5	2	3	6.00
5-9	4.5-9.5	1	1	2.00
		N = 50		

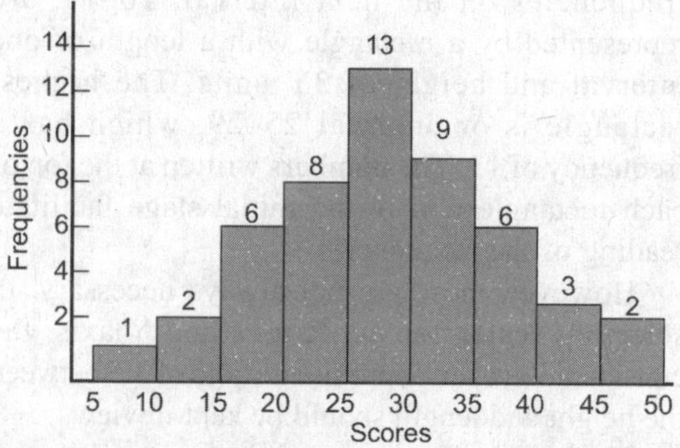

Fig. 5.23: Histogram of the 50 scores given in Table 5.13

1. Convert the data in the exclusive series if it is given in the inclusive series. For example, if it is given in the form. For example:

Age (years):	10-19	20-29	30-39	40-49
No. of cases:	1	0	1	10

Here the given data in inclusive series. Transform it into exclusive series of the form:

Age (years):	9.5-19.5	19.5-29.5	29.5-39.5	39.5-49.5
No. of cases:	1	0	1	10

2. The scores in the form of actual limits as 9.5, 19.5, 29.5 etc. are taken in the construction of a histogram rather than the written class limits as 10, 19, 20, 29.
3. It is customary to take two extra intervals (classes) one below and other above the given grouped intervals or classes low (with zero frequency). In the case of the frequency distribution of above data, we take 0.5–9.5 and 49.5–59.5 as two required class intervals.
4. Now we take the actual lower limits of all the class intervals (including the extra intervals) and plot them on the X-axis. The lower limit of the lowest interval (one of the extra intervals) is taken at the intersecting point of X-axis and Y-axis.
5. Each class or intervals with its specific frequency is represented by a separate rectangle. The base of each rectangle is the width of the class interval and the height is the respective frequency of that class or interval.
6. Frequencies of the distribution are plotted on the Y-axis.
7. Care should be taken to select the appropriate units of representation along the X-axis and Y-axis. Both X-axis as well as Y-axis should not be too short or too long.

Types of Histograms

There are two types of histograms:

a. Histograms with equal class intervals
b. Histograms with unequal class intervals

Histograms with equal class intervals: The sizes of class intervals are drawn on X-axis with equal distances and their respective frequencies on Y-axis. Class and its' frequency taken together form a rectangle. The graph of rectangles is known as histogram.

For example: The monthly profits in rupees of 100 clinics distributed as follows:

Profit per clinics	*No. of clinics*
0-100	12
100-200	18
200-300	27
300-400	20
400-500	17
500-600	6

This is the case of histogram with equal frequencies (Fig. 5.24).

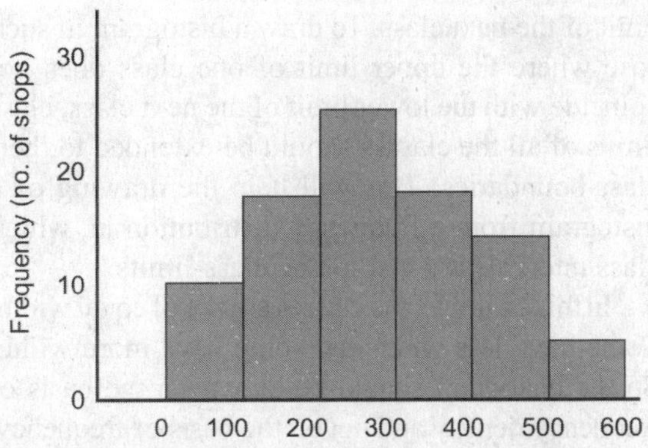

Fig. 5.24: Histogram showing monthly profits

Another example: Draw the histogram of the following frequency distribution and show the area on your graph which represents the total number of earning members in the family, in the age-group 19–32 years:

Age group	*No. of earning members*
14-15	60
16-17	140
18-20	150
21-24	110
25-29	110
30-34	100
35-39	90

Solution: Here the class intervals have been marked by class-limits. As a result the upper limit of one class does not coincide with the lower limit of the next class. In order to draw a histogram the upper limit of one class must coincide with the lower

Class-interval (Age group)	*Class-boundary (Age group)*	*Class-width*	*Frequency No. of wage-earners*	*Frequency density*
14-15	13.5-15.5	2	60	80
16-17	15.5-17.5	2	140	70
18-20	17.5-20.5	3	150	50
21-24	20.5-24.5	4	110	27.5
25-29	24.5-29.5	5	110	22
30-34	29.5-34.5	5	100	20
35-39	34.5-39.5	5	90	18

limit of the next class. To draw a histogram in such case where the upper limit of one class does not coincide with the lower limit of the next class, class limits of all the classes should be extended to their class-boundaries. This will help the drawing of a histogram from a frequency distribution in, which class intervals are marked by class-limits.

In this example, the classes are not of equal width. Some have less width and some have more width. So the histogram should be drawn on the basis of frequency density and not on the basis of frequency.

The graph has been shaded showing the area which is represented by the total number of wage-earners in the age-group 19–32 years (Fig. 5.25).

Frequency Polygon

It is the curve obtained by joining the middle points of the tops of the rectangles in a histogram by straight lines. It is generally used in a frequency distribution in which the class-intervals are equal and have a common width. It is particularly useful in representing a simple and ungrouped frequency distribution of discrete variable. It has no special significance, but it gives a fair idea about the shape of the frequency distribution. In order to complete the drawing of a frequency polygon, the two end points of it are joined to the base-line at the mid-points of the empty class of both ends of the frequency distribution.

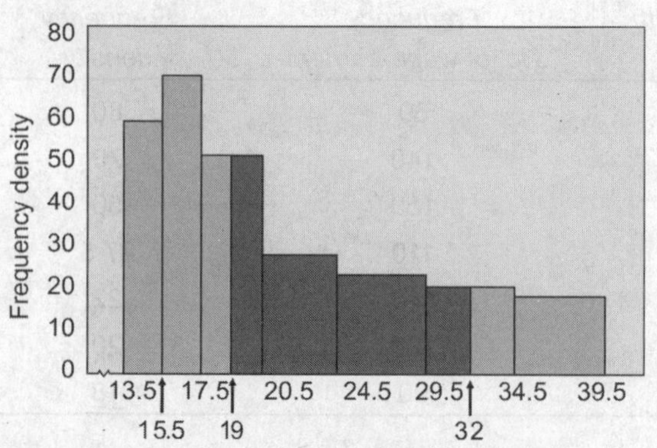

Fig. 5.25: Histogram showing the number of earning member

A polygon is defined as a many-sided figure. When a many-sided figure is drawn on the basis of frequencies given in a frequency distribution, the figure is called a frequency polygon. Construction of all graphic figures requires the selection of a good graph paper with cross-sections. For polygons, a graph paper rules into heavy lines one inch apart each way and sub-divided into tenths of an inch more lightly drawn will be more convenient.

Since a polygon is a complete figure, its ends should touch the baseline. For this purpose, at each end of the distribution, assume one additional class interval with zero frequency. In Table 5.13, there are in all nine class intervals and with the assumption two additional class intervals, this number will go up to eleven. By allowing ½ inch to each class interval, the distribution will spread over an extent of 5½ inch which is sufficiently large for easy readability. Since there are five scores in each class interval, the total units would be 5×No. of Class intervals, i.e. 5×11=55. Hence, 1/5 in of space (two subdivisions) will be allowed to each unit. On the base line, every fifth line will be labeled with a multiple of five such as, 0, 10, …, 50, 55.

The height of the figure should be roughly 3/5 to 3/4 or 60-75 percent of the total width. Our total

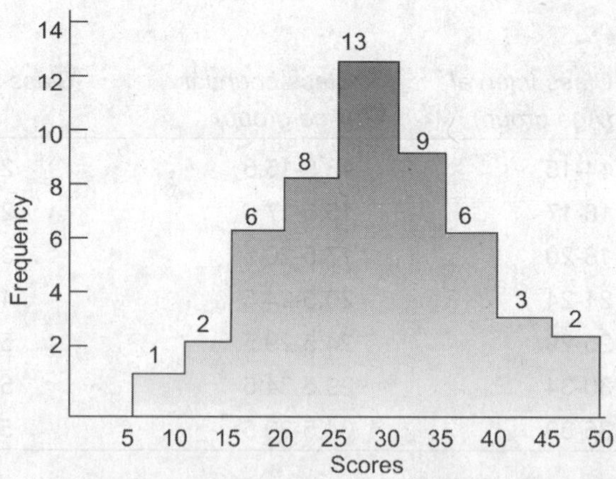

Fig. 5.26: A histogram with sides of rectangles not projected to the baseline

width is 5.5". Hence, a height of 5.5 inches × 3/5 to 5.5 inches × 3/4 (or 3.3 inches to 4.2 inches) will be appropriate. We may choose 4.2 inches as it will be divisible by the maximum frequency of 13 of our data. Hence, four small squares (2/5 in.) on the Y-axis will represent one limit of frequency. This will satisfy the general convention about the ratio of width to the height of the polygon.

The next step is to locate the mid-points of the class intervals. It can be done by averaging either the exact or the stated limits of each class intervals. In our case for class interval, 5-9, the mid-point is (5+9)1/2 or 7; and for 10-14, it is (10+14)1/2 or 12.

Now we have to plot the dots for the frequency polygon. For the first class interval (additional one), 0–4, the frequency is zero. Hence, the dot is placed at the mid-point of the class interval on the baseline. For the next class interval of 5–9, the dot is placed exactly above the score seven and at a perpendicular distance from the relevant frequency of one. Dots for the other class intervals are to be plotted in the same manner keeping the relevant frequency in view. The dot for the last (additional) class interval will be on its mid-point on the baseline.

Now join the dots with straight lines. The curve so drawn is the frequency polygon as shown in Figure 5.27.

A frequency polygon can also be constructed by joining the mid-points of horizontal lines of a histogram. Figure 5.28 illustrates the procedure of the same.

A frequency polygon is generally preferred to a histogram because of several reasons: (i) The former gives much better conception of the contour of the distribution; (ii) Another important merit is that it gives a more accurate impression that the cases are more frequent near the central tendency, mode; (iii) We can also plot two or more polygons overlapping on the same baseline for the purpose of comparison. If N in each case is unequal, the frequencies of both the distribution should be converted into percentages by multiplying each frequency by 100/N. here, N stands for the total number of cases in the relevant

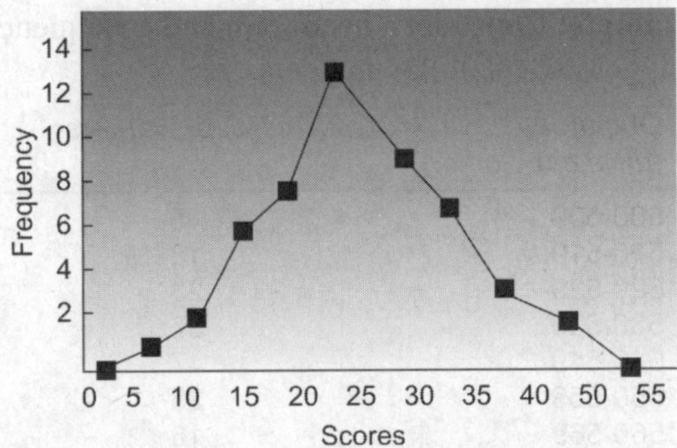

Fig. 5.27: A frequency polygon for the data in Table 5.13

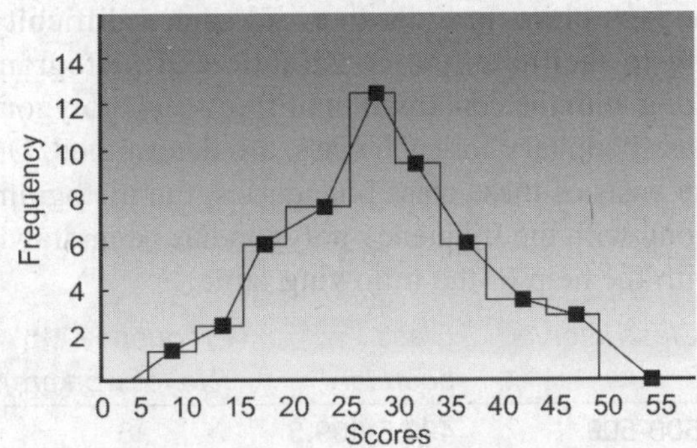

Fig. 5.28: A frequency polygon conustructed from a histogram given in Figure 5.27

distribution. If Ns are equal, conversion into percentages is not required and frequencies can be plotted straightway.

Example: Construct a histogram and frequency polygon for the following data (Figure 5.29):

100-150	150-200	200-250	250-300	300-350
4	6	13	5	2

Solution: We have the case of equal class interval (Fig. 5.29).

Class interval	*Frequency*	*CF*
100-150	4	4
150-200	6	10
200-250	13	23
250-300	5	28
300-350	2	30

Example: Construct a histogram and a frequency polygon for the following data:

Output (units per worker)	*No. of workers*
500-509	8
510-519	18
520-529	23
530-539	37
540-549	47
550-559	26
560-569	16

Solution: Here we notice that the upper limit of one class does not coincide with the lower limit of the next class. In order to avoid such a difficulty and to facilitate, the construction of histogram along with the construction of frequency polygon, class boundary for each class, are determined. On the basis of these class boundaries, the histogram along with the frequency polygon has been drawn with the help of the following table:

Class interval	*Class boundary*	*Frequency (No. of workers)*
500-509	499.5-509.5	8
510-519	509.5-519.5	18
520-529	519.5-529.5	23
530-539	529.5-539.5	37
540-549	539.5-549.5	47
550-559	549.5-559.5	26
560-569	559.5-569.5	16

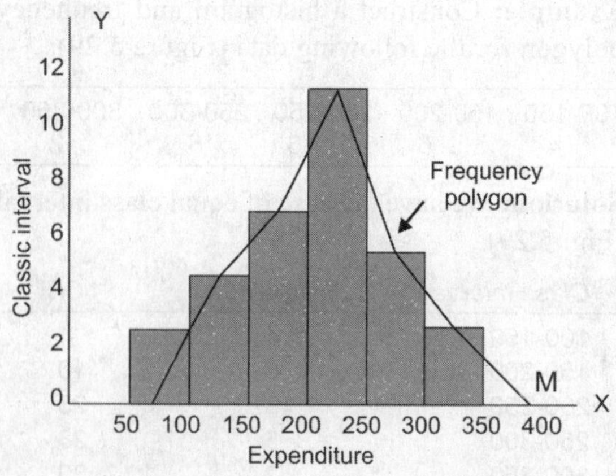

Fig. 5.29: Histogram and frequency polygon

Smoothed Frequency Polygon

When the sample is small and frequency distribution somewhat irregular, the frequency polygon tends to be jagged in its shape. Hence, with a view to iron out chance irregularities and obtain a better picture of how the figure would look like if the data were more numerous, the frequency polygon may be smoothed. The process involves taking of 'moving' or 'running' averages to determine the smoothed polygon. These are later plotted to form the smoothed polygon. In Table 5.14, Col. (4), process of taking the "running averages" and the smoothed frequencies so obtained have been shown. To find out 'smoothed' or 'adjusted' frequencies, we add the f on the given interval and f's on the two adjacent intervals (the interval just below and the interval just above) and divide the sum by 3. To find the smoothed f's for the two extreme intervals, namely 5–9, and 45–49 it is presumed that there are zero frequencies below the interval 5–9 and also above the interval 45–49. In Figure 5.30, a frequency polygon based on the original frequencies and another based on smoothed frequencies have been given.

Original and Smoothed Frequency Polygons based on data in Table 5.14.

Smoothing can be done twice to improve the outline of the frequency polygon and make it more flowing. However, so much adjustment of frequencies

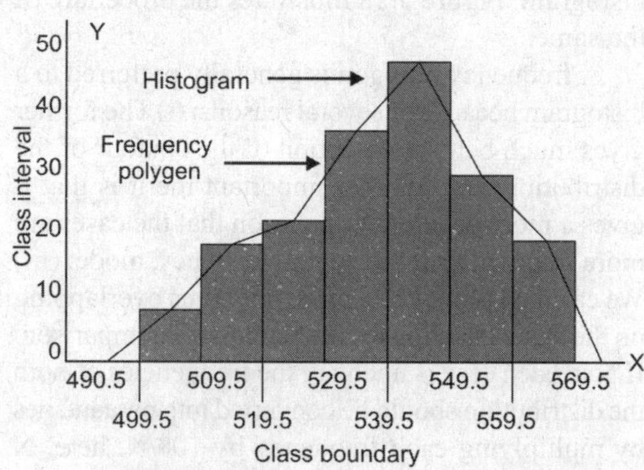

Fig. 5.30: Histogram and frequency polygon

Table 5.14

Smoothed frequencies

Class interval (1)	*Mid-points (2)*	*f (3)*	*Smoothed f (4)*
45-49	47	0	(3+0+0)/3=1.00
40-44	42	3	(6+3+0)/3=3.00
35-39	37	6	(12+6+3)/3=7.00
30-34	32	12	(13+12+6)/3=10.33
25-29	27	13	(8+13+12)/3=11.00
20-24	22	8	(6+8+13)/3=9.00
15-19	17	6	(2+6+13)/3=5.33
10-14	12	2	(0+2+6)/3=2.67
5-9	7	0	(0+0+2)/3=0.67
	N = 50		50.00

is seldom warranted. The original polygon must also be presented along with the smoothed one so that the extent of adjustment can be gauged by the reader. If N is large, smoothing may not largely improve the shape of the polygon. Moreover, smoothing is desirable with continuous variables; or distribution based on small samples, and the total area in both the polygons should be equal.

Comparison between the Histogram and the Frequency Polygon

Although both histogram and frequency polygon are used for the graphic representation of frequency distribution are alike in many respects, yet they possess points of difference. Some of these differences are cited below:

- Where histogram is essentially the bar graph of the given frequency distribution, the frequency polygon is a line graph of the distribution.
- In comparison to the histogram, frequency polygon gives a much better conception of the contours of the distribution. With a part of the polygon curve, it is easy to know the trend of the distribution, but a histogram is unable to tell such a thing.
- In comparing two or more distributions by plotting two or more graphs on the same axis, frequency polygon is more useful and practicable than the histogram.
- In frequency polygon, it is assumed that the frequencies are concentrated at mid-points of class-intervals. It points out merely the graphical relationship between mid-points and frequencies and thus is unable to show the distribution of frequencies within each class-interval. But the histogram gives a very clear and accurate picture of the relative proportions of frequency from interval to interval.

Frequency Curve

It is drawn by free hand through various points of the polygon in such a way that the area included is just the same as that of the polygon. The basic object of drawing a frequency curve is to present graphically, the area covered by histogram in a more symmetrical manner. It is also known as smooth frequency curve.

For example: Draw a histogram, a frequency polygon and a smoothed frequency curve from the following data relating to marks secured in

Nursing foundation by school students in a house-test.

Marks	No. of students	Marks	No. of students
0-5	3	25-30	14
5-10	7	30-35	10
10-15	13	35-40	7
15-20	25	40-45	4
20-25	40	45-50	2

Solution: The required curves are shown in Figure 5.31.

Cumulative Frequency Curve or Ogive

It is a graph which represents the data of a cumulative frequency distribution. An Ogive, when it is drawn, is in the form of a curve. The curve drawn from the data cumulated downward is known as less than ogive and the curve drawn from the data cumulated upward as more than ogive. An Ogive is used to find median, quartiles, deciles and percentiles, etc.

It is also used to find the number of observations which are expected to lie between two given values.

A cumulative frequency curve or Ogive is obtained by plotting the successive cumulative frequencies on the graph paper and joining them by a free hand. An Ogive is drawn with the following points in mind:

- The upper limits of the classes are represented along X-axis
- The cumulative frequency of a particular class is taken along the Y-axis
- The points corresponding to cumulative frequency at each upper limit of the classes are joined by a free hand curve. This curve is called a cumulative frequency curve or an Ogive. The Ogive is always monotonically increasing because cumulative frequency increases as we move from one class to the next class.

The main difference between the construction of a frequency graph and the Ogive is that in the case of the former the frequencies must be plotted at the mid-points of the class but in the case of an Ogive, the cumulative frequency is plotted at the upper limit of the class.

Example: Draw a cumulative frequency graph and estimate the number of persons between the ages 32–42 in the following table:

Age	No. of persons
20-25	50
25-30	70
30-35	100
35-40	180
40-45	150
45-50	120
50-55	70
55-60	59

Solution: A cumulative frequency distribution table, showing cumulative frequency 'less than Ogive', has been prepared and on the basis of the

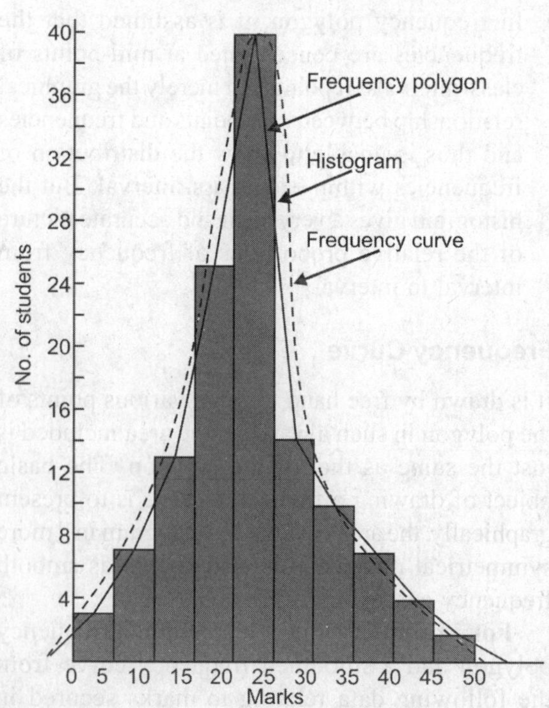

Fig. 5.31: Frequency polygon, histogram and frequency curve

same a 'less than Ogive', cumulative frequency graph has been drawn as shown in the Figure 5.33.

The graph has been drawn showing the age on the horizontal line and the number of persons on the vertical line. It is seen from the graph that the number of persons up to the age of 32 years is 140 and the number of persons up to the age of 42 is 440 as is disclosed on the vertical line of the graph. So the estimated number of persons between the ages 32–42 is 440-140 = 300 (Fig. 5.32).

Table 5.15

Class (Age)	*Class (Age)*	*Frequency (No. of persons)*	*Cumulative (Less than Ogive)*
	20	0	0
20-25	25	50	50
25-30	30	70	120
30-35	35	100	220
35-40	40	180	400
40-45	45	150	550
45-50	50	120	670
50-55	55	70	740
55-60	60	59	799
		799	

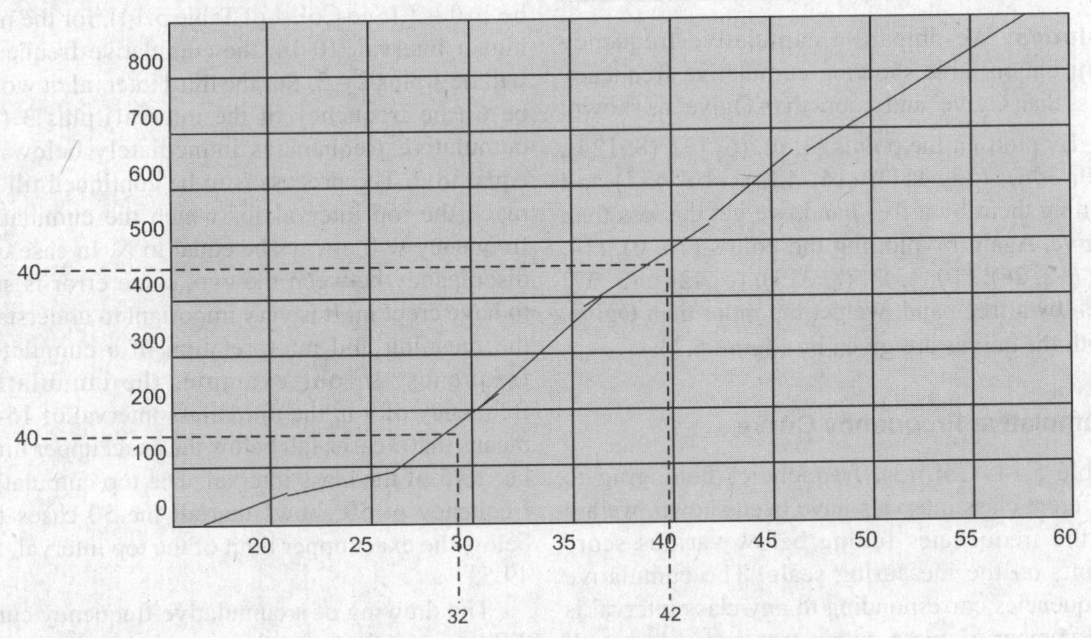

Fig. 5.32: Cumulative frequency graph (Less than Ogive)

Table 5.16

Class interval (Cost of production)	Class boundary (No. of farms)	Frequency	Cumulative frequency (Less than Ogive)	(More than Ogive)
	4	0	0	437
4-6	6	13	13	424
6-8	8	111	124	313
8-10	10	182	306	131
10-12	12	105	411	26
12-14	14	19	430	7
14-16	16	7	437	0
		437		

Example: Plot less than Ogive and more than Ogive for the following data:

Cost of production	No. of farms
4-6	13
6-8	111
8-10	182
10-12	105
12-14	19
14-16	7

Solution: We prepare a cumulative frequency distribution table showing cumulative frequency 'less than Ogive' and 'more than Ogive' as shown:

By plotting the points (4, 0), (6, 13), (8, 124), (10, 306), (12, 411), (14, 430), (16, 437) and joining them by a free hand, we get the less than Ogive. Again by plotting the points (16, 0), (14, 7), (12, 26), (10, 131), (8, 313), (6, 424), (3, 37) then by a free hand, we get the more than Ogive. Both the curves are given by Figure 5.33.

Cumulative Frequency Curve

Table 5.14, Col. (3), frequencies belonging to different class intervals have been shown, we are in the frequencies falling below various score points on the measuring scale. The cumulative frequencies corresponding to any class interval is the number of cases within that interval plus all the cases in intervals lower to it on the scale. In Table 5.14, cumulative frequencies have been shown in Col. (4). The method of calculating cumulative frequencies is very simple and requires successive additions of ordinary or non-cumulative frequencies. The cumulation starts from the bottom. For example, in our case, there is a frequency of one in the lowest interval of five to nine; and there are no frequencies below it. Hence, the cumulative frequency for this class interval will be 1+0 = 1 (See Col. 4 of Table 5.14). for the next higher interval, 10-14, the cumulative frequency will be 1 plus 2 = 3. For the third interval, it would be 6 (the frequency of the interval) plus 3 (the cumulative frequencies immediately below it), equal to 9. The process is to be continued till we reach the top interval for which the cumulative frequency will always be equal to N. In case of a discrepancy between the two, some error is sure to have crept in. It is very important to understand the meaning and interpretation of a cumulative frequency. In our example, the cumulative frequency of 9 in the third class interval of 15-19 means that 9 cases fall below the exact upper limit, i.e. 19.5 of the class interval. The top cumulative frequency of 50 shows that all the 50 cases fall below the exact upper limit of the top interval, i.e. 49.5.

The drawing of a cumulative frequency curve differs from that of a frequency polygon in two aspects:

i. Instead of plotting above the mid-points of the class intervals, we plot them above the exact upper limits of the class intervals
ii. Instead of using ordinary frequencies for plotting the points, we use cumulative frequencies.

In plotting the cumulative frequency distribution of Table 5.14, we would plot the cumulative frequency of 1 above the exact upper limit 9.5, the lowest class interval, five to nine. The cumulative frequency of 3 would be plotted over the exact upper limit, 14.5 of the next higher class interval, 10-14. For this purpose, the exact upper limit, instead of the mid-points, are to be marked on the baseline. A cumulative frequency curve based on the data of Table 5.14 has been plotted in Figure 5.33.

It may be noted that the general trend of the cumulative frequency curve is progressively rising; there are no inversions or setbacks. The upward rise is not a straight line. When the distribution of frequencies is symmetrical, the cumulative distribution curve is usually S-shaped. The zero frequency does not lead to any inversion in the curve but may show up as plateau where the height of the curve remains constant.

Cumulative Percentage Curve or Ogive

There are occasions when cumulative frequencies become more meaningful and convenient, when converted into cumulative percentages. This process makes a comparison of two or more distribution possible, when N differs. This leads to a standardization of N at 100. The determination of percentiles and percentile ranks becomes possible and the need of calculation is eliminated.

In Table 5.14, Col. (5) cumulative percentages corresponding to various cumulative frequencies have been given. The process of conversion is simple. Cumulative percentage for any cumulative frequency can be obtained by multiplying the later by 100/N. In our example, N = 50. For the cumulative frequency of 1, the cumulative percentage would be $1 \times 100/50 = 2$. For the third interval, the cumulative percentage is $9 \times 100/50 = 18$.

A cumulative percentage curve or Ogive based on the data of Table 5.13 is shown in Figures 5.34 and 5.35.

Arithlog or Ratio Diagrams

This diagram has the added diagrams that both relative and absolute changes can be determined

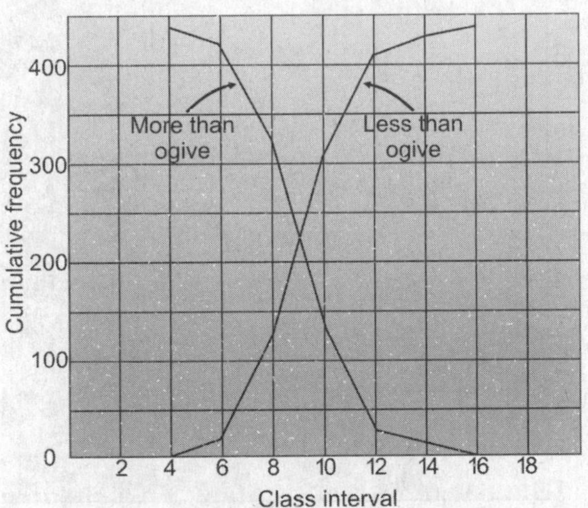

Fig. 5.33: Cumulative frequency diagram

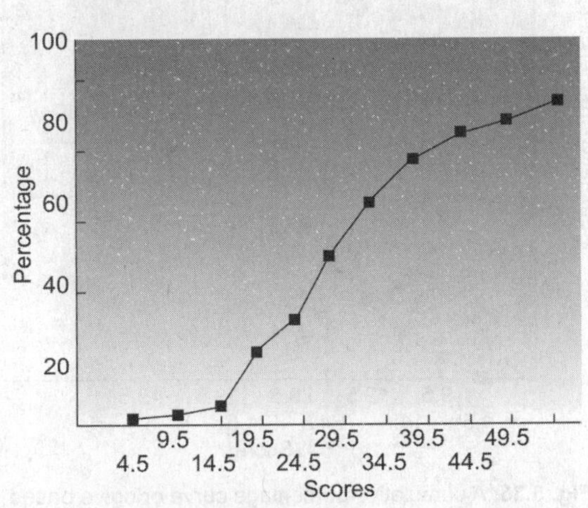

Fig. 5.34: Cumulative percentage curve

from it. It is not necessary to calculate percentages. The basis of the construction is the use of a special paper known as Arithlog or ratio paper which has scales so drawn that the same ratio between two numbers will always be represented by the same increment on the scale. For example, in Figure 5.36 the distance on the vertical scale between 8 and 4 is the same as that distance between 16 and 8 or between 80 and 40, since in each case, the first number is twice the second. It will be seen that line A, which starts at 16 and ends at 8, is parallel to line A, which starts at 6 and ends at 3. This indicates that the same proportional change has occurred in the variable represented by line a as has occurred in the variable represented by line C. Line B, which shows a change from 20 to 5, has a much sharper decline showing that the proportional change in the variable represented has been much greater than in the variables of lines A and C. This is true since the numbers indicate not a two fold decrease as in the first lines but a fourfold decrease.

This Arithlog or ratio paper is provided in various sizes, depending on the multiples of ten that are shown. Each multiple of ten is commonly known as a cycle. Hence, if the data to be presented include numbers in the tens, hundreds and thousands, a paper with three cycles would be used. The tens would be plotted in the first cycle, the hundreds in the second cycle and the thousands in the third cycle. The vertical scale would be labeled the same as in the ordinary arithmetic line diagram.

The horizontal scale on this type of paper is the same as on arithmetic paper that is, equal increments represent equal units of measure. Therefore, the same labeling of the horizontal scale will be used. The diagram is plotted by the same method as in the arithmetic line diagram (Fig. 5.36).

A comparison of the identical data plotted by these three types of line diagrams at first glance, shows that the infant deaths per 1,000 livebirths have decreased more rapidly than have the maternal deaths per 1,000 livebirths. In absolute numbers this is true as there has been an absolute decrease of 20.4 infant deaths per 1,000 livebirths as compared with an absolute decrease of 3.2 maternal deaths per 1,000 livebirths. The diagram on arithmetic paper should be used only when comparisons of absolute number are to be made. Should the proportional change diagram or the

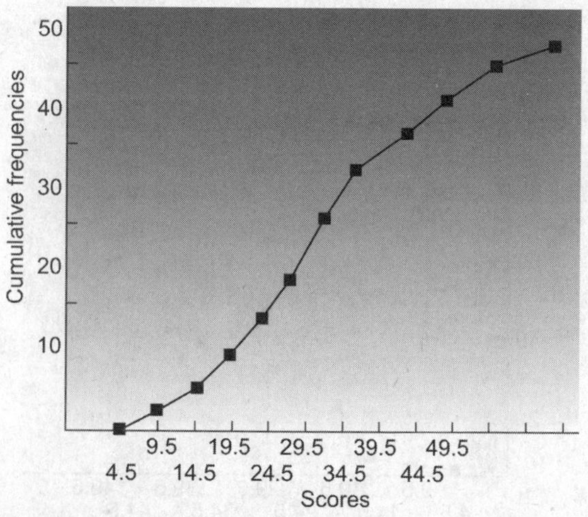

Fig. 5.35: A cumulative percentage curve or ogive based on the frequency distribution in Table 5.13

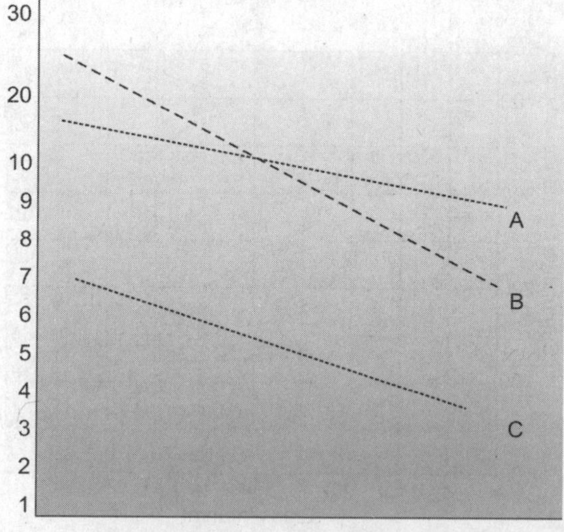

Fig. 5.36: Illustration of arithlog diagram

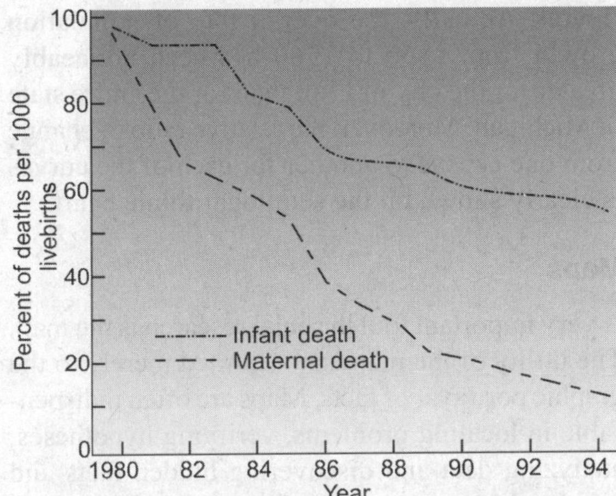

Fig. 5.37: Percentage change in number of infant and maternal deaths per 1,000 livebirths in a city, 1980–1994

diagram on ratio paper be used, if the relative change is of importance? This will be true usually when comparing variables in which the measurements are of different magnitudes. The ratio paper is simpler to use but is not so easily understood by the untrained person.

Proportional Change Diagram

When comparing two or more sets of figures, it is in many instances more important to show the relative change in the variables than absolute change. This is especially true when the figures to be compared are markedly different in magnitude. This may be done by two different techniques. The first of these is easily understood since it involves a proportional change concept. The value for any given year, usually the first year in the series, is selected as a base. The value of 47.0 deaths per 1,000 livebirths for the year 1980 was selected as a base. The value of 45.3 deaths per 1,000 livebirths for the year 1981 was then calculated to the 96.4 percent of this value by the following method: 45.3 × 47.0 × 100. This is repeated for each year. The resulting percentages are then plotted on the vertical scale in place of the absolute values (see Fig. 5.37). This scale must be labeled, therefore, percent of deaths per 1,000 livebirths in base period—in this case 194. If the change is a decrease in the rate, it is common to start the vertical scale with 0. If, however, the change is an increase, the zero of the scale should be shown, although the values between 0 and 100 may be omitted by indicating a break in the scale.

There are two main objectives to this type of diagram. First, both lines start at the same point 100 percent. This may give the reader the first impression that the values for the two or more variables for this particular year are the same even though a study of the scales will show this is not to be true. Secondly, the process of calculating the necessary series of percentages may become very time consuming, if one does not have mechanical equipment available.

Semilogarithmic charts: Because of its simplicity, accuracy and adaptability, the semilogarithmic chart is of greatest importance in social research. In general, the semilogarithmic scale is superior to either the natural or the percentage scale, for it can show very clearly both relative and absolute changes. In fact, it combines the advantages of both the natural and percentage scales without the disadvantages of either.

To the fresh student the term "logarithmic" may sound formidable, but a knowledge of logarithms is not essential in order to understand and use this type of chart. Semilogarithmic paper may be purchased already ruled. With a little practice this type of chart can be used effectively. The principles of constructing and interpreting these charts are relatively easy to understand.

The essential features of the semilogarithmic chart are a logarithmic vertical scale and an arithmetic horizontal scale (or vice versa). Therefore the chart is called semilogarithmic or sometimes arithlog. In the arithmetic scale equal spaces indicate equal values and the divisions are determined accordingly. The logarithmic scale, on the other hand, is ruled entirely differently, since the divisions are based on logarithms. Figure 5.37 shows a three-cycle semilogarithmic chart.

1. The vertical axis consists of one or more sets of rulings graduated in accordance with series of logarithmic values of 1 to 10.
2. Each complete set of rulings is referred to as a deck or a cycle. Theoretically a chart may have an indefinite number of decks or cycles. Figure 5.38 has three cycles. In practice more than five cycles are seldom used.
3. The rulings for each deck are the same but the scale values change from one to the other. For example, if the first cycle runs from 1 to 10, the adjacent deck above will vary from 10 to 100, the third from 100 to 1,000, the fourth from 1,000 to 10,000, the fifth from 10,000 to 100,000. On the other hand, the adjacent cycle below the one from 1 to 10 would vary from 0.1 to 1.0. The logarithmic scale can thus be extended either upward or downward indefinitely.
4. No matter how far the logarithmic scale is extended downward, zero is never reached. There is no zero line on a semilogarithmic scale.

The interpretation and significance of the semilogarithmic chart can be further elucidated by comparison with a rectilinear coordinate chart. The differences between the rectilinear and the semilogarithmic graphs as well as superiority of the latter. The curves in both panels represent the growth of populations of the city. Curves in both panels represent the growth of populations of the city of Flint and the entire state of Michigan.

An examination of both sets of curves shows that the rectilinear scale conceals and distorts the rate of change of these two series. The conclusion one naturally draws from the arithmetic chart is that the rate of growth is greater for the state than for the city. The slope of the curve for the state is very sharp and definite, whereas the slope of the curve for the city of Flint is very gradual. Since, however, the figures for the entire state are relatively so large, the changes are greatly exaggerated on the arithmetic scale. By contrast, the semilogarithmic chart reliably indicates rates of change regardless of the absolute size of the figures. Actually, the overall rate of population growth from 1860 to 1960 has been noticeably greater for the city of Flint than for the entire state of Michigan. Moreover, the relative ratio of change from one census to another for each of the curves is clearly shown on the semilogarithmic chart.

Maps

A very important tool in social research is the map. The utility of the map is not limited merely to the graphic portrayal of facts. Maps are often indispensable in locating problems, verifying hypotheses, analyzing data and discovering hidden facts and relationships.

Our primary interest in discussing maps is to describe their functions and applications as well as their limitations in social research. Very little space will be devoted to the actual mechanics of drawing maps. The present survey will be confined largely to the following fundamental types:

- Base map
- Spot map
- Cross-hatched map
- Maps with one or more types of graphic forms superimposed, such as bars, columns, curves, flow diagrams, or pictorial symbols. All of these fundamental types are capable of wide variation and adaptation for special purposes.

Base Maps

Of the several types of maps used in social research the base map is perhaps the most useful. The main distinguishing characteristic is the underlying facts of the physical and social environment which it portrays. Maps of this kind provide an important background or framework for primary data which are superimposed upon it and in this way greatly elucidate as well as facilitate analysis of the spatial patterning of social phenomena. In the construction of a base map a careful selection is made of the features of the physical and man-made environment which are of fundamental importance in conditioning the spatial distribution of social phenomena. These facts are then clearly indicated on the base maps by means of coloring, cross-hatching, or some other suitable technique. Characteristics of the physical environment which are often included on maps of this kind are rivers, lakes, ravines, prominent hills and other topographical features. Some of the factors of the cultural environment which possess special ecological significance are railroads, railway yards, canals, boulevards, industrial areas, commercial sections, vacant property, heavily traveled thoroughfares, parks, schools and cemeteries.

In actual practice it may be necessary to forego a detailed presentation of all of these characteristics, unless the base map is drawn to a very large scale and its' use is limited entirely to research purposes. Maps to be published usually have to be reduced to such a small scale that only a relatively fewer details can be included. This fact should be kept in mind in connection with other types of maps.

In planning a base map for an urban community that is not to be used for publication, a blue-line or black-line street map varying in scale from 500 to 1,000 feet to the inch - depending upon the area of the city—should be procured from the city engineer or city planning commission. If, in addition, access can be had to a complete, accurate and up-to-date land utilization map, very little field or laboratory work will be required to compile the basic data for the base map. With the appropriate kinds of colored inks or cross-hatching, it is a relatively simple task to transpose certain amount of the data from the land utilization map to the sociological base map. It is very important to discriminate cultural environment. A map cluttered up with too many inconsequential details is confusing and misleading. In constructing a map of this kind it is important not to make the basic features too heavy, since they may visually overshadow the primary data which later may be superimposed. If colors are used, it is generally most satisfactory to use pastel shades or tints of water colors or diluted drawing ink. If hatching is used, the scheme should be simple and the lines drawn very lightly.

Spot Maps

A very commonly used technique of portraying the geographic location or frequency of social phenomena is by means of dots, discs, squares, or other symbols. Maps of this general type are frequency referred as 'spot' or 'point symbol' maps. There are five different types of 'spot' maps. Although in actual practice these types tend to overlap, there is nevertheless in any particular case an emphasis on the:

1. Size
2. Number
3. Density
4. Shade
5. Form of the dots or other kinds of point symbols.

In the first type of spot map mentioned, the size of each symbol is proportional to the number or frequency represented. The symbol employed may be either two or three-dimensional (plane or solid). If a circle is used, then the area is made in proportion to the magnitude or frequency that is to be represented. If on the other hand a sphere is used, the volume indicates the magnitudes or frequency portrayed.

It was pointed out earlier in the chapter that the beginner should be very careful in using area or volume charts. As a general rule, charts of this type should be avoided because of the difficulties of visualizing area or volume and making reliable evaluations and comparisons. In spite of their limitations, charts of this type do have their functions for certain purposes.

In the second type of spot map the basic criterion is not size, but rather number or frequency. All the dots which are of uniform size have a definite value assigned to them. The purposes of this type of map is to show countable frequencies for a given area. With a well constructed map of this kind, it is possible to ascertain at a glance whether the one geographic area contains more or fewer dots than another and if one desires to make exact comparisons between two or more areas, it is very easy to count the dots and compare results. As a general rule the smallest geographical area on the map will determine the size of the dot and the number of units of frequency to be represented by each dot. The size of the dot chosen as well as the arrangement on the map should fairly be accurate to the estimates of the total number of cases.

The purpose of the third type of 'spot' map is to portray comparative densities of distribution. Like the map just discussed, it is of the multiple dot variety, but the emphasis is on the density of the dots rather than on the actual number of dots. Very frequently densities or degrees of concentration are much more important than actual numbers. The symbol used for this type of map is invariably uniform black dots of relatively small size.

The density of the dots indicates the relative distribution over the entire area. In certain areas very pronounced clustering of dots may give the impression of almost solid black, whereas in other sections there may be a complete absence of dots. Maps of this type are useful in showing population densities and the distribution of various population groups. A simple glance gives a clear impression of the population distribution.

The main criterion of the fourth type of spot map is shading and not size, number or density. The amount of shading within each symbol indicates different values. The most common form is based on a quarter-section shading scheme. The largest frequency or magnitude is represented by a solid symbol, three-quarter, one-half, one-quarter, and possibly other divisions indicating smaller amounts.

The main criterion of the fifth type of spot map is in the form of the symbol. This type of map is primarily qualitative in contrast to the other types of spot maps which are fundamentally quantitative. The attributes of the data determine the form of the symbols. If, for example, a distinction is to be made on the basis of sex, one symbol will indicate males and another symbol females. If several different kinds of institutions, such as schools, churches, libraries, settlement houses and hospitals are plotted on the same map, each type of institution will be represented by a different symbol.

In this type, the distribution of the disease frequency is represented in the form of dots or spots, each dot representing an unit number of 10, 20, 30 etc. in the area map prepared. Number of dots will indicate the frequency in units. Such maps show at a glance areas of high frequency (clustering of spots) or low frequency. Clustering of spots may indicate a common source of infection or a common risk factor shaped by all the cases. This is how John Snow of England, in 1854, was able to find out that the particular water pump in Broad Street of London was the source of infection of cholera. Thus he was able to hypothesize that cholera was a water borne disease, much before the bacilli were isolated by Robert Koch. It was with the spot-map, Maxcy (1922-25) hypothesized rodent as the reservoir of typhus fever (Fig. 5.38). Thus spot-map help the epidemiologist to study the place distribution, source/reservoir of infection and behavior of a disease.

Two different colored dots may be marked on the map to show attacks and deaths, in the area.

Maps prepared on weekly or monthly basis help in monitoring changes in the magnitude of epidemics over a period of time and also the direction of their spread.

Cross-hatched or Shaded Map

In social research, many of the data are expressed in the form of rates and ratios. By far the best technique of portraying data of this kind is the cross-hatched or shaded map. In the case of spot maps the emphasis is placed largely on absolute frequencies and densities, whereas in cross-hatched maps the emphasis is on relative frequencies and rates. In constructing a cross-

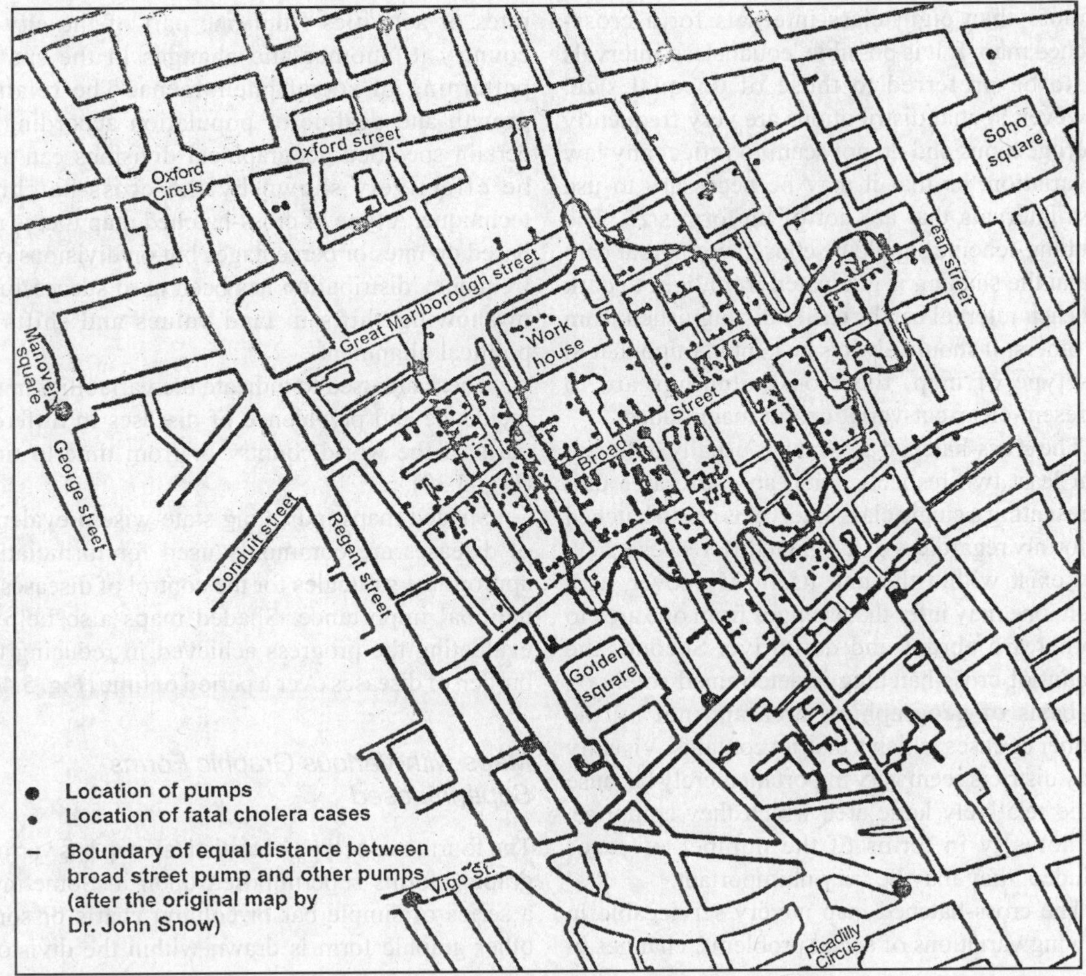

Fig. 5.38: Spot map Asiatic cholera in London

hatched map the rates or ratios for various geographical units are grouped into a small number of classes, each represented by an appropriate type of cross-hatching.

The fundamental principle underlying the cross-hatching technique is to arrange the density of lines or stippling in such a way as to give an optical effect from light to dark in intensity of tone or pattern. At the same time the shadings should be sufficiently different to be easily identified from a legend on the client. The smallest values are usually represented by light hatching or stippling; the highest values are represented by full back; and the hatchings for the intervening values are graduated accordingly.

The first step in constructing a cross-hatched map is to make an array or frequency distribution with relatively small, equal class-intervals. From this preliminary tabulation it is possible to group the data into relatively few class-intervals so as to bring out the essential features of the data. In actual practice there usually should not be less than four or more than eight class-intervals for a cross-hatched map. If it is possible, equal class-intervals are to be preferred to those of unequal size. However, spatial distributions are very frequently heterogeneous and do not seem to reflect any law of variation, so that it may be necessary to use class-intervals that are not of uniform size. The hatching scheme should be chosen with great care so that the shading is graduated from light to dark and each interval can be easily distinguished from the others. It should always be kept in mind that in this type of map, the cross-hatchings are to represent clear-cut-variations in magnitudes.

The cross-hatched area map is usually deficient in at least two respects. First, an entire area unit representing a single class-interval is cross-hatched uniformly regardless of the great differences which may exist within the unit itself. Moreover, as a result, one may infer that changes from one area to another are abrupt and definitive. Second, the amount of cross-hatching is determined solely on the basis of geographical area and not by the number of cases which a district contains. Visually many districts seem very important merely because of the relatively large area which they comprise, but actually in terms of the number of cases included, they may be very unimportant.

The cross-hatched map is very serviceable in showing variations of social problems, changes in rates of activities from one part of the city or country to another and changes in the spatial patterning of social phenomena. The relative growth and decline of population according to certain specified geographical divisions can also be effectively shown by the cross-hatching technique. A type of cross-hatched map that is not based on rates or percentages but on divisions of a frequency distribution has been used successfully in showing shifts in land values and shifts in political alignment.

These are used to indicate the variability in the incidence and prevalence of diseases in different parts of the world/country or from time to time (Fig. 5.39).

Shaded maps indicating state-wise prevalence of diseases are commonly used for formulating appropriate strategies for the control of diseases of national importance. Shaded maps also help in evaluating the progress achieved in reducing the burden of diseases over a period of time (Fig. 5.40).

Maps with Various Graphic Forms Superimposed

The fourth major type of statistical map has various graphic forms superimposed upon it. Sometimes a series of simple bar or column charts or some other graphic form is drawn within the divisions

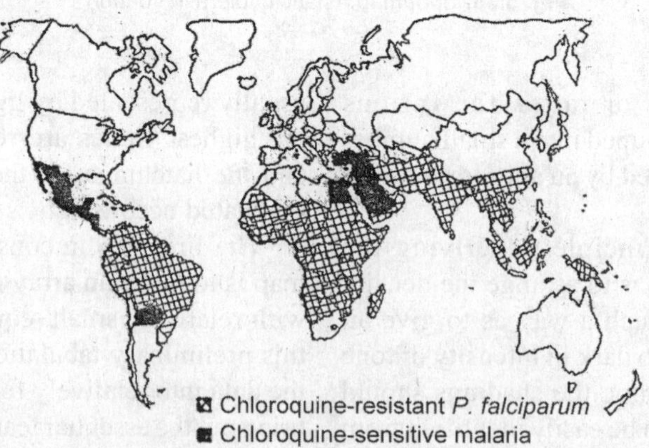

Fig. 5.39: Shaded map showing distribution of malaria and chloroquine-resistant *Plasmodium falciparum* (1993)

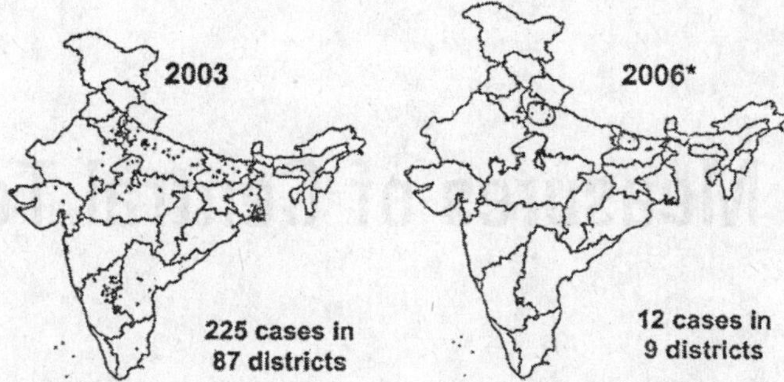

Fig. 5.40: Location of polio-virus in India. 2003-06 *Data as on 10th March 2006: *Source*. National Polio Surveillance Project: GOI and WHO

of the map. In such instances the map, of course, provides a more exact and meaningful geographical orientation to the series of graphs. Another interesting and significant illustration of this type of map is the flow chart. In the social sciences, for example, the flow map has been widely used to show volume and direction of population movements.

EXERCISES

1. Construct a single table and draw a bar diagram for population of different countries as given below
   a. India 120 Crores
   b. China 130 Crores
   c. Indonesia 21 Crores
   d. USA 28 Crores
   e. Pakistan 15 Crores
   f. Srilanka 2 Crores
2. Program a Pie diagram for following data of diseases occuring in a year some below
   a. Malaria 50 Cases
   b. Flaria 42 Cases
   c. Dengue fever 34 Cases
   d. Diarrhea 28 Cases
   e. ARI 39 Cases
   f. Diphtheria 29 Cases
3. Weights of 50 Nursing students in given. Tabulate the data in appropriate class intervals using tally mark system (wt are gram in kgs)
   51, 53, 52, 39, 58, 48, 45, 56, 62, 64, 66, 67, 42, 48, 43, 44, 45, 47, 52, 54, 50, 49, 38, 39, 32, 34, 36, 33, 34, 36, 42, 43, 48, 49, 50, 51, 52, 30, 30, 31, 32, 45, 45, 47, 46, 48, 49, 58.

CHAPTER

6 Measures of Central Tendency

Introduction

Measures refers to ascertain signs, amounts or degree of something by comparison with a standard unit or with an object or known size of population. The phrase **measures of central tendency** or sometimes **measures of location**, refers to the set of measures that reflect where on the scale the distribution is centered. These measures differ in terms of how much use they make of the data, particularly of extreme values. The three major measures of central tendency are the mode, which is based on only a few data points, the median, which ignores most of the data and the mean, which is calculated from all of the data.

Frequency distributions are extremely valuable for summarizing large masses of data, but the process of summarization can be carried much further by compressing the characteristics of an entire series into one or almost a few significant figures. These figures are known as averages and they represent typical values of a variable. Averages hold a very important place in all types of statistical work. In fact, statistics has been referred to as "the science of averages". For example when considering the achievement scores of nursing students of a class and arrange them in a frequency distribution, the teacher will find that there are very few students who either score very high or very low. The marks of most of the student's lie somewhere between the highest and the lowest scores of the whole class. This tendency of a group distribution is named as 'Central tendency or average'. The typical score lying between the extremes and shared by most of students is referred to as "measures of central tendency".

Measures of central tendency is a sort of average or typical value of the items in the series and its function is to summarize the series in terms of this average value. A single expression representing the whole group is selected which may convey a fairly adequate idea about the whole group. This single expression in statistics is known as the average. Averages are generally, the central part of the distributions and, therefore they are also called the measures of central tendency.

The word 'average' has been defined differently by different authors; to quote as given below:

- Average is an attempt to find one single figure to describe whole of figures (Clarks)
- An average value is a simple value within the range of the data that is used to represent all of the values in the series. Since an average is somewhere within the range of the data, it is also called a measure of central value (Croxton and Cowder).

Thus, an average is a single value that represents as group of values. Such a value is of great significance because it depicts the characteristics of the whole group. Since an average represents the data it is called as the "measure of central tendency".

Objectives of Measures of Central Tendency

There are two main objectives of the study the measures of central tendency, which include:

- To get simple value that describes the characteristics of the entire group. Measures of central tendencies, by condensing the mass of data in single value, enable us to get a bird's eye view of the entire data. Thus one value can represent thousands, lakhs or even millions of values
- Reducing the mass of data to one single figure. This enables comparison to be made. Comparison can be made either in point of time or over a period of time.

Needs for Measures of Central Tendency

The collected data as such are not suitable to draw conclusions about the mass from which it has been taken. Some inferences about the population can be drawn from the frequency distribution of the observed values. This process of condensation of data reduces the bulk of data, and the frequency distribution is categorised by certain constants known as parameters. Generally, a distribution is categorized by two parameters, viz the location parameter (central values) and the scale parameter (measures of dispersion). Hence, in finding a central value, the data are condensed into a single value around which the largest number of values tend to cluster. Commonly, such a value lies in the center of the distribution and is termed as central tendency.

RA Fisher has rightly said, "The inherent inability of the human mind to grasp entirely a large body of numerical data, compels us to seek relatively few constants that will adequately describe the data."

Two series of observations are not comparable because of the unsystematic variation generally present in the series, but the constants make it possible to compare the series easily. In this chapter we will continue the discussion of the measures of central values. There are three popular measures of central tendency namely:

1. Mean
2. Median
3. Mode.

Each of these will be discussed in detail here. Besides these, some other measures of location are also dealt with, such as quartiles, deciles and percentiles.

Most of the observations in the Universe are subject to variability and it is more predominant with biological observations. In the case of many biological characteristics, the values or sizes of the observations are not equal, but it can be noticed that a general tendency. There is for such observations to cluster around a particular level. In such situations it may be preferable to characterize each group of observations by such a level, which is called "central tendency of the group". This single value of that group, this level around which the observations tend to cluster, may vary from group to group.

It is a known fact that the biological observations like those of height, weight, pulse, blood counts of the groups similar with respect to age, sex, health status, etc. differ from person to person. In order to make sensible definitions of the group or to identify the group with reference to the observations it is required to express the observations in a precise manner. That is to say, that the observations are to be expressed as a single estimate, so that this estimate summarizes the observations. This is useful not only as a precise estimate of the series of data, but also useful to compare two or more series of data.

As already seen, a frequency distribution can be compared within itself in terms of the frequencies in various class intervals. To a certain extent two or more distributions can be compared with reference to different class intervals. But when it is a question of overall comparisons of the distributions, comparing them in terms of frequencies within class intervals is not advantageous and the only alternative way is to compare them in terms of single estimate of the series of the observations of the data. Such single estimates of the series of data which summarizes the distributions are known as 'Parameters' of distribution. These parameters define the distribution completely. One such parameter is the "measures of central tendency".

Characteristics of Measures of Central Tendency

Measures of central tendency as the name itself indicates gives an estimate of the center of distribution. The concept of the center may be different in different contexts. In one context it may be some mathematical estimate of the center. While in the other it may be the exact central observation in the order of magnitude or it may be the value of the observation with maximum frequencies. Based on these contexts three common measures of central tendency have been defined. These three measures of central tendency are – Mean, Median and Mode. Each of them in its' own way, can be called a representative of the characteristics of the whole group and thus the performance of the group as a whole can be described by the single value which each of these measures are given. The values of mean or median or mode also help us in comparing two or more groups or frequency distributions in terms of typical frequency performance.

The characteristics of an ideal measure of central tendency are given below:

There are various measures of central tendency. The difficulty lies in choosing the measure as no hard and fast rules have been made to select any one. However, some norms have been set which work as a guide line for choosing a particular measure of central tendency. A measure of central tendency is good or satisfactory if it possesses the following characteristics.

- It should be based on all the observations
- It should not be affected by the extreme values
- It should be as close to the maximum number of observed values as possible
- It should be defined rigidly which means that it should have a definite value. The experimenter or investigator should have no discretion
- It should not be subjected to complicated and tedious calculations, though the advent of electronic calculators and computers has made it possible to overlook this aspect
- It should be capable of further algebraic treatment. By algebraic treatment, we mean that these measures can be used further in the formulation of other formulae. For instance, a mean can be used to calculate the pooled mean of two or more series
- It should be stable with regard to sampling. This mean that if a number of samples of the same size are drawn from a population, the measure of central tendency having the minimum variation among the different calculated values should be preferred
- It should be rigidly defined so that different persons may not interpret it differently
- It should be easy to understand and easy to calculate
- It should be based on observation of all the data
- It should be easily subjected to further mathematical calculations
- It should be least affected by the fluctuations of the sampling
- It should not be unduly affected by extreme values
- It should be easy to interpret.

Accordingly, measure of central tendency should have the following:

- It is desirable that an average is such that it is readily understood
- It should not only be easy to understand but also simple enough to compute so that it can be used widely
- It should depend upon each and every item of the series; if any item is dropped the average will be altered
- Each and every item should influence the value of the average
- It should be properly defined by the algebraic formula. So that it has one and only one

interpretation if it is computed by different people
- It should get a value which has statistical stability.

Types of Measures of Central Tendency

When a person is asked to state the one value that would best capture and communicate the distribution as a whole, in obtained distribution of numerical scores, the answer is to find the score value which is in a good 'bet' about any randomly selected case for distribution. Such as score may not be exactly correct for any given case but it should be a fairly good guess about the obtained score for that case. However, these are three different ways to specify what is meant by a 'good bet' about any case and will include:
1. The arithmetic average of the distribution.
2. The point exactly midway between the top and bottom halves of the distribution and
3. The most frequently occurring score or the mid points of the most frequent measurement class.

The first of these ways of defining the central tendency leads to the familiar measure known as the average or the mean; the second leads to the median of the distribution and the third is known as the mode. All these three, as a class, are known as measures of central tendency. So these three are the important types of averages mostly used in statistical work, i.e. Mean, Median, Mode.

Diagrammatic Presentation of Measures of Central Tendency

Average is a vague term and when applied to salaries may do little justice to the worker with a low salary (Fig. 6.1). This lay average is correctly described as the *mean* and is calculated by dividing the total by the number of observations. The *median* divides the curve into equal parts (Fig. 6.2) and the *mode* shows what occurs most frequently and, in the curve, is the frequency density at its maximum. All of these—mean, median and mode—coincide on a curve with a perfectly symmetrical distribution (Fig. 6.3). Sometimes the sides of the curve may not come down fairly sharply as in a bell but tail off as, for example, may happen with certain biochemical estimations of the constituents of blood.

Means

Mean is the sum of scores divided by the number of cases i.e. individual observations are first added together and then divided by number of observations.

There are three types of means which are suitable for a particular type of data. They are:
1. Arithmetic mean or average
2. Geometric mean
3. Harmonic mean.

Arithmetic Mean

It is also popularly known as average. If mean is mentioned, it implies arithmetic mean, as the other means are identified by their full names. It is the most commonly used measure of central tendency.

Sum of the observed values of a set divided by the number of observations in the set is called a mean or an average.

Mean gives an estimate of the center in terms of averages. The simplest average is the arithmetic average and in common usage, the 'mean' refers to the arithmetic average or arithmetic mean. Similarly, there are other averages like geometric mean and harmonic mean. But mean or the arithmetic mean has the highest utility in branches of statistics and so wherever the word 'mean' occurs, unless specified otherwise, always refers to arithmetic mean.

The arithmetic mean of a group is the simple arithmetic average of the observations. This is calculated by dividing the total of all the observations by the number of observations. In the case of grouped data (frequency distribution) arithmetic mean is miscalculated assuming that each observation in a class interval is equal to the midpoint of that class interval.

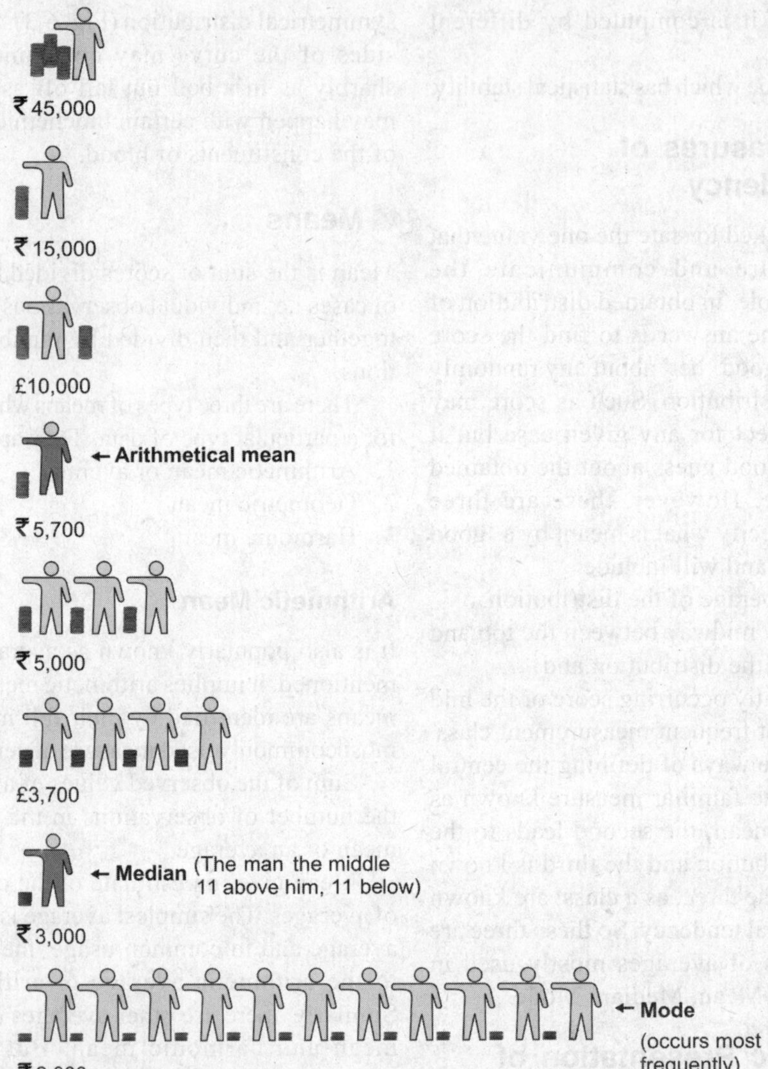

Fig. 6.1: The term average (mean) does little justice to the worker with a low salary. Mode shows that occurs most frequently

Mean is calculated from the formula:

$$\text{Mean} = \frac{\text{Sum of all the observations of the data}}{\text{Number of observations in the data}}$$

The procedure in calculating the mean from ungrouped data can be expressed. In algebraic terms by the following formula,

$$\bar{X} = \frac{\Sigma fx}{n}$$

$\bar{X}$ is the mean

Σ (Greek Capital S or sigma) in the conventional summation sign

x is the mid-point of the class interval or is the value of each observation in the data

n is the total number of observations in the data.

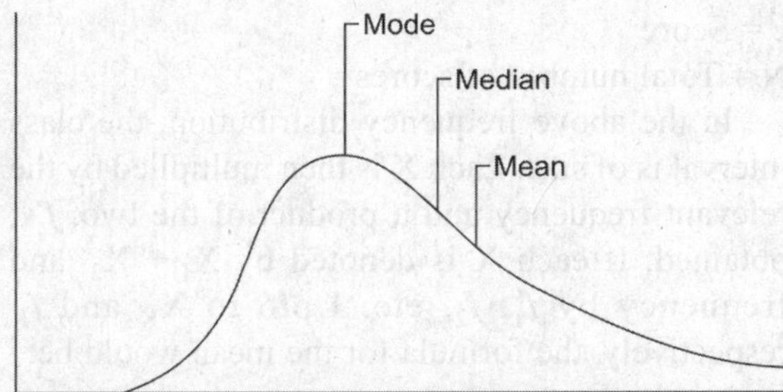

Fig. 6.2: Curve of frequency density to illustrate mean, median and mode

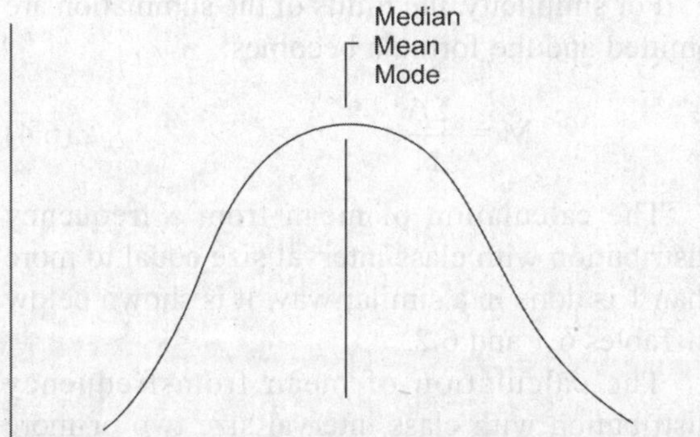

Fig. 6.3: As the curve is perfectly symmetrical, the mean, median and mode coincide (normal, Gaussian, parametric, unimodal)

Characteristics of the Mean

- The mean is the best known and most frequently used average. Aftertimes it may be advantageous to use the mean merely because it is so well understood
- The mean is affected by the value of every case in the series. As a result, undue weightage sometimes may be given to extreme and erratic items. For example the mean wage of a group may actually be misleading if these are extreme on typical items at either end of the scale
- From an algebraic standpoint, the mean is superior to either the median or mode.

Advantages

- Mean can be easily calculated and is easy to understand
- Mean calculation is based on all the observations
- Mean is rightly defined by sampling fluctuation
- Mean is the best measure to compare two or more series (data)
- Mean is the average obtained by calculations and it does not depend upon any position.

Disadvantages

- Mean may not be represented in actual data so it is theoretical
- Mean is affected by extreme values
- Mean cannot be determined for qualitative data such as love, beauty, honesty, etc.
- Mean may lead to fallacious conditions or the absence of original observations.

Uses

Mean is useful in following situations or events:

- When scores are symmetrically or nearly symmetrically distributed around a central point
- When the situation warrants a measure of central tendency, having the greatest stability
- When the researchers wishes to compute SD, co-efficient of correlation and other statistics which are based upon mean
- Common man uses means for calculating average
- It is extensively used in statistics
- Estimates are always obtained by mean
- Useful for all businessmens and professionals.

Calculation of the Mean

The most used and familiar index of central tendency for a set of raw data or a distribution is the mean. *The mean is a simple arithmetic average.* It is common place knowledge that to take the average of a set of raw scores, *we simply add all the scores up and divide by the total number of scores, N.* Consider the following scores or measurements: 8, 14, 23, 10, 12, 5. The sum of these scores is 72. The arithmetic mean is, therefore, 72 divided by 6, i.e., 2. In general, if N measurements are represented by the symbols, X_1, X_2,

X_3......, X_N, the arithmetic mean in algebraic language is

$$M = \frac{X_1 + X_2 + X_3 + ... + X_N}{N} = \frac{\sum_{i=1}^{N} X_i}{N} \quad ...(6.1)$$

The Greek letter sigma Σ describes the operation of summing the N measurements. The summation extends from $i = 1$ to $i = N$. Generally the arithmetic mean is written simply as

$$M = \frac{\Sigma X}{N} \quad ...(6.2)$$

The limits of the summation are omitted. The summation is understood to extend over all available values of X. Sometimes X (bar upon X) is used to denote the mean of X series; Y to denote the mean of Y series. In this text, M will be used as a generalized term for mean. However, for a distinction between the two different series of scores, M_x, M_y, etc. will be used. The student should note another fact about the mean:

$$M = \frac{\Sigma X}{N}$$

By cross multiplication, we obtain

$$\Sigma X = NM \quad ...(6.3)$$

Thus, the sum of a variable X is N times the mean of X. It is a useful concept and is used in a variety of situations.

Calculation of Mean from Frequency Distribution

When scores or measurements have been arranged in the form of a frequency distribution showing class intervals and frequencies, the following methods are used:

Calculation of Mean by Long Method

Symbols

Σ = Sum of

F = Frequency

x = Score

N = Total number of scores

In the above frequency distribution, the class interval is of size. Each X is then multiplied by the relevant frequency and a product of the two, fX, obtained. If each X is denoted by $X_1 + X_2$, and frequency by f_1, f_2, etc. Upto to X_K and f_K respectively, the formula for the mean would be:

$$M = \frac{f_1X_1 + f_2X_2 + f_3X_3 + \cdots f_KX_K}{N} = \frac{\sum_{i=1}^{K} f_iX_i}{N}$$

For simplicity, the limits of the summation are omitted and the formula becomes:

$$M = \frac{\Sigma fx}{N} \quad ...(6.4)$$

The calculation of mean from a frequency distribution with class interval size equal to more than 1 is done in a similar way. It is shown below in Tables 6.1 and 6.2.

The calculation of mean from frequency distribution with class interval size two or more as shown in Table 6.2.

Formula

$$\text{Mean} = \frac{\Sigma fx}{N}$$

Substituting the values in the formula:

$$\text{Mean} = \frac{1120}{50} = 22.40$$

The steps in the calculation of mean by the long method are as follows:

- Calculate the mid-points of each class interval and call them x (Col. 2)
- Multiply f and x (Col. 2 × Col. 3) to obtain fx (Col. 4)
- Add fx values in Col. 4 to obtain Σfx
- Divide this sum, Σfx, by N to obtain the mean.

Calculation of Mean by the Short Method or Assumed Mean Method (Table 6.3)

The long method of calculating mean as shown above is an accurate and straightforward method.

Table 6.1

Calculation of mean from frequency distribution with class interval of size 1.

Class interval x	Frequency f	Frequency × mid-point	Computation formula
16	2	32	$M = \frac{\Sigma fx}{N}$
15	3	45	
14	4	56	$\Sigma fx = 266$
13	5	65	$N = 20$
12	3	36	
11	2	22	$M = \frac{266}{20} = 13.3$
10	1	10	
	20	266	

Table 6.2

Calculation of mean from frequency distribution with class interval size of two or more.

Class interval	Mid-point (x)	Frequency (f)	Frequency × Mid-point (fx)
45 – 49	47	2	94
40 – 44	42	3	126
35 – 39	37	2	74
30 – 34	32	6	192
25 – 29	27	8	216
20 – 24	22	8	176
15 – 19	17	7	119
10 – 14	12	5	60
5 – 9	7	9	63
		N = 50	$\Sigma fx = 1120$

However, it very often involves the handling of large numbers and requires tedious calculations. Hence, to overcome these difficulties, the "Assumpted Mean" method or simply the short method has been devised for the computation of mean from the frequency distribution. The same is illustrated below:

Assumed mean, AM = 27; $\Sigma fx' = -46$

Correlation, $C = \frac{\Sigma fx'}{N} = \frac{-46}{50} = -0.92$

Size of class interval, $i = 5$.

Formula

Mean = AM + CI ...(6.5)

= 27 + (–0.92 × 5) (substituting the values)

= 27 – 4.6 = 22.40

In the short method, people "guess" or assume a mean and later apply a correction to the assumed mean (AM) in order to obtain the actual mean (Table 6.3).

The steps involved in the calculation of mean by the short method are as below:

Table 6.3

Calculation of mean from a frequency distribution by short method or assumed mean method

Class Interval	*Mid-point*	*Frequency*	*Deviation of (X) from A in units of CI*	
(1)	*(2)*	*(3)*	*(4)*	*(5)*
	(x)	*(f)*	*(x′)*	*(fx′)*
45 – 49	47	2	+4	+8
40 – 44	42	3	+3	+9
35 – 39	37	2	+2	+4
30 – 34	32	6	+1	+6
25 – 29	27	8	0	0
20 – 24	22	8	–1	–8
15 – 19	17	7	–2	–4
10 – 14	12	5	–3	–15
5 – 9	7	9	–4	–36
	N = 50			+ 27 –73 $\Sigma fx' = -46$

1. Tabulate the scores into a frequency distribution and find out the midpoint of the class intervals (Cols. 1–3).
2. Take the midpoint of an interval somewhere near the center of the frequency distribution and if possible, the interval should contain the largest frequency. This is for convenience of computation as it would involve working with smaller values (If any other class interval is assumed, the value of mean will remain the same). It is assumed, the class interval, 25–29, is considered and its midpoint, 27 is taken as assumed mean.
3. The x' values as in Col. 4 are the *deviations from the assumed mean in units of class interval*. The midpoint of class interval, 25–29, is 27 and deviates 0 units from the AM and hence zero is placed in the Col. x' against this interval. As we go up, we find the class interval, 30–34, deviates +1 unit, from the assumed mean.

$\left(x' = \dfrac{\text{Mid-point} - \text{AM}}{\text{Size of CI}} = \dfrac{32-27}{5} = +1\right)$. This value is placed opposite to this class interval in the x' column. The process is repeated to obtain values of +2, +3 and +4 for other class intervals above the class interval 30–34. Let us come back to the class interval 25–29, which was assigned $x' = 0$. The value of x' for the class intervals below it are calculated in the manner as shown below:

CI	x'
20-24	$\dfrac{22-27}{5} = -1$
15-19	$\dfrac{17-27}{5} = -2$ and so on

The other x's thus are –3, –4 and –5.

However, the student will be able to see the simple way in which x' values can be assigned almost mechanically. Starting with $x' = 0$ for the class interval having the AM, go up assigning x' values of +1, +2, +3, etc. till you reach the uppermost class interval. Once again starting from $x' = 0$, go down assigning x' values of –1, –2, –3, etc till you reach the lowest class interval. This is possible because all class intervals are of uniform size.

1. fx' in Column 5 is the product of f and x' (Col. 3x Col. 4). While multiplying f and x' values

the algebraic sign is to be kept intact and noted alongwith the values in Column 5. It may be that all fx' values in intervals above the AM are positive; and all fx' values below the AM are negative.

2. Obtain $\Sigma fx'$, the sum of fx' values by summing up algebraically the fx' values in Col. 5. For convenience, sum up separately the negative values and the positive values and obtain the absolute difference of the two sums. Give this difference, the sign of the larger sum. In our example, sum of x' with plus sign is 27; that of minus sign is –73; the difference of the two sums is –46 with sign of the larger sum kept intact.
3. The value of correction, C, is obtained by dividing $\Sigma fx'$ by N. In our example, –46 is divided by 50 to obtain C = –0.92 (the sign of the value is very important). Multiply C by I to obtain CI = –0.92 × 5 = 4.6. Substituting these values in the formula, M = AM + C_i, we obtain M = 27 + (–4.6) = 22.40.

Short-cut Method: For Mean of ungrouped data, short-cut method is applied when the frequencies and the values of the variables are quite large and it becomes very difficult to compute the arithmetic mean as in the case of the above example. In a frequency table of such a type the provisional mean is taken as that values of x (mid value of the class interval) which corresponds to the highest frequency or which comes near the middle value of the frequency distribution. This number is called the **Provisional Mean or Assumed Mean.** Also the deviations of the variates from this provisional mean. Then the arithmetic mean is given by the formula:

(i) In the case of **ungrouped data**

$$\overline{x} = a + \frac{\Sigma d}{n}, \text{ where}$$

a = assumed mean, n = number of items,
d = x-a = deviations of any variate from a.

Working Rule for Short-Cut method for Ungrouped Data

Step I. Denote the variable of the discrete series by x or X.

Step II. Take any item of series, preferably the middle one and denote it by a. This number a is called the **assumed mean or provisional mean**.

Step III. Take the difference $x - a$ and denote it by d or dx or $d' = x - a$, where d' is the deviation of any variate from 'a'.

Step IV. Find the sum of Σd.

Step V. Use the following formula to calculate the arithmetic mean:

$$\overline{x} = a + \frac{\Sigma d}{N}$$

(i) In the case of **grouped data**

$$\overline{x} = a + \frac{\Sigma fd}{N}, \text{ where}$$

fd = product of the frequency and the corresponding deviation
N = Σf = the sum of all the frequencies.

Working Rule for Short-Cut method for Grouped data

Step I. In the case of discrete series, denote the variable by x of X and the corresponding frequency by f (But in the case of continuous series x is the mid value of the interval and f the frequency corresponding to that interval).

Step II. Take any item x series, preferably the middle one and denote it by 'a'. This number 'a' is called the **assumed mean or provisional mean**.

Step III. Take the differences $x - a$ and denote it by d or dx or $d' = x - a$ = deviation of any variate x from a, the assumed mean.

Step IV. Multiply the respective f and d and denote the product under the column fd.

Step V. Find Σfd.

Step VI. Use the following formula to calculate the arithmetic mean.

$$\overline{x} = a + \frac{\Sigma fd}{\Sigma f}$$

Properties

The mean possess several properties which make it very useful. Some of them are described as:

The Mean as a "Center of Gravity" of a One Distribution

The mean of a distribution parallels the physical idea of a center of gravity, or balance point, of ideal objects arranged in a straight line. For example, imagine an ideal board having zero weight. Along this board are arranged stacks of objects at various positions. The objects have uniform weight and differ from each other only in their positions on the board. The board is marked off in equal units of some kind, and each object is assigned a number according to its position as shown below in Figure 6.4.

Now given this idealized situation, at what point would a fulcrum placed under the board create a state of balance? That is, what is the point at which the "push" of objects on one side of the board is exactly equal to the push exerted by the objects on the other side? This is found from the mean of the positions of the various objects.

$$M = \frac{3+3+9+11+11+11+16+16+19+21}{10} = 12$$

Here, the board would exactly balance if a fulcrum were placed at a position marked 12. It may be noted that this center of gravity has been found in exactly the same way as for the mean of a distribution. The position of an object of uniform weight (midpoint of the class interval) was, in effect, multiplied by the number of objects at that position (the frequency). These values were summed and divided by the number of objects (the total frequency or N).

Deviations in one Direction of the Mean Exactly Equal the Deviations in the Other Direction

This characteristic emerges from property No.1 of the mean as mentioned above. Since mean is the center of gravity or the balance point, the sum of deviations in one direction of the mean exactly equals the sum of the deviations in the other direction. This leads us to a further conclusion that the *sum of deviations about the mean in any distribution is always zero.* This is illustrated in Table 6.4.

It can also be shown that the sum of deviations taken from any other arbitrary value will not be zero. Σx for arbitrary means of 3 and 6 are +5 and –10 respectively.

The Principle of Least Squares

Another property that emerges from the first two mentioned above is that the *sum of the squared deviations of all the scores about the mean is less*

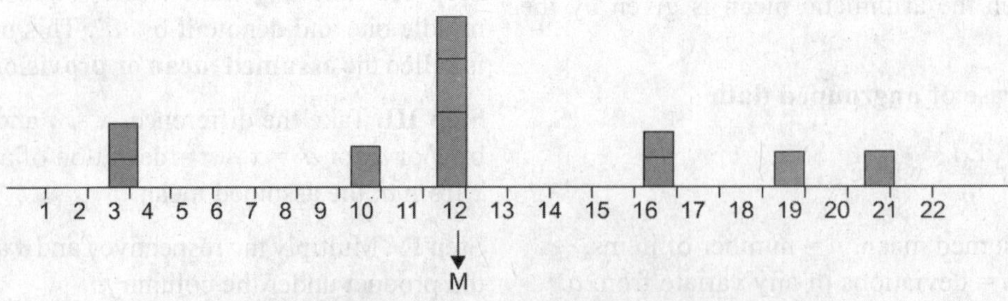

Fig. 6.4: Mean as center of gravity of a frequency distribution

Table 6.4

Deviations from the mean

Score (X)	Deviations (x)	Squares of deviations (x^2)
6	+2	4
5	+1	1
4	0	0
3	–1	1
2	–2	4
$\Sigma X = 20$ $M = 4$	$\Sigma x = 0$	$\Sigma x^2 = 10$

than the sum of the squared deviations about any other value. This is called the principles of least squares. For example, in the above illustrations (Table 6.4), the sum of the squared deviations about the mean equals 10. The M was 4. If 3 and 6 are taken as arbitrary values of the mean, the value of Σx^2 becomes, 15 and 30 respectively. Thus the sum (10) taken about the mean is less than any other of these examples and it can be shown that it always will be less than any other value. Hence, the essential property of mean is that *it is closer* (in terms of squared deviations) to the individual scores over the entire group than is any other single value. This is a highly useful concept that enters into several other statistical methods like regression and prediction. If we were told to guess the score of some case picked at random from a distribution, we may guess the mean for that and every other case so picked. It may not be true that the mean is exactly the same as any obtained. The overall signed error, on the average, will be zero and the sum of the squared errors will be least.

The mean has the property that for most distributions, it is a more accurate, or more efficient estimate of the population.

If a constant is added to each of a distribution, the value of the mean will increase by the value of that constant. The subtraction of a constant from each score of a constant. The multiplication and division will also lead to a result equal to the product of mean and the constant; and the quotient obtained by dividing the mean by that constant, respectively. An algebraic proof of this will be attempted later. However, a numerical example is given in Table 6.5 to demonstrate the above.

Combined Mean (M_{comb})

A combined mean for two or more samples can be calculated if the M's and N's of those groups are available. This would avoid the necessity of combining the raw scores of all the samples and calculating the average in the normal way. For example, see Table 6.6.

Formula

$$M_{comb} = \frac{N_1M_1, \text{etc} + N_2N_2 + \cdots N_nM_n}{N_1 + N_2 + \cdots + N_n} \quad ...(6.6)$$

Substituting the numerical values,

$$= \frac{(40 \times 50) + (30 \times 45) + (20 \times 35)}{40 + 30 + 20}$$

$$= \frac{2000 + 1350 + 700}{100}$$

$$= \frac{4050}{100} = 40.5$$

When *only two groups are involved,* the formula becomes

$$M_{comb} = \frac{N_1M_1 + N_2M_2}{N_1 + N_2} \quad ...(6.7)$$

Table 6.5

Effect of a constant on mean

Original score	*Adding 2 to each score*	*Subtracting 2 from each score*	*Multiplying each score by 2*	*Dividing each score by 2*
4	6	2	8	2
5	7	3	10	2.5
6	8	4	12	3
7	9	5	14	3.5
8	10	6	16	4
------	-----	-----	-----	-----
Σ30	40	20	60	15.0
6	8	4	12	3.0
Effect	(6 + 2)	(6 – 2)	(6 × 2)	(6/2)

Table 6.6

Calculation of combined mean

Group	*K*	*M*	*Symbols*
I	40	50	M_{comb} = Weighted arithmetic mean obtained from combining groups.
II	30	45	N_1, N_2, etc. Number of cases in groups I, II, etc.
III	20	35	M_1, M_2, etc. Means of Groups I, II, etc.

When N is equal, the formula reduces to

$$M_{comb} = M_1M_2 + ... + M_n \qquad ...(6.7a)$$

(Where n is the number of groups)

For example, for the three groups having means of 10, 15 and 35 respectively and equal N's the $M_{comb} = (10+15+35)/3 = 20$.

Problems and Solutions

1. Find the arithmetic mean from the frequency table

Marks obtained	52	58	60	65	68	70	75
No. of Nursing students	7	5	4	6	3	3	2

Solution. Let x be the marks and f be the frequency so that we have the following table:

x	f	Σfx
52	7	364
58	5	290
6	4	240
65	6	390
68	3	204
70	3	210
75	2	150
Total	**30**	**1848**

Here $N = \Sigma f = 30$ and $\Sigma fx = 1848$

$$\therefore \quad \text{Mean} = \bar{x} = \frac{1848}{29} = \frac{616}{10} = 61.6$$

2. Calculate the arithmetic mean for the following data

Class-interval	*Frequency*
10 – 20	2
20 – 30	7
30 – 40	17
40 – 50	29
60 – 70	10
70 – 80	3
80 – 90	2
90 – 100	1

Solution. While calculating the arithmetic mean for such a tabular data, it is assumed that all the observations in any particular class interval have the same value. The value is the middle value or midpoint of the class interval, i.e. we replace the classes by the mid-values and proceed as above:

Class interval	Mid values (x)	Frequency (f)	fx
10 – 20	15	2	30
20 – 30	25	7	175
30 – 40	35	17	595
40 – 50	45	29	1305
50 – 60	55	29	1595
60 – 70	65	10	650
70 – 80	75	3	225
80 – 90	85	2	170
90 – 100	95	1	95
Total		**100**	**4840**

Here $N = \Sigma f = 100$ and $\Sigma fx = 4840$

$$\therefore \quad \bar{x} = \frac{\Sigma fx}{\Sigma f} = \frac{4840}{100} = 48.4$$

3. Find, by short-cut-method, the mean height of the following 8 nursing students whose height in centimeter are

59, 65, 71, 67, 61, 63, 69, 73

Solution. Let us take 65 as assumed mean, i.e. $a = 65$. Let us prepare the following table (*i*)

x	d = x – 65
59	–6
65	0
71	+6
67	+2
61	–4
63	–2
69	+4
73	+8

Total deviation $= \Sigma fd = 8$

Here $a = 65$, $n = 8$, $\Sigma fd = 8$

$$\therefore \quad \bar{x} = a + \frac{\Sigma fd}{n} = 65 + \frac{8}{8} = 66 \text{ cm.}$$

4. Ten coins were tossed together and the number of tails resulting from were observed. The operation was performed 1,050 times and the frequencies thus obtained for different number of tails (x) are shown in the following table. Calculate the arithmetic mean by the shortcut method

x	0	1	2	3	4	5	6	7	8	9	10
f	2	8	43	133	207	260	213	120	54	9	1

Solution. Let 5 be the assumed mean, i.e. $a = 5$. let us prepare the following table in order to calculate the arithmetic mean:

x	f	d = x – 5	fd
0	2	–5	–10
1	8	–4	–32
2	43	–3	–129
3	133	–2	–266
4	207	–1	–207
5	260	0	0
6	213	1	+213
7	120	2	+240
8	54	3	+162
9	9	4	+36
10	1	5	+5
	Σf = 1050	**Σfd = 12**	

$$\therefore \quad \text{Arithmetic mean} = \bar{x} = a + \frac{\Sigma fd}{\Sigma f}$$

$$= 5 + \frac{12}{1050}$$

$$= 5 + 0.0114$$

$$= 5.0114$$

Step deviation method. When the class intervals in a grouped data are equal, then the calculations can be simplified further by taking out the common factor from the deviations. This common factor is equal to the width of the class-interval. In such cases, the deviation of variates x from the assumed mean '*a*' (i.e. $d = x - a$) are divided by the common factor. The arithmetic mean 0 is then obtained by the following method:

$$\bar{x} = a + \frac{\Sigma fd}{N} \times i, \qquad \text{...(6.8)}$$

where a = assumed mean or Provisional Mean,

Marks	Mid-value	$d = \frac{x-35}{10}$	No. of students	fd
0 – 10	5	– 3	42	–126
10 – 20	15	– 2	44	– 88
20 – 30	25	– 1	58	– 58
30 – 40	35	0	35	0
40 – 50	45	1	26	26
50 – 60	55	2	15	30
			N = 220	**Σfd = –216**

$d = \frac{x-a}{i}$ = the deviation of any variate from a,

i = the width of the class interval,
N = the number of observations

5. Calculate, by step deviation method, the arithmetic mean of the following marks obtained by students in Fundamentals of Nursing

Solution. Let $a = 20$ and $i = 5$.

X	f	dx = x – a	dx′ = dx/i	fdx′
5	20	–25	–5	–100
10	43	–20	–4	–172
15	75	–15	–3	–225
20	67	–10	–2	–134
25	72	–5	–1	–72
30	45	0	0	0
35	39	5	1	39
40	9	10	2	18
45	8	15	3	24
50	6	20	4	24
	Σf = 384			**Σfdx′ = –598**

Now $\bar{x} = a + \frac{\Sigma fdx'}{N} \times i$

$= 30 - \frac{598}{384} \times 5$

$= 30 - 1.56 \times 5$

$= 30 - 7.80 = 22.2$

6. Calculate the average marks, by the step deviation method, from the following data

Marks obtained	No. of students
0 – 10	42
10 – 20	44
20 – 30	58
30 – 40	35
40 – 50	26
50 – 60	15

Solution

Here $a = 35$, N = 220, $\Sigma fd = -216$, $i = 10$

$\therefore \quad x = a + \frac{\Sigma fd}{N} \times i$

$x = 35 + \frac{-216}{220} \times 10$

$= 35 + -098 \times 10$

$= 35 - 9.81$

$= 25.19$

Geometric Mean

In algebra, geometric mean (GM) is calculated in case of geometric progression, but in statistics we need not bother about the progression. Here, it is the particular type of data for which the geometric mean is of importance because it gives a good mean value. If the variate values are measured as ratios, proportions or percentages, geometric mean gives a better measure of central tendency than other means.

Geometric mean of N variate values is the Nth root of their product. Like arithmetic mean it also depends on all observations. It is affected by the extreme values but not to the extent of average. However, there is one great drawback with it, that it can not be calculated if any one or more values are zero or negative. In case an even number of observations are negative, an absurd value of geometric mean will be available from a practical point of view. Hence, if there is a zero or negative value in the set of variate values, it should not be used.

Geometric mean is also/useful under certain conditions. It is defined as the *n*th root of the values of *n* items in a given series. Symbolically, we can put it thus:

Geometric mean (GM)

$$= \sqrt[n]{\Pi X_i} \qquad ...(6.9)$$

$$= \sqrt[n]{X_1, X_2, X_3 \cdots X_4}$$

Where

GM = geometric mean

n = number of items

X_i = ith value of the variable X

Π = conventional product notation

For instance, the geometric mean of the numbers 4, 6, and 9 is worked out as

Geometric mean (GM)

$$= \sqrt[3]{4.6.9}$$

$$= 9$$

the most frequently used application of this average is in the determination of average percent of change, i.e. it is often used in the preparation of index numbers or when we deal in ratios.

Harmonic Mean

In algebra, harmonic mean (HM) is found out in the case of harmonic progression only. But in statistics harmonic mean is a suitable measure of central tendency when the data pertains to speed, rates and time.

Harmonic mean is the inverse of the arithmetic mean of the reciprocals of the observations of a set.

Harmonic mean is defined as the reciprocal of the average of reciprocals of the values of items of a series. Symbolically, we can express it as under:

Harmonic mean (HM)

$$= \text{Rec.} \frac{\Sigma \text{Rec } X_i}{n}$$

$$= \text{Rec.} \frac{\text{Rec } X_1 + X_2 + \cdots + \text{Rec } X_n}{n} \qquad ...(6.10)$$

Where

HM = harmonic mean

Rec = reciprocal

X_i = ith value of the variable X

n = number of items

For instance, the harmonic mean of the numbers 4, 5, and 10 is worked out as

$$\text{HM} = \frac{\text{Rec } \frac{1}{4} + \frac{1}{5} + \frac{1}{10}}{2}$$

$$= \frac{\text{Rec } \frac{15+12+6}{60}}{3}$$

$$= \text{Rec}\left(\frac{33}{60} \times \frac{1}{3}\right)$$

$$= \frac{60}{11} = 5.45$$

Harmonic mean is of limited application, particularly in cases where time and rate are involved. The harmonic mean gives largest weight to the smallest item and smallest weight to the largest item. As such it is used in cases like time and motion study where time is variable and distance constant.

From what has been stated, time is variable, we can say that there are several types of statistical averages. These researcher has to make a choice for some average. There are no hard and fast rules for the selection of a particular average in statistical analysis for the selection of an average mostly depends on the nature, type and objectives of the research study. One particular type of average cannot be taken as appropriate for all types of studies. The chief characteristics, and the limitations of the various averages must be kept in view, discriminate use of average is very essential for sound statistical analysis.

Median

Median was defined as the point in a distributions with an equal number of cases on eitherside of it, i.e. the individual measures can be arranged from low to higher value, the middle observation in "median".

It has been pointed out that mean cannot be calculated whenever there is frequency distribution with open end intervals. Also the mean is to a great extent affected by the extreme values of the set of observations. Hence in such cases, there has been a search for some better measure of central tendency. For instance, there are eight persons getting daily wages as Rs 150, 225, 240, 260, 275, 290, 300 and 1500. The mean daily wage of the persons involved is Rs 405. This value is not a good measure of central tendency because out of the eight people, seven get Rs 300 or less. Hence, some better measure is preferable and median is one of them.

It means:

- In a distribution, median is the value of the variable which divides it into two equal halves.
- In an ordered series of data, median is an observation lying exactly in the middle of the series.
- In a set of observations, median is the value of a variable that have half of the number of observations below it and remaining half above it.

The median for a set of observations can easily be found out after arranging them in ascending or descending order.

The median is another simple average or measure of central tendency. Many statisticians define the median as the size of the middle item when the items are arranged in their order of magnitude. This means, of course, that there are as many items above or larger than the middle one, as there are below or smaller than it. If the number of items in the series is even, the median is taken as the arithmetic mean of the middle items, misconcepts which are discussed should not be considered as genuine median, but rather as the value of the mid-item or mid-case. The concept median should be reserved for frequency distributions and not simple arrays. If such distinction is made, then the median may be defined as that point on the scale of the variable (the point on the *x*-scale on a frequency graphs) which divides the distribution into two equal parts.

The **median (Med)** is the score that corresponds to the point at or below which 50 percent of the scores fall when the data are arranged in numerical order. By this definition, the median is also called the 50th percentile.[†] For example, consider the numbers (5 8 3 7 15). If the numbers are arranged in numerical order (3 5 7 8 15), the middle score would be 7 and it would be called the median. Suppose, however, that there were an even number of scores, for example (5 11 3 7 15 14). Rearranging, we get (3 5 7 11 14 15) and no score has 50 percent of the values below it. That point actually falls between 7 and 11. In such a case the average (9) of the two middle scores (7 and 11) is commonly taken as the median.[‡]

A term that we will need shortly is the median location. The median location of N numbers is defined as follows:

$$\text{Median location} = \frac{N+1}{2}$$

Thus, for five numbers the median location = (5 + 1)/2 = 3, which simply means that the median is the third number in an ordered series. For 12 numbers the median location = (12 +1)/2 = 6.5; the median falls between and is the average of, the sixth and seventh numbers.

Median is the value of the middle item of series which is arranged in ascending or descending order of magnitude. It divides the series into two halves, in one half all items are less than median, whereas in the other half all items have values higher than median. If the values of the items arranged in ascending order are: 60, 74, 80, 88, 90, 95, 100, then the value of the 4th item viz 88 is the value of the median. It may also be stated as:

$$\text{Median (M)} = \text{value of} \left(\frac{n+1}{2}\right)^{\text{th}} \text{terms}$$

Median is a positional average and used in the contact of qualitative phenomena, for example, in estimating intelligence, etc. which are often encountered in psychosocial fields. Median is not useful where items need to be assigned relative importance and weights. It is not frequently in sampling statistics.

Median refers to the middle value in a distribution. In case of median one-half of the items in the distribution have a value the size of the median value or smaller and one half have a value the size of the median value or larger. The median is just the 50th percentile value below which 50 percent of values in the sample fall. It splits the observation into the halves. In short, when the variables are arranged in either ascending or descending order, the middle observation is known as median. It implies the middle value of a series. Median is also called as "positional average" as the term position refer to place of value in a series. The place of median in a series is such that an equal number of items lie on either side of it.

Characteristics

- The median is not influenced by the size of the extreme items. It is based on the values lying immediately on either side of it. The median can be used very effectively in which extreme items are likely to have an unduly disproportionate influence on the mean
- The median is easily calculated
- The median is generally less reliable than the mean and is not so well adapted to algebraic manipulations.

Properties

- Median is a positional average and hence it is not influenced by the extreme values
- Median can be calculated even in the case of open end intervals
- Median can be located even if the data are incomplete
- It is not a good representative of data if the number of items is small
- It is not amenable to further algebraic treatment
- It is susceptibe to sampling fluctuations.

Advantages

- Median is easily understood
- Median is not affected by extreme values
- Median can be located graphically
- Median is the best measure for qualitative data such as love, beauty, intelligence, etc
- Median can be easily located even if the class intervals in the series are unequal
- Median can be determined even by inspection of many cases.

Disadvantages

- Median is not subjected to algebraic treatments
- Median cannot represent the irregular distribution series
- Calculating median necessitates to arrange the data, other averages do not need any arrangement
- Median in some cases cannot be computed exactly as the mean
- Median is erratic if the number of item is large.

Uses

Median is Useful

- When the exact mid-point separating the distribution into two equal halves is wanted i.e. where the exact midpoint of the distribution is wanted
- When extreme scores are present in the distribution. Extreme scores affect the mean more than the median
- When the number of scores above or below the central tendency is known, but not their exact values

- When the upper exact limit of the top class interval (or when it is desired that certain scores should influence the mean, but we only know whether they are below or above the number of lower exact limit of the lowest class interval) is not known, i.e. the frequency distribution is not complete.

The median also symbolized by Md, is the point that divides the distribution into two parts such that an exactly equal number of scores fall above and below the point. It means that 50 percent of the scores will be above the median and the remaining 50 percent below it.

Computational examples: The computation of the median varies under different circumstances. The same is given below:

Ungrouped Data

When there is an odd number of scores in the distribution.

From distribution which have an odd number of scores but no duplication of scores near the median, *the median is the middle score.* The series is to be arranged in an ascending or descending order. *For example:* Consider the distribution 6, 4, 8, 7, 10. Arranging the scores in ascending order: 4, 6, 7, 8, 10, we find that the middle value, 7, is the median. It divides the distribution into two equal halves.

When there is an even number of scores in the distribution.

When there is an even number of scores and there is no duplication of scores near the median, the average of the middle two scores is taken as the median. The scores must be arranged in ascending or descending order.

For example: Consider the distribution 6, 4, 8, 7, 10, 5.

Arranging the scores in ascending order: 4, 5, 6, 7, 8, 10.

$$\text{Median} = \frac{\text{Sum of the middle two scores}}{1}$$

$$= \frac{6+7}{2} = 6.5$$

This convention applies even if the scores near the median are not adjacent.

For example: In a series of scores 4, 5, 6, 10, 11, 14.

The median is the average of the two middle scores.

$$\text{Median} = \frac{6+10}{2} = 8$$

Where there is a duplication of scores near the median

When more than one instance of a score value falling near the median exits, the median is obtained by interpolation.

Even Number

Example: *Consider the distribution 4, 5, 6, 6, 7, 7, 8.*

The situation is diagrammed below in Figure 6.5. The scores occupying the space on the scale of measurement between their real limits have been shown. Since four of the eight scores are required to be below the median, the median must fall within the interval 5.5–6.5. Since two scores already fall below that interval, two of the three scores existing between 5.5 and 6.5 are required to be below the median. Therefore, two-thirds or 0.67 of the one unit interval is added to its lower limit: 5.5 + .67 = 6.17. Examine Figure 6.5 carefully and consider

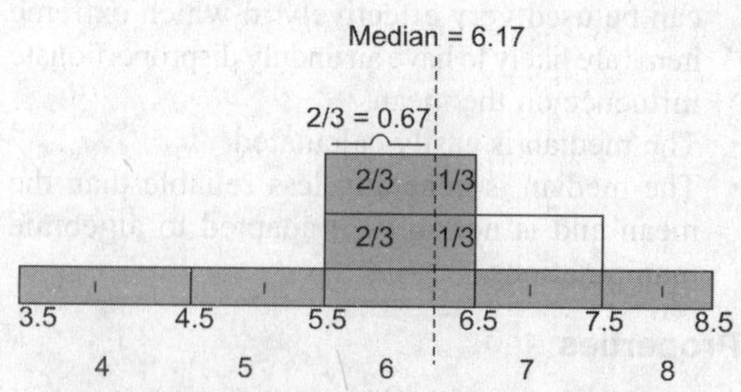

Fig. 6.5: Computation of the median when there is duplication of scores (even number)

the fractions of frequencies and you will notice that the distribution is divided in half at the point 6.17.

Odd Number

Example: *When there is an odd number of scores, the solution proceeds in the same manner as above.*

Suppose a distribution contains the following nine scores: 4, 5, 6, 6, 6, 7, 7, 8, 8. The median falls within the score interval 5.5 to 6.5. In the diagram shown below (Fig. 6.6) the scores occupying on the space of measurement between their real limits have been shown. Since there are, in all, 9 scores in the distribution, 4½ of them must be below the median. Again two scores exist below 5.5 and therefore 2½ of the three scores in one interval 5.5 – 6.5 must fall below the median.

That is $\frac{2\frac{1}{2}}{3} = \frac{5/2}{3} = \frac{5}{6} = 0.83$ of the one-unit interval must fall below the median. Therefore, the median = 5.5 + 0.83 = 6.33.

The student may notice that in Figure 6.6, the point 6.33 divides the distribution into exact two halves.

The procedure and the logic presented above is quite simple and follows a layman's approach to such problems. We can also have a formula for the calculation of median in such situations:

Formula

$$\text{Md} = \text{L} + \left(\frac{\text{N}/2 - \text{F}_b}{\text{F}_w}\right)i \quad ...(6.11)$$

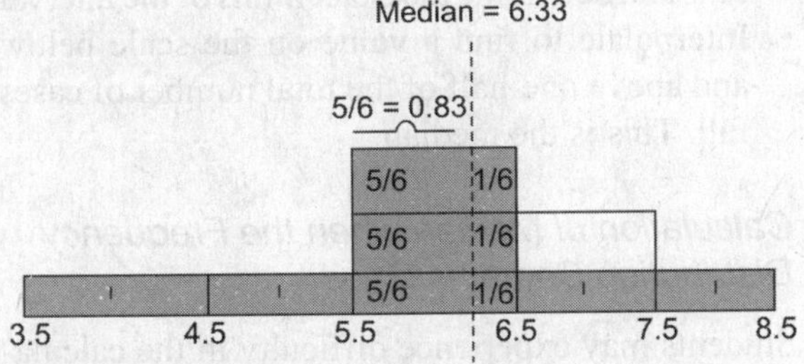

Fig. 6.6: Computation of median when there is duplication of scores (odd number)

In which symbols,

L = the lower limit of the interval containing the Md

N = the number of scores in the total distribution

F_b = the number of cases falling below the lower limit of interval containing the median

F_w = the number of scores within the interval containing the median

i = the size of the class interval

Substituting the values in the formula, we have:

$$\text{Md} = \text{L} + \left(\frac{9/2 - 2}{3}\right) \times 1$$

$$= 5.5 + \frac{5/2}{3}$$

$$= 5.5 + 0.83$$

$$= 6.3$$

Calculation of Median from a Frequency Distribution

In calculating the median from data grouped in the form of a frequency distribution, the problem is to determine a value of the variable such that one half the observations fall above this and the other half below. The fundamental logic calculation remains the same as already described above in relation to the ungrouped data. The method will be illustrated with reference to the data in Table 6.7.

Formula

$$\text{Median} = \text{L} + \left(\frac{\text{N}/2 - \text{F}_b}{\text{F}_w}\right)$$

Where, L = exact lower limit of the CI in which median lies

F_b = cumulative frequency below the CI containing median

F_w = frequency within the CI containing median

I = size of class interval

Table 6.7

Calculation of median

Class interval (1)	*Exact items* (2)	*Frequency* (3)	*Cumulative frequency* (4)
45 – 49	44.5 – 49.5	2	50
40 – 44	39.5 – 44.5	3	48
35 – 39	34.5 – 39.5	2	45
30 – 34	29.5 – 34.5	6	43
25 – 29	24.5 – 29.5	8	37
20 – 24	19.5 – 24.5	8	29 Md. Lies in this CI
15 – 19	14.5 – 19.5	7	21
10 – 14	9.5 – 14.5	5	14
5 – 9	4.5 – 9.5	9	9
		N = 50	

Here, $L = 19.5$

$F = 21; F_w = 8; i = 5.$

$$\text{Median} = 19.5 + \left[\frac{50/2 - 21}{8}\right] \times 5$$

$$= 19.5 + \left[\frac{25 - 21}{8}\right] \times 5$$

$$= 19.5 + \left(\frac{4}{8}\right) \times 5$$

$$= 19.5 + 2.5 = 22.$$

Computational Steps

First, record the cumulative frequencies as shown in column 4.

Second, determine $\frac{N}{2}$, one half the number of cases, in this example, $\frac{50}{2} = 25$.

Third, identify the class interval in which the 25th case, the middle case, falls. In this example, it is in class interval 20 – 24 exact limits 19.5 – 24.5.

Fourth interpolate between the exact limits of the interval to find a value above and below which 25 cases lie. Observe that 8 cases fall within the limits 19.5–24.5. We assume that these 8 cases are uniformly distributed in rectangular fashion between these exact limits. Now to arrive at the 25th or middle case we require 4 of the 8 cases within this interval because the cumulative frequency below this interval is 21 which shows that 21 cases have been covered up to 19.5, the upper limit of CI 15–19. This means that we find a point between 19.5 and 24.5 such as 4 cases fall below and 4 cases fall above it. The proportion of the interval we require is 4/8 which is 4/8 × 5 units of scores, or 2.5. We add this to the lower limit of the interval to obtain median, which is 19.5 + 2.5 = 22.00.

The formula and the calculation shown in Table 6.7 are quite easy and the student can follow the same with convenience. However, the steps mentioned above are summarized below:

- Compute the cumulative frequencies
- Determine N/2 or one-half of the cases
- Find the class interval in which the middle case falls and determine the exact limits of the interval
- Interpolate to find a value on the scale below and above one-half of the total number of cases fall. This is the median.

Calculation of Median when the Frequency Distribution Contains Gaps

Students may experience difficulty in the calculation of Median when there are gaps or zero frequency upon one or more intervals near the center of the distribution. The method to be followed in such cases is shown in Table 6.8.

$$\text{Median} = L + \frac{N/2 - \text{Cum } F_b \times i}{F_w}$$

$$= 9.5 + \frac{10-8}{2} \times 10$$

$$= 9.5 + 10 = 19.5$$

Value of I in this case is 10, the size of the extended class interval of 10–19.

Since N = 20, N/2 = 10, count up the frequency column 10 scores from below. Ordinarily 14.5, the upper limit of CI 10–14 should have been taken as the median. However, by counting down 10 scores from the frequency Col, we arrive at 24.5, the lower limit of CI 25–29. To resolve this discrepancy in the value of the median by the two approaches of counting up from below and counting down from above, we extend the middle class intervals. Here, the CI 10–14 is extended upto 19 with a new size of 10; the CI 25–298 is extended down to 20, with a new size of 10. Lengthening of these intervals removes the zero frequency on the adjacent intervals by spreading the numerical frequency over to CIs having zero frequencies and creating

Table 6.8

Computation of the median from distribution with Gaps

Class intervals (scores)	*f*	
35 – 39	3	
30 – 34	5	
25 – 29	2	20 – 29
20 – 24	0	
15 – 19	0	10 – 19
10 – 14	2	
5 – 9	4	
0 – 4	4	
	N = 20	
	N/2 = 10	

confusion in the correct calculation of the median. Now counting up from below, we complete 10 frequencies at 19.5 the upper limit of CI 10–19. Counting down from above also gives a median of 19.5, the lower limit of CI 20–29. Computation from the two ends of the distribution with extended CIs near the median, as shown in Table 6.8 now gives consistent results.

In cases where there is only one zero frequency exactly at the center of the distribution, the midpoint of the interval having zero will be the median. The same logic can be used in cases having three or more zeroes.

Mode (Mo)

Mode is a variable value which occurs most frequently in a set of value. It is most frequently occurring observation in a series.

The **mode (Mo)** can be defined simply as the most common score, that is, the score obtained from the largest number of subjects. Thus, the mode is that value of X that corresponds to the highest point on the distribution. If two *adjacent* times occur with equal (and greatest) frequency, a common convention is to take an average of the two values and call that the mode. If, on the other hand, two *non-adjacent* reaction times occur with equal (or nearly equal) frequency, we say that the distribution is bimodal and would most likely report both modes. For example, the distribution of time spent playing electronic games is roughly bimodal with peaks at the intervals of 0–9 minutes and 40–49 minutes. (You might argue that it is trimodal, with another peak at 120+ minutes, but that is a catch all interval for "all other values," so it does not make much sense to think of it as a modal value.)

The reaction time data presents us with a very minor problem. There are actually two modal values (at 62 and 67, with 14 scores falling at each of these times). These points are too close to really call the distribution "biomodal", but too far apart to feel good about averaging them. Preference would be to either report both values or to simply say that the modal value is "in the 60s," and leave it at that. When many data points are examined in an ungrouped fashion, there is probably so much unimportant variability from one value to another that it does not make much sense to worry about the mode or to be very concerned with bimodality.

Mode is the most commonly or frequently occurring value in a series. The mode in a distribution is that item around concentration. Mode is defined as that value in series which occurs most frequently. In a frequency distribution mode is that variate which has the maximum frequency. In these words, mode represents that value which is most frequent or typical or predominant.

In a simple series, the mode is the size of the measurement that occurs most frequently. In the following series of values; 15, 17, 18, 22, 25, 25, 25, 28, 28, 30 and 31, the mode is 25, because 25 occurs more often than any other measure. In a frequency distribution the mode is that point on the scale of the variable where the frequency is greatest. In general, mode is the size of the item which has the maximum frequently. At times such an item may not be mode. An account of the effect of the frequencies of the neighboring items. Like median, mode is a positional average and is not affected by the values of extreme items. It is therefore, useful in all situations where we need to eliminate the effect of extreme variations.

In practice it will be found that frequency distributions often have more than one mode. Distributions which have one mode are referred to as being unimodel, those with two modes are described as bimodal, those with three, trimodal or more generally multimodal.

Characteristics

- The mode, like the median, is a positional average, and is not affected by extreme items. It is therefore, useful in those cases in which it is desirable to eliminate the effects of extreme variations
- The mode is frequently very difficult to locate
- The mode possesses little significance unless there is a distinct central tendency and unless it is applied to a relatively large sample
- The mode is not susceptible to algebraic manipulation.

Advantages

- When quick and approximate measure of central tendency, wanted
- When measure of central tendency should be most typical value.

Disadvantages

- The value of mode cannot always be determined
- It is not capable of algebraic manipulation
- It is not a rigidly defined measure, as there are various formulae to calculate median which usually give somewhat different answer.

Uses

- Mode is useful when a quick measure is all what is wanted
- When an approximate measure of central tendency would do
- When only the most typical value is required
- Mode is particularly useful in the study of popular sizes. For example shirts and shoes.

Mode is the value which occurs with a greater frequency. This is obtained simply by obtaining the frequencies of the scores and locating the one with the highest frequencies. In short it is the most repetitive number in a series of observations. It is rarely used in health sciences including nursing.

The mode is the most frequently occurring score. When a frequency distribution is used, the mode is the midpoint of the interval with the largest number of cases or frequencies. If two adjacent scores have the same frequency and the frequencies are the highest in the distribution, then the mode is the sum of the two scores divided by two. When there are two non-adjacent scores with the same frequency and they are the highest in the distribution, each score may be referred to as the "mode" and the distribution is *bimodal.* Consider the following sets of scores to understand the method of calculation of mode from each.

Scores	f
35 – 39	3
30 – 34	4
25 – 29	6
20 – 24	7
15 – 19	9
10 – 14	6
5 – 9	5
	40

Mode is the mid-point of class-interval 15 – 19 which has the largest frequency of 9.

$$\text{Hence Mode} = \frac{\text{Lower limit + Upper limit}}{2}$$

$$= \frac{15+19}{2} = 17$$

Set I

Scores : 5, 5, 10, 10, 10, 11, 11, 11, 13, 13, 13, 13, 14, 14, 15, 15.

Mode = Since score 13 occurs the largest number of times ($f = 4$), it is the value of the mode.

Set II

Scores : 5, 5, 10, 10, 12, 12, 12, 13, 13, 13, 14, 14, 15, 15.

Mode = The adjacent scores of 12 and 13 have the largest but equal frequency of 3 each, hence, the average of these two values will be the mode which is (12 + 13)/2 = 12.5.

Set III

Scores : 5, 5, 10, 10, 12, 12, 12, 13, 13, 14, 14, 14, 15, 15.

Mode = The non-adjacent values of 12 and 14 have the largest but equal frequency of three each. Hence, this set of scores has two modes, 12 and 14. It can thus be called as *bimodal.*

Set IV

Scores : 7, 7, 8, 8, 10, 10, 11, 11, 13, 13, 16, 16.

Mode = Here all values occur with a frequency of 2, hence do not permit the calculation of a model value. In this case, mode is interminate. It is a rectangular shaped distribution with equal frequency on all the score points.

Calculation of Mode in a Frequency Distribution

When scores are grouped in frequency distribution, the mode is the midpoint of the interval with the largest frequency. Consider the following frequency distribution.

This is also called the *crude mode* or the *empirical mode.* It may be distinguished from the *true mode* which is the point (or peak) of the greatest concentration of scores in the distribution. The crude mode is approximately equal to the true mode and serves most of the practical purposes. A formula for approximately the true mode from the symmetrical or not badly skewed distribution is

Mode = 3 Median – 2 Mean

In the frequency distribution given above,

Median = 19.5; and Mean = 20.4

Hence, Mode = (3 × 19.5) – (2 × 20.4)

= 17.7

The mode is a measure of very limited practical value. It does not lend itself readily to further algebraic manipulations. It does not, in general, enter into the calculations of further statistical measures. It may acquire meaning if the number of measurements under consideration is fairly very large.

Comparison of the Mean, Median and Mode

The essential difference between the mean and the median is that the mean reflects the values of each score in the distribution whereas the median is based largely on the score where the midpoint of the distribution falls without regard for the particular of many of the scores. For example, consider the following illustration:

Scores	*Mean*	*Median*
2, 3, 4, 5, 6	4	4
2, 3, 4, 6, 36	10	4
2, 3, 4, 5, 76	16	4

In the above table, only the last number differs from one distribution to the other. The mean reflects these differences but the median does not. The median is the midpoint of the distribution and has equal number of cases falling on both sides of it. The value of the extreme scores does not matter but only the fact of their existence is taken into consideration. The numerator of the formula for M, ΣX shows that each score is to be summed up. Thus changing a score value will change the value of the mean.

The mode is a simple measure of central tendency and reflects only the most frequently occurring score. Its' use is restricted to very few problems in social sciences.

The mean, median and mode are sensitive to different aspects of a group of scores, generally they are not the same in a given distribution.

The relative position of mean, median and mode in different types of distribution:

a. Symmetrical unimodal
b. Symmetrical bimodal
c. Positively skewed
d. Negatively skewed.

1. If the distribution is symmetrical and unimodal (having one mode only), the mean, mode and median fall at the same point i.e., they have the same value.
2. If the distribution is symmetrical but *bimodal* (having two modes), the mean and the median fall at the same point but the values of the modes are different.
3. If the scores are bunched on the lower side of mean (*positively skewed distribution)* the value of the mean is higher than that of median.
4. If the scores are bunched on the upper side of the mean (*negatively skewed distribution)* the value of the median is higher than that of the mean.

Guidelines for the Use of Various Measures of Central Tendency

The following simple rules may prove helpful to the puzzled student as to when to use the various measures of central tendency.

Mean is Useful

- When scores are symmetrically or nearly symmetrically distributed around a central point
- When the situation warrants a measure of central tendency, having the greatest stability
- When the researcher wishes to compute standard deviation (SD), coefficient of correlation and other statistics which are based upon the mean.

Of the three principal measures of central tendency, the mean is by far the most common. It would not be too much of an exaggeration to say that for many people statistics is (unfortunately) nearly synonymous with the study of the mean.

As we have already seen, certain disadvantages are associated with the mean. It is influenced by extreme scores, its value may not actually exist in the data, and its' interpretation in terms of the underlying variable being measured requires at least some faith in the interval properties of the data. You might be inclined to politely suggest that if the mean has all the disadvantages that has just been ascribed to it, then maybe it should be quietly forgotten and allowed to slip into oblivation along with statistics like the "critical ratio," a statistical concept that hasn't been heard of for years. The mean, however, is made of sterner stuff.

The mean has several important advantages that far outweight its' disadvantages. Probably the most important of them from a historical point of view (though not necessarily from your point of view) is that the mean can be manipulated algebraically.

In other words, we can use the mean in an equation and manipulate it through the normal rules of algebra, specifically because we can write an equal that defines the mean. Since you cannot write a standard equation for the mode or the median, you have no real way of manipulating those statistics using standard algebra. Whatever the mean's faults, this accounts in large part for its' widespread application. The second important advantage of the mean is that it has several desirable properties with respect to its use and an estimate of the population mean. In particular, if we drew many samples from some population, the sample means that resulted would be more stable (less variable) estimates of the central tendency of that population than would the sample medians or modes. The fact that the sample mean is in general a better estimate of the population mean that is the mode or the median is a major reason that it is so widely used.

Median is Useful

- When the exact midpoint separating the distribution into two halves is wanted
- When extreme scores are present in the distribution. Extreme scores affect the mean more than the median
- When the number of scores above or below the central tendency is known but not their exact values
- When the upper exact limit of the top class interval (or the lower exact limit of the lowest class interval) is not known, i.e. the frequency distribution is not complete.

The major advantage of the median, which it shares with the mode, is the fact that it is unaffected by extreme scores. Thus, the medians of both (5 8 9 15 16) and (0 8 9 15 206) are 9. Many experts find this characteristic to be useful in studies in which extreme scores occasionally occur but have no particular significance. For example, the average trained rat can run down a circuit runway in approximately 1 to 2 seconds. Every once in a while this same rat will inexplicably stop halfway down, scratch himself, poke his nose at the photocells and lie down to sleep. In that instance it is of no practical significance whether he takes 30 seconds or 10 minutes to get to the other end of the runaway. It may even depend on when the experimenter gives up and pokes him with a pencil–a common practice when stamping your feet, blowing on the rat and tapping on the runway, all fail. If we ran a rat through three trials on a given day and his times were (1.2, 1.3, and 20 seconds), that would have the same meaning to us—in terms of what it tells us about the rat's knowledge of the task—as if his times were (1.2, 1.3, and 136.4 seconds). In both cases the median would be 1.3. Obviously, however, his daily *mean* would be quite different in the two cases (7.5 versus 46.3 seconds). It is this problem that frequently induces experimenters to work with the median rather than the mean time per day.

The median has another point in its' favor, when contrasted with the mean, which those writers who get excited over scales of measurement like to point out. The calculation of the median does not require any assumption about the interval properties of the scale. With the numbers (5, 8, and 11), the object represented by the number 8 is in the middle, no matter how close or distant it is from objects represented by 5 and 11. When we say that the *mean* is 8, we may be making the implicit assumption that the underlying distance between objects 5 and 8 is the same as the underlying distance between objects 8 and 11. Whether or not this assumption is reasonable is up to the experimenter to determine. It is preferred to work on the principle that if it is an absurdly unreasonable assumption, the experimenter will realize that, and take appropriate steps. If it is not absurdly unreasonable, then its practical effect on the results most likely will be negligible (This problem of scales of measurement was discussed in more detail earlier.)

A major disadvantage of the median is that, it does not enter readily into equations and is thus more difficult to work with, than the mean. It is also not as stable from sample to sample, as we will see shortly.

Mode is Useful

- When a quick measure is all what is wanted
- When an approximate measure of central tendency would do
- When only the most typical value is required. For example, the most typical size of the shirt or shoes worn by an average man.

The mode is the most commonly occurring score. By definition, then, it is a score that actually occurred, whereas the mean and sometimes the median may be values that never appear in the data. The mode also has the obvious advantages of representing the largest number of people. Someone who is running a small store would do well to concentrate on the mode. If 80 percent of your customers want the giant economy family size and 20 percent want the teeny-weeny, single-person size, it wouldn't seem particularly wise to aim for the mean and stock only the regular size.

Related to these two advantages is the fact that, by definition, the probability that an observation drawn at random (X_i) will be to the mode is greater than the probability that it will equal to any other specific score. Expressing this algebraically, we can say.

$$p\,(X_i = \text{mode}) > p\,(X_i = \text{any other score})$$

Finally, the mode has the advantage of being applicable to nominal data, which if you think about it, is obviously not true of the median or the mean.

The mode has its' disadvantages, however. We have already seen that the mode depends on how we group our data. Another disadvantage is that it may not be particularly representative of the entire collection of numbers. This advantages is illustrated in the electronics game data, in which the modal interval equals 0–9, which probably reflects the fact that a number of people do not play video games (difficult as that may be to believe). Using that interval as the mode would be to ignore all of those people who do play.

EXERCISES

1. Calculate mean, median and mode from the following ungrouped scores.
   a. 2, 8, 7, 10, 5, 2, 1
   b. 20, 15, 14, 14, 16, 13, 12
   c. 10, 12, 13, 15, 14, 15
2. Calculate mean, median and mode from the following frequency distribution.

Class interval (a)	*f*	*Class interval (b)*	*f*	*Class interval (c)*	*f*
80 – 89	6	190 – 199	2	45 – 49	2
70 – 79	9	180 – 189	4	40 – 44	3
60 – 69	10	170 – 179	15	35 – 39	6
50 – 59	25	160 – 169	11	30 – 34	9
40 – 49	25	150 – 159	38	25 – 29	13
30 – 39	10	140 – 149	8	20 – 24	8
20 – 29	5	130 – 139	6	15 – 19	6
10 – 19	7	120 – 129	2	10 – 14	2
0 – 9	3	110 – 119	7	5 – 9	1
		100 – 109	7		
	N = 100		N = 100		N = 50

3. What do you understand by a measure of central tendency? Explain with examples.
4. Under which circumstances, would you use the following instead of any other measure of central tendency?
   a. Mean
   b. Median
   c. Mode
   d. Geometric mean
   e. Hormonic mean
5. Name different kinds of average and discuss their merits and demerits.
6. Find out the arithmetic mean, mode and median for the following distribution:

Mid-points (weight no. lb)	*No. of nursing student*
95	4
105	2
115	18
125	22
135	21
145	19
155	10
165	3
175	2

7. The following table gives the monthly income of twelve families in a given community:

S No	*1*	*2*	*3*	*4*	*5*	*6*	*7*	*8*	*9*	*10*	*11*	*12*
Income	2800	1800	960	980	1040	750	800	940	1000	750	6000	2000

Calculate the arithmetic mean, the median and the mode of the income.

CHAPTER 7

Measures of Variability/ Dispersion

Introduction

In the previous chapter we considered several measures related to the center of a distribution. However, an average value for the distribution (whether it be the mode, the median or the mean) fails to give the whole story. We need some additional measure (or measures) to indicate the degree to which individual observations are clustered about or equivalently, deviate from that average value. The average may reflect the general location of most of the scores or the scores may be distributed over a wide range of values and the average may not be very representative of the full set of observations. Probably everyone has had experience with examinations in which all students received approximately the same grade and with examinations in which the scores ranged from excellent to dreadful. Measures that refer to the differences between these two types of situations are what we have in mind when we speak of dispersion or variability, around the median, the mode or any other point we wish. In general we will refer specifically to dispersion around the mean.

Variability is an important concept in the statistics. The fact that there is need for an average or a measure of central tendency shows that there is variation among the observations. Variation which is another characteristic of a group of observations has to be considered for describing the group more satisfactorily. The concept of variation also has been variously designated 'dispersion', 'scatteration', 'spread' or 'deviation'.

When describing a set of scores, it is often significant to report how variable the scores are, how much, they spread out from right to the low scores. For example, the groups of children, both with a median age of 10 years, would represent quite different educational situations, if one had a spread of ages from 9 to 11, while the other ranged from 6 to 14. A measure of this spread is important for describing a group.

Measures of variability of observations help to find how individual observations are dispersed around the mean of a large series. It is the measure of the variation of the items. In other words it is the degree of the scatter or variations of the variable about a central value.

Need for the Measure of Variability

Measure of central tendency is useful for defining a distribution in a concise manner. But by knowing only the mean, median or mode it is not possible to fix the distribution completely. It is also essential to know how far these observations are scattered. Variations are known as measures of variation. By knowing these measures of variations along with measure of central tendency, most of the biological distribution can be completely defined and thereby they can be easily compared with each other.

It was understood that measurement of central tendency was useful for defining a distribution in a concise manner. But by knowing only the mean, median and mode, it is not possible to fix the distribution completely. For example, there are 2 groups of Kabaddi teams, having their diastolic pressures (in mm of Hg) as:

Team A—92, 90, 88, 88, 88, 86, 84, 84, 84, 82, 80

Team B—100, 98, 96, 94, 90, 86, 82,78, 76, 74, 72.

It is seen that both the groups have their mean as 86 mm Hg. At the same it is also seen that the range as well as the diastolic pressures of the two groups are different. Hence, two sets of data with a common mean need not be same with regard to various individual values of the observation.

Purposes of Measures of Dispersion

Various measures of dispersion are calculated with the following purposes.

1. **To have an idea about the reliability of central value:** In a way, it is a measure of degree of scatteredness. If scatter is large, an average is less reliable. If the value of dispersion is small, it indicates that a central value is a good representative of all the values in the set.
2. **To compare two or more sets of values with regard to their variability:** Two or more sets can be compared by calculating the same measure of dispersion having the same unit of measure. A set with smaller value possess lesser variability.
3. **To provide information about the structure of a series:** A value of measure of dispersion gives an idea about the spread of the observations. Further one can surmise about limits of expansion of values in a set.
4. **To control the variation:** In many situations a measure of dispersion provides the basis for controlling the causes which lead to greater variation. For instance, one tries to have minimum error variance in experiments by controlling nuisance variables. In an industry, a production mananger will like to maintain his product having negligible variability. If it is more, he will find ways to check it.
5. **To pave way to the use of other statistical measures:** Measures of dispersion, especially variance and standard deviation lead to many statistical techniques like correlation, regression, analysis of variance, etc.

Properties of a Good Measure of Dispersion

There are certain requisites of a good measure of dispersion in general. The same are expounded here.

1. It should be based on all values of a series.
2. It should not be susceptible to fluctuations of sampling.
3. It should be capable of further algebraic treatment.
4. It should be rigidly defined, i.e. each investigator should arrive at the same value for the same set of data.
5. It is preferable that the unit of measurement of dispersion should be same as the unit of measurement of observations.
6. It should be calculable with reasonable ease, i.e. the formula should be such that it does not complicate the computation of a measure of dispersion.
7. It should be least affected by extreme values.

Each of the measures of dispersion is adequately elucidated in the subsequent discussion.

Measures of variation serve following purposes:

- To determine the reliability of an average
- To serve as a basis for the control of the variability
- To compare two or more series with regard to their variability
- To facilitate the use of other statistical measures.

Since the measure of variability give an average of the differences of various items from an average, they are also called averages of the second order, and possess the following properties.

Measures of variability should be:

- Simple to understand
- Easy to compute

- Rigidly defined
- Based on each and every item in the distribution
- Useful for further statistical treatment
- Have sampling stability
- Unaffected by extreme items.

Methods of Studying Variability/ Dispersion

Like different measures of central tendency, there are also different measures of variation. But each of them has its merits and demerits. The measures commonly used to describe such variability are:

- Range
- Interquartile range
- Mean or average deviation
- Standard deviation
- Coefficient of variation.

Range

Range is the simplest possible measure of dispersion and is defined as the difference between the values of the extreme items of a series. The range of a group of observations is the interval between the smallest and the biggest observations. The value of the range is dependent only upon two extreme observations in the group and does not consider the other observations. The occurrence of rare observations in the group greatly influences the value of the range and so it is not considered ideal as a measure of dispersion even though it is used in certain circumstances. This can be calculated easily and can be understood by the layman very easily.

The range or total range is the distance given by the highest score minus lowest score in the distributions. Thus,

$$\text{Range} = X_{Max} - X_{Min} \quad ....(7.1)$$

Range = (Highest value of an item in a series) – (Lowest value of an item in a series).

The ranges in the three sets of scores given in Table 7.1 can be calculated as follows:

Table 7.1

Calculation of range

Sl. No	*Highest score*		*Smallest score*	*Range*
1	5	Minus	5	= 0
2	13	Minus	7	= 6
3	19	Minus	1	= 18

Interpretation, Set 1 = All scores are covered within a score distance of zero units.

Set 2 = All scores are covered within a score distance of six units.

Set 3 = The student may interpret this result himself/herself.

The utility of range is that it gives an idea of the variability very quickly, but the drawback is that range is affected very greatly by fluctuations of sampling. Its value is never stable, being based on only two values of the variable and is not considered as appropriate measure in serious research studies.

Limitations

Technically, the range should probably be defined as the difference between the upper real limit of the largest score minus the lower real limit of the smallest score. Since the range is at best an approximate index of variability, it does not seem appropriate to insist upon this level of accuracy. As evident from Formula 7.1, range takes into account the extremes of the scores only and ignores others, it suffers from the following limitations:

- It is unreliable when N is small or when there are gaps (i.e. zero f's) in the frequency distribution
- A change in the value of either of the highest score or the lowest score leads to a change in its values
- It does not consider the value of the scores between the highest and the smallest scores and does not reflect the change if made in them
- Further statistical analysis are difficult to make.

Range is the difference between the largest and the smallest observations in a set. If we denote the largest observation by L and the smallest observation by S, the formula is:

$$\text{Range} \qquad R = L - S \qquad ...(7.2)$$

A relative measure known as *coefficient of range* is given as,

$$\text{Coefficient of range} = \frac{L - S}{L + S} \qquad ...(7.3)$$

Lesser the range or coefficient of range, better the result.

Properties

- It is the simplest measure and can easily be understood.
- Besides the above merit, it hardly satisfies any property of a good measure of dispersion, e.g. it is based on two extreme values only, ignoring the others. It is not liable to further algebraic treatment.

Example: The population in eighteen panchayat sammities of a district is as given below.

Population ('000 number)

77,	76,	83,	68,	57,	107,	80,	75,	95
100,	113,	119,	121,	121,	83,	87,	46,	74

We can find the range by the formula (7.1)

$$L = 121 \text{ and } S = 46$$

The range, $R = 121 - 46 = 75$

Some people also write the range as, i.e. 46 – 121. Also,

$$\text{Coefficient of range} = \frac{121 - 46}{121 + 46} = \frac{75}{167} = 0.449$$

Uses of Range

However, range can be used with profit in the following situations:

- When a quick and crude estimate of variability is all what is desired.
- When data are too scant or too scattered and a more precise measure of variability is not warranted.
- When the knowledge of only the extreme scores or of total spread is required.
- When the phenomenon is prone to wide fluctuations such as, range of fluctuating temperature of a patient, the daily fluctuating values of a stock and the annual range of temperature values for a particular geographical region.
- When ease of computation is an important consideration.

Although range is easy to compute and its units are the same as the units of the variable being measured, the range does not take into account the number of observations in the sample, only takes into consideration the largest observations and the smallest observation, whatever they may be because people expect large samples to include occasional extreme values and expected a large range. A measure of variability should not depend on the number of observations used in the sample. Observations between the smallest and largest in a set are used only to determine which observations are smallest and largest. Some use of the actual value of interviewing observations seem desirable. The range also suffers from dependants upon extreme observations.

Despite serious limitations, range is useful in the following cases:

- In order to test the quality control of a drug
- In order to check the fluctuations in the blood pressure, temperature, heart rate, pulse rate, respiration of the patients
- Range is used in everyday life, for example to know the maximum and minimum temperature.

For example, Table 7.2 gives hemoglobin level of nursing students.

According to Table 7.2, it is evident that 237 or 61.6 percent nursing students are having a Hb of 11.1 to 13.0 gm. Thus, the Table helps in a quick understanding of the number of persons with particular ranges of Hb level. It can be seen from the table that the hemoglobin level ranges between

Table 7.2

Hemoglobin level of nursing students

Hb level (grams %)	*Number of students*	*Percentage*
9.1 – 10.0	10	2.6
10.1 – 11.0	21	5.5
11.1 – 12.0	67	17.4
12.1 – 13.0	170	44.2
13.1 – 14.0	84	21.8
14.1 – 15.0	29	7.5
15.1 – 16.0	4	1.0
Total	385	100.0

9.1 to 16.0. In other words the minimum or maximum values of the variable are noted in the cases. This measure of the scatter of the values of the variables is known as the range. The range thus gives the two extreme values of the variable, but no information about the values which lie in between the extreme values. This method is simple to comprehend as well as to calculate, but is useful only on certain occasions. Range is misleading when the extreme values are of unusual occurrence.

Range is the interval between the lowest and the highest of the values. Thus range gives the values of the extremes but does not give any information about the values in between the extreme values.

In the above example, the range in team A is 12 and in team B is 28. The values are scattered or dispersed around the mean 86 in both the groups.

Range usually defines the limits of normalcy. However, it will be misleading when the extreme values are of unusual occurrence.

Sometimes, instead of knowing the range between all the observations, it may be necessary to know the range within which a certain percentage of observations lie. Such a range is called "percentile range". For example, the range between Q_1 and Q_3 (Fig. 35.15) includes middle-half of observations in an ordered series. It is also called as "Interquartile range". This give little more information about the distribution of the individual observations than range. It will indicate whether the concentration is more at the extremes or in the middle or the observations are evenly distributed.

The Semi-interquartile Range or Q

Instead of knowing the range between all the observations the person may be interested to know the range within which a certain percentage of observation lies. Such a range is called as the percentile range. Percentile can also be calculated from zero to any percentage of observations. Suppose if we note down the value of the variable covering upto the first 25th percent of the observations, it is called as 75th percentile. Incidentally it may be noted that median is the 50th percentile value of the variable. These three values of the variables are also known as 'quartile', as they divide the distribution into quarters.

Interquartile Range

The difference between the third quartile and first quartile is called interquartile range (IR). Symbolically,

$$IR = Q_3 - Q_1 \quad \text{...(7.4)}$$

Quartile Deviation (QD)

This is half of the interquartile range, i.e.

$$QD = \frac{Q_3 - Q_1}{2} \quad \text{...(7.5)}$$

Also the coefficient of quartile deviation is given by the formula,

$$\text{Coefficient of QD} = \frac{Q_3 - Q_1}{Q_3 + Q_1} \quad \text{...(7.6)}$$

Coefficient of quartile deviation is an absolute quantity (unitless) and is useful to compare the variability among the middle 50 percent observations.

Properties

- It is a better measure of dispersion than range in the sense that it involves 50 percent of the mid values of a series of data rather than only two extreme values of a series.

- Since it excludes the lowest and highest 25 percent values, it is not affected by the extreme values.
- It can be calculated for the grouped data with open end intervals.
- It is not capable of further algebraic treatment.
- It is susceptible to sampling fluctuations.
- This measure does not take into account the individual values occurring between Q_1 and Q_3. It means that no idea about the variation of even 50 percent mid values are available from this measure. Anyhow, it provides some idea if the values are uniformly distributed between Q_1 and Q_3.
- It is not considered a good measure of dispersion as it does not show the scattering of the central value. In fact, it is a measure of partitioning of distribution. Hence, it is not commonly used.

Another measure of variation based on the values of quartile is the quartile deviations or the semi-interquartile deviation. It is one-half of the distance from the third Quartile (Q_3) and the first Quartile (Q_1). One semi-interquartile range is commonly symbolized by 'Q'.

The formula for the semi-interquartile range is:

$$Q = \frac{Q_3 - Q_1}{2} \qquad ...(7.5)$$

This measure gives a little more knowledge about the distribution than does the range. It includes the middle half of the measurements in the series/sets, the distributions being first divided into quarters; using the same principle as is used in calculation of the median.

The semi-interquartile range which is also known as quartile deviation can be defined as half of the difference between the 75th percentile and the 25th percentile. Hence, it is one half the scale between the 75th and 25th percentiles in a frequency distribution. The 25th percentile is Q_1 or the first quartile on the score scale. The 75th percentile is Q_3 or the third quartile on the score scale. Hence, the formula for the calculation of Q is

$$Q = \frac{Q_3 - Q_1}{2} \text{ or } \frac{P_{75} - P_{25}}{2} \qquad ...(7.6)$$

Hence to find out Q_1, it is essential to calculate the values of Q_3 (or P_{75}) and Q_1 (or P_{25}). Their calculation follows the same procedure as the calculation of median as explained in the previous chapter.

These formulas are:

$$Q_1 \text{ (or } P_{25}) = L + \frac{\left(\frac{N}{4_1} - \text{Cum } f_b\right)}{f_q} \times 1 \qquad ...(7.7)$$

$$Q_3 \text{ (or } P_{75}) = L + \frac{\left(\frac{N}{4_1} - \text{Cum } f_b\right)}{f_q} \times I \qquad ...(7.8)$$

In which,

L = The exact lower limit of interval in which the quartile falls

i = The size of the class interval

Cum f_b = Cumulative f below the interval which contains the quartile; f_q = the f on the interval which contains the quartile (Table 7.3).

Calculation of Q_1

Here, L = 9.5; Cum $f_b = 9, f_q = 5$; $i = 5$, N = 50.

Substituting these values in formula (7.7), we have

$$Q_1 = 9.5 + \frac{\left(\frac{50}{4} - 9\right)}{5} \times 5 = 9.5 + 3.5 = 13.00$$

Calculation of Q_3

Here, L = 29.5; Cum $f_b = 37, f_q = 6$; $i = 5$; N = 50

Substituting these values in formula (7.8), we have

$$Q_1 = 29.5 + \frac{\left(3 \times \frac{50}{4} - 37\right)}{6} \times 5$$

$$= 29.50 + 0.42 = 29.92$$

Table 7.3

Calculation of Q_1, Q_3 and quartile deviation

Class interval (1)	*Frequency* (2)	*Cumulative frequency (Cum f)* (3)	
45 – 49	2	50	
40 – 44	3	48	
35 – 39	2	45	
30 – 34	6	43	Q_3 lies in this CI
25 – 29	8	37	
20 – 24	8	29	
15 – 19	7	21	
10 – 14	5	14	Q_1 lies in this CI
5 – 9	9	9	
	N = 50		

Calculation of Q

Substituting the values of Q_1 and Q_3 in formula (7.6), we have:

$$Q = \frac{29.92 - 13.00}{2} = \frac{16.92}{2} = 8.46$$

Properties and Uses of Q or Semi-interquartile Range

- In a distribution which is symmetrical around the mean or when it is normal — Q marks off the 25 percent cases just above and the 25 percent cases just below the median.
- It is a measure of the variability of the middle 50 percent cases and ignores the 25 percent cases in each of the two tails
- It should be used when a measure of dispersion of the concentration of 50 percent of the cases around the median is required
- It should be used when the measure of central tendency to be used is the median
- It is a better measure, when there are scattered or extreme scores which would influence the SD disproportionately
- Q is known as the Probable Error (PE) in a normal distribution.

Mean Deviation or Average Deviation (AD)

Mean deviation (MD) is the average distance between the mean and the scores in the distribution. It is the arithmetic mean of all the deviations when algebraic signs are disregarded.

Mean deviation is the average of difference of the values of items from some average of the series. Such difference is technically described as deviation.

The deviation is defined as the distance of the score from the mean of the distribution. Scores larger than the mean will have positive or plus signs, and those smaller than the mean, negative or minus signs. Scores which coincide with the mean will have zero deviation. Algebraically, deviation can be defined, $x = X - M$ (A deviation of a score from the mean, where X = original score and M = arithmetic mean.

The measures of dispersion discussed so far are not satisfactory in the sense that they lack most of the requirements of a good measure. Mean deviation is a better measure than range and QD.

MD is the average of the absolute deviations taken from a central value, generally the mean or median.

Mean deviation (MD): It is the mean or average of the deviations. The deviation (new value) is obtained by deducting the arithmetic mean from each observations. The average of all the deviations in called as "Mean deviation". It is calculated by the following procedure.

- The "mean" of the observations is calculated.
- Then the mean is subtracted from each of the observations to calculate the deviation.
- The mean (or average) of these deviations is then calculated by totaling the differences from the mean and divide by the number of observations without considering the sign of the deviation, which gives mean deviation.

MD is given by the formula,

$$\text{MD} = \frac{\Sigma |x_i - \bar{x}|}{n}$$

Where MD = mean deviation,

Σ = Summation

|| = vertical bracket (modulus) refers to absolute value, ignoring + or – sign (because if the signs are considered, the total value becomes zero).

x_i = Individual value of observation.

$\bar{x}$ = The mean of observations.

n = Number of observations.

Though calculation of mean deviation is simple and easy, it is not used in statistical analysis being of less mathematical value, particularly in drawing inferences.

Properties

1. Mean deviation removes one main objection of the earlier measures, that it involves each value of the set.
2. It is not affected much by extreme values.
3. Its main drawback is that algebraic negative signs of the deviations are ignored which is mathematically unsound.
4. Mean deviation is minimum when the deviations are taken from median.

Note: If the deviations are taken from mean and the signs of the deviations are taken into consideration, the sum of the deviations is zero, i.e. $Z_i\ (X_i - \bar{X}) = 0$

In calculating mean deviation, people ignore the minus sign of deviation, while taking their total for obtaining the mean deviation. Mean deviation is, thus, obtained as given below:

Mean Deviation

1. From Mean $(\delta \bar{X}) = \dfrac{\Sigma X_i - \bar{X}}{n}$ ...(7.9)

If deviation d or $X_i - \bar{X}$, are obtained from arithmetic mean

Or

Mean deviation

2. From median $(\delta \text{m}) = \dfrac{\Sigma X_i - \text{M}}{n}$ ...(7.10)

If deviation d or X_i – M, are obtained from median

Mean deviation

3. From mode $(\delta \delta_2) = \dfrac{\Sigma X_i - Z}{n}$ ...(7.11)

If deviation d or $X_i - Z$, are obtained from mode, where,

Σ = Summation

δ = Symbol of mean deviation (pronounced as delta)

X_i = ith values of the variable X from score

N = Number of items

$\bar{X}$ = Arithmetic mean or average

M = Median

Z = Mode

d = Deviation for

The mean deviation or average deviation as it is frequently called, is the mean of the sum of the deviations (irrespective of signs) from some measure of central tendency. The mean is usually taken as the standard although the median or mode is sometimes used. Care should always be taken to specify the particular average that is chosen for computing the mean deviation. To illustrate the calculation of the mean deviation, let us consider the following simple series of values:

m, series of values: 2,3,5,7,11,12,13,14,16,17
d, the deviation
from the mean: 8,7,5,3,0,1,2,3,4,6,7

$$\bar{X}\, m = \frac{100}{10} = 10$$

$$\bar{X}\, d = \frac{46}{11} = 4.18$$

It will be observed that the mean of the series was first derived by adding the numbers together and dividing by 10. The deviations of each value from the mean of the series ($\bar{X}\, m = 10$) are indicated in the second line. The mean deviation is the sum of these deviations (disregarding signs) from the mean divided by the number of cases in the series or 46/11 = 4.18.

When the mean deviation is calculated from a frequency distribution the following procedure can be followed:

- Compute the measure of central tendency that is to be used as a standard
- Indicate in a separate column the midpoint of each class-interval in the distribution
- In the next column tabulate the deviations (*d*) from the standard that has been selected to the midpoints of the several class-intervals.
- In the last column tabulate the products of the frequencies of each class-interval times the deviation (*fd*).
- Add the figures in the *fd* column, disregarding signs (Σfd).
- Divide Σfd by the number of cases in the distribution

$$\text{MD} = \frac{\Sigma fd}{\text{N}} \quad ...(7.12)$$

In actual practice it will be found that the mean deviation is of little value and very seldom used in social research. The main justification therefore, in devoting so much space to the mean deviation is to assist the student in obtaining a clearer understanding of the concept of variability and especially the standard deviation, which is much more widely used and is far superior, in every way, to the mean deviation.

It is always better to find the deviation of the individual observations with reference to a certain value in the series of observations and then an average of these deviations. This deviation is usually measured from mean or median, but mean is more commonly used for this measurement. This index of variation is known as the mean deviation or average deviation.

Thus, the mean deviation can be defined as the average of the differences between the mean and each of the values of the observation in the series of data. This is calculated by the following procedure.

First the mean of the observations is calculated. Then the mean is subtracted from each of the observations.

The mean of these deviations is then calculated by averaging all these deviations without considering the sign of the deviation which gives mean deviation.

Mathematically it is written as:

$$\text{MD} = \Sigma \frac{|(\text{X}_1 - \bar{\text{X}})|}{n} \quad ...(7.13)$$

where MD refers to mean deviation
X_1 refers to individual values of the observations in the mean
N is the number of observations
And | | refers to the absolute the value and termed as modulus

The mean deviation of the data of systolic blood pressure given in following example is calculated in Table 7.4.

$$\Sigma|\text{X}_i - \bar{\text{X}}| = 22$$

$$\frac{\Sigma|\text{X}_i - \bar{\text{X}}|}{n} = \frac{22}{10} = 2.2$$

Incidentally, it may be noted that $\Sigma|(\text{X}_i - \bar{\text{X}})|$, i.e. the sum of deviations taking signs into consideration is zero and hence the absolute values of these differences are taken.

Table 7.4

Calculating mean deviation (MD)

X_i	$(X_1–\bar{X})$
115	115–119 = –4
117	117–119 = –2
121	121–119 = +2
120	120–119 = +1
118	118–119 = –1
122	122–119 = +3
123	123–119 = +4
116	116–119 = –3
118	118–119 = –1
120	120–119 = +1

In a grouped data, mean deviation is calculated using the formula:

$$MD = \frac{[\Sigma|(X_i - \bar{X})| f_i]}{n}$$

where X_i refers to the middle point of the class interval and f_i the frequency in the class interval. The other symbols have the usual meaning.

The mean deviation is the average difference between the items in the distribution and the median or mean of the series. It is concerned with the extent to which the values are dispersed about the mean or the mode or the median. It is found by averaging all the deviations from the central tendency. Here these deviations are taken by ignoring the signs. Theoretically, the deviation of items are taken preferably from the median instead of mean or mode, as median the suitable central tendency for calculating deviations.

The advantages of mean deviation include the following:

- It is rigidly defined and easy to compute and understand
- It is less affected by extreme values of variables is compared to SD
- As deviations are taken from central value, comparison about formation of differences can easily be made

The disadvantage of the mean deviation are as follows:

- This method may not give an accurate result. It gives the best result when deviation is from median, but, median is not satisfactory measure when the degree of variability in series is very high
- It is not capable of further algebraic or statistical treatment
- It is not a satisfactory measure. When the deviations are taken from this mode
- It is not suitable when the class intervals are open ended.

Mean deviation is not a commonly used statistic. It will be replaced by standard deviation, which is the commonly used statistics.

Standard Deviation

Standard deviation (SD) is an improvement of the mean deviation. In the calculation of the mean-deviation, the signs of the deviation (+ or –) of the observations from the mean was not taken into consideration. In order to avoid this discrepancy, instead of the actual values of the deviations, the squares of the deviations are considered for calculation and then the average of the squares in taken, which is known as "Variance". As this variance is a square, square-root of the variance is considered as a measure of variation of the observations. The square-root of the variance is known as "Standard deviation".

In otherwords, standard deviation is the square-root of the mean of the squared deviations of the individual observations from the mean. It is also called as "Root mean square deviation".

Of all the measures of dispersion, standard deviation is the most important one, and is the best measure of dispersion of observations. It is most widely used in statistical methodologies. It is one of the important parameters of the standard distributions like normal distribution and skewed (i.e., asymmetrical) distributions, which are described later.

Further, standard deviation is useful in testing of significance or in measurement of correlation between two sets of data and other statistical methodologies (explained below).

It is conventional to represent the standard deviation of a sample by "S" and that of a population by "s" (pronounced as "sigma") and it is expressed in the same unit as that of original observations.

Standard deviation is computed by the following steps:

a. Mean of the observations is calculated.
b. Mean is subtracted from each of the observation to calculate the deviation (i.e., difference of observation).
c. Square the differences of observations (deviations) from the mean, which removes the problem of signs + or –.
d. Total (adding) of the squared values to get "sum of squares".
e. This sum is divided by the number of observations minus one (n = 1) to get "mean-squared deviation", called "Variance".
f. Finally square-root of this variance is obtained to get "root-mean squared deviation", called standard deviation (having squared the original, reverse step of taking square-root must finally be taken).

Formula:

$$SD = \frac{\sqrt{\Sigma(x_i - \bar{x})^2}}{n-1}$$

Where SD = Standard deviation,
$\sqrt{\ }$ = Square root of,
Σ = Summation of,
x_i = Value of each observation,
$\bar{x}$ = mean of observation,
$x_i - \bar{x}$ = Deviation from the mean
n = Number of observations
$n - 1$ = when 'n' is less than 30

The drawbacks of variance are overcome in this measure of dispersion.

Definition: The positive square root of the variance is called standard deviation.

$$SD = \sqrt{\sigma^2} = \sigma \qquad ...(7.14)$$

For a sample,

$$SD = \sqrt{s^2} = s \qquad ...(7.15)$$

In simple words, we can say that standard deviation explains the average amount of variation on either side of the mean.

Example: The pulse rate per minute of 10 students in a class are as follows:

80, 90, 96, 80, 94, 72, 84, 92, 82, 90

Mean of the observations = 86

The standard deviation of the pulse rate for the group is calculated as follows:

x_i	$(x_i - \bar{x})$		Deviation	$(x_i - \bar{x})^2$
80	80-86	=	– 06	36
90	90-86	=	+04	16
96	96-86	=	+10	100
80	80-86	=	–06	36
94	94-86	=	+08	64
72	72-86	=	–14	196
84	84-86	=	–02	04
92	92-86	=	+06	36
82	82-86	=	–04	16
90	90-86	=	+04	16

$$\text{Mean } x = \frac{\Sigma x_i}{n} = \frac{860}{10} = 86 \quad \Sigma x_i - \bar{x} = 520,\ n = 10$$

$$\therefore \quad S = \frac{\sqrt{\Sigma(x_i - \bar{x})^2}}{n-1} = \frac{\sqrt{520}}{9}$$

$$= 57.78 = 7.60 \text{ per minute.}$$

Properties

- Standard deviation is considered to be the best measure of dispersion and is used widely.
- There is however one difficulty with it. If the unit of measurement of variables of two series is not the same, then their variability cannot be compared by comparing the values of standard deviation.
- An empirical relation between QD, MD and SD is,

6 QD = 5 MD = 4 SD ...(7.16)

Measures QD, MD and SD are classified as methods of averaging deviations.

Standard deviation is the most widely used measure of dispersion of series. The concept of standard deviation was introduced by Karl Pearson in 1823. The standard deviation is always computed from the mean. It provides a more refined and statistically important measure of variability than the mean deviation. In the calculation of mean deviation the signs of the deviation of the observations from the mean was not taken into consideration. In order to avoid this discrepancy instead of the actual values of the deviations, if the squares of the deviations are considered for calculations, a quantity known as variance can be calculated by arranging the squares of the above deviation. As this, by quantity in a square root of the variance is considered as a measure of variation of the observations. The square root of variation is known "standard deviation". In other words, standard deviation is the square root of the mean, of the square deviations, of the individual observations from the mean. It is also called as 'root mean square deviation'.

$$\sigma = \frac{\sqrt{\Sigma fd}}{N}$$

The standard deviation is symmetrical by observations SD, but much more frequency by s, the small Greek Letter 's'. The standard deviation measures the absolute dispersion for variability of the greater the standard deviation for the greater will be the magnitude of the deviation of the values from their mean. A small standard deviation means a high degree of uniformity of the observations as well as homogeneity of a series. A large standard deviation means just the opposite.

Variance and Standard Deviation

A more stable index that reflects the degree of variability in a group of scores is the variance and its derivative, the standard deviation.

In a previous section, it was shown that in any frequency distribution, the mean deviation from the mean must be zero. Hence the device to get around the difficulty is to take the square of each deviation from the mean and then to find the average of these squared deviations:

$$\text{Variance, } \sigma^2 = \frac{\Sigma(X - M_x)^2}{N} = \frac{\Sigma X^2}{N} \quad ...(7.17)$$

Here the symbols are Σ = Summation; X = Any raw score; M_x = Mean of X scores; N = Number of cases; X^2 = Square of deviation from the mean; Σ = Greek letter sigma.

In a grouped distribution, for each interval, the deviation of the midpoint from the mean is squared and multiplied by the frequency for that interval. When this has been done for each interval, the average of these products is the variance.

The formula thus becomes:

$$\text{Variance, } \sigma^2 = \frac{\Sigma fx^2}{N} \quad ...(7.18)$$

where f stands for the frequency in each class interval; other symbols, as above.

Standard Deviation is derived from the variance by taking the square root of the latter. The formula for the calculation of the standard deviation is thus as follows:

$$\text{SD or } \sigma = \sqrt{\text{Var}} = \frac{\sqrt{\Sigma x^2}}{N} \quad ...(7.19)$$

(σ, is pronounced as sigma' and used to denote SD).

Although variance is an adequate way of describing the degree of variability in a distribution, it does have one drawback. The variance is a quantity in squared units of measurement. For example, if measurements are taken in inches then the mean is some number of inches and a deviation from the mean is a difference in inches. However, the square of a deviation is a square-inch unit and thus the variance, being a mean squared deviation, must also be in square inches. Thus, the problem of obtaining an index of variability in original units arise. This has been taken care of by further calculating the square root of the mean square deviation. This process converts the index of variation from the square to the linear measure and gives us the root mean square deviation or the standard deviation. Hence, standard deviation is the square of the variance or square root of the mean squared deviation and is an index of variability in the original units.

In the calculation of SD, deviation is always taken from the mean, never from the median or mode. The value of SD is always positive.

Standard deviation has been termed so because it provides a standard unit for measuring distances of various scores from their mean.

The standard deviation (SD) is located on the curve at the point where it changes from concave to convex; approximately 68 percent of all observations will lie within this segment (Fig. 7.1). Furthermore, if one measures off twice the distance, approximately 95 percent of all observations will lie within the enlarged segment. These intervals are known respectively as 1 and 2 standard deviations. Since the segment covering 2 standard deviations embraces 95 percent of the observations it follows that the remaining 5 percent are outside these limits and have a 5 percent probability of occurrence ($p = 0.05$). However, the standard deviation can be calculated from the observations and the steps are as follows:

1. First list the observations and calculate the mean.
2. Alongside the listed observations write the difference between each value in turn and the mean.
3. These figures are now squared and added up, producing the sum of squares.

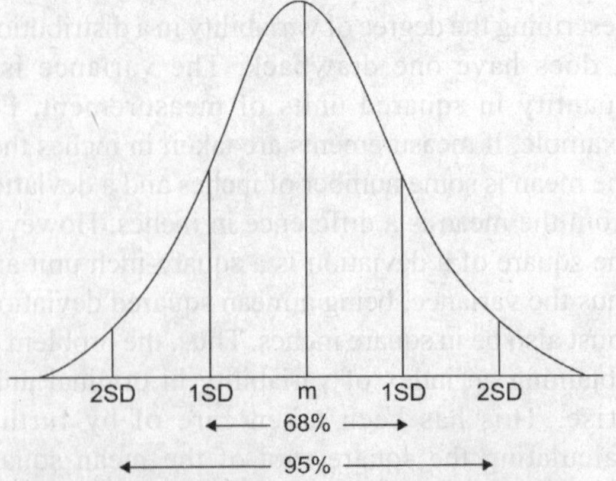

Fig. 7.1: Curve to illustrate standard deviation (SD)

4. This sum of squares is divided by one less than the number of observations to produce the mean sum of squares or variance.
5. By taking the square root of the variance one obtains the standard deviation, which can lie on either side of the mean.

Calculations using the height of ten subjects for standard deviation are shown in Table 7.5. The standard deviation is usually shown as mean $\pm$ 2 SD as follows:

This mean, and the scatter of values around it as described by two standard deviations, is a much better way of expressing the results than just giving the range of values. Also the two values which describe the limits of two standard deviations in either direction from the mean are 95 percent probability limits. Normal values for the laboratory data are commonly expressed in this way. In clinical pharmacology blood levels of drugs from limited number of subjects should also show the standard deviation to give the best idea of the total scatter of results.

Calculation of SD

Methods of Calculating Variance and Standard Deviation from Ungrouped Data

The conceptual definitions of the variance and the SD are based on the formulas which incorporate the deviation soccer method as shown in formulas

Table 7.5

Calculations using the height of ten subjects for determining the standard deviation

Height (in)	*Difference from mean*	*Square*
68	0	0
71	3	9
66	–2	4
60	8	64
67	–1	1
65	–3	9
75	7	49
70	2	4
68	0	0
70	2	4
680		144 = sum of squares

7.11 to 7.13 in this chapter. However, to avoid inconvenience of working with fractional values and when a calculating machine is available, the following formulas which are mathematically equivalent to them are also available. In the example solved below the use of both the types of formulas has been made:

$$\text{Mean } (\bar{x}) = \frac{680}{10} = 68 \text{ in}$$

$$\text{SD} = \sqrt{\sum \frac{(x - x)^2}{n-1}} = 4$$

Mean = 68 in

SD = 4

Therefore 68 ± 8 is mean ± 2SD

Steps in the Computation of SD

Deviation Score Method

- Calculate mean
- Calculate deviation of each score from the mean
- Square each deviation
- Sum of the squared deviation to obtain Σx^2
- Substitute the values in the formula and solve.

Raw Score Method

- List up the scores, X
- Sum up the scores to obtain ΣX
- Square each score
- Sum up the squared scores
- Substitute the values in the formula and solve (Table 7.6).

$$M = \frac{40}{5} = 8$$

N = 5

$$\text{Variance} = \frac{\Sigma X^2}{N}$$

Substituting the values

$$\text{Variance} = \frac{10}{5} = 2$$

$$\sigma = \sqrt{2} = 1.414$$

Formula:

$$\text{Variance} = \Sigma X^2 - \frac{(\Sigma x^2)}{N} \bigg/ N \quad \text{...(7.20)}$$

$$\sigma = \sqrt{\frac{\Sigma x^2 - \frac{(\Sigma x^2)}{N}}{N}} \quad \text{...(7.21)}$$

$$= \sqrt{\frac{330 - \frac{(40)^2}{5}}{5}} = \sqrt{\frac{10}{5}} = \sqrt{2}$$

$$\sigma = \sqrt{2} = 1.414$$

Substituting the values.

Interpretation: The scores, on the average, vary or deviate 1.414 units from their mean.

Table 7.6

Calculation of SD from ungrouped scores

	Deviation score method		*Raw score method*	
Score	*Deviation from the mean (x) X – M(x)*	*Squared deviation x^2*	*Score x*	*Squared Score X^2*
10	+2	4	10	100
7	–1	1	7	49
9	+1	1	9	81
6	–2	4	6	36
8	0	0	8	64
ΣX = 40	(Σx)	$\Sigma x^2 = 10$	40	$\Sigma X^2 = 330$

Calculation of SD from the Grouped Data

When scores are arranged in the form of score bands or class intervals and frequencies are shown against each class interval calculation of SD can be undertaken by using a long method or a short method. Both of these methods are demonstrated below with the help of solved examples.

Long Method

See Table 7.7.

Steps in the Computation of SD by Long Method

- Write down the class intervals and frequencies as shown in Cols 1 and 3
- Find out the midpoint of each class interval
- Calculate mean by using any method described in a previous chapter
- Obtain deviations from mean, (mid-point – mean) as in Col. 4
- Multiply *f* and *x*, [Col. (3) X Col. (4)] to obtain *fx*.
- Multiply *fx* and *x*, i.e. Col. (4) and (5) to obtain fx^2 as in col. (6)
- Sum up Col. (6) to obtain S fx^2.

Short Method

When large values of scores are involved, it is better to use the short method for calculating SD. In this method, like the calculation of mean by the assumed mean method, deviations are taken from the assumed mean (Table 7.8). The detailed procedure is given below:

In which, *i* stands for the size of class interval; and C, for correction.

Here: $i = 5$; $\Sigma fx^2 = 256$; $N = 50$; and

$$C = \frac{\Sigma fx}{N}$$

Substituting the values in the formula

$$C^2 = \left(\frac{4}{50}\right)^2 = 0.0064$$

$$\sigma = \sqrt{\frac{256 - 0.0064}{50}} = 11.31$$

Table 7.7

Calculation of SD by long method (using real mean)

Class interval (1)	*Mid point* *X* (2)	*Frequency* *f* (3)	*Deviation of (X) from mean* *x* (4)	*fx* (5)	*fx²* (6)
45–49	47	2	24.6	49.2	1210.32
40–44	42	3	19.6	58.8	1152.48
35–39	37	2	14.6	29.2	426.23
30–34	32	6	9.6	57.6	552.96
25–29	27	8	4.6	36.8	169.28
20–24	22	8	–.40	–3.2	1.28
15–19	17	7	–5.40	–37.8	204.12
10–14	12	5	–10.40	–52.0	540.80
5–9	7	9	–15.40	–138.6	2134.44
Mean = 22.40	N = 50				6392.00

$$\sigma = \sqrt{\frac{\Sigma fx^2}{N}} = \sqrt{\frac{6392.00}{50}} = \sqrt{12784} = 11.31$$

Table 7.8

Calculation of SD by Short Method (Deviations taken from Assumed Mean)

Class interval	*Mid-point*	*Frequency*	*Deviation of (X) from Mean*			
	X	*f*	*x*	x^2	*fx*	fx^2
(1)	*(2)*	*(3)*	*(4)*	*(5)*	*(6)*	*(7)*
45 – 49	47	2	5	25	10	50
40 – 44	42	3	4	16	12	48
35 – 39	37	2	3	9	6	18
30 – 34	32	6	2	4	12	24
25 – 29	27	8	1	1	8	8
20 – 24	22	8	0	0	0	0
15 – 19	17	7	–1	1	–7	7
10 – 14	12	5	–2	4	–10	20
5 – 9	7	9	–3	9	–27	81
		50 (N)		$\Sigma x^2 = 69$	4 (Σfx)	256 (Σfx^2)

Computational Steps

- Arrange the scores and *f's* as in Cols. (1) and (3)
- Find out the midpoints of all the class intervals and write in Col. (2)
- Take a midpoint as an assumed mean. This point should be close to the middle of the distribution and as far as possible should have the largest *f's*
- Deviations (x) are taken from the assumed mean (here, 22) in units of class interval. It can be a mechanical process. Assign 0 to the class interval in which the assumed mean lies. Go on assigning +1, +2, +3, etc. to the class intervals above the mean and –1, –2, –3, etc. to those below the mean (Col. 4).
- Multiply cols. (3) and (4) to obtain *fx* and sum up to obtain $\Sigma fx'$
- Multiply cols. (4) and (5) to obtain fx^2 and sum up to obtain Σfx^2
- Find out the value of C which is $\frac{\Sigma fx^2}{N}$
- Substitute these values in the formula and solve

Some other formulas for the calculation of SD are given below:

$$\sigma = \frac{\sqrt{\Sigma X^2 - M^2}}{N} \quad ...(7.22)$$

$$\sigma = \frac{\sqrt{N\Sigma X^2 - (\Sigma X)^2}}{N} \quad ...(7.23)$$

The symbols are as explained in the previous formulas.

Note: When sample SD is to be used as an estimate of the population SD, the denominator of the formulas will have N – 1, instead of N, as the former is considered as an unbiased estimate.

Properties and Uses of Variance and SD as Measures of Variability

- The variance of proportional to the average squared deviation of each score form every other score. Hence, it indeed reflects the variability of the scores
- Since all deviations are squared, the variance will always be positive. The SD is the positive

square root of variance and hence will always be positive

- If there is no variability among the scores, that is, all the scores in the distribution are identical, the value of variance and also of SD will be zero. As variability of scores increases and the scores of SD increases
- Variance and SD are more sensitive to variability in a group of scores and are less variable in themselves
- The variance and SD are frequently used in other statistical analysis and manipulation and hence are more important than the other measures of variability
- The variance can be partitioned into different parts attributed to different sources and hence find its' use in analysis of multivariate factorial designs
- Variance and SD is used when statistic of the greatest stability is sought
- Variance and SD should be used when extreme deviations are likely to exercise a proportionally greater effect upon the variability.

Example of Calculations of SD

The standard deviation, like the mean deviation, represents a mean of deviation items. It is different, however from the mean deviation in that the deviations are squared before being assumed, the sum of the squared deviations is divided by the total number of observations (cases) in the distribution and the square root is extracted from this quotient. The standard deviation is always computed from the mean, whereas the mean deviation may be computed from the mean, the median or sometimes the mode. Algebraically these steps may be represented by the following formula:

$$\sigma = \frac{\sqrt{\Sigma fd}}{N} \quad ...(7.24)$$

In computing the standard deviation from a frequency distribution, the following procedure is the one most generally used. It is known as the short method:

- It will be observed from the illustrative problem in Table 7.9 that the first column contains the class-intervals and the second column, the frequencies. The total number of cases (N) is 265.
- Select as an arbitrary origin, the interval in which the mean is most likely to occur and mark off the deviations in terms of intervals above (plus) and below (minus), the assumed mean. The interval 140 to 149 was chosen as the zero interval.
- Multiply the frequency of each class by its corresponding deviation (*fd*) and enter the products in the fourth column. Find Σfd. The procedure thus far is identical with that followed in computing the mean.
- In the fifth column tabulate the products of (*fd*) (*d*), that is, the fd^2 values.
- Obtain Σfd^2. It will be observed that there are never any minus quantities in the fd^2 column. In the problem, $\Sigma fd^2 = 931$.
- The correction (c), which is $\Sigma fd/N$, is squared. In the problem,

$$\frac{\Sigma fd}{N} = \frac{99}{265} = 0.374 \text{ and } (0.374)^2 = 0.1396$$

It will be observed that c is expressed in terms of the class-interval and not in the original scale unit.

- The next step is to make the proper substitutions in the complete formula of the standard deviation.

$$\sigma = \frac{\sqrt{\Sigma fd}}{N} = C^2 \quad ...(7.25)$$

It will be observed that C^2 is always subtracted. After the calculations have been made under the radical sign, the square root is extracted and the results multiplied by the size of the class-interval (i). In the illustration in Table 7.8 the standard deviation is 18.4. In order to check the accuracy of the calculations a different guessed mean can be chosen and the problem recomputed accordingly.

Table 7.9

Calculation of the standard deviation(s). Data represent weights of 265 nursing students at the Rajarajeswari College of Nursing, Bengaluru, Karnataka, India

Class interval (Weight)	*f*	*d*	*fd*	*fd²*
90 – 99	1	–5	–5	25
100 – 109	1	–4	–4	16
110 – 119	9	–3	–27	81
120 – 129	30	–2	–60	120
130 – 139	42	–1	–42	42
140 – 149	66	0	0	0
150 – 159	47	1	47	17
160 – 169	39	2	78	156
170 – 179	15	3	45	135
180 – 189	11	4	44	176
190 – 199	1	5	5	25
200 – 209	3	6	18	108
N = 265			Σ*fd* = 99	Σ*fd*² = 931

$$\sigma = \sqrt{\frac{\Sigma fd^2}{N} - \left(\frac{\Sigma fd}{N}\right)^2} \quad \text{(i)}$$

$$= \left(\sqrt{\frac{931}{265} - \left(\frac{99}{265}\right)^2}\right)(10)$$

$$= \left(\sqrt{3.5132 - 0.1396}\right)(10)$$

$$= \left(\sqrt{3.5132}\right)(10)$$

$$= (1.8367)(10)$$

$$= 18.37 \text{ or } 18.4$$

Relationship Between Sum of Squares, Variance and SD

The concepts of sums of squares (Σx^2), variance (V), and standard deviation (SD), are very closely related with each other. These concepts are also very important in all statistical work. Hence, this section is devoted to explain them.

In verbal terms, a standard deviation is the square root of the arithmetic mean of the squared deviations of scores from their mean. It can thus rightly be termed as *root-mean-square-deviation.* Consider Table 7.8 shown. In column (4), we have the deviations of each score from the mean. The sum of these deviations is always zero. In column (5), we have the squares of these deviations (x^2). The sum of these squared deviations (Σx^2), is briefly called as *sum of squares,* From the formula, variance is 12.57; the SD is the square root of variance which in this case is:

$$\text{SD} = \sqrt{12.57} = 3.55$$

A geometrical representation of the above ideas is shown, as usual, in the form of a straight line extending from left to right. The original score values have also been marked below the relevant points. The mean score of 12 has been shown as deviation equal to zero and taken as the main reference point. All seven persons have been shown to retain their relative positions, in correct rank order and at the same separations as in original scores.

The deviations have been represented by linear distances. Hence, the squared deviations as shown have been represented in terms of *areas* namely squares.

The sum of squares would be represented geometrically as an area equal to a composite of all the squares. This could also be shown as a square or as a rectangle. Its surface will have 88 units, each unit equal in size to those representing persons C and E. The apportioning of the total area (Σx^2) equally among the seven individuals amounts to taking the arithmetic mean of it. The baseline of this square has units equal to those in the larger diagram (Fig. 7.2). The length of its side is the square root of its area and represents the standard deviation. The inter-relationships of sum of squares, variance and standard deviation can also be shown algebraically as follows:

Standard deviation, $\sigma = \sqrt{\frac{\Sigma X^2}{N}} = \sqrt{V}$

$$\text{Variance} = \frac{\Sigma X^2}{N} = \sigma^2 \qquad \text{...(7.26)}$$

Sum of squares, $\Sigma X^2 = NV = N\sigma^2$

Both V and s are indicators of amount of variability or dispersion in a distribution. V or σ^2 is said to measure variance and *s*, to measure variability. V and σ also form familiar indicators of the extent of individual differences which form the basis of all psychological and educational testing.

Applications of SD

1. A standard deviation (SD) is the universally accepted unit of dispersion of values from the mean value (*x*).

 In a normal distribution series, a confidence interval of $\bar{x} \pm 1$ SD encloses 68.27 percent values, an interval of $\bar{x} \pm 2$ SD encloses 95.45 percent values and an interval of $\bar{x} \pm 3$ SD encloses 99.73 percent values, for purpose of simplicity, a confidence limit of X + 2SD is treated as including 95 percent values. In other words, six standard deviations, three on either side of the mean cover almost the entire range of a quantitative series (explained under "normal curve").
2. SD summarises the variation of a large distribution in one figure and defines the normal limits of variation.
3. SD measures the position or distance of observation from the mean (i.e., to measure individual variability).
4. SD indicates whether the variation of difference of an individual from the mean is by chance (natural or real) due to some special reasons.
5. SD is used to calculate Standard Error (SE) of mean and SE of difference between two means.
6. SD helps in finding the size of the sample.
7. SD is used for calculation of "relative deviate" or "Z score". It is the difference of a specific observation from the mean in terms of the SD. Its formula is:

$$Z = \frac{x - \text{mean}}{SD}$$

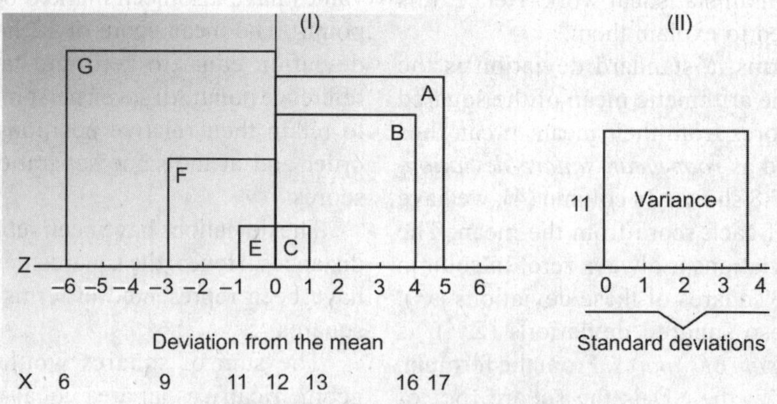

Fig. 7.2: Comparison of standard deviation and variance

where Z = relative deviate,
x = the observation in question;
Example: The mean height of college students is 150 cms with SD of 10 cms. A particular student's height is 165 cms. Z-score (relative variate) of his height is calculated as follows:

$$Z = \frac{165 - 150}{10} = \frac{15}{10} = 1.5 \text{ cms}$$

8. SD is used in the calculation of "coefficient of variation" (CV)

$$CV = \frac{SD}{Mean} \times 100$$

Relationship between the Mean Deviation, Standard Deviation, and Semi-Interquartile Range

It will be recalled that the mean, median and mode represent points or values on the X-scale and that the average deviation, standard deviation and semi-interquartile range represent distances on the X-scale. In a normal frequency distribution: (1) What proportion of the area or the cases is included within the limits of the respective measures of variability? (2) What is the relationship between the average deviation, the standard deviation and the semi-interquartile range? In a perfectly normal distribution the AD (X or X ± AD) defines the limits of the middle 57.5 percent of the cases; the *s* (X ± σ) marks the range of the middle 68.26 percent of the cases; and the Q (X ± Q) indicates the middle 50 percent of the items.

It will be observed that in a perfectly symmetrical distribution, or in a distribution that varies from this type only moderately, the mean deviation is approximately four-fifths of the standard deviation and the semi-interquartile range is about two-thirds of the standard deviation.

Table 7.10 presents more exactly the relationship between these three measures of variability.

As an illustration for interpreting a measure of variability let us take the standard deviation of the distribution in Table 7.11.

Table 7.10

Relationship between the mean deviation, standard deviation, and semi-interquartile range as found in normal frequency distributions

Measure	*Relationship*
σ	1.2533 AD
σ	1.4825 Q
AD	0.7979 σ
AD	1.1843 Q
Q	0.6745 σ
Q	0.8453 AD

The standard deviation was found to be 18.4. In a perfectly normal distribution the standard deviation, when measured off above and below the mean, includes within this range approximately 68.26 percent of the cases in the distribution. This fact is also approximately true for distribution which are almost normal.

Coefficient of Variation

The standard deviation of any two quantitative groups (series) in the same group, cannot be compared if the attributes are different (like SD of Ht and SD of Wt) and even if the values pertain to the same attribute (like height only) comparison can not be made if the units of measurement are different in the two groups, for example cms and inch. This limitation of SD is satisfactorily removed by converting standard deviation into "coefficient of variation" (CV).

All the measures of dispersion discussed so far have units. If two series differ in their units of measurement, their variability cannot be compared by any measure given so far. Also, the size of measures of dispersion depends upon the size of values. Hence in situations where either the two series have different units of measurements, or their means differ sufficiently in size, the coefficient of variation should be used as a measure of dispersion. It is a unitless measure of dispersion and also takes into account the size of the means of the two series. It is the best measure to compare

Table 7.11

Data illustrating sum of square (Σx^2), variance (V) and standard deviation (SD)

Person	*Score x*	*Deviations x*	*Deviations squared x^2*
(1)	*(2)*	*(3)*	*(4)*
A	17	+5	25
B	16	+4	16
C	13	+1	1
D	12	0	0
E	11	−1	1
F	9	−3	9
G	6	−6	36
Sum	84	$0 = \Sigma x$	$88 = \Sigma x^2$
Mean	12.0	0.0	12.57 = V
Standard deviation			$3.55 = \sigma$

Table 7.12

Means, standard deviations and coefficients of variation of the age distributions of four groups of mothers who gave birth to one or more children in the city from 2001 to 2005

Classification	$\bar{X}$	σ	*CV*
Arranged married mother	28.2	6.0	21.3
Not arranged married mother	29.5	6.0	20.3
Unmarried mother	23.4	5.8	24.8
Unwed unmarried	21.7	3.7	17.1

the variability of two series or sets of observations. A series with less coefficient of variation is considered more consistent or stable.

Coefficient of variation of a series of variate values is the ratio of the standard deviation to the mean multiplied by 100.

If σ is the standard deviation and $\bar{X}$ is the mean of the set of values, the coefficient of variation is,

$$CV = \frac{\sigma}{\bar{X}} \times 100 \quad ...(7.27)$$

This measure was given by Professor Karl Pearson.

Note: In case of sample studies, we use s, the sample SD and x, the sample mean instead of σ and $\bar{X}$ respectively.

The CV is the standard deviation expressed as the "percentage of the mean". Thus while SD is expressed in different units of measurement, coefficient of variation is an unitless number. Therefore CV is well suited for all types of dissimilar measurements such as Ht and Wt or Hb and Wt or pulse rate and midarm circumference.

Formula:

$$CV = \frac{SD \times 100}{Mean}$$

As an example, the variation of Hb level of a group of persons and the variation of their body weight, which are expressed in different units like gm percent and kgs respectively, will have different means and different standard deviation. Coefficient of variation helps to compare the deviations in two sets of dissimilar measurements in the same group or one character in two groups.

Example 1: Example for two characters in the same group. The mean and standard deviation of Hb level of a group is 12.6 gm percent and 1.5 gm percent respectively while the mean and standard deviation of the body weight of the same group is 50 kgs and 2.2 kg respectively.

To compare the deviations of these two sets of observations coefficient of variation is calculated for each data.

$$\text{CV of Hb level} = \frac{1.5 \times 100}{12.6} = 11.9\%$$

$$\text{CV of body weight} = \frac{2.2 \times 100}{50} = 4.4\%$$

It is seen that the variation is greater for Hb level than for body weight of the same group.

Example 2: Example for one character in two groups. In two series of boys and girls of the same age of 20 years, following values were obtained for the height. Find which sex shows greater variation.

Sex	*Mean Ht (cms)*	*SD (cm)*
Boys	163.25	6.25
Girls	150.35	5.25

$$\text{CV of boys} = \frac{6.25}{163.25} \times 100 = 3.83\%$$

$$\text{CV of girls} = \frac{5.25}{150.35} \times 100 = 3.49\%$$

Thus it is seen that the height in boys shows slightly greater variation than in girls being in the ratio of 3.83:3.49 = 1.1:10.

Properties

- It is one of the most widely used measure of dispersion because of its virtues.
- Smaller the value of CV, more consistent are the data and vice versa. Hence, a series with smaller CV than the CV of other series is more consistent, i.e. it possesses less variability.
- For field experiments, CV is generally reported. If CV is low, it indicates more reliability of experimental findings.
- It is a relative measure of variability.

The mean deviation, the standard deviation, and the semi-interquartile range represent measures of absolute variability. It is also frequently necessary to measure the relative variability of two or more frequency distribution. Table 7.12 is listed the respective mean ages, standard deviations and coefficients of variation of four groups of women who gave birth to one or more children in one of the city during the five-year period 2001 to 2005.

Which group shows the relatively highest degree of variability and which the least? By merely examining the standard deviations it would be impossible to say. When, however, the standard deviations of the several distributions are related to their corresponding means, it is possible to determine the relative amount of variability of a number of frequency distributions. Karl Pearson has worked out a simple measure of relative variability which is generally known as the coefficient of variation.

$$\text{CV or V} = \frac{\sigma}{X}\ \frac{(100)}{1}$$

In Table 7.12, it will be seen that the unwed unmarried mothers show the least relative variability (17.1) in age and the unmarried, the highest (24.8). The coefficient of variation for the problem in Table 7.8 is:

$$\text{CV} = \left(\frac{18.367}{148.736}\right)\left(\frac{100}{1}\right) = 12.3\%$$

EXERCISES

1. What does variation indicate about the data? Why is this important?
2. Which measures of variation do you consider the best and why?
3. Define and discuss the following:
   a. Range b. Quartile deviation c. Mean deviation
   d. Variance e. Coefficient variates
4. Explain why standard deviation is considered supreme to the other measures of variations.
5. Discuss the relative merits of range, standard deviation and mean deviations.
6. What is meant by variation? What are the methods of computing measure of variation? Illustrate the presented utility of these methods.

CHAPTER 8 Probability

Introduction

The word 'Probable' is used very commonly in everyday language to denote something which is very likely or has a very good chance to happen. People use the word probability in conversation, have a vague idea about its meaning. Such vague and general description is not of much help to quantify the chance of occurrence of an event. It needs a more precise definition to quantify chance. The concept of probability fills this need adequately.

The concept of 'Probability' is used widely in biological science, including medical and nursing sciences. It is used in the presentation of research findings as well as in drawing conclusions. For example, a nurse researcher works to make inferences or draw conclusions from experimental data. This process is not simple and straight forward because the experimental results pertain to a particular experiment or sample, whereas, the inferences made from samples have an element of uncertainty associated with it. However, knowledge and action of researcher to a large extent is based on inferences made from studies of sample. This is true in everyday life as well as in scientific research. An understanding and application of the concepts of probability will help the interpretation of the statistics in skillful way.

Probability theory originated from gambling theory. A large number of events/sports exist even today which are based on the game of chance. Few of these are spinning a roulette wheel, throwing dice, tossing a coin, playing cards, etc. Here the outcome of a trail is unpredictable. However, it is recognized that even though the outcome of any particular trail may be uncertain, there is a predictable long-term outcome. The utility of probability in business and economics is most emphatically revealed in the predications of future. People can anticipate consequences of the each of these plans and finally it helps for comparing the results.

Uncertainty plays an important role in business and probability is a concept which measures the degree of uncertainty and that of certainty also as a corollary. In the same way uncertainty and probability are also very useful in the field of health sciences, including nursing. For example, it is uncertain whether an offspring will be a male or a female, but in the long run it is known approximately what percent of offspring's will be males and what percent what will be females. The long-term regularity provides us with a measure of the amount of chance to a particular trail in the subject. This measure of chance is denoted as Probability. Now probability has become a fundamental tool of scientific thinking. In general, the interpretation of experiments is in probabilistic terms.

Definition

Probability is the chance of occurrence of certain events when expressed quantitatively. The probability of a given event is an expression of likelihood or chance of occurrence of an event. The chance is measured on a probability scale having zero at one end and unity at the other. The top end of the scale marked unity represents an absolute certainty. The bottom end scale marked zero, represents "absolute impossibility". The other points on the probability scale falling between '0' and '1' would indicate the relative chance of occurrence of the outcome. So a probability is a number which ranges from 0–1. Zero (0) for an event which cannot occur and one (1) for an event that is certain to occur. How the number assigned would depend on the interpretation of the term 'Probability', however, its interpretation is associated with nebulous and mystic ideas.

Probability can be defined in three approaches:

- Subjective or personalistic approach
- Mathematical approach
- Statistical approach.

1. *Subjective approach* is based on the statement. For example: The probability is high that terrorists may attack Bengaluru because attacks have happened in Hyderabad, Mumbai, and Jaipur.
2. *Mathematical approach* is that probability of an event which can be defined as the ratio of the number of cases for the particular event to the total number of cases both favorable and unfavorable to this event. For example considering the event of enumerating the persons who had an attack of a disease in a community. The probability of coming across a person with the history of attack of the disease is the ratio of the number of persons with the history of attack to the total number of persons in the community. Thus,

   Probability of any event

   $$= \frac{\text{Number of favorable cases of the event}}{\text{Total number of cases}}$$

   This denoted as $P(A) = \frac{n}{N}$. ...(8.1)
3. *Statistical approach*: This is the empirical relative frequency approach considering relative frequencies as the basis of predictions. If a series of 'N' trails is male and given event occurs 'n' times, then $\frac{n}{N}$ is the relative frequency. The relative frequency in a sample observation is an estimate of that parameter.

The three approaches stated above to probability are not incompatible. All three, must of necessity and coexist. While the personalistic probability may be an interesting topic of psychological inquiry, the other two approaches are widely used in statistical work, the relative frequency approach, being the complement of the formal mathematical one.

Probability means a chance factor for the occurrence of a specific event e.g. Chances of winning a lottery, chances of being selected, chances of getting a male child in the first pregnancy etc. This chance factor is associated with uncertainty, because information in the happenings is not available. This uncertainty or mathematical quantity which depends upon the occurrence of the favorable or unfavorable event, is numerically expressed as "probability".

The probability of a particular event can be defined as the ratio of the number of favorable cases for the particular event to the total number of cases both favorable and unfavorable to the particular event.

For example, if the probability of a patient leaving the hospital against medical advice during a year's time is to be computed, then this will be the ratio of the number of patients (n) who left the hospital against medical advice during a year's time to the total number of patients (N) admitted to the hospital during that year.

$$\text{Formula} = P = \frac{n}{N} = \frac{\text{Number of favorable cases}}{\text{Total number of both favorable and unfavorable cases}}$$

Example: Suppose there are 100 students in a class, 90 boys and 10 girls, then the probability of a student chosen at random to be a girl is

$$= \frac{\text{Number of girls in the class (n)}}{\text{Total number of students (both boys and girls) N}} = \frac{10}{90+10}$$

$$= \frac{10}{100} = 0.1$$

The probability scale varies from the lowest value "0" (zero) to the highest value "1" (one). In other words if none of the cases are favorable, i.e. when the numerator is zero, then the probability of the event will be zero on the contrary, if all the cases are favorable for the event, then both the numerator (n) and the denominator (N) will be equal, then the probability of that event will be 1. As in the above example, if there are no girl students and all are boys, then the probability of a student to be a girl in zero and the probability of a student to be a boy is one. Thus zero indicates no occurrence and one implies 100 percent certainty.

When there are only two complimentary events of occurrence, then the probability of one event will be equal to (1-probability of the other event).

As seen in the above example, the probability of selecting a boy at random.

$$= \frac{90}{100} = 0.9$$

= (1 – probability of selecting a girl)
= (1 – 0.1)

The probability of an event becomes more and more consistent when the number of observations is increased.

Basic Notions

The concepts which are basic to the understanding of probability are described below:

In day-to-day life, one comes across many statements which create doubt about certain happenings and one may want to determine the chance of occurrence of a particular happening, e.g. if one desires to know the chance of rain based on some meteorological observations. In the case of coin tossing, one wants to know what will be the chance of winning if a person always stakes for head in a fixed number of tossings; in the game of bridge what is the chance that a hand will have all the aces. For a production unit one wants to know what would be the chance of a defective item being manufactured. There can be unnumberable such queries which one would like to make and meanwhile evaluate mathematically the chance of the occurrence of such possibilities. This invoked the need of probability theory. The theory of probability came into existence when problems of games were referred to mathematicians like Karl Pearson, Laplace and others.

If an experiment or trial can be repeated any number of times under similar conditions and it is possible to enumerate the total number of outcomes, but an individual outcome is not predictable, such an experiment is called a *random experiment*. For instance, if a fair coin is tossed three times, it is possible to enumerate all the possible eight sequences of head (H) and tail (T). But, it is not possible to predict which sequence will occur at any occasion. This is one example of a random experiment. Many more can be thought of.

Each conceivable outcome of a random experiment under consideration is said to be a sample point. The totality of all conceivable sample point is called a *sample space*. Sample space of a trial conducted by three tossings of a coin is, HHH, HHT, HTH, HTT, THH, THT, TTH, TTT.

In the above experiment it is simple to note that anyone sequence of H and/or T is a sample point whereas all the possible eight sample points constitute the sample space.

Any subset of the sample space is an *event*. In other words, the set of sample points which satisfy certain requirement(s) is called an event.

For example, in the event, that there are exactly two heads in three tossings of a coin, it would consist of three points HTH, HHT and THH.

Possible Outcomes

In tossing a coin, the number of possible outcomes are two—either a head or a tail, i.e. H or T. In tossing two coins, the four possible outcomes are:

First coin	*Second coin*	*Description*	*Symbols*
Head	Head	Both coins heads	HH
Head	Tail	First coin head, Second tail	HT
Tail	Head	First coin tail, Second head	TH
Tail	Tail	Both coins tails	TT

Similarly, in tossing three coins, the possible outcomes are:

HHH, HHT, HTH, THH, HTT, THT, TTH, and TTT.

When a die is thrown, the possible outcomes are six: 1, 2, 3, 4, 5, 6.

When two dice are thrown, the number of possible outcomes are 36 and can be listed as shown in Table 8.1.

In drawing a single card from a deck of 52 cards the number of possible outcomes are 52. But in drawing one card from one deck of 52 cards and another card from a different deck, the possible outcomes are 52 × 52 = 2,704.

With most coins, dice and cards, the basic assumption of equal likelihood of all possible outcomes is justifiable. The truth of the statement can be checked by experiment (Table 8.2). The probability of an event is denoted by *P* (event). For instance, the probability of one head in the one coin example will be *P* (H), and of one tail *P* (T).

Probability can be regarded as the ratio of the number of favorable cases to the total number of equally likely cases. The following examples may be viewed with profit (Table 8.2).

The total probability for all the possible events as shown above is always unity or 1.00 and can be obtained by adding up the probabilities of the individual events. We may also remember that the probability of an event occurring plus that it will not occur also equals 1.00 if no third possibility was there. In the above examples, we were able to deduce the probabilities associated with the given events, on the basis of the equally likely cases. However, sometimes the estimation of the probability requires the empirical approach. For example, to know the probability of a person chosen at random from the population of Bengaluru to be over 50 years of a age would require the use of census data.

Classical Definition

This definition of probability is credited to Laplace. If there are N mutually exclusive and equally likely outcomes of a random experiment, and out of these N outcomes, only *n* are favorable to an attribute, i.e. *n* sample points constitute an event E under consideration, the probability of the event E is,

$$P(E) = \frac{n}{N} \quad \text{...(8.2)}$$

Table 8.1

List of 36 possible outcomes when two dice are thrown

*I	II	I	II	I	II	I	II	I	II	I	II
1	1	2	1	3	1	4	1	5	1	6	1
1	2	2	2	3	2	4	2	5	2	6	2
1	3	2	3	3	3	4	3	5	3	6	3
1	4	2	4	3	4	4	4	5	4	6	4
1	5	2	5	3	5	4	5	5	5	6	5
1	6	2	6	3	6	4	6	5	6	6	6

*I and II stand for first and second dice.

Table 8.2

Calculation of probability in different situations

Event	*Number of favorable cases*	*Total number Equally likely*	*Probability Col. (2)/Col. (3)*
One coin example			
One head	1	2	½ = 0.5
One tail	1	2	½ = 0.5
			Total = 1.0
Two coins example			
Two heads	1	4	¼ = 0.25
Two tails	1	4	¼ = 0.25
One head, one tail	2	4	2/4 = 0.50
			Total = 1.00
Three coins example			
Three heads	1	8	1/8 = 0.125
Three tails	1	8	1/8 = 0.125
Two heads, one tail	3	8	3/8 = 0.375
One head, two tails	3	8	3/8 = 0.375
			Total = 1.00
One die example			
Number 1	1	6	1/6 = 0.167
Number 2	1	6	1/6 = 0.167
Number 3	1	6	1/6 = 0.167
			Total = 0.167

In the trial of tossing a coin three times, N = 8 and for the event E that there are exactly two heads, n = 3. It means that there are only three points favorable to E. Thus, the probability of event E is 3/8. Similarly if for the event E_1 if there are at least two heads in tossing up 3 coins, n = 4. The probability of the event E_1 is 4/8, i.e. 1/2. Students will come across a number of examples later in this chapter.

The above definition of probability is widely used, but it cannot be applied under the following situations:

- If it is not possible to enumerate all the possible outcomes for an experiment.
- If the sample points (outcomes) are not mutually independent.
- If the total number of outcomes is infinite.
- If each and every outcome is not equally likely.

It is clear that the above drawbacks of a classical approach restrict its use in practical problems. Yet this is still widely used for problems concerning the flipping of coin(s), throwing of dice, games of cards and roulette wheel, etc. The probability by classical approach cannot be discovered in the situations like an electric bulb will fuse before it is used for 100 hours, a patient will die if operated for an ailment, a student will fail in a particular examination. Some of the drawbacks of a classical probability are removed in another definition given below, i.e. statistical definition.

Example for the classical definition of probability: If an experiment has n mutually extensive, equally likely and exhaustive cases, out of which m are favorable to the happening of the event A, then the probability of the happening of A is denoted by P(A) and is defined as:

$$P(A) = \frac{m}{N} = \frac{\text{Number of cases favorable to A}}{\text{Total (exhaustive) number of cases}}$$

N = Total (exhaustive) number of cases

Example: What is the probability of getting an even number in a single throw with a dice?

The possible cases in the throw of a dice are six, viz., 1, 2, 3, 4, 5, 6.

Favorable cases are those which are marked with 2, 4, 6 and these are three in number.

$\therefore$ Probability of getting an even number $= \frac{3}{6} = \frac{1}{2}$.

Notes:

1. Probability of an event which is certain to occur is I and the probability of an impossible event is zero.
2. The probability of occurrence of any event lies between 0 and 1, both inclusive.

Example: What is the probability of getting tail in a throw of a coin?

When we toss a coin, there are two possible outcomes viz., Head or Tail. In this case the number of possible cases $n = 2$.

Number of favorable cases $= m = 1$.

($\therefore$ The outcome of tail is a favorable event)

$\therefore$ Probability of getting a tail $= \frac{m}{n} = \frac{1}{2}$

Example: A bag contains 6 white balls, 9 black balls. What is the probability of drawing a black ball?

The total number of equally likely and exhaustive cases $= n = 6 + 9 = 15$.

Number of favorable cases $= m = 9$.

($\therefore$ Number of black balls = 9)

$\therefore$ Probability of drawing a black ball $= \frac{9}{15} = \frac{3}{5}$

Example: What is the probability that if a card is drawn at random from an ordinary pack of cards, it is (i) a red card, (ii) a club, (iii) one of the court cards (Jack or Queen or King)?

Number of exhaustive cases = 52.

(i) There are 26 red cards and 26 black cards in an ordinary pack.

$\therefore$ Favorable cases $= n = 26$ (number of red cards)

$\therefore$ Probability of getting a red card $= \frac{26}{52} = \frac{1}{2}$

(ii) Number of clubs in a pack = 13

$\therefore$ Favorable cases = 13

$\therefore$ Probability of getting a club $= \frac{13}{52} = \frac{1}{4}$

(iii) There are $4 \times 3 = 12$ court cards in a pack of cards

$\therefore$ Number of favorable cases $= m = 12$.

Number of exhaustic cases $= n = 52$.

$\therefore$ Probability of getting a court card

$$= \frac{12}{52} = \frac{3}{13}$$

Example: What is the probability that a leap year, selected at random, will have 53 Sundays?

There are 366 days in a leap year and it has 52 complete weeks and 2 days over. These two extra days can occur in following possible ways:

i. Sunday and Monday
ii. Monday and Tuesday
iii. Tuesday and Wednesday
iv. Wednesday and Thursday
v. Thursday and Friday
vi. Friday and Saturday
vii. Saturday and Sunday

$\therefore$ Number of exhaustive cases = 7.

$\therefore$ Number of favorable cases = 2.

($\therefore$ There are two cases which have Sunday [(i) and (vii)]

$\therefore$ Probability $= \frac{2}{7}$

Example: A card is drawn from an ordinary pack of playing cards and a person bets that it is a spade or an ace. What are the odds against his winning this bet?

In a pack of 52 cards, 1 card can be drawn in 52 ways. Since there are 13 spades and 3 aces (one ace is also present in spade), therefore, the favorable cases $= m = 13 + 3 = 16$.

Number of exhaustive cases $= n = 52$.

Probability of getting a spade or an ace

$$=\frac{16}{52}=\frac{4}{13}=\frac{4}{9+4}$$

∴ Odds against winning the bet are 9 to 4.

Statistical Definition

If out of a large number of trials, only n of them are conducted and out of these n outcomes under each trial, only k outcomes are favorable to an event E, then the probability of E is,

$$P(E)=\lim_{n\to\infty}\left(\frac{k}{n}\right) \qquad ...(8.3)$$

The above definition of probability involves a concept which has a long-term consequence. This approach was initiated by von Mises. Moreover n is not equal to infinity. Thus, in this case, the probability is the limit of relative frequency. Whether such a limit always exists, is not definite. Hence, statistical definition of probability is also not very sound. The probability calculated by conducting an actual experiment is called a posteriori probability, whereas the probability specified by logic or based on some prior information is called a priori probability.

Statistical or empirical definition. Von Mises has given the following statistical or empirical definition of probability.

'If the experiment be repeated a large number of times, under essentially identical conditions, the limiting value of the ratio of the number of times the event A happens to the total number of trials of the experiment as the number of trials increases indefinitely is called the probability of happening of the event A'.

Symbolically, let P(A) denote the probability of the occurrence of A. Let m be the number of times in which an event A occurs in a series on n trials, then:

$$P(A)=\lim_{n-\infty}\frac{m}{n} \qquad ...(8.4)$$

Provides the limit is finite and unique.

Laws of Probability of Independent Events

Any subset of sample space is an event.

The complement of an event A, means non-occurrence of A and is denoted by A or A^c, $\bar{A}$ contains those points of the sample space which do not belong to A.

The set of sample points which satisfy certain requirement called an event.

An event having only one sample point is called an elementary event or simple event.

Mutually Exclusive Events

Two events E_1 and E_2 are said to be mutually exclusive if the occurrence of E_1 precludes the occurrence of E_2 and vice versa. In other words if there is no sample point in E_1 which is common to the sample points in E_2, i.e. $E_1 \cap E_2 = ø$, the events E_1 and E_2 are said to be mutually exclusive. For example, if we flip a fair coin, the coin will display either head or tail. Hence, the two events that the coin displays head E_1 or tail E_2 are mutually exclusive. Further, in a city a dealer has cars of three models namely, Maruti, Santro and Chevrolet, and another dealer has four models of scooters namely, Scorpio, Xylo, Indica and Ikon. Let us denote the event E_1 as Maruti, Santro and Chevrolet and event E_2 as Scorpio, Xylo, Indica and Ikon. It is obvious that a buyer will select a car either from E_1 or E_2. Hence, the two events E_1 and E_2 are mutually exclusive.

Independent Events

Two events E_1 and E_2 are said to be independent if the occurrence of E_1 has no bearing on the occurrence of E_2, i.e. the knowledge that the event E_1 has occurred gives no information about the occurrence of the event E_2. Formally, two events E_1 and E_2 are independent if and only if.

$$P(E_1 \cap E_2) = P(E_1)\,P(E_2) \qquad ...(8.5)$$

The intersection, $(E_1 \cap E_2)$, between two events E_1 and E_2 is known as joint event. For example, a bag contains balls of two different colors say, red and white. The two balls are drawn successively. First a ball is drawn from one bag and replaced after noting its color. Let us presume that it is white and is denoted by the event E_1. Another ball is drawn from the same bag and its color is noted. Let this event be denoted by the event E_2. The result of the second draw is independent of the first draw. Hence, the events E_1 and E_2 are independent. Let us consider another example. A state Director declares that each lottery ticket will have the chance of winning prizes at two draws at the intervals of one month. The event that a ticket wins a prize at the first draw is denoted by E_1, and the event that a ticket wins a prize at the second draw is denoted by E_2. It is obvious that the winning of a prize of any ticket at the first draw has no bearing on any ticket that wins a prize at the second draw. Hence, the events E_1 and E_2 are independent.

There are two important laws of probability which are useful in finding out probabilities in complex situation where the events concerned are independent.

1. Additional theorem or theorem on total probability
2. Multiplication theorem or theorem on compound probability.

1. Additional law or theorem on total probability: If an event can occur in any one of the several mutually exclusive ways, the probability of that event is the sum of the individual probabilities of the different ways is the probability of getting 2 or 4 or 6 in a throw of die?

The probability of 2 = 1/6

The probability of 4 = 1/6

The probability of 6 = 1/6

The probability of 2 or 4 or 6 is 1/6 + 1/6 + 1/6 = 3/6 =1/2

If the events are more exclusive, then the probability of happening of any one of them is equal to the sum of the probabilities of the happening of the events, i.e. in other words, if, E_1, E_2, E_3, ……, E_n be *n* events and $P(E_1)$, $P(E_2)$, their respective probabilities, then

$$P(E_1 + E_2 + E_3 + \ldots + E_n) = P(E_1) + P(E_2) + P(E_3) \quad \ldots(8.6)$$

Example 1: A dice is rolled. What is the probability that a number 1 or 6 may appear on the upper face?

The probability of appearing the number 1 on the upper face = $\frac{1}{6}$

The probability of appearing 6 on the upper face = $\frac{1}{6}$

∴ The probability of 1 or 6 may appear on the face = $\frac{1}{6} + \frac{1}{6} = \frac{1}{3}$

Example 2: If the probability of the horse A winning the race is $\frac{1}{5}$ and the probability of the horse B winning the same race is $\frac{1}{6}$, what is the probability that one of the horses will win the race?

Probability of the winning of the horse A = $\frac{1}{5}$.

Probability of the winning of the horse B = $\frac{1}{6}$.

$$\therefore \quad P(A + B) = P(A) + P(B)$$

$$= \frac{1}{5} + \frac{1}{6} = \frac{11}{30}$$

The addition theorem states that the *probability that anyone of a number of mutually exclusive events will occur is the sum of the probabilities of the separate events*. Events that cannot happen at the same time are mutually exclusive. In a one-coin toss problem, the occurrence of a head is mutually exclusive with the occurrence of a tail as both cannot happen at a time. In a throw of a dice, the probability of obtaining each of a 1, 2, 3, 4, 5, or 6 is 1/6; what is the probability of obtaining either a 1 or 2 or 4 in a single throw? This can be obtained by adding up the probabilities associated with 1, 2 and 4, i.e. 1/6 + 1/6 + 1/6 = 3/6 or ½. In tossing two coins, four possible events, HH, HT, TH, and TT are possible. What is the probability of obtaining either two heads or two tails? The probability of each of these events is ¼. Hence, the probability of obtaining either two heads or two tails is ¼ + ¼ = ½.

2. Multiplication law or theorem compound probability: The probability of the simultaneous occurrence of 2 or more independent events is the product of the individual probabilities. For example, in tossing the 2 coins the probability of head in one coin $= \frac{1}{2}$

The probability of head another coin $= \frac{1}{2}$

Thus, the probability of the heads in both coins $= \frac{1}{2} \times \frac{1}{2} = \frac{1}{4}$.

In multiplicative, before we proceed further in stating and proving this theorem, we require the following definitions:

Simple and compound events: A single event is called a **simple event**, whereas when two or more then two simple events occur in connection with each other, then their simultaneous occurrence is called a **compound event.** If A and B are two simple events, the simultaneous occurrence of A and B is called a compound event and is denoted by AB.

Conditional probability: The probability of the happening of an event A, when it is known that B has already happened, is called the **conditional probability** of A and is denoted by P(A/B), i.e. P(A/B) ⇒ conditional probability of A given that B has already occurred.

Similarly, P(B/A) ⇒ conditional probability of B given that A has already happened.

Laws of Probability of Mutually Independent Events

An event A is said to be independent of the event B if P(A/B) = P(A), i.e. the probability of the happening of A is independent of the happening of B.

The multiplication theorem *states that the probability of the joint occurrence of two or more independent events is the product of their separate probabilities.* When a single coin is tossed twice, the probability of getting a head on the first is ½, and on the second toss, ½. The probability of getting two heads is therefore ½ × ½ = ¼. In the same manner, we could determine that the probability of getting three heads from tossing a single coin three times would be ½ × ½ × ½ = 1/8. What is the probability of obtaining 6's in rolling two dice? The probability that the first die is a 6 is 1/6. The probability that the second dice is a 6 is also 1/6. Hence the probability that both dice are 6's is 1/6 × 1/6 = 1/36.

Theorem on Compound Probability

The probability of the simultaneous occurrence of the two events A and B is equal to the probability of one of the events multiplied by the conditional probability of other, given the occurrence of the first, i.e.,

$$P(AB) = P(A) \cdot P(B/A) = P(B) \cdot P(A/B)$$

Example 1: A card is drawn from a pack of 52 cards and then a second is drawn. What is the probability that both the cards drawn are queen?

First draw. Probability of getting a queen $= \frac{4}{52} = \frac{1}{13}$

Second draw. After drawing the first queen, we are left with 51 cards having 3 queens.

∴ Probability of getting a queen in second draw $= \frac{3}{51} = \frac{1}{17}$

∴ Probability that the cards are queen $= \frac{1}{13} \times \frac{1}{17} = \frac{1}{221}$.

Example 2. A bag contains 5 white and 3 black balls. Two balls are drawn at random one after the other without replacement. Find the probability that both the balls drawn are black.

Let P(A), P(B/A) denote the probability of drawing a black ball in the first and second attempt respectively.

∴ Probability of drawing a black ball in the first attempt is P(A), where

$$P(A) = \frac{\text{Favorable cases}}{\text{Total exhaustive cases}}$$

$$= \frac{3}{5+3} = \frac{3}{8}$$

Probability of drawing the second black ball given the first ball drawn is black, is

$$P(B/A) = \frac{\text{Favorable cases}}{\text{Total number of exhaustive cases}}$$

$$= \frac{2}{5+2} = \frac{2}{7}$$

$$\therefore \quad P(AB) = P(A)\,P(B/A)$$

$$= \frac{3}{8} \times \frac{2}{7} = \frac{3}{28}$$

Additional Theorem for Compatible Events

Theorem. The probability of the occurrence of at least one of the events A and B is given by

P (A+B) = P(A) + P(B) – P (AB)

Conditional Probability

In some situations, the chance of occurrence of a particular event depends on some other event. The multiplication law explained above is not applicable in case of *dependent* events. For example, the chance that a patient with some disease survives the next year depends, of course, on his having survived to the present time and the current status of his disease. Such probability is called conditional probability.

Let P (A) represents the probability of occurrence of event A, and P (B) that of event B. Let (AB) represent the probability of the simultaneous occurrence of events A and B.

Then, by definition, the probability that event A occurs, given that even B has already occurred, P(A/B), is given by

$$P(A/B) = \frac{P(AB)}{P(B)} \qquad \text{...(8.7)}$$

Basic Properties of Probability

1. The probability of an event E lies between 0 and 1, i.e. $0 \leq P(E) \leq 1$. If an event is certain not to occur, its probability is zero and if it is certain to occur, its probability is one.
2. The assignment of probability to each outcome of an experiment is a rule to assign a non-negative number such that the sum of these numbers to all possible outcomes 'Ω' is unity, i.e. P (Ω) = 1.
3. Any two equivalent events will be assigned the same probability.
4. If two events E_1 and E_2 are mutually exclusive, the probability of occurrence of either E_1 or E_2, i.e. of $(E_1 \cup E_2)$ is given as the sum of the individual probabilities, symbolically,

$$P(E_1 \cup E_2) = P(E_1) + P(E_2) \qquad \text{...(8.8)}$$

Venn diagram (Fig. 8.1) shows the mutually exclusive events E_1 and E_2. This property of probability is known as general additive property of probability or addition law. This theorem may

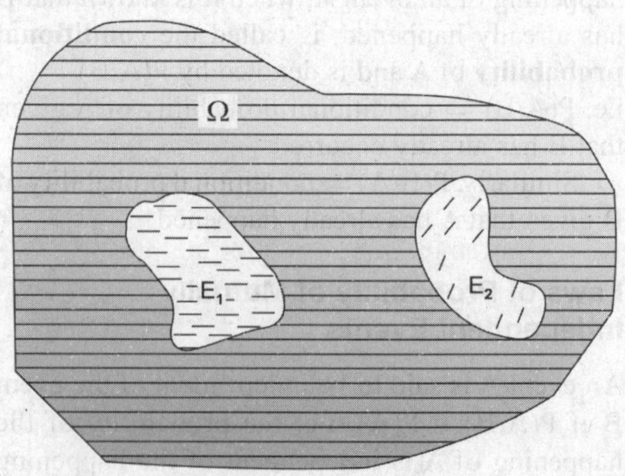

Fig. 8.1: Venn diagram

be extended to any number of mutually exclusive events. If E_1, E_2, ...E_k are k mutually exclusive events, the probability,

$$P(E_1 \cup E_2 \cup ... \cup E_k) = P(E_1) + P(E_2) + ... + P(E_k) \quad ...(8.9)$$

Example 1: If we draw a card from a pack, what is the probability that the card is either ace or a king? The events that the card drawn is either an ace or a king are mutually exclusive. Let the event of the ace card drawn be denoted by E_1 and the king card drawn be denoted by E_2. A pack consisting of 52 cards will have 4 aces and 4 kings, hence,

$$P(E_1) = \frac{4}{52} \text{ and } P(E_2) = \frac{4}{52}$$

$$P(E_1 \cup E_2) = P(E_1) + P(E_2)$$

$$= \frac{4}{52} + \frac{4}{52} = \frac{2}{13}$$

Readers will come across many other problems in which the additive property will be used.

The general rule of multiplication in its modified form in terms of conditional probabilities become

$$P\ (A \text{ and } B) = P\ (B) \times P\ (A/B)$$

$$\text{or } P\ (A) \times P\ (B/A) \quad ...(8.10)$$

Example 2: From past experience with the illnesses of his patients, a doctor has gathered the following information in a population:

5 percent feel that they have cancer and do have cancer;

15% feel that they have cancer and do not have cancer;

Denoting the events as

A when the patient feels he has cancer

B when the patient has cancer,

$$P\ (AB) = 0.05$$

$$P\ (A) = 0.5$$

$$P\ (B) = 0.15$$

The probability that a patient has cancer, given that he feels he has it, is given by:

$$P\ (B/A) = \frac{P(AB)}{P(A)} = \frac{0.05}{0.5} = 0.1$$

The probability he feels he has cancer, given that he does have it is given by

$$P\ (A/B) = \frac{P(AB)}{P(B)} = \frac{0.05}{0.15} = 0.33$$

Bayes Theorem

The principle given by Thomas Bayes in 1763 was reprinted in *Biometrika* (1958). His contention was that in absence of any idea about the prior probability of an event occurring, out of all possible events, one may assume that all the values of the probabilities are equal. Then on the basis of the experimental results (outcomes), one modifies his equally likely probabilities giving the posteriori probabilities. Briefly, assuming certain a priori probabilities, the posteriori probabilities are obtained. That is why Bayes probabilities are also called posteriori probabilities.

Usually the physician knows the conditional probability of a particular symptom (or positive test) for a particular disease. However, it is important that he knows the conditional probability of the disease for an individual patient, given the particular symptom (or positive test). A theorem attributed to Thomas Bayes (1702-61) provides the means to derive the latter probability from the former probability. This theorem is illustrated by an example.

An example to develop Bayes theorem, this example concerns bacteriuria, and pyelonephritis in pregnancy. Suppose it is known that roughly 6 percent of pregnant women attending a prenatal clinic at a large urban hospital have bacteriuria (bacteria in the urine).

Consider the two events A a pregnant woman has bacteriuria, and $\bar{A}$ she does not have bacteriuria.

Since A and $\bar{A}$ are mutually exclusive and complementary, then

P (A) = 0.06, and

P ($\bar{A}$) = 1 – 0.06 = 0.94

Suppose it is further known that 30 percent of bacteriuric and 1 percent of non-bacteriurica pregnant women proceed to develop this disease.

Using B to denote the occurrence of pyelonephritis, and $\bar{B}$ its absence, then

Notation	Event	Probability
B/A	Pyelonephritis given that the pregnant woman was bacteriuric	0.30
B/$\bar{A}$	Pyelonephritis given that the pregnant woman was non-bacteriuric	0.01

1. With these definitions consider the following probability questions:
   i. What is the chance a pregnant woman will have both bacteriuria and pyelonephritis?
   Using multiplicative law:
   P (A and B) = P (B/A) P (A)
   = (0.30) (0.06) = 0.0180.
   ii. What is the chance a pregnant woman will not have bacteriuria but will have pyelonephritis?
   Using multiplicative law:
   P ($\bar{A}$ and B) = P (B/$\bar{A}$)
   = (0.01) (0.94) = 0.0094
2. What is the chance of pyelonephritis?
   In this particular example, pyelonephritis can happen in two mutually exclusive ways, with or without bacteriuria. Hence, application of the additive law to the probabilities determined in 1(i) and 1(ii) gives
   P (pyelonephritis)
   = P (B)
   = P (A and B) + P ($\bar{A}$ and B)
   = 0.0180 + 0.0094 = 0.0274
3. Finally, with the knowledge that a pregnant woman has developed pyelonephritis, what is the chance she had been bacteriuric?

Using the notation developed, the question asks for the probability of A/B, i.e. the presence of bacteriruia given that the pregnant woman has pyelonephritis. From the alternative form for the multiplicative law of the preceding section and the answers to 1 (i) and 2 above:
P (A/B) = 0.0180/0.0274 = 0.6569

In other words, if a pregnant woman has developed pyelonephritis there is a 65.7 percent chance that she had been bacteriuric.

From the above illustration of Bayes theorem, we find that knowledge of the chances of pyelonephritis when bacteriuria is present and when it is absent along with knowledge of the relative frequency of bacteriruia among pregnant women has permitted the determination of a conditional probability, namely the chance that the pregnant woman had been bacteriuric given that she has developed pyelonephritis.

Substituting letters for numbers and working backward from the expression in the answer to question 3, it may be seen that

$$P\,(A/B) = \frac{P(A \text{ and } B)}{P(B)}$$

$$= \frac{P(A \text{ and } B)}{P(A \text{ and } B) + P(\bar{A} \text{ and } B)} \quad ...(8.11)$$

The last expression is the usual formulation of Bayes theorem.

Bayes theorem is frequently applied in evaluating the performance of a diagnostic test intended for use in screening program.

With the knowledge of (1) the sensitivity, P(A/B), and the specificity, 1 – P(A/B), of the test and (2) the overall case rate, P (B), the false positive rate and the false negative rate for the test can be determined.

Applied Probability

Since its humble beginning at the gambling tables in the 17th century, probability theory has been developed and employed to treat and solve many weighty problems. It is the foundation of the classical decision procedures of estimation and testing of hypothesis. Probability theory has enriched and enlarged our knowledge of several biological phenomena. Two main areas of application of probability theory are:

1. Description of empirical phenomena through specific probability distributions or models;
2. Predictions of events based on pertinent theoretical (probabilistic, stochastic) considerations.

Examples of specific uses may be found in the descriptions of population dynamics and estimates of population growth, determination of risks and competing factors in fertility or mortality, description of the course of epidemics and epidemic processes and in the documentation of clinical and biologic processes such as those encountered in human physiology, pathology or therapeutics.

Thus Yule (1924), Furry (1937), Feller (1939) and others have postulated population growth models based on certain assumptions regarding the initial population levels, rates of input (or birth), and decay (or death). Likewise, Hodgkin and Huxley (1952) and other physiologists have described nerve conduction in terms of probability of movement of ions and their concentration at the relevant place on the axon membrane. Pharmacologists have followed up these ideas by describing in probability terms the actions of drugs, especially by invoking receptors connected with the pharmacological response. The clinical process refers to the passage of an individual through the various stages of a disease in probability terms. Disease is a dynamic pathological process reversible in its' early stages. Alling (1958), Pesky and Tautu (1971) and others have built models of the evolution of pulmonary tuberculosis by defining various stages and the differential probabilities of movement from one stage to another. Arley (1972) and others have tried to describe the mechanism of tumour growth using probabilities for continued genotype variation, adaptation and selection within the genetic mosaic of cell clones constituting a tumour. Probability theory is applied in human genetics, such as in the prediction of specific phenotypes of the offspring, outcomes of mating patterns, mutation and selection of genes, the discussion about sex of an unborn baby, etc.

Mendel (1866) postulated that there were certain entities, now called genes, responsible for flower color and passed on from the plants to their progeny. The present example involves two types of genes, which we may denote by A and a. Each plant has two genes so that there are three kinds of plants, or genotypes: AA, Aa, and aa. A plant (AA), both of whose genes are of type A, will have red flowers. Finally, a plant (Aa) with one gene of each type will have pink flowers. Each offspring obtains one gene from each parent to make up its own pair. When we cross an AA plant with another AA plant, the offspring must also be AA. Similarly, (aa) × (aa) → (aa), and (AA) × (aa) → (Aa). The varying results are now also explained: in the (AA) × (Aa) cross, the offspring is sure to get A from the first parent, but may receive either A or a from the other, and thus may be either AA or Aa. Similarly, the (Aa) × (Aa) cross may produce each of the three types (Table 8.3).

To explain the suitable frequencies, we now introduce probability assumptions into the model. We suppose that:

- From an (Aa) parent, an offspring has probability ½ of receiving each of the genes A and a.
- The genes obtained by an individual from his two parents are unrelated.

Breeding experiments also justify another assumption of unrelatedness:

- The genes passed on by a parent to different offspring's are unrelated.

With these simple assumptions, all the Mendelian frequencies are explained. Thus, in an

Table 8.3

Probabilities of genotypes

Mother/Father	AA		Aa		aa	
AA	AA	1	AA	½	AA	0
	Aa	0	Aa	½	Aa	1
	aa	0	aa	0	aa	0
Aa	AA	½	AA	½	AA	0
	Aa	½	Aa	½	Aa	½
	aa	0	aa	½	aa	½
aa	AA	0	AA	0	AA	0
	Aa	1	Aa	½	Aa	0
	aa	0	aa	½	aa	1

(Aa) × (Aa) cross, the probability is ¼ that the offspring will be (AA), since there is probability ½ of obtaining the A gene from each parent and by assumption (2) these probabilities are to be multiplied. Table 8.3 shows the nine possible crosses, and the probabilities of each of the three possible offspring in each case.

Probability theory has become an indispensable tool for all types of formal studies that involve uncertainty. It should be noted that the concept of probability is employed not only for various types of scientific investigations, but also for many problems in everyday life. It is difficult to explain satisfactorily the basic idea of probability and its' applications without resource to some algebra and calculus. Also, in figuring out the 'total' of probabilities, we need to be familiar with the idea of permutations and combinations. Combinations concern forming of groups without any reference to the order within the group, while in permutations, we take the arrangement into account. We shall not go into this aspect now and the reader who is interested may refer to other textbooks.

We will conclude this chapter with one instance of the application of the basic concepts of probability, in the formation of probability distributions. Let us consider the problem of finding out the probabilities of getting different total points when we throw two dice. There are 36 (i.e. 6 × 6) equally likely and mutually exclusive outcomes. According to multiplication law, each outcome has a probability, 1/6 × 1/6 = 1/36.

The lowest total points of 2 can occur in only one way (1, 1) out of the total 36 outcomes. It has, therefore, a probability 1/36. A total of 3 points can occur in two ways (1, 2; 2, 1); and the probability of that outcome is 1/36 + 1/36 = 2/36 (according to the addition law). Similarly, we can find out the probabilities of other total points. Table 8.4 shows the probabilities corresponding to the different total points.

Table 8.4 gives the probability distribution in the case of a simple model. There are some important models which are very close approximations to actual situations. Their probabilities are tabulated in sufficient detail and made available for use.

Permutations and Combinations

Sometimes questions of the following kind are asked. In how many ways can five books be arranged on a shelf? In how many ways can six persons be seated at a table? The answer lies in calculating the number of possible arrangements. *Any arrangement is called a permutation.* Order is the essential idea here and a different order is a different permutation. With two objects A and B,

Table 8.4

Probability distribution for different total points when two dice are thrown

Total point	*Probability*
2	1/36
3	2/36
4	3/36
5	4/36
6	5/36
7	6/36
8	5/36
9	4/36
10	3/36
11	2/36
12	1/36
Total	1

two arrangements or permutations are possible, AB and BA. Three objects A, B, C can provide six arrangements or permutations — ABC, ACB, BAC, BCA, CAB and CBA. In general, if there are n distinguishable objects, the number of permutations of these objects taken *n* at a time are given by *n*! read as *n* factorial. Factorial of any number is the product of all integers from that number to 1, e.g. 4! = 4 × 3 × 2 × 1 = 24. The value of *n* in the three objects example is 3. Hence the number of permutations equals 3! or 3 × 2 × 1 = 6. The number of possible arrangements or permutations of 5 books equals 5! or 5 × 4 × 3 × 2 × 1 = 120; and of six persons, 6! or 6 × 5 × 4 × 3 × 2 × 1 = 720.

If arrangements require *r* to be taken at a time, when *r* is less than *n*, then the formula for the calculation of permutations is:

$$^{n}P_{r} = n(n-1)\ldots(n-r+1) = \frac{n!}{(n-r)!} \quad \ldots(8.12)$$

For example, the number of arrangements of ten objects taken three at a time is

$$^{n}P_{r} = \frac{10!}{(10-3)!} = \frac{10!}{7!}$$

$$= \frac{10\times9\times8\times7\times6\times5\times4\times3\times2\times1}{7\times6\times5\times4\times3\times2\times1}$$

$$= 720$$

Combinations are the arrangements of objects when the order in which they are arranged is ignored.

Given the objects A, B, C and D, the number of permutations of two from this set is 4!/(4 – 2) = 12. These are AB, BA, AC, CA, AD, DA, BC, CB, BD, DB, CD and DC. It is evident that each arrangement occurs in two different orders. If the order of arrangement of each pair of objects is ignored, we have the number of combinations. Obviously, the number of combinations, in this example, would be reduced. In general, the formula for calculating the number of combinations is:

$$^{n}C_{r} = \frac{n!}{r!(n-r)!} \quad \ldots(8.13)$$

Read as: *n* factorial upon *r* factorial into (*n* – *r*) factorial. $^{n}C_{r}$ stands for the number of combinations of *n* things taken *r* at a time; other terms are factorials. The number of combinations of 10 things taken 2 at a time is 10!/2/(10 – 2)! = 45. The number of combinations of *n* things taken *n* at a time is obviously 1, because there is only one way of picking all *n* objects if the order of their arrangement is ignored.

CHAPTER 9 Standard Distributions

Introduction

Most of the variables when classified into a frequency distribution follow a certain fixed pattern. This pattern becomes more and more consistent with the increase in the number of observations. That is to say that when a certain characteristic of a biological variate is measured or noted on a sufficiently large sample and the frequency distribution of these measurements are plotted in frequency polygon, the curve tends to take a particular common shape for all the samples of observation. This curve may be different for different characteristics of the data. The shape of these curves are governed by certain mathematical laws. The probability of occurrence of different values of observation can be depicted in terms of mathematical laws. These laws are known as probability distributions laws of the variable from the distributions of the number or the percentage of observation lying at a particular value of observation or beyond a value can be estimated. In any frequency distribution, if the frequencies are plotted against the various values of the variable, the area under the curve up to any value of the variable is a function of the cumulative probability of occurrence of that particular value of the variable. So when the exact distribution law of any variable is known as the shape of the curve, the probability of occurrence of the various values of observations etc. can be known.

Observations

Observations are always taken about a factor or character under study, which can take different values and the factor or character is termed as variable. The observations may be the number of certain items or objects or their measurements. These observations vary even though the experiment is conducted under identical conditions. Hence, we have a set of outcomes (sample points) of a random experiment. A rule that assigns a real number to each outcome (sample points) is called random variable. The rule is nothing but a function of the variable, say, X, that assigns a unique value to each sample point of the sample space.

So, it is clear that there is a value for each outcome, which it takes with certain probability. Hence, a list of values of a random variable together with their corresponding probabilities of occurrence, is termed as probability distribution. As a tradition, probability distribution is used to denote the probability mass or probability density of either a discontinuous or a continuous variable.

A **random variable** X is a real valued function, X (x), of the elements of the sample space Ω where x is an element of the sample space. It should be noted that the range of the random variable will be a set of real numbers.

Generally, a random variable is denoted by capital letters like X, Y, Z, U, V, ..., whereas the values of the random variable are denoted by the corresponding small letters like x, y, z, u, v....

Illustration (i) if we flip a coin and denote the head by 1 and tail by 0, then the random variable X takes only two values 1 and 0. Symbolically, the random variable.

$$X(x) = \{x{:}x = (1, 0) \in \Omega\}$$

where $\in$ is a connotation for 'belongs to'.

Illustration (ii) if we measure the height of people, the random variable.

$$X(x) = \{x{:}x \text{ is any real positive number}\}$$

Random variables are of two types: (i) Discrete random variable and (ii) Continuous random variable.

Discrete Random Variable: A random variable X, which can take only a finite number of values in an interval of the domain is called discrete random variable. A few examples are: (i) if we throw two dice at a time and note the sum of spots which turn up on the upper face, the discrete random variable.

$$X(x) = \{x{:}x = (x_1 + x_2) = 2, 3, ..., 12\}$$

where x_1 is the number of spots on the upper face of one dice and x_2 is the number of spots on the other dice. (ii) The random variable denoting the number of students in a class is:

$$X(x) = \{x{:}x \text{ is any positive integer}\}$$

Continuous Random Variable: A random variable X, which can take any value in the domain or when its range 'R' is an interval or the union of intervals on the real line, is called a continuous random variable.

Note that the probability of any single x, a value of X, is zero, i.e.

$$P(X = x) = 0$$

Example: (*i*) The height of students in India lies between 3 and 6 feet. The continuous random variable.

$$X(x) = \{x{:}3 \le x \le 6\}$$

(*ii*) The maximum life of electric bulbs is 2000 hours. The continuous random variable.

$$X(x) = \{x{:}0 \le x \le 2000\}$$

Distribution Function

The distribution of a random variable X is a function $F_x(x)$ for a real value x which is the probability of the event $(X \le x)$, i.e.,

$$F_x(x) = P(X \le x) \qquad ...(9.1)$$

It is evident from the expression that the distribution function is the probability that X takes a value in the interval $(-\infty, x)$.

Discrete Probability Distribution

If a random variable is discrete, its distribution will also be discrete, except in some exceptional situations. For a discrete random variable X, the distribution function or cumulative distribution is given by P(x) and is same as given by (6.1), i.e.

$$p(x) = P(X \le x) \qquad ...(9.2)$$

Discrete Probability Function

The probability function is the probability of a discrete random variable X, which takes the value x and is denoted by $p(x)$, i.e.

$$p(x) = P(X = x) \qquad ...(9.3)$$

The probability function always possesses the following properties:

(i) $p(x) \ge 0$ for all x in sample space Ω

(ii) $\sum_{\text{all } x} p(x) = 1$

Mathematical Expectation

The expected value of a random variable X is given as:

$$E(X) = \sum_{\text{all } x} x\, p(x) \qquad ...(9.4)$$

E(X) is also known as theoretical average value. In general, the expected value of a function H(X) of a discrete random variable X is given as,

$$E\{H(X)\} = \sum_{\text{all } x} H(x)\, p(x) \qquad ...(9.5)$$

Some Results on Expectation

If X and Y are two variates defined over the same sample space and if E(X) and E(Y) exist, then

$$E(X + Y) = E(X) + E(Y) \quad ...(9.6)$$

Also if X and Y are independent, then

$$E(XY) = E(X) E(Y) \quad ...(9.7)$$

Consider a variable X and a constant C. The expected values of X in relation to C are as follows:

$$E(C) = C \quad ...(9.8)$$

$$E(CX) = CE(X) \quad ...(9.9)$$

$$E(X + C) = E(X) + C \quad ...(9.10)$$

If X and Y are two variables and C_1 and C_2 are any constants, then

$$E(C_1X + C_2Y) = C_1E(X) + C_2E(Y) \quad ...(9.11)$$

If $X \leq Y$, then

$$E(X) \leq E(Y) \quad ...(9.12)$$

The operations given from (9.8) to (9.12) are also true for functions of X and Y.

Binomial Distribution

It is one of the most popular discrete distributions. The origin of binomial distribution lies in Bernoulli's trails. A Bernoulli's trial is an experiment having only two possible outcomes, i.e. success or failure. In other words, the results of the trial are always dichotomous. For example, if we flip a coin, it will show either head or tail on the upper face. The sex of an expected baby will either be male or female (excluding exceptions). A manufactured item will either be defective or non-defective. A person will either be healthy or sick.

Frequency distributions are tables or histograms constructed from a series of records of individuals—whatever the characteristics measured—to show the frequency with which these occur. With discrete events such as the occurrence of heads or tails on frequent tossing of a coin histograms can be drawn, producing what is known as the *binomial distribution.* Figure 9.1 shows the distribution of events with eight tosses of a coin, four heads and four tails being the most common. A curve of sorts can be superimposed. However, if a large number of measurements is available, such as the height of 200

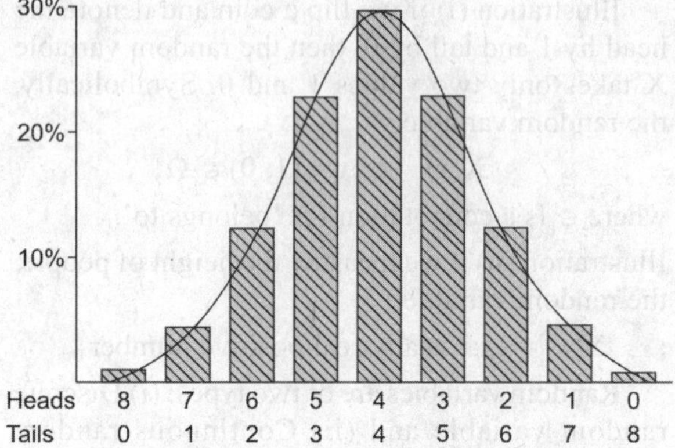

Fig. 9.1: Histogram with superimposed curve to show a frequency distribution

people attending a lecture, then it should be possible to describe a normal or *Gaussian distribution*—a mathematical definition given by Carl Gauss, a German mathematician, when he was 17 years old. This distribution has interesting properties and from it the standard deviation can be calculated as an estimate of the variability of any characteristic under study.

When the population under observation can be divided into twoi distinct groups, one with a certain characteristic of observation and the rest without this characteristic, the distribution of the occurrence of the characteristic in the population is called as "Binomial distribution".

For example, suppose it is required to define the distribution of prevalence of certain disease, then the entire population can be divided into two groups, one with the disease and the other without the disease. If the probability of a person having the disease is "p" and not having the disease is "q" (i.e. $1 - p$) then the distribution of various probabilities, i.e., the probability of finding name, one, two, three, four .... Persons with the disease in a group of "n" persons is given by the successive terms of the binomial distribution $(q + p)^n$. (If the sample is divided into multiple classes like blood group A, B, AB and O groups, that sample is called "multinomial").

Mean Features of the Binomial Distribution

- Mean number of frequencies with the characteristic is given by "*np*", where "*n*" is the number of observations and "*p*" is the probability of occurrence of the characteristics.
- Standard deviation is *npq*, where $q = 1 - p$.
- If '*p*' and '*q*' are equal, i.e. each equal to 0.5, the curve will be symmetrical.
- If '*p*' and '*q*' are not equal, then the curve will be skewed (asymmetrical).
- For any fixed value of '*p*' and '*q*', if '*n*' is increased to a sufficiently lare quantity, binomial distribution becomes more symmetrical and tends to be normal distribution.

Since a Bernoulli's trial has been considered, certain conditions for the application of binomial distribution are obvious. For clarity, (i) the probability of a success (or failure) remains same in each trial, (ii) trials must be independent, (iii) number of trials must be finite, (iv) the sum of probabilities of success and failure is sone, (v) the probability of success *vis-a-vis* failure is not very low. A dichotomous variable X, which has the probability function.

$$P_X(x) = \binom{n}{x} p^x q^{n-x} \quad \text{for } x = 1, 2, ..., n$$
$$= 0 \quad \text{otherwise} \qquad ...(9.13)$$

is said to have binomial distribution. In the binomial function,

n = number of trials; p = probability of a success; q = probability of a failure and $p(x)$ = probability of getting exactly x successes in n trials.

The distribution given is called binomial distribution since it is the $(x + 1)$th term in the binomial expansion of $(q + p)^n$.

Properties of Binomial Distribution

1. Binomial distribution has two parameters, *n* and *p* (or *q*).
2. The mean of the binomial distribution is *np* and variance is *npq*.
3. The moment generating function is $(q + pe^t)^n$.
4. The characteristic function is $(q + pe^{ii})^n$.
5. Binomial distribution tends to normal distribution as *n* increases. The normal approximation is correct enough if the mean *np* is greater than 15 for $p = 1/2$.

The binomial distribution is also known as *Bernoulli distribution* is associated with the name of a Swiss mathematician James Bernoulli. Binomial distribution is a probability distribution expressing the probability of one set of *dichotomous* alternative, i.e. success or failure or 'Yes' or 'No'. Very often people are interested in knowing what proportion of individuals in a population possess a particular character. For example, the proportion of persons in a locality who are sick at a particular point of time.

When the population under observation can be divided into two distinct groups—one with a certain characteristic of observation and the rest without this characteristic, the distribution of the occurrence of the characteristic in the population is defined by the binomial distribution. Usually an estimate of this proportion is calculated on the basis of a suitably drawn sample from this population and the corresponding sampling distribution. In this type of problem the sampling distribution is given by a theoretical frequency distribution known as *binomial distribution*.

Suppose, we have the hypothesis that, a student taking a true-false test will respond to each item by tossing a coin. Adding to it, we assume that 50 percent of the times the toss will result in correct answers and the rest of the 50 percent times, in an incorrect answer. The probability of correct answer is ½ and is equal to the probability to making an incorrect answer which is also ½. Suppose further, that the test contains 10 true-false items. The questions that may be asked are: what is the probability of the student with 7 answers correct and 3 answers incorrect. In such situations, binomial distribution provides the answer. To answer the last question, we may use the formula:

$$^{n}C_{r}p^{r}q^{n-r} = \left(\frac{n!}{(n-r)!\,r!}\right)(p)^{r}(q)^{n-r} \quad ...(9.14)$$

where ${}_nC_r$ is the number of combinations of n things taken r at a time:

p is the probability of getting a correct answer
q the probability of getting an incorrect answer
n is the total number of questions
r is the number of correct answers desired

Substituting the numerical values in the formula, we obtain

$${}^{10}C_7(1/2)^7(1/2)^{10-7} = \frac{10!}{(10-7)!(7)!}(1/2)^7(1/2)^3$$

$$= \frac{120}{1024} = 0.117$$

Similarly, we could use the above formula to obtain the probability of the student getting any particular score, ranging from 10 to 0 correct answers.

The binomial for n things can be expanded as follows:

$$(p+q)^n = p^n + np^{n-1}q + \frac{n(n-1)}{(1)(2)}p^{n-2}q^2 +$$

$$\frac{n(n-1)(n-2)}{(1)(2)(3)}p^{n-3}q^3 + ... + q^n \quad ...(9.15)$$

For the problem of 10 true-false items mentioned above, the binomial expansion will be as given below:

$$(p+q)^{10} = p^{10} + 10p^9q + 45p^8q^2 + 120p^7q^3 + 210p^6q^4 + 252p^5q^5 + 210p^4q^6 + 120p^3q^7 + 45p^2q^8 + 10pq^9 + q^{10}$$

The value of p and q which is ½ in each case can also, be inserted. The fourth term then would be $(120)(1/2)^7(1/2)^3$.

The exponent of p in each of the terms of the binomial expansion as in formula (9.15) indicates the number of items correct (successes) and that of q indicates, the number of items incorrect (failures). The numerical coefficients represent the number of ways in which each of the combinations of successes and failures may occur.

The rules for expanding the binomial $(p + q)^n$ are summarized below:

1. Each term in the binomial consists of the product of a numerical coefficient and a power of p and power of q.
2. The first term always has a numerical coefficient of 1 which is understood and hence not written; the power of p in the first term is always n and the power of q is zero; since $q^0 = 1$, q does not appear. Thus, the first term always is p^n.
3. In each succeeding term, the power of p decreases by 1 in regular order, while the power of q increases by 1 in regular order until the final term, q^n, is obtained.
4. The product of the numerical coefficient and the power of p in any given term, divided by 1

Table 9.1

The binomial coefficients of $(p + q)^n$ (Pascal's triangle)

n	*Binomial coefficients*																					*Sum*
1										1		1										2
2									1		2		1									4
3								1		3		3		1								8
4							1		4		6		4		1							16
5						1		5		10		10		5		1						32
6					1		6		15		20		15		6		1					64
7				1		7		21		35		35		21		7		1				128
8			1		8		28		56		70		56		28		8		1			256
9		1		9		36		84		126		126		84		36		9		1		512
10	1		10		45		120		210		252		210		120		45		10		1	1024

plus the power of q in that term, will give the numerical coefficient of the term that follows.

For example, the numerical coefficient 45, of the third term, has been obtained by multiplying the coefficient of the second term by its' power of p and then dividing by one plus the power of q. Thus

$$\frac{(10)(9)}{1+1} = \frac{90}{2} = 45$$

The numerical coefficient for any combination of correct and incorrect answers can be obtained by the formula:

$$^{n}C_{r} = \frac{n!}{(n-r)!(r)!} \quad ...(9.16)$$

In the above example, with $n = 10$ items; and number of correct answers, $r = 3$, the numerical coefficient will be

$$^{10}C_{3} = \frac{10!}{(10-3)!(3)!} = 45$$

The coefficients for n up to 10 are given in Table 9.1. It may be noted that entry in a given row consists of the sum of the coefficients to the right and left of the entry in the row directly above. Thus, the entries for $n = 11$ can be obtained from the entries for $n = 10$. They would be 1, 11, 55, 165, 330, 462, 462, 330, 165, 55, 11 and 1. Since the binomial is symmetric, the values of the numerical coefficients to the left and to the right of the middle term/terms are equal.

If we tested N students with our true-false test and if we still assume that each student answered each item by flipping a coin, that is, by chance, then we may readily determine the number of students expected to obtain each possible score formula (9.13) would thus become:

$$\text{N}(p+q)^n = \text{N}p^n + \text{N}\left(\frac{n(n-1)}{(1)(2)}p^{n-2}q^2\right)$$

$$+\,\text{N}\left(\frac{n(n-1)(n-2)}{(1)(2)(3)}p^{n-3}q^3\right) + \text{N}q^n \quad ...(9.17)$$

N in which: N = The number of students tested; n = the number of items in the test; p = probability of a correct response to a single item; $q = 1 - p$.

Since the sum of the numerical coefficients for $n = 10$, as given in the Pascal's triangle is 1,024, we can, for simplicity, take N = 1,024. The probabilities and N's for various events are given in Table 9.2.

The mean of the binomial distribution is given by the formula

$$m = np \quad ...(9.18)$$

where,

m = the mean number of correct responses of the binomial $(p+q)^n$

n = the exponent of $(p+q)$

p = the probability of having an item correct

In our case, where $n = 10$,

$$m = (10)(0.5) = 5.0$$

The variance and standard deviation of the binomial are given by the formulas

$$\sigma^2 = npq \quad ...(9.19)$$

$$\sigma = \sqrt{npq} \quad ...(9.20)$$

Where σ^2 = the variance of the distribution $(p+q)^n$

n = the exponent of $(p + q)$

p = the probability of having an item correct

$q = 1 - p$ or the probability of having an item incorrect

Substituting our values in the above formulas, we have

$$\sigma^2 = (10)(.5)(.5) = 2.5$$

$$\sigma = \sqrt{(10)(.5)(.5)} = \sqrt{2.5} = 1.58$$

The above formulas are in terms of n or frequency of correct responses or in terms of the scores of col. (1) of Table 9.2.

Examples

Let us consider the following example. In a morbidity survey in a village it is found that the proportion of sick persons is 40 percent. A sample of 4 persons can be any one of the five types having no sick person in the sample or having 1, 2, 3, or 4 sick persons. Assuming random sampling, there

Table 9.2

The binomial distribution $(p+q)^n$ and $N(p+q)^n$ with p = 5, n = 10 and N = 1024

Score number correct	*Score proportion correct*	*Probability*	*Expected number of students, f*
10	1.0	1/1024=0.001	1
9	0.9	10/1024=0.010	10
8	0.8	45/1024=0.044	45
7	0.8	120/1024=0.117	120
6	0.7	210/1024=0.205	210
5	0.6	252/1024=0.246	252
4	0.5	210/1024=0.205	210
3	0.4	120/1024=0.117	120
2	0.3	45/1024=0.044	45
1	0.2	10/1024=0.010	10
0	0.1	1/1024=0.001	1
S	0.0	1.000	1024

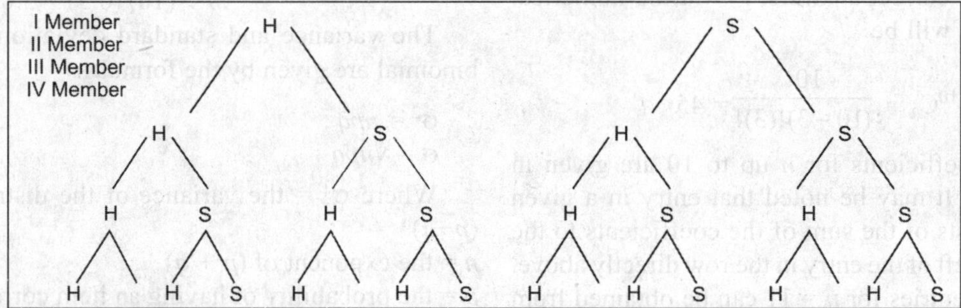

are sixteen ways in which we will get such a sample as shown in the following diagram.

H stands for a healthy person and S for a sick person. The first member selected may be either a healthy person or a sick person. The second also may be either a healthy or a sick person and so on. All such possibilities are listed in this diagram. If we follow each line starting from the first either H or S we get one composition. So we get 16 such compositions. The probability of a sick person being chosen is 0.4 and the probability of a healthy person being chosen is 0.6. The probabilities of the various compositions are got by using the addition and multiplication theorems on probability (Table 9.3).

In the last column of the above table are shown the probabilities of getting the five types of samples when the proportion of sick in the population is 40 percent. This type of distribution is called *binomial distribution*. The individual probability of each type of sample is given by the formula,

$$\left(\frac{n}{x}\right) p^x q^{n-x} \qquad \text{...(9.21)}$$

where x is the number of occurrences of the event, p is the probability of occurrence of the event, q is the probability of non-occurrence of the event and n is the size of the sample.

$\left(\frac{n}{x}\right)$ indicates the number of ways in which x occurrence can appear in a sample of size n.

Table 9.3

Calculation of probabilities for a binomial distribution

Composition of the sample	*Ways of occurring*	*Probability of occurrence*	*Probability of getting such sample*
No Sick Persons	HHHH	0.6 × 0.6 × 0.6 × 0.6	0.1296
1 Sick and	SHHH	0.4 × 0.6 × 0.6 × 0.6	
3 Healthy	HSHH	+0.6 × 0.4 × 0.6 × 0.6	
Persons	HHSH	+0.6 ×0.6 × 0.4 × 0.6	
	HHHS	+0.6 × 0.6 × 0.6 × 0.4	0.3456
2 Sick and	SSHH	0.4 × 0.4 × 0.6 × 0.6	
2 Healthy Persons	SHSH	+0.4 × 0.6 × 0.4 ×0.6	
	SHHS	+0.4 ×0.6 × 0.6 × 0.4	
	HSSH	+0.6 × 0.4 × 0.4 × 0.6	
	HSHS	+0.6 × 0.4 × 0.6 × 0.4	
	HHSS	+0.6 × 0.6 × 0.4 × 0.4	0.3456
3 Sick and	SSSH	+0.4 × 0.4 × 0.4 × 0.6	
1 Healthy Persons	SSHS	+0.4 × 0.4 × 0.6 × 0.4	0.1536
	SHSS	+0.4 × 0.6 × 0.4 × 0.4	
	HSSS	+0.6 × 0.4 × 0.4 × 0.4	
All Sick Persons	SSSS	0.4 × 0.4 × 0.4 × 0.4	0.0256

A useful notational device for the binomial probability uses the symbol P $(x'; n, p)$ for the probability that the total number of successes is x in n independent trials with success probability p on a single trial. For example, with four patients and single patient cure probability 0.6,the probability of exactly two cures is B (2;4,0.6) = 0.3456. Formally,

$$P(x; n, p) = {}^{n}C_{x} p^{x} (1 - p)^{n-x} \quad ...(9.22)$$

The construction of tables giving binomial probability can be simplified by taking advantage of the property that

$$P(x; n, p) = B(n - x; n, 1 - p) \quad ...(9.23)$$

It is as easy to establish this relation semantically, as it is analytically. The statement says that, the probability of x successes in n independent trials when the probability of success on a single trial is p is the same as the probability of $n - x$ failures in n independent trials when the probability of failure on a single trial is $1 - p$. The designation of one kind of outcome as success and the other as failure is, as we have noted is purely arbitrary. The tables can be interchanged, provided we remember that if the probability of one outcome is p, then the probability of the other is $1 - p$. This relation makes it unnecessary to tabulate binomial probabilities for values of p larger than 0.5. If, for example, we want P (6;10,0.8), we notice that it is numerically equal to P (4;10,0.2).

Example: Suppose that the probability of a single human birth producing a male infant is 0.5, ignoring twins and other multiple births (Infact, this probability is slightly greater than 0.5). Assuming that different deliveries are independent with respect to sex, find the probability that a family of five children will include: (a) exactly three boys, (b) at least one boy, (c) at most one boy.

Solution

a. P (exactly 3 boys) = B (3; 5, 0.5) = 0.3125
b. P (at least 1 boy) = 1 – p (no boys) = 1 – p (0; 5, 0.5) = 1 – 0.0312 = 0.9688
c. P (at least 1 boy) = P (exactly 0 boys or exactly 1 boy)
= P (0; 5, 0.5) + P (1; 5, 0.5)
= 0.0312+0.1562 = 0.1874

The Poisson Distribution

If in a binomial distribution, the value of 'p' or 'q' becomes indefinitely small and 'n' the number of observations becomes very large, so that the product 'np', the mean number of events is always finite, then the binomial distribution tends to be "Poisson distribution". Here, the occurrence of an event at any point of time is independent of previous event.

The main features of poisson distribution are:

- Mean = m
- Variance = mean = m
- Standard deviation = $\sqrt{m}$
- The distribution can be defined in terms of the mean only.

Another important discrete distribution is the Poisson Distribution. It is the distribution of a random variable taking values 0, 1, 2,.......... and is useful in a wide variety of applications dealing with counts. However, not all variables arising from counting applications follow this distribution.

Before we know the distribution, it becomes necessary to understand what is a Poisson random variable. A variable which can take only one discrete value in an interval of time, howsoever small, is known as Poisson variable, some of the well known examples of Poisson variable are:

- Number of mistakes in a typed page;
- Number of cars parked at a place in an hour, say between 10:00 am and 11:00 am;
- Number of defects in the insulation of a fifty meter length of wire;
- Number of suicides in a certain period in a city or town, etc.

If we consider a Poisson's process for a unit length of interval (time, length, space, etc.), the number of occurrences are a random variable which follow Poisson distribution. It has been named after its inventor, Simeon D Poisson, a French probabilist of 19th century. It is one of the most important discrete distributions. Poisson distribution is a classical approximation to binomial distribution, in which case n, the number of trials, is comparatively large and p, the probability of an occurrence, is small.

Let X be the number of occurrences in a Poisson process and μ be the actual average number of occurrences of an event in an unit length of interval, the probability function for Poisson distribution is,

$$P_x(x) = \frac{e^{-\mu}\mu^x}{x!} \quad \text{for } x = 0, 1, 2, \ldots \qquad \ldots(9.24)$$

$$= 0 \text{ otherwise}$$

If we consider the length of interval as d instead of unit length, the average number of occurrences in d length of interval is μd. Thus, the probability function in this situation is

$$P_x(x) = \frac{e^{-\mu d}(\mu d)^x}{x!} \quad \text{for } x = 0, 1, 2, \qquad \ldots(9.25)$$

$$= 0 \text{ otherwise.}$$

Properties of Poisson Distribution

1. Poisson distribution as given has mean μ and its variance is also μ. It is the only distribution known so far, of which the mean and variance are equal.
2. Poisson distribution possesses only one parameter (μ).
3. The moment generating function of a Poisson variate or equivalently the Poisson distribution is $e^{\mu(e^t-1)}$.
4. The characteristic function of Poisson distribution is $e^{\mu(e^{it}-1)}$.

If x is of a particular value, then the probability from the Poisson distribution that this value will occur is:

$$P(x) = \frac{e^{-\mu}\mu^x}{x!} \quad \text{...(9.26)}$$

$$\text{for } x = 0, 1, 2, \ldots\ldots\ldots\ldots$$

The quantity e in the formula above is a constant with value approximately equal to 2.71828.

In the expression for the Poisson probability, the quantity μ is a parameter that can take any value greater than zero. We have used the symbol μ because it is, in fact, the mean of the distribution. Notice that in contrast binomial distribution, which required knowledge of the values of n an p before probabilities could be calculated, the Poisson distribution requires knowledge of μ alone. We sometimes say that the binomial is a two-parameter family of distribution, while the Poisson is a one-parameter family.

The Poisson distribution can be a reasonably adequate representative of such diverse quantities as radioactive counts per unit time, the number of calls arriving at a busy telephone switchboard during certain time periods, the number of raisins per cookie in a batch of cookies from a bakery, the number of plankton per aliquot of seawater, the number of deaths by horse kick per year of Prussian army officers, or the count of bacterial colonies per petri plate in a microbiological study.

Two general models can be shown to lead directly to the Poisson probability. The first considers a large quantity of some medium such as seawater, air, serum, or cookie dough in which are found a large total number of discrete small entities, such as plankton, bacteria, granulocytes or raisins. The material is thoroughly mixed to overcome clumping or social instincts. The mixing must guarantee a uniform density of entities throughout the medium. Then, when a small quantity of the median is examined, the probability that x of the entities will be found in the examined portion is the Poisson probability.

The other model producing Poisson probability concerns events occurring in time. These events might be emissions of radioactive particles, calls arriving at a switchboard or patients entering a waiting line at a hospital out-patient registration desk. Suppose that the events occur independently and that the probability an event will occur in a short interval of length Δt is proportional to the length of interval—in other words, the probability is $c\Delta t$ where c is some constant. Suppose, further that Δt is short enough, the probability that more than one event occurs in an interval of such a length is negligible. Then, the probability that x events occur in an interval of some fixed length is the Poisson probability.

We are concerned that you might think nearly everything is Poisson distributed. Notice that both models require a kind of independence—the first by speaking of thorough mixing or uniform density, the second by stating that events occur independently in time. This is an important and essential assumption. The Poisson distribution cannot be expected to fit counts of entities that tend to aggregate or clump, and it similarly cannot be expected to fit arrivals at a waiting line when the length of the line tends to stimulate new arrivals perhaps in search of bargain or alternatively to repel them because of the possibility of a long wait. Similarly, the number of cases of streptococcal infection in schoolrooms should not follow the Poisson distribution because of the effect of contagion.

The Poisson probabilities can be derived as limits of binomial probabilities when p get very small (that is, close to zero) and n gets very large in such a way that np remains constant. A demonstration that the first model dealing with entities in a medium produces Poisson probabilities proceeds by examining the binomial probability under these circumstances. The probability p that a given entity enters the examined aliquot is very small under our assumptions of a large total volume of medium compared to the sampled volume. We assume then n, the total number of entities, is large, and the assumption of thorough mixing without clumping or aggregation guarantees that the long-term average number of entities per aliquot *np* will remain constant.

These considerations that *np*, the binomial mean, should equal *m*, the parameter of the Poisson distribution, which, as we have stated, is its' means. They also allow us to determine the variance of the distribution. The variance of the corresponding binomial distribution is $np(1-p) = m(1-p)$. But as *p* approaches 0, $(1-p)$ approaches 1 and the variance approaches *m*, an interesting fact about the Poisson distribution emerges: Its' mean and variance are both equal to the quantity *m* appearing in the expression for the Poisson probability. Remember that the Poisson distribution is important in its own right and should not be regarded solely as a limiting form of the binomial. The purpose of discussing this relationship is to show the connection between these two important distributions.

As an example of a set of data to which the Poisson distribution provides a reasonably good fit, we show in Table 9.4 observed and Poisson expected frequencies for a set of 100, 0.1-minute radiologic counts from a single source. The counts were made by John Nehemias. The expected frequencies are obtained by calculating the Poisson probabilities for a distribution having the same mean, 2.2, as the observed data. These probabilities are tabulated in Table A-3 for a variety of values of m. If any member of the Poisson family of distributions is to fit the data, we would expect the best fit from the distribution with $m = x$ the sample mean of the data.

The probabilities needed for the data in Table 9.4 are $P(x=0) = 0.110803$, $P(x=1) = 0.243767$, $P(x=2) = 0.268144$, $P(x=3) = 0.196639$, $P(x=4) = 0.108151$, $P(x=5) = 0.047587$, and $P(x=6) = 0.024909$. These values are found from an extended version of Table A-3 which includes = 2.2.

Because a probability can be regarded as a kind of long-term relative frequency, we multiply each probability by 100, the sample size, to get the expected frequency. These expected frequencies will not necessarily be whole numbers, since they represent the long run average frequencies for repeated samples of size 100 from a Poisson distribution with $\mu = 2.2$. The general agreement of observed and expected frequencies can be seen from the Table 9.4. We do not expect perfect agreement because of sampling variation and because the underlying distribution is probably not exactly Poisson. Remember that the Poisson distribution is simply a mathematical model useful as an idealization of natural phenomena. We never expect an exact fit of any such model. We will examine a class of statistical procedures for investigating the adequacy of fit of a set of expected or theoretical frequencies to a set of observed frequencies.

The probability distribution of a random variable X is said to have a **Poisson Distribution** if it takes only non-negative values and if its distribution is given by

$$P(X = x) = \frac{m^x e^{-m}}{x!}; \quad x = 0, 1, 2, \ldots\ldots..$$

where *m* is the parameter.

Hence, the probability of 0, 1, 2, 3, ..., *x*, ... successes are given by

$$e^{-m}, \frac{e^{-m} m}{1!}, \frac{e^{-m} m^2}{2!}, \ldots, \frac{e^{-m} m^x}{x!}, \ldots \text{ respectively}$$

Table 9.4

Observed and Poisson expected frequencies for 100 0.1-minute radiologic counts

Count	*Observed*	*Poisson expected frequency*
0	11	11.1
1	20	24.4
2	28	26.8
3	24	19.7
4	12	10.8
5	5	4.8
6 and over	0	2.5

where m is called the parameter of the Poisson distribution and

$$e = 2.7183 = \frac{1}{1!} + \frac{1}{2!} + \frac{1}{3!} + \ldots\ldots$$

Some examples of Poisson distribution

- The number of cars passing through a certain street (say Janpath) in a time t.
- The number of deaths in a city in one year by a rare disease
- The number of defective screws per box of 100 screws
- The number of suicides or deaths by heart attack in time t.
- The number of printing mistakes in each page of the first proof of a book
- The emission of radioactive (alpha) particles
- The number of air accidents in India in one year
- The number of pieces of a certain merchandise sold by a Super Bazaar in time t
- The number of telephone calls received at a particular telephone exchange in some units of time
- The number of defective material in a packing material manufactured by a good concern
- The number of fragments received by a surface area t from a fragment atom bomb.

The Poisson distribution can be derived from Binomial distribution under the following conditions:

- p, the probability of the occurrence of the event is very very small
- n is very large, where n is the number of trials
- np is a finite quantity, say $np = m$, then m is called the parameter of the Poisson distribution. In Poisson distribution probability of r success is given by $P(r)$.

Example 1: Suppose that the chance of an individual coal-miner being killed in a mine accident during a year is $\frac{1}{1400}$. Use the Poisson distribution to calculate the probability that in mine employing 350 miners, there will be at least one fatal accident a year.

(Use $e^{-0.25} = 0.78$)

Solution. Here $p = \frac{1}{1400}$, $n = 350$,

$$\therefore \text{Mean} = m = np = \frac{350}{1400} = 0.25$$

Then Poisson distribution is

$$P(r) = \frac{e^{-0.25}(0.25)^r}{r!}$$

Probability of zero fatal accident

$$= P(0) = \frac{e^{-0.25}(0.25)^0}{0!}$$

$$P(0) = e^{-0.25} = 0.78$$

Or

$\therefore$ P (at least one fatal accident) $= 1 - P(0) = (1 - 0.78) = 0.22$.

Example 2: Suppose a book of 585 pages contains 43 typographical errors. If these errors are randomly distributed throughout the book. What is the probability that 10 pages, selected at random, will be free from errors? (Use $e^{-0.735} = 0.4795$)

Solution. Here $n = 10$, $p = \frac{43}{585} = 0.0735$,

mean $= np = 0.735$

Then Poisson distribution is given by

$$P(r) = \frac{e^{-m} m^r}{r!} = \frac{e^{-0.735} \times (0.735)^r}{r!}$$

$\therefore$ Probability of zero error

$$= P(0) = \frac{e^{-0.735} \times (0.735)^0}{1000} = e^{-0.735} = 0.4795$$

Example 3: The mortality rate for a certain disease is 7 in 1,000. What is the probability for just 2 deaths on account of this disease in a group of 400? (Given $e^{-0.28} = 0.06$).

Solution. Here $p = \frac{7}{1000}$ and $n = 400$.

$$\therefore m = np = 400 \times \frac{7}{1000} = 2.8.$$

Now the required probability is given by

$$P(2) = \frac{m^2}{2!} e^{-m} = \frac{(2.8)^2}{2!} e^{-2.8}$$

$$= \frac{2.8 \times 2.8 \times 0.06}{2} = 0.235$$

Example 4: A car hire firm has two cars, which it hires out day by day. The numbers of demands for a car on each day is distributed as Poisson distribution with mean 1.5. Calculate the proportion of days on which neither car is used and the proportion of days on which some demand is refused [$e^{-1.5} = 0.2231$].

Solution. Since the number of demands for a car on each day is distributed as Poisson distribution with mean 1.5 therefore, the probability of having r demands a day is given by $P(r) = \dfrac{(1.5)^r e^{-1.5}}{r!}$

Thus, the proportion of days on which neither car is used

= Probability of no demand = $P(0) = e^{-1.5} = 0.2231$

And the proportion of days on which some demand is refused

= Probability of more than two demands in a day

$= 1 - [P(0) + P(1) + P(2)]$

$= 1 - [e^{-1.5} + 1.5e^{-1.5} + \dfrac{(1.5)^2}{2} e^{-1.5}]$

$= 1 - 0.2231 \times 3.625 = 0.1913.$

The Multinomial Distribution

The binomial distribution we have just examined is a special case of a more general distribution, the multinomial distribution. In binomial distributions, we deal with events that can have only one of two outcomes—a coin could land heads or tails, a wine could be judged as more expensive or less expensive, and so on. In many situations, however, an event can have more than two possible outcomes—a roll of a die has six possible outcomes; a maze might present three choices (right, left, and center); political opinions could be classified as For, Against, or Undecided. In these situations, we must invoke the more general multinomial distribution.

If we define the probability of each of k events (categories) as p_1, p_2, ...p_k and wish to calculate the probability of exactly X_1 outcomes of event$_1$, X_2 outcomes of event$_2$, ..., X_k outcomes of event$_k$, this probability is given by

$$p(x_1, x_2, ..., X_k) = \frac{N!}{X_1!X_2!...X_k!} p_1^{x_1} p_2^{x_2} ... p_k^{x_k} \quad ....(9.27)$$

where N has the same meaning as in the binomial. Note that when $k = 2$ this is in fact the binomial distribution, where $p_2 = 1 - p_1$ and $X_2 = N - X_1$.

As a brief illustration, suppose we had a die with two black sides, three red sides and one white side. If we roll this dice, the probability of a black side coming up is 2/6 = 0.333, the probability of a red is 3/6 = 0.500, and the probability of a white is 1/6 = 0.167. If we roll the die 10 times, what is the probability of obtaining exactly four blacks, five reds, and one white? This probability is given as

$$p(4,5,1) = \frac{10!}{4!5!1!}(0.333^4)(0.500^5)(0.167^1)$$

$$= 1260(0.333^4)(0.500^5)(0.167^1)$$

$$= 1260(0.000064)$$

$$= 0.081$$

Comparison between Binomial and Poisson Distribution

We have discussed two discrete distributions, each dealing with counts, the binomial and the Poisson. An interesting contrast between these distributions is provided by comparing the relative size of their mean and variance.

The binomial distribution, giving the probability of x successes in n independent trials with probability p of success in a single trial has, as we have seen, mean np and variance npq. Because q is the probability of failure in a single trial, its value is less than 1 and the variance is the mean, np multiplied by q. therefore, the variance is less than the mean.

As we have seen, the Poisson distribution has the same quantity, *m*, for its mean and variance. That is, its mean equals its variance.

Binomial: Variance less than mean

Poisson: Variance equal to mean.

This can provide clues as to the possible applicability of the two distributions. If you are in a situation in which you can collect several random samples, by calculating the mean and variance of each and comparing their relative size you can choose an appropriate distributional model. Of course, you must be dealing with counts in order to be faced with such a choice. Furthermore, conditions of observation may lead directly to only of the distributions.

Normal Distribution

The Binomial and Poisson distributions deal with the occurrence of distinct events such as the number sick, number of accidents, number of cells, number of coins, etc. There are many situations in which the quantity that is studied is continuous in magnitude. Body temperature, intelligence quotient, height, weight, etc. are examples of quantities that vary continuously. For such characteristics many populations and also their sampling distributions are very close to a pattern of frequency distribution known as Normal (Gaussian) Distribution. The mathematical function that generates the probabilities is,

$$\frac{1}{\sigma.\sqrt{2\pi}} \; e^{\frac{1}{2\sigma^2}(x-\mu)^2} \qquad ....(9.28)$$

where *x* is the variable in question (characteristic studied), *m* is the mean and *s* is the standard deviation.

An example of normal distribution is given in Table 9.5 and some of the interesting properties are enumerated.

Normal distribution is a frequency distribution, in which a large number of observations of any variable biological characteristic such as Hb,

Table 9.5

Example of A Normal Distribution – Distribution of 1000 Men in a village according to their heights

Height in Inches	*Number of men of given height*			
61-	2			
62-	5			
63-	17			
64-	43			
65-	86			
66-	152			
67-	193	690	955	997
68-	197			
69-	148			
70-	91			
71-	45			
72-	16			
73-	4			
74-75	1			
Total	1000			

Ht, Wt, pulse, BP etc. are made with a small class interval. Such a distribution will have the following characteristics.

a. Half the measurements lie above the mean and half below.
b. Most of the measurements (observations) are concentrated around the mean.
c. All the observations are symmetrically distributed on each side of the mean; i.e., if they are arragned in an order, the highest frequencies will be seen in the middle around the mean and the lowest at the extremes, decreasing smoothly on both sides. This is called "central tendency" or concentration of observations around the central value or mean.

Such distribution is called "Normal distribution" or "Gaussian distribution" and when plotted graphically it is called Normal curve or Gaussian curve, named after a famous mathematician and astronomer Karl Gauss (Fig. 9.2a). The term "normal" is not used in medical sense. By "normal" is meant usual and not "not abnormal".

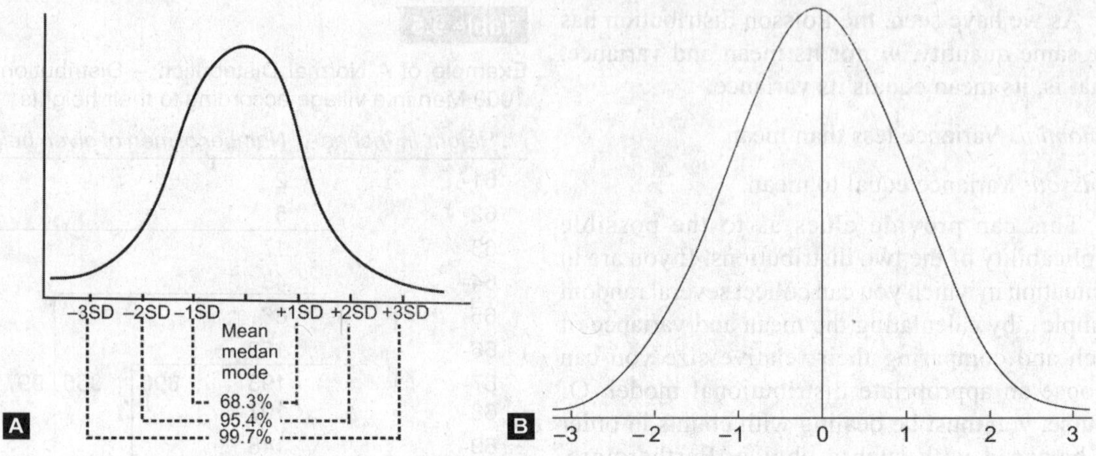

Figs 9.2A and B: (A) Normal distribution curve; (B) Standard normal curve

Normal distribution is the most popular and commonly used distribution. It was discovered by De Moivre in 1733, about twenty years after Bernoulli gave binomial distribution. A random variable X is said to follow normal distribution, if and only if, its probability density function (pdf) is

$$fX(x) = \frac{1}{\sigma\sqrt{2\pi}} e^{\frac{-1}{2\sigma^2}(x-\mu)^2} \quad ...(9.29)$$

where x is the real value of X, i.e. $-\infty < x < \infty$.

The variable x is said to be distributed normally with mean μ and variance σ^2, i.e. $X \sim N(\mu, \sigma^2)$.

The density function given has two parameters, namely μ and σ. Here μ can take any real value in the range $-\infty$ to ∞, where σ is any positive real value, i.e. $\sigma > 0$.

Since the probability can never be negative,

$fX(x) \geq 0$ for all x.

In case $\mu = 0, \sigma = 1$, the density function for X is

$$fX(x) = \frac{1}{\sqrt{2\pi}} e^{-\frac{1}{2}x^2} \quad ...(9.30)$$

where $-\infty < x < \infty$. Notationally, $X \sim N(0, 1)$.

In this situation the variable x is called the standardized normal variate and the distribution given is called the standardized normal distribution.

Properties of Normal Distribution

- If we plot the curve for the values of the standard normal variate X and the corresponding probabilities, it is of the shape given in Figure 9.2b.

  The curve is bell-shaped and symmetrical about the vertical line at $x = 0$. For the random variable $X \sim N(\mu, \sigma^2)$, the curve is symmetrical about the mean μ. Symmetry implies $fX(x) = fX(-x)$.
- The vertical line at $x = 0$ cuts the curve at its highest point i.e. $fX(x)$ at $x = 0$ is maximum. The value of $fX(x)$ decreases as the value of x is other than zero (or the mean μ).
- The area under the normal curve within the limits $-\infty$ to ∞ is unity, i.e.

$$\frac{1}{\sigma\sqrt{2\pi}} \int_{-\infty}^{\infty} e^{-\frac{1}{2\sigma^2}(x-\mu)^2} dx = 1$$

If μ=0, σ=1, then

$$\frac{1}{\sqrt{2\pi}} \int_{-\infty}^{\infty} e^{-\frac{1}{2}x^2} = 1$$

- On either side of the mean μ, the frequency decreases more rapidly within the range (μ ± σ) and gets slower and slower as it goes away from the mean. The frequencies are extremely small beyond the distance of ± 3σ. As a matter of fact 99.73 percent units of the population lie within the range μ ± 3σ.
- Theoretically the curve never touches the X-axis.
- As the value of σ increases, the curve becomes more and more flat and vice-versa.
- The moment generating function of the general normal distribution is

$$m_x(t) = e^{\left(\mu t+\frac{1}{2}\sigma^2 t^2\right)}$$

- All central moments of odd order are zero.
- The characteristic function of the general normal distribution is

$$\phi x(t) = e^{\left(\mu it-\frac{1}{2}\sigma^2 t^2\right)}$$

Normal distribution is most widely used in statistics despite the fact that theoretically a population hardly follows the exact normal distribution. This is due to various reasons which are as follows:

- Convenience is a strong support for its use in statistics. Extensive tables have been prepared and provided for ordinates and area under the normal curve. This has facilitated the job of the scientist immensely.
- If the variable does not follow normal distribution, it can be made to follow after making a suitable transformation like square root, arcsine, logarithm, etc.
- The most important and convincing reason is that whatever be the original distribution, the distribution of sample mean can, in most of the cases, be approximated to normal distribution, when the sample size is sufficiently increased.

The graphical presentation of the data as shown in Figure 9.3 follows a normal distribution not entirely but fairly closely.

The characteristics of an ideal normal distribution are as follows:

- The curve of the distribution is bell shaped and symmetrical around the mean of the distribution.

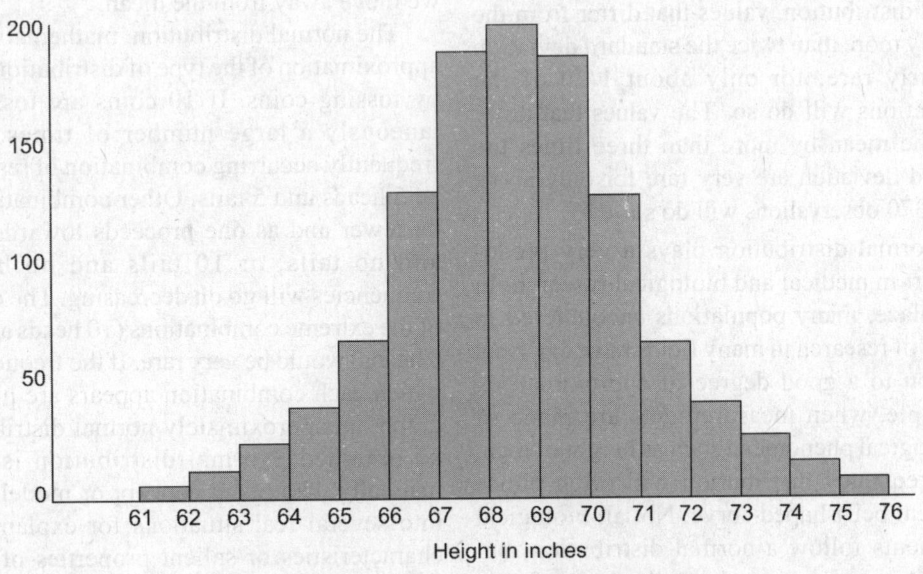

Fig. 9.3: Graphical presentation of normal distribution

We can define symmetry as that property where the total frequencies on either side of the mean value are the same; also the frequencies at equal distances from the mean on either side are same.

- The mean, median and mode of the distribution coincide.
- If we consider a certain number of standard deviations from either side of the mean, we can theoretically state the proportion of frequencies that lie within these limits. To be more specific, we have about 68.27 pecent of the observations lying within one standard deviation of either side of the mean, 95.45 pecent of the observations lie within 2 standard deviation from either side of the mean and about 99.73 pecent of the observations lie within 3 standard deviations from either side of mean. From the example that we have presented, we notice that nearly 1/3 of the observations are to the complement of the proportion within one standard deviation. Similarly, if we consider the number of observations outside 2 standard deviations, we notice that it is 100 percent – 95 percent = 5 percent, and also only three in a thousand differ from the mean by more than three times the standard deviation. Thus in a normal distribution, values that differ from the mean by more than twice the standard deviation are fairly rare; for only about 1/20 of the observations will do so. The values that differ from the mean by more than three times the standard deviation are very rare for only about one in 370 observations will do so.

The normal distribution plays a very predominant part in medical and biological research. In the first place, many populations encountered in the course of research in many fields have a normal distribution to a good degree of approximation. For example, when measurements are made of some biological phenomena such as height of men, etc. the frequency distribution will often plot a symmetrical bell-shaped curve. Not all biological measurements follow a normal distribution, but many do so and we could make use of this particular feature in the statistical theory. The other consideration which favors the normal distribution is the fact that sampling distributions of the statistics calculated from samples taken from the parent (population) normal distribution are, in most of the cases, known. The third consideration, of course, is that we have a mathematical basis for calculation of various descriptive measures. When the distribution is normal, the mean and standard deviations describe the distribution completely. If the distribution is approximately normal, no essential details are lost by considering it to be normal. The particular use of this normal distribution is made whenever, we have a large sample since many other theoretical distributions approximate to a normal curve.

The normal distribution is a special case of the binomial distribution with p = 0.5, and a sufficiently large N. As N grows infinitely large, the normal and binomial probabilities become identical for any interval. It also depicts a tendency that test scores always tend to be distributed around the averages. On a test with items of average difficulty level, many students of an unselected group, will obtain average or near average scores. The number of students in the two tails of the distribution go on decreasing, as we move away from the mean.

The normal distribution, mathematically, is an approximation of the type of distribution generated by tossing coins. If 10 coins are tossed simultaneously a large number of times, the most frequently occurring combination of results would be 5 heads and 5 tails. Other combinations would be fewer and as one proceeds towards 10 heads and no tails, or 10 tails and no heads, the frequencies will go on decreasing. The occurrence of the extreme combinations (10 heads and 10 tails, 0 heads) would be very rare. If the frequencies with which each combination appears are plotted on a graph, an approximately normal distribution will be obtained. Normal distribution is a mathematically theoretical concept or model, yet it fits into several real situations for explanation. The characteristics or salient properties of the curve are given below:

DeMoivre (1733) first developed the equation of the curve. This concept was further developed and perfected by Gauss and Leplace.

The Normal Probability Curve

- It is a bell-shaped curve because of its characteristic roundness at the top and infections on each side.
- The tails of the curve are asymptotic to the base line. It means that the tails of the curve theoretically approach the baseline but never touch it.
- The mean, mode and median, in a normal curve coincide or fall at the same point. They have the same numerical values. It means in a normal curve, Mean = Median = Mode (Figure 9.4).
- It is symmetrical about the mean and hence the area below the mean is equal to the area above the mean. Thus, it is bilateral.
- For practical purposes, the baseline of the curve is divided into six sigma distances from –3σ to +3σ. Most of the cases (i.e. 99.73%) are covered, within ± 3σ from the mean. Very few cases deviate by more than 3σ above or below the mean.
- The curve is unimodal.
- The maximum ordinate of the curve occurs at the mean or where Z = 0. The highest of the ordinate at this point is 0.3989. The heights of the ordinates at 1σ, 2σ, 3σ are 0.2420, 0.0540 and 0.0044 respectively.

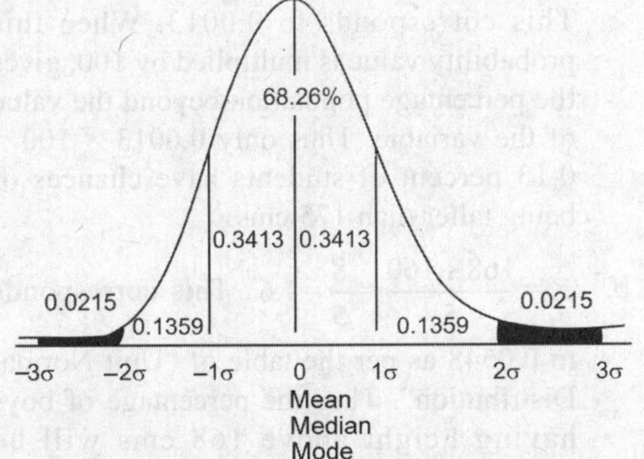

Fig. 9.4: Different proportions of area under the normal curve

- The area under the curve represents the total frequency (N) of the distribution.
- The points of inflection of the curve occur at points plus and minus one s unit above and below the mean. It means the curve changes from convex to concave in relation to horizontal axis at these points.
- In a normal curve,
  Quartile deviation,
  Q = Probable error = 0.6745 σ
  Mean deviation, AD = 0.7979 σ
  Skewness = 0
  Kurtosis = 0.263
- The normal curve is defined by the equation:

$$Y = \frac{N}{\sigma\sqrt{2\pi}} e^{-x^2/2\sigma^2} \qquad \text{...(9.31)}$$

(Symbols explained in the next section).

The features of a normal curve are:

i. It is a smooth curve, resembling the shape of a bell.
ii. It is symmetrical about the middle point.
iii. The rim of the bell does not rest on the abscissa but is separated from it by a gap.
iv. All the three measures of central tendency, i.e. mean, median and mode coincide, i.e. a perpendicular drawn from the peak of the curve to the abscissa, that point on the abscissa is the mean, median and the mode. The mean divides the area under the curve into two equal halves.
v. Maximum number of observations are at the value of the variable correspondig to the mean and the number of observations on both sides of this value gradually decrease and there are few observations at the extreme points.
vi. The area under the curve is proportional to the frequency.
vii. The area under the curve (number of observations) can be represented in terms of relationship between the mean and the standard deviation. The relationship is expressed as follows.

a. Mean ± 1 SD includes 68.3 percent of (roughly (2/3rds) of all observations. 1/3rd of the values (34.13 percent) lie on either side of the mean.
b. Mean ± 2 SD includes 95.4 percent of all observations.
c. Mean ± 3 SD includes 99.7 percent of all observations.

Thus it is seen that almost all the values of observations will be within the range mean ± 3 SD and most of the values are within the range mean ± 2 SD. This relationship is useful for fixing the confidence intervals of the varieties. The confidence interval is the limit upto ± 3SD on either side of the mean (i.e., the limits upto ± 3SD on either side of the mean are called as "Confidence limits").

viii. The distance of the value X from the mean ($\bar{x}$) of the curve in terms of standard deviation is called "Relative deviate" or "Standard Normal Variate" (SNV). It is expressed as a ratio between difference of a given observation and the mean and the standard deviation and is denoted by "Z" and is calculated by the formula,

$$Z = \frac{\text{Observation} - \text{mean}}{\text{SD}} = \frac{x - \bar{x}}{\text{SD}}$$

It gives the proportion of individuals who do not exceed this value in nature. If this ratio value is more than two, it is significant and if more than 3, it is considered as highly significant. It is based on the assumption that sample values are normally disturbed. In case of small samples, instead of *Z*, '*t*' ratio is used.

ix. The properties of a normal distribution and a normal curve form the basis of various tests of significance.

x. Values larger and smaller than mean ± 3SD will be rare (less than 1%) in nature and those larger and smaller than mean ± 2 SD will occur less than 5 percent. In otherwords, suppose we say that the confidence limit is 99 percent, that means 99 percent of the values are distributed within the range of x ± 3 SD and the probability of occurrence fo any value falling outside this range is only 1 percent ($p = 0.01$). Similarly, suppose we say that the confidence limit is 95 percent, that means 95 percent of the values are distributed within the range of x ± 2 SD and the probability of occurrence of any value falling outside or beyond this range is only 5 percent ($p = 0.05$).

The practical application of the above procedure is illustrated in the following example.

The mean height of 500 students is 160 cms and the SD is 5 cms.

- What are the chances of heights above 175 cms being normal if height follows normal distribution?
- What percentage of boys will have height above 168 cms.
- What number of boys will have height between 168 and 175 cms.

a. First, the SNV is calculated for the given value of the variable.

$$\text{i.e. } Z = \frac{x - \bar{x}}{\text{SD}} = \frac{175 - 160}{5} = \frac{15}{3} = 3$$

To this calculated value 3, the probability level is noted by referring to the table of "Unit Normal Distribution" (Annexure I). This corresponds to 0.0013. When this probability value is multiplied by 100, gives the percentage population beyond the value of the variable. Thus only 0.0013 × 100 = 0.13 percent of students have chances of being taller than 175 cms.

b. $Z = \frac{168 - 160}{5} = \frac{8}{5} = 1.6$. This corresponds to 0.0548 as per the table of "Unit Normal Distribution". Thus the percentage of boys having height above 168 cms will be = 0.0548 × 100 = 5.48 percent.

c. The number boys having height above 168 and below 175 cms will be 0.0548 – 0.0013 = 0.0535 out of 1. Thus only 5.35 percent of students will have height within the range of 168–175 cms.

The Equation for the Normal-Distribution Curve

The normal distribution curve is described by the following general mathematical equation:

$$Y = \frac{N}{\sigma\sqrt{2\pi}} e^{-x^2/2\sigma^2} \quad ...(9.32)$$

Where, Y = frequency for any given point of the baseline

N = number of observations

σ = SD of the distribution

π = 3.1416 (Approx.); A mathematical constant

e = 2.718 (Approx.) A mathematical constant

x = deviation of a score from the mean; $(X - \overline{M})$

The equation leads to the following features of the curve:

- With N and σ fixed, all elements, except x, are constants
- Since x is squared, the negative or the positive values of x will yield the same value of Y, hence leading to the symmetry of the curve
- Since x^2 has a negative sign, as x increases, the exponent of e decreases and Y also decreases
- If $x = 0$, exponent of e becomes zero and the value of e with the exponent 0 reduces to 1. The equation then reduces to

$$Y = \frac{N}{\sigma\sqrt{2\pi}} e^{-x^2/2\sigma^2}$$

The value of Y is at a maximum at this point.

The Unit Normal Curve

Table of areas of normal curve have been prepared based on N = 1 and s = 1.0. The equation in these circumstances reduces to

$$Y = \frac{N}{\sqrt{2\pi}} e^{-(z^2)/2} \quad ...(9.33)$$

The total area is considered to be unity or one and all frequencies are proportions. The mean of distributions remains at zero.

Area Under the Normal Curve

The normal curve tables (Table 9.6) are generally limited to the areas under the Unit Normal Curve, with N = 1, s = 1. In case when the values of N and s are different from these, the measurements or scores should be converted into sigma scores or standard scores or Z-scores. The process is as follows:

Table 9.6

Normal probability curve area values for given Z values

Z values	*Area from mean proportion*	Percentage	*Z values*	*Area from mean proportion*	Percentage
+0.5	0.1915	19.15	– 0.5	0.1915	19.15
+1.0	0.3413	34.13	– 1.0	0.3413	34.13
+1.5	0.4332	43.32	– 1.5	0.4332	43.32
+2.0	0.4772	47.72	– 2.0	0.4772	47.72
+2.5	0.4938	49.38	– 2.5	0.4938	49.38
+3.0	0.4987	49.87	– 3.0	0.4987	49.87

Normal curve area tables shown only positive values of Z.

$$Z = \frac{x}{\sigma_x} = \frac{X - M_x}{\sigma_x} \quad ...(9.34)$$

In which, Z = standard score

X = deviation of the raw score from the mean

M_x = mean of X scores

σ_x = SD of X scores

The tables of areas of Normal curve are then consulted to find out the proportion of area between mean of the curve and the Z. *While consulting Normal Curve Area tables, the following points should always be kept in mind to avoid error:*

- Everything, i.e. scores or observations must be converted into standard measures, i.e. Z scores and above.
- The mean of the curve is always the reference point and all the values of areas are given in terms of distances from the mean which is zero
- The area in terms of proportion can be converted into percentage by multiplying it by 100 or by simply shifting the decimal two places to the right.
- While consulting tables, absolute value of Z (ignoring sigma) should be taken. However, a negative value of Z shows that the score and the area lie below the mean and this fact should be kept in mind while doing further calculations on the area. A positive value of Z shows that the score and hence the area also lies above the mean. Figure 9.3 shows the distribution of areas under the normal curve within the limits of some selected s units on the baseline.

Table 9.6 depicts the proportions of area between mean and various Z scores and the learner should study it carefully and see the various relationships, that exist in these values. The areas for the positive and negative values of a Z score are the same. Proportions of areas have been converted into percentages simply by shifting the decimal points two places to the right. While the baseline distance from one Z value to the next is equal, the relative differences in the areas are not equal.

Study Table 9.7 also carefully and visualize the various relationships in terms of Z values and areas.

Problems and Numericals on Normal Distribution

Normal distribution has been found to be very useful in problems involving inferences. Several types of problems can be solved by using normal curve as a theoretical model. However, the following five types of problems will be illustrated through numerical solutions:

1. Determination of the percentage of cases within given limits of scores
2. Determination of the limits of scores which include a given percentage of cases [converse of type (1) above].
3. Comparison of two distributions in terms of overlapping
4. Determination of the relative difficult of test questions, problems and other test items
5. Division of a given group into subgroups, when trait is normally distributed.

Table 9.7

Area under normal probability curve between given limits

Limits (in Z-scores)	*Area (in percentage)*
Above +1.0	(50-34.13) = 15.87
Below +1.0	50+34.13) = 84.13
Between +0.5 and +0.75	(27.34–19.15) = 8.19
Between –0.5 and +0.5	(19.15+19.15) = 38.30
Above +0.75	(50.00–27.34) = 22.66
Below +2.00	(50.00+47.72) = 97.72
Above +2.00	(50.00+47.72) = 2.28
Below +2.5	(50.00+49.38) = 99.38
Above +2.5	(50.00-49.38) = 0.62
Between –2.0 and +1.5	(47.72+43.32) = 91.04
Between +0.4 and –0.2	(15.54+7.93) = 23.47
Between +0.8 and –0.6	(28.81–22.57) = 6.24
Between –1.65 and –1.25	(45.05–39.44) = 5.61

Cases within Given Score Limits

Generally three types of cases are encountered under this type-percentage of cases below a score point; percentage of cases above a score point; and percentage of cases within two score limits.

Example: Given a normal distribution of 500 scores with M = 40, and σ = 8, what percentage of cases lie (a) between scores of 36 and 42 (b) above a score of 48 and (c) below a score of 52?

Solution (Fig. 9.5)

Score limits	Equivalent	Normal curve table reading	% Area or % Cases
36	(36-40)/8 = –0.5	0.1915	19.15
42	(42-40)/8 = +0.25	0.0987	9.87
			29.02

Cases out of N = % area × N/100

$$\text{Hence cases out of } 500 = \frac{29-02\times 500}{100}$$

$$= 145.10 \text{ or } 145 \text{ cases}$$

i. The two score limits have been converted into equivalent Z's by using the formula (X – M)/s and algebraic signs also noted (see Col.2)

ii. Normal curve area tables consulted to find out readings equivalent to Z's (see Col.2)

iii. Since the two Z values have different signs, the one with a negative sign falls 0.5s units below the mean and the other falls 0.25s units above the mean. Hence, the two percentages of the area are to be added.

iv. The percentage of area can be converted into number of cases by using formula.

v. In cases where the two values of Z have the same sign or fall in the same half (i.e. only in the lower half, or only in the upper half), the smaller area is to be subtracted from the larger one. See Figure 9.6 which has been constructed on the basis of score limits of 52 and 48, both of which fall in the upper half.

Percentage of Area above a Score of 48

Raw score	Exact upper limit of score	Z score	Table reading	% Area
48	48.5	(48.5-40) 8 = +1.06 (Rounded)	0.3554	35.34

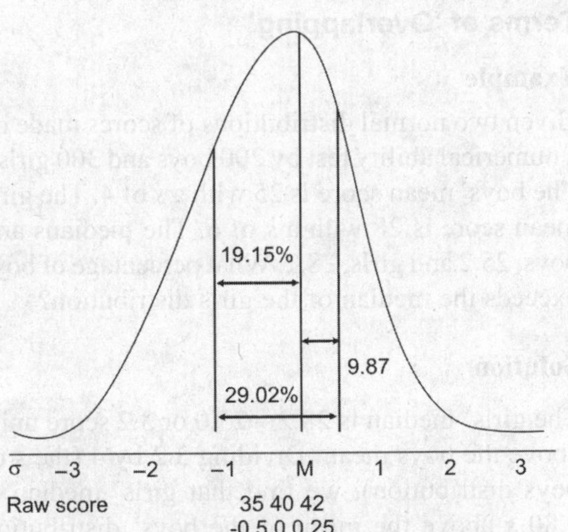

Fig 9.5: Calculation of area when *X* limits fall on both sides of the Mean

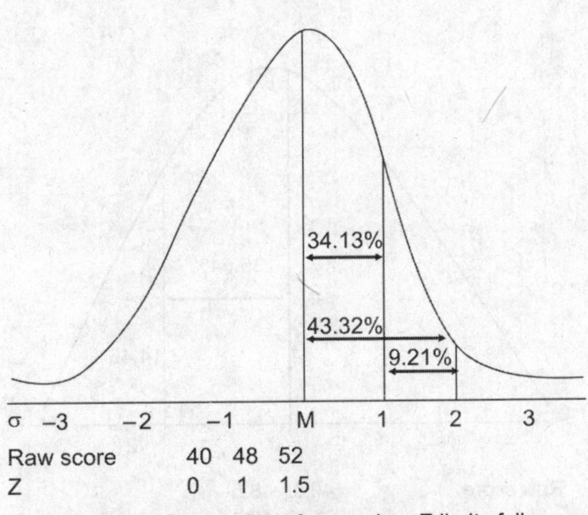

Fig. 9.6: Calculation of area when Z limits fall in the same half

Since the total area in the upper half is 50 percent and the area between Mean and 1.06Z is 35.34 percent, the area above AZ of 1.06 is obtained by subtracting 35.34 percent from 50.00. Hence the area above a score of 48 is equal to 50.00 percent –35.54 percent = 14.46 percent and the corresponding number of cases out 500 are = 14.46 × 500/100 = 72.30 or 72 cases (Fig. 9.7).

Percentage of Area below a Score of 52

Raw score	Exact upper limit of score	Z score	Table reading	% Area
52	51.5	(51.5 – 40.00)/8 = +1.44 (Rounded)	0.4251	42.51

The area below a Z of 1.44 would include the whole of the lower half, i.e. 50 percent, i.e. from mean to Z = 1.44 (Fig. 9.8). Hence, by adding, we obtain 50.00 + 42.51 = 92.51 percent or

$$\frac{92.51 \times 500}{100} = 462.55 \text{ or } 463 \text{ cases out of } 500.$$

Limits of Scores which include a given Percentage

Example: Given a normal distribution of 500 scores with a mean of 50 and s of 10. What score limits would include the middle 60 percent cases?

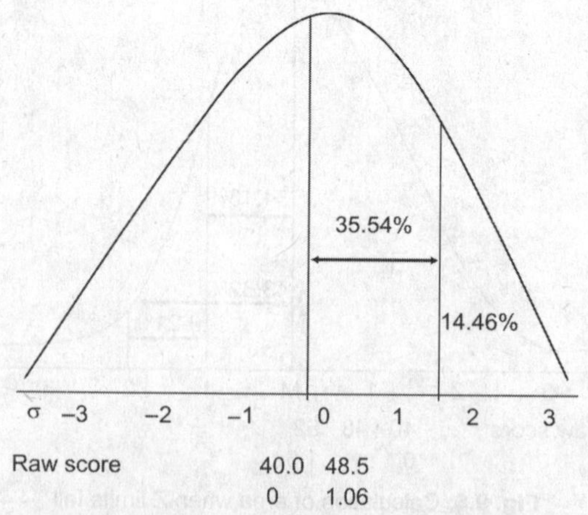

Fig. 9.7: Calculation of area above a given score

Solution: To obtain the middle 60 percent cases, one has to find out the score limits which combine 30 percent cases below the mean and 30 percent cases above the mean. Hence, the normal curve area tables are to be consulted in a reverse manner. Locate the 30 percent area in Table A and read Z equivalent to it. Then use the following formula to obtain the score limits:

$$\text{Raw score} = M + Z \times \sigma$$

The procedure is illustrated (Fig. 9.9) here:

Area percentage	Equivalent × with sign	Z × σ	Raw score M + Zσ
30% below	M-0.84	= 0.84 × 10 = –8.4	50+(–8.4) = 41.6
30% above	M+0.84	= 0.84 × 10 = 8.4	50+8.4 = 58.4

The Z values below the mean will carry minus signs and those above the mean, plus signs. Thus, the score limits of 41.6 – 58.4 include the middle 60 percent cases. In a similar manner other score limits can be calculated.

Comparison of Two Distributions in Terms of 'Overlapping'

Example

Given two normal distributions of scores made on a numerical ability test by 200 boys and 300 girls'. The boys' mean score is 25 with a *s* of 4. The girls mean score is 28 with a *s* of 6. The medians are: boys, 25.2 and girls, 28.2. What percentage of boys exceeds the median of the girls distribution?

Solution

The girls' median is 28.2 – 25.0 or 3.2 score units above the boys mean. Dividing 3.2 by 4 (the *s* of boys distribution), we find that girls' median is 0.80 *s* above the mean of the boys' distribution (Fig. 9.10). From the normal curve area table, we find that 22.57 percent of the normal distribution

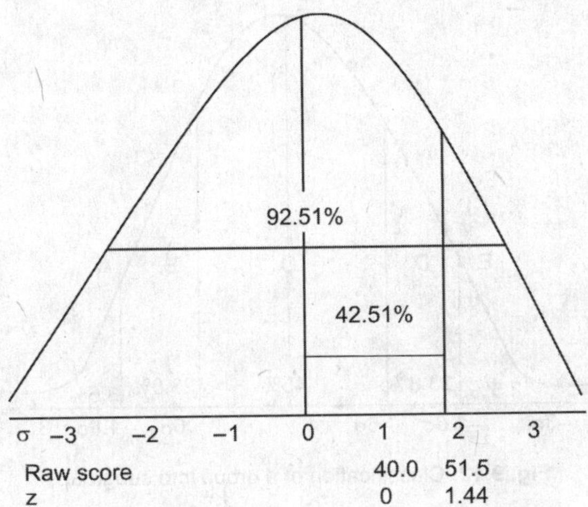

Fig. 9.8: Calculation of area below a given score

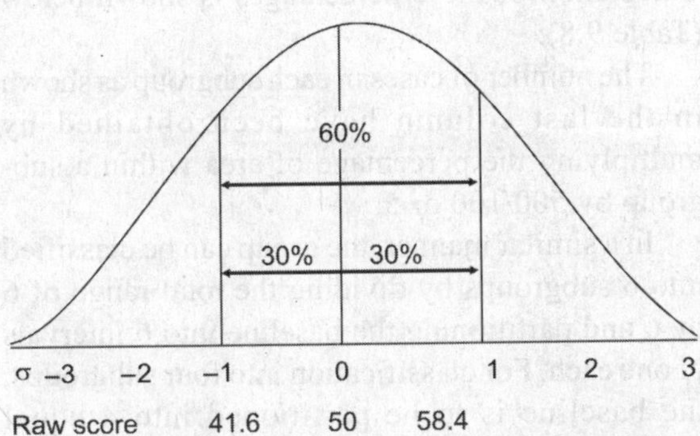

Fig. 9.9: Score limits equivalent to middle 60 and cases

lies between the mean and 0.60 σ. Hence, 27.43 percent of the boys (50 percent – 22.57 percent) exceed the girls' median.

Determination of Relative Difficulty of Test Items

Example: A test item is answered correctly by 20 percent of a large unselected group; a second item, solved correctly by 30 percent of the same group; and a third problem solved by 40 percent. Assuming normal distribution of capacity to solve test problems, what is the relative difficulty of items, 1, 2, and 3?

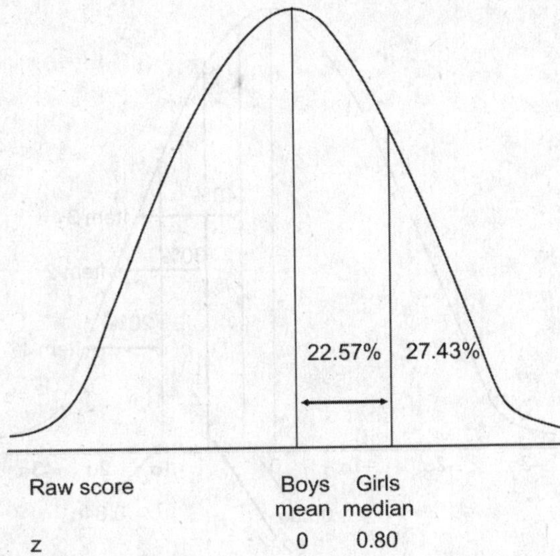

Fig. 9.10: Percentage of cases exceeding a particular score

Solution: First of all, we shall find out the cut off points of the baseline of the curve, which show top 20 percent, top 30 percent and top 40 percent of the cases (Fig. 9.11). Since all the distances are to be taken from the mean, the areas to be looked up in the Normal curve table are (50–20) = 30 percent; (50–30) = 20 percent; and (50–40) = 10 percent.

Now find out the Z's equivalent of these three percentages:

Item	*Passed by*	*Z*	*Z difference*
1	20%	0.84σ	--
2	30%	0.52σ	0.32 σ
3	40%	0.25 σ	0.27σ

We may now compare the three items on the difficulty level based on Z's. Item 1 has a difficulty value of 0.32 higher than item 2 and item 2 has a difficulty value of 0.27 higher than item 3. Thus, the difference in difficulty value of item 2 and 3 is about ¾ of the difference in difficulty value of item 1 and 2. Thus the difference in percentages (which is equal to 10 percent in each case here) is not good an index of differences in difficulty as the difference is.

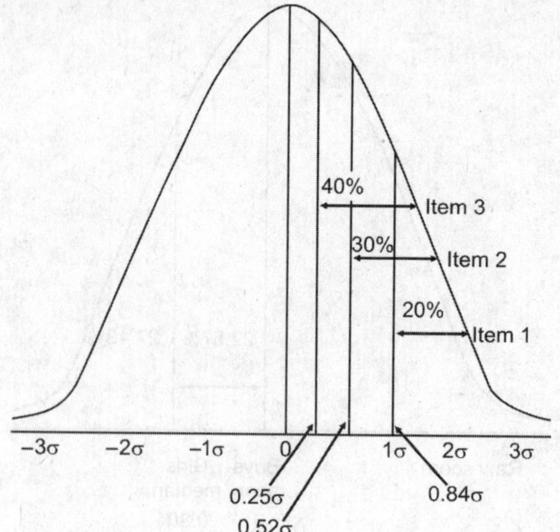

Fig. 9.11: Comparison of relative difficulty value of test items based on sigma differences

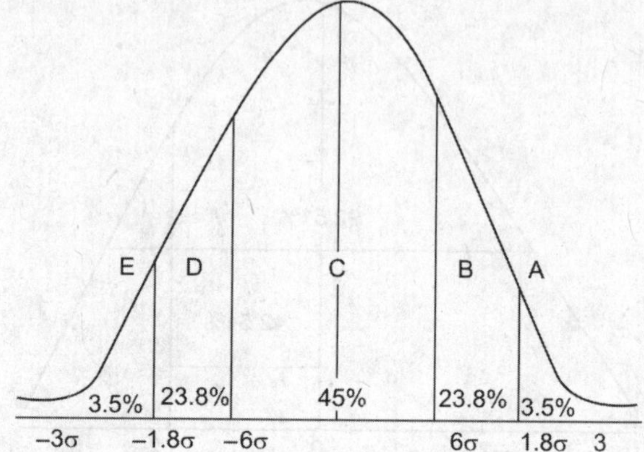

Fig. 9.12: Classification of a group into subgroups

Division of a Group into Subgroups

Example: Given a group of 500 college students who have been administered a general mental ability test. We wish to classify our group into five subgroups. A, B, C, D and E according to ability, the range of ability being equal in each sub-group. It is assumed that the trait is normally distributed in the application. Calculate the number of students that can be placed in groups A, B, C, D and E.

Solution: The baseline of a normal curve is considered to extend from −3 to +3 that is over a range of 6. Dividing this range by 5 (the number of subgroups) we obtain 1.2. Each group is to be allotted an equal extend of 1.2 on the baseline. The five intervals, thus formed, have been shown in Figure 9.12.

Group A covers the upper 1.2; group B the next 1.2; group C has 0.6 to the right and 0.6 to the left of the mean; Groups D and E occupy the same relative positions in the lower half of the curve that B and A occupy in the upper half. The next step is to find the percentage of the area that falls in the upper and lower limits of each subgroup. Calculation of these percentages is shown below (Table 9.8):

The number of cases in each subgroup as shown in the last column have been obtained by multiplying the percentage of area within a sub-group by 500/100 or 5.

In a similar manner, the group can be classified into 6 subgroups by dividing the total range of 6 by 6 and partitioning the baseline into 6 intervals of one each. For classification into four subgroups, the baseline is to be partitioned into 4 equal intervals of 1.5 inch (6/4 = 1.5).

Importance of the Normal Distribution

The normal distribution is by far the most used distribution in inferential statistics. There are some very important reasons for the same.

- *A good fit to many phenomena:* Sufficient evidence has accumulated to show that the normal distribution provides a good fit to describe the frequency of occurrence of many variable facts in biological statistics (sex ratio in births in a country over a number of years); in anthropometrical data (height, weight, etc.) in social and economic data (rates of births, marriages or deaths); in psychological measurements (intelligence, perception span

Table 9.8

Calculation of percent area and number of cases in each sub-group

Subgroup	*Upper* σ	*Limit* %	*Lower* σ	*Limit* %	*% In subgroup*	*Cases out of 500*
A	+ 3.0	49.86	+ 1.8	46.41	49.86–46.41 = 3.45	18
B	+ 1.8	46.41	+ 0.6	22.57	46.41–22.57 = 23.84	119
C	+ 0.6	22.57	– 0.6	22.57	22.57+22.57 = 45.14	226
D	– 0.6	22.57	– 1.8	46.41	46.41–22.57 = 23.84	119
E	– 1.8	46.41	– 3.0	49.86	49.86–46.41= 3.45	18

reaction time, educational test scores); and in errors of observation (chance errors which cause observations of heights and weights to deviate above or below their true value).

- It may be convenient, on mathematical grounds alone, to assume a normally distributed population. The normal function has important mathematical properties shared by no other theoretical distribution. Assuming a normal distribution gives the statistician an extremely rich set of mathematical consequences that he can use in developing methods.
- The normal distribution can be used as a good approximation to a number of other theoretical distributions like the binomial and can allow the calculation of probabilities that are either laborious or impossible to work out exactly.
- There is a very intimate connection between the size of sample and the extent to which a sampling distribution approaches the normal form. The central limit theorem states that many sampling distributions based on large N follow the normal curve even though the population distribution is definitely non-normal. This is one of the most remarkable and useful principles used in inferential statistics.

Divergence from Normality

Measures of a Symmetry or Skewness

When frequency distribution or a frequency curve is not symmetrical about the peak it is said to be skewed.

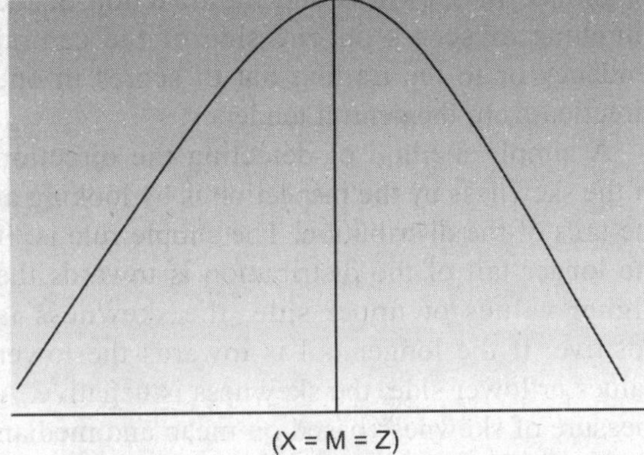

Fig. 9.13: Curve showing no skewness in which case we have X = M = Z

In other words one tail of the curve will be longer than the other in skewed curve. This skewness can be either to the right or left of the peak.

When the distribution of items in a series happens to be perfectly symmetrical, we then have the following type (Figure 9.13) of curve for the distribution:

Such a curve is technically described as a *normal curve* and the relating distributions as normal distribution. Such a curve is a perfect bell-shaped curve in which case the value X or M or Z is just the same and skewness is altogether absent.

But if the curve is distorted (whether on the right side or on the left side), we have asymmetrical distribution which indicates that there is skewness. If the curve is distorted on the right side, we have positive skewness but when the curve is distorted towards left, we have negative skewness as shown here under.

When distribution of scores is not symmetrical, it is said to be asymmetrical or skewed. By skewness, then, we mean the degree of its departure from symmetry. The frequency distribution of a set of scores is called symmetrical about the mean if the number of frequencies at any point on the upper side of the mean is exactly the same at a point equidistant from the mean on the lower side. Measures of skewness indicate two things—the magnitude of skewness and the direction of the bunching of scores on one side of the central tendency or to the trailing out of scores in one direction from the central tendency.

A simple method of detecting the direction of the skewness by the inspection is by looking at the tails of the distribution. The simple rule is: if the longer tail of the distribution is towards the higher values or upper side, the skewness is positive; if the longer tail is towards the lower values or lower side, the skewness is negative. A measure of skewness based on mean and median is given by the formula:

$$\frac{1}{\sigma\sqrt{2\pi}} \int_{-\infty}^{\infty} e^{-\frac{1}{2\sigma^2}(x-\mu)^2}$$

Another measure of skewness based on percentiles is given by the formula:

$$\phi x(t) = e^{\left(\mu i t - \frac{1}{2}\sigma^2 t^2\right)}$$

The two measures are not mathematically equivalent. A normal curve has SK=0. Deviations from normality can be in negative and positive directions leading to negatively skewed and positively skewed distributions respectively.

Skewness is, thus, a measure of asymmetry and shows the manner in which the items are clustered around the average. In a symmetrical distribution, the items show a perfect balance on either side of the mode, but in a skew distribution the balance is thrown to one side. The amount by which the balance exceeds on one side measures the skewness of the series. The difference between the mean, median or the mode provides an easy way of expressing skewness in a series. In case of positive skewness, we have $Z < M < \overline{X}$ and in case of negative skewness we have $\overline{X} < M < Z$. Usually, we measure skewness in this way:

Skewness = $\overline{X} - Z$ and its coefficient (j) is worked

Out as $j = \beta_2 = \frac{\mu_4}{\mu_2^2} \alpha_4$

In case Z is not well defined, then we work out skewness as under:

Skewness = 3 ($\overline{X} - M$) and its coefficient (j) is worked out as

$$j = \beta_2 = \frac{\mu_4}{\mu_2^2} \alpha_4 \text{ or } \gamma_2 = (\beta_2 - 3)$$

The significance of skewness lies in the fact that through it one can study the formation of series and can have the idea about the shape of the curve, whether normal or otherwise, when the items of a given series are plotted on a graph.

Kurtosis is the measure of flat-toppedness of a curve. A bell-shaped curve or normal curve is Mesokurtic because it is kurtic in the center, but if the curve is relatively more peaked than the normal curve, it is called Leptokurtic whereas, a curve is more flat than the normal curve, it is called Platykurtic. In brief, Kurtosis is the humpedness of the curve and points to the nature of distribution of items in the middle of a series.

It may be pointed out here that knowing the shape of the distribution curve is crucial to the use of statistical methods in research analysis since, most methods make specific assumptions about the nature of the distribution curve.

In actual practice, frequency distributions are rarely symmetrical; rather they show varying degrees of asymmetry or skewness. In a perfectly symmetrical distribution, the mean, median and mode coincide, whereas this is not the case in a distribution that is asymmetrical or skewed. Figures 9.14 and 9.15 present illustrations of curves that are noticeably skewed. The one on the left is skewed negatively and the one on the right is skewed positively. It will be observed that in the curve with negative skewness the mean is less than the mode, whereas in the curve with positive skewness the mean is greater than the mode. The mode is not affected by either the size or the number of extreme items in a frequency distribution, but the mean is.

Coefficients of skewness have been devised which measure the direction of the skewness as well as the degree, either absolutely or relatively. A commonly used but only rough measure of skewness is merely the difference between the mean and the mode $= \frac{\mu_4 - 3\mu_2^2}{\mu_2^2}$. The sign indicates the direction of skewness and the difference, the amount. The distribution of the weights of 265 university students shows a slight positive skewness for $\mu = A + \frac{\Sigma_i f_i d_i}{N} \times I = 148.74$ and $\Sigma = 145.28$ and $148.74 - 145.28 = +3.46$.

A more satisfactory measure of skewness in which the degree of variability is given due weight is:

$$\frac{-11}{60}$$

Since the true mode is frequently difficult to determine, another formula developed by Karl

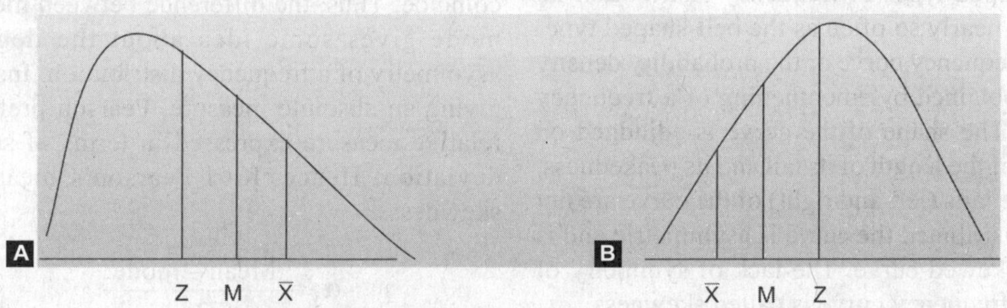

Figs 9.14A and B: Illustration of curves that are negatively skewed

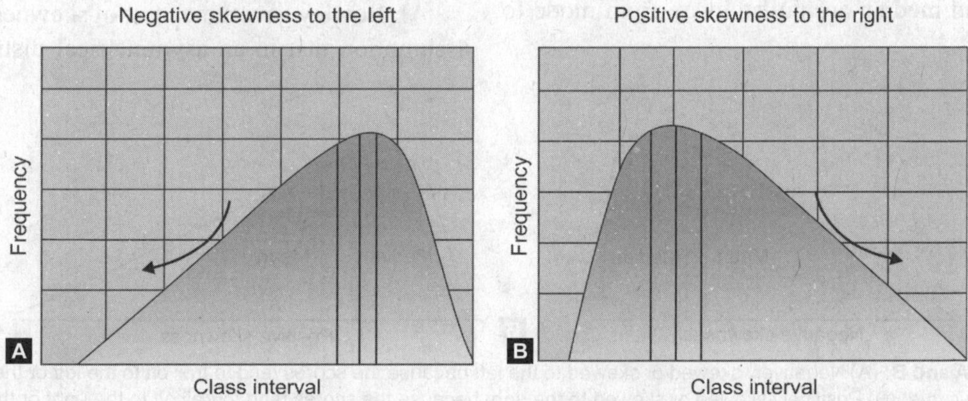

Figs 9.15A and B: Illustrations of skewed curves

Pearson for indicating skewness can be applied, especially, if the series is only moderately skewed. According to this formula,

$$\text{Mode} = I_0 + \frac{\Delta_1}{\Delta_1 + \Delta_2} \times I$$

The frequency distributions which have been considered thus far have been the common type in which the frequencies are relatively low at the ends and high towards the middle. In addition to this type, there are frequency curves which show a tendency constantly to increase or decrease. These curves possess the general characteristics of a capital "J" and are known as J-shaped curves. There is also another type of irregular distribution in which the frequencies are relatively high at the two ends and low toward the middle. This type is referred to as U-shaped curves. Both the J-shaped and U-shaped types of frequency distribution do not occur nearly so often as the bell-shaped type.

The frequency curve or the probability density curve is obtained by smoothening of a frequency polygon. The shape of the curve is adjudged on the basis of the length of its tail and its peakedness. If both the tails (left and right) of the curve are not equally distributed the curve is asymmetric and is called a skewed curve. The lack of symmetry of tails of a frequency curve is called skewness.

If the left tail of the frequency curve is longer than the right tail, the curve is said to be negatively skewed as shown in Figure 9.16A. In this case, mean and median are pulled away from mode to the left.

On the other hand, if the right tail is more elongated than the left tail, the curve is said to be positively skewed as shown in Figure 9.16B. The mean and median are pulled away from mode towards right hand side. In the case where we are given some frequency distribution, the idea of skewness can be perceived through a frequency curve. The measure of skewness is an indicator of lack of symmetry. This also gives an idea as to whether dispersal of observations about a central value is symmetrical or not. The curve can give some vague idea but the numerical measurement of skewness gives an exact idea of distribution. Different formulae for the measure of skewness, denoted by α_3, are as follows:

Karl Pearson's method of measurement of skewness is based on the assumption that in an asymmetrical distribution, mean and mode never coincide. Thus, the difference between mean and mode gives some idea about the degree of asymmetry of a frequency distribution. Instead of giving an absolute measure, Pearson preferred a relative measure expressed in terms of standard deviation. Hence, Karl Pearson's measure of skewness.

$$\alpha_3 = \frac{\text{Mean} - \text{mode}}{\text{SD}} \qquad ...(9.35)$$

Obviously formula (9.35) is good when it is easy to find out the mean, mode and standard deviation.

AL Bowley gave a measure of skewness on the assumption that in an asymmetrical distribution,

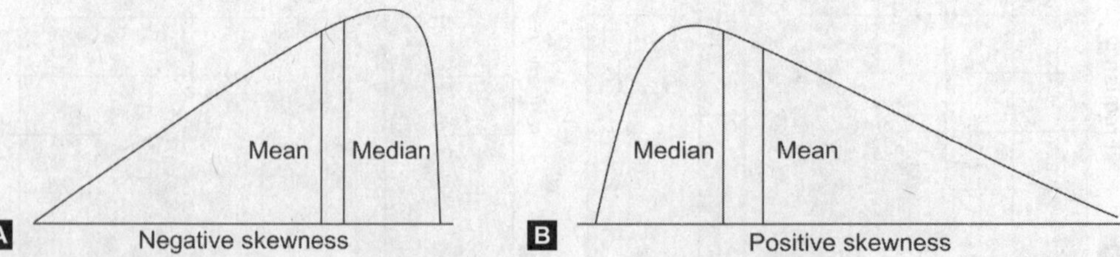

Figs 9.16A and B: (A) Negatively skewed or skewed to the left because the scores tend to trail off to the left or the negative end of the curve; (B) Positively skewed or skewed to the right because the scores tend to trail off to the right or the positive end of the curve

the second quartile is not equidistant from the first and the third quartile.

Thus, Bowley's formula for the measure of skewness, is

$$\alpha_3 = \frac{Q_3 + Q_1 - 2Q_2}{Q_3 - Q_1} \quad ...(9.36)$$

Another formula for α_3 in terms of moments is,

$$\alpha_3 = \frac{\mu_3}{(\mu_2)^{3/2}} \quad ...(9.37)$$

Value of α_3 by any formula is a pure number, i.e. α_3 has no physical unit. For a symmetrical curve $\alpha_3 = 0$. If $\alpha_3 = 0$, mean, median and mode coincide. The sign of α_3 is same as the of μ_3. If α_3 is negative, i.e. $\alpha_3 < 0$, then the curve is negatively skewed which means that the curve has an elongated left tail. If α_3 is positive, i.e. $\alpha_3 > 0$, then the curve is positively skewed which indicates that the right tail of the frequency curve is longer than the left tail (Figs 9.17 and 9.18).

Some other coefficients of skewness based on moments are Beta coefficient and Gamma coefficient. Their relation with each other is also given below:

$$\beta_1 = \frac{\mu_3^2}{\mu_2^3} \quad ...(9.38)$$

or $$\sqrt{\beta_1} = \frac{\mu_3}{\mu_2^{3/2}} = \alpha_3 \quad ...(9.38.1)$$

Also, $$\gamma_1 = \sqrt{\beta_1} = \alpha_3 \quad ...(9.39)$$

Karl Pearson introduced the concept of Beta coefficients which are known as Pearsonian coefficients. Gamma notations were introduced by RA Fisher. The interpretation of γ_1 remains the same as that of α_3. It is a fact that median always lies between mean and mode in an asymmetrical distribution. Hence, the following relation between mean, median and mode based on experience and intuition holds good for a moderately asymmetrical distribution.

Mean – Mode = 3 (Mean – Median) ...(9.40)

Mode = 3 Median – 2 Mean ...(9.40.1)

When a distribution of scores is not symmetrical, it is said to be asymmetrical or skewed. By skewness, then, we mean the degree of its' departure from symmetry. The frequency distribution of a set of scores is called symmetrical about the mean, if the number of frequencies at any point on the upper side of the mean is exactly the same at a point equidistant from the mean on the lower side. Measures of skewness indicate two things—the magnitude of skewness and the direction of skewness. The symmetry of a curve is disturbed

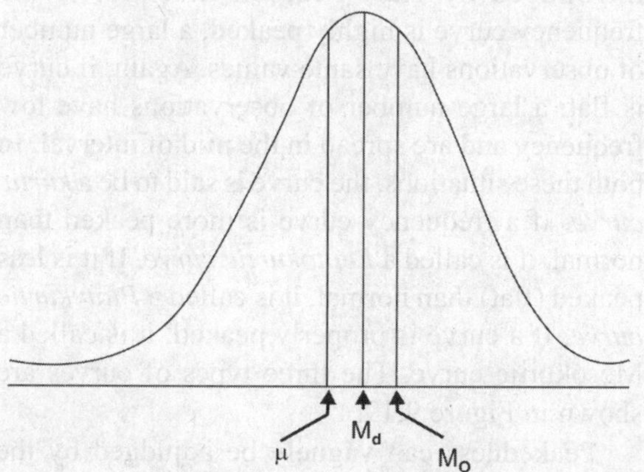

Fig 9.17: Negative skew curve

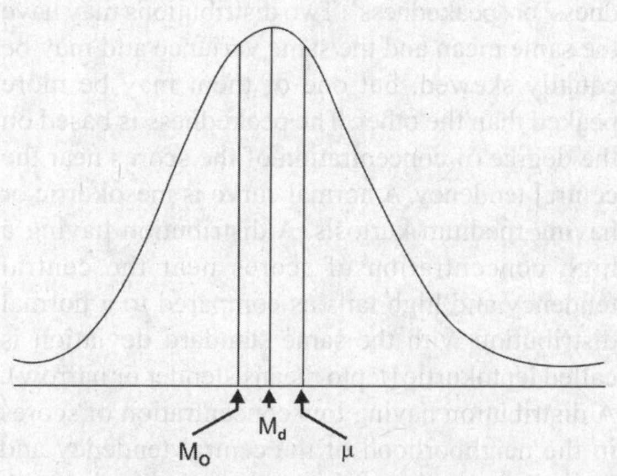

Fig. 9.18: Positive skew curve

by the bunching of scores on one side of the central tendency or to the trailing out of scores in one direction from the central tendency.

A simple method of detecting the direction of skewness by inspection is by looking at the tails of the distribution. The simple rule is: if the longer tail of the distribution is towards the higher values or upper side, the skewness is positive; if the longer tail is towards the lower values or lower side, the skewness is negative. A measure of skewness based on mean and median is given by the formula:

$$SK = \frac{3\,(\text{mean} - \text{median})}{\sigma} \quad ...(9.41)$$

Another measure of skewness based on percentiles is given by the formula:

$$SK = \frac{(P_{90} + P_{10})}{2} - P_{50}$$

These two measures are not mathematically equivalent. A normal curve has SK = 0. Deviations from normality can be in negative and positive directions leading to negatively skewed and positively skewed distribution respectively (Figs 9.17 and 9.18).

Kurtosis

The Kurtosis of a distribution refers to its 'curvedness' or 'peakedness'. Two distributions may have the same mean and the same variance and may be equally skewed, but one of them may be more peaked than the other. The peakedness is based on the degree of concentration of the scores near the central tendency. A normal curve is mesokurtic or having medium kurtosis. A distribution having a high concentration of scores near the central tendency and high tails as compared to a normal distribution with the same standard deviation is called leptokurtic (lepto means slender or narrow). A distribution having low concentration of scores in the neighborhood of the central tendency and low tails as compared to a normal distribution with the same standard deviation is called platykurtic (platy means flat, broad or wide).

Several rough methods can be used for judging whether a distribution lacks normal symmetry or peakedness. It may ordinarily be detected by inspection of the frequency polygon. However, apparent peakedness may result from choice of dimensions for the polygon. Another way of detecting kurtosis is by seeing whether the percentages of cases in various quartile or standard deviation intervals included normal percentages of cases. If these percentages are not normal, the distribution is either skewed or abnormally peaked.

Kurtosis can be measured by the following formula based on percentiles:

$$KU = \frac{Q}{(P_{90} - P_{10})}$$

where, Q = quartile deviation,

P_{90} and P_{10} = 90th and 10th percentiles respectively.

A normal distribution has KU = 0.263. If KU is less than 0.263, the distribution is leptokurtic; and if KU is greater than 0.263, the distribution is platykurtic.

As already mentioned, the other criterion for determining the shape of a unimodal frequency curve is its peakedness. Kurtosis is a Greek word and it means bulginess. The term 'kurtosis' was introduced by Karl Pearson in 1906. If the frequency curve is highly peaked, a large number of observations have same values. Again, if curve is flat. a large number of observations have low frequency and are spread in the mid of interval. In both these situations, the curve is said to be a *kurtic curve*. If a frequency curve is more peaked than normal, it is called a *Leptokurtic curve*. If it is less peaked (flat) than normal, it is called a *Platykurtic curve*. If a curve is properly peaked, it is called a Mesokurtic curve. The three types of curves are shown in Figure 9.19.

Peakedness can vaguely be adjudged by the curve but it can be better ascertained by the mathematical measure known as the measure of kurtosis. The formula for the measure of kurtosis is,

$$\alpha_4 = \frac{\mu_4}{\mu_2^2} \quad ...(9.42)$$

$$= \frac{\mu_4}{\sigma^4} \quad ...(9.42.1)$$

It is apparent from (9.42) that α_4 is always positive, as it is the ratio of two positive quantities. α_4 has no physical unit. For leptokurtic curve, $\alpha_4 > 3$ and for a platykurtic curve $\alpha_4 < 3$. If $\alpha_4 = 3$, the curve is a mesokurtic. The quantity $(\alpha_4 - 3)$ is called the excess of kurtosis. α_3 and α_4 given an exact idea only, if the population constants (moments) are known or the size of the sample is substantially large.

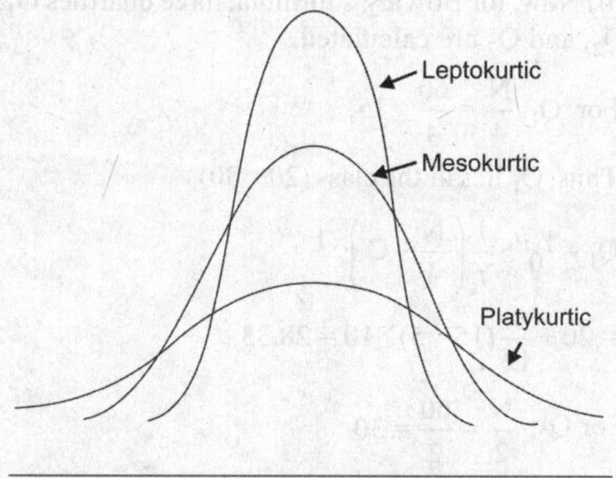

Fig. 9.19: Kurtic curves

Note: In case moments and other population constants are not known, then the estimated values are substituted to get an idea of the shape of frequency curve.

As in the case of skewness, the measure of kurtosis in terms of Beta and Gamma coefficients are also given. These coefficients are the expressions in terms of moment ratio and are given below. Interrelationship between them have also been given.

$$\beta_2 = \frac{\mu_4}{\mu_2^2} \alpha_4 \quad ...(9.43)$$

$$\gamma_2 = (\beta_2 - 3) \quad ...(9.44)$$

$$= \frac{\mu_4 - 3\mu_2^2}{\mu_2^2} \quad ...(9.44.1)$$

Different values of γ_2 give information about the peakedness of the frequency curve.

If $\gamma_2 = 0$, the curve is properly peaked, i.e. mesokurtic curve.

If $\gamma_2 > 0$, the curve is more peaked than normal, i.e. leptokurtic cruve.

First prepare the following table:

Marks	*Mid values (x)*	$d = \frac{(X-45)}{10}$	*freq (f)*	*cu freq*	*fd*	*fd*^{2}	*fd*^{3}	*fd*^{4}
0-10	5	– 4	2	2	– 8	32	– 128	512
10-20	15	– 3	3	5	– 9	27	– 81	243
20-30	25	– 2	12	17	– 24	48	– 96	192
30-40	35	– 1	8	25	– 8	8	– 8	8
40-50	45	0	10	35	0	0	0	0
50-60	55	1	17	52	17	17	17	17
60-70	65	2	4	56	8	16	32	64
70-80	75	3	3	59	9	27	81	243
80-90	85	4	1	60	4	16	64	256
		0	60		– 11	191	– 119	1535

If $\gamma_2 < 0$, the curve is less peaked than normal, i.e., platykurtic curve. For a normal curve, $\gamma_1 = 0$ and $\gamma_2 = 0$.

Example 9: Given the following distribution of marks in physics of 60 students of undergraduate class, the skewness and kurtosis of the frequency curve can be determined as follows:

Marks	*Frequency*
0-10	2
10-20	3
20-30	12
30-40	8
40-50	10
50-60	17
60-70	4
70-80	3
80-90	1

To clarify the method of calculation, the skewness has been calculated by all the three formulae, and kurtosis by the method of moments.

(i) To find out the coefficient of kurtosis, first the mean, mode and standard deviation are calculated.

We know,

$$\mu = A + \frac{\Sigma_i f_i d_i}{N} \times I$$

for $i = 1, 2, ..., 9$

Here we have taken $A = 45, I = 10$.

Also $N = 60$ and $\Sigma f_i d_i = -11$

Therefore, $\mu = 45 + \frac{-11}{60} \times 10 = 43.17$

$$\text{Mode} = I_0 + \frac{\Delta_1}{\Delta_1 + \Delta_2} \times I$$

In the given distribution model class is (50–60),

$$\Delta_1 = 7, \Delta_2 = 13 \text{ and } I = 10$$

Therefore,

$$\text{Mode} = 50 + \frac{7}{7+13} \times 10 = 53.5$$

We know,

$$\sigma = \sqrt{\frac{1}{N}\left\{\Sigma_i f_i d_i^2 - \frac{(\Sigma_i f_i d_i^2)}{N}\right\}} \times I$$

In the above table $\Sigma f_i d_i^2 = 191$

Therefore,

$$\sigma = \sqrt{\frac{1}{60}\left\{191 - \frac{(-11)^2}{60}\right\}} \times 10 = 17.75$$

$$\alpha_3 = \frac{\text{Mean} - \text{Mode}}{\text{SD}} = \frac{43.17 - 53.5}{17.75} = -0.58$$

(ii) Now, for Bowley's formula, three quartiles Q_1, Q_2, and Q_3 are calculated.

For $Q_1, \frac{N}{4} = \frac{60}{4} = 15,$

Thus, Q_1 lies in the class $(20-30)$

$$Q_1 = I_0 + \frac{1}{f}\left(\frac{N}{4} - C\right) \times I$$

$$= 20 + \frac{1}{12}(15-5) \times 10 = 28.33$$

For $Q_2, \frac{N}{2} = \frac{60}{2} = 30$

Thus, Q_2 lies in the class (40 – 50).

$$Q_2 = I_0 + \frac{1}{f}\left(\frac{N}{2} - C\right) \times I$$

$$= 40 + \frac{1}{10}(30-25) \times 10 = 45.00$$

Similarly for, $Q_3, \frac{3N}{4} = \frac{3 \times 60}{4} = 45$

Hence, Q_3 ies in class (50–60)

$$Q_3 = I_0 + \frac{1}{f}\left(\frac{3N}{4} - C\right) \times I$$

$$= 50 + \frac{1}{17}(45-35) \times 10 = 55.88$$

Bowley's formula for measure of skewness is

$$\alpha_3 = \frac{Q_3 + Q_1 - 2Q_2}{Q_3 - Q_1}$$

$$\alpha_3 = \frac{55.88 + 28.33 - 2\times 45}{55.88 - 28.33} = \frac{5.79}{27.55} = -0.21$$

Measure of skewness from moments can be calculated by the formula,

$$\alpha_3 = \frac{\mu_3}{\alpha^3}$$

We know,

$$\mu_3 = \frac{1}{N}\Sigma_i f_i\ (X_i - \bar{X})^3 \ \text{ for } i = 1, 2, \ldots, 9$$

$$= \frac{1}{N}\left\{\Sigma_i f_i (d_i - \bar{d})^3\right\}\times I^3$$

$$= \left[\left\{\frac{1}{N}(\Sigma_i f_i d_i^3 - 3\bar{d}\,\Sigma_i f_i d_i^2 + 3\bar{d}^2\,\Sigma_i f_i d_i - \bar{d}^3)\times I^3\right]\right.$$

where,

$$\bar{d} = \Sigma_i f_i d_i / N$$

$$= \left[\frac{1}{60}\left\{\frac{1}{60}(-119)\left(\frac{-11}{60}\right)\times 191 + 3 \left(\frac{-11}{60}\right)^2(-11) - \left(\frac{-11}{60}\right)^3\right\}\right]\times 10^3$$

$$= \left\{\frac{1}{60}(-119) - 105.05 - 1.11 + 0.006\right\}\times 10^3$$

$$= -\,0.2509 \times 1000 = -\,250.90$$

$$\sigma^3 = (17.75)^3 = 5592.36$$

Thus,

$$\alpha_3 = \frac{-250.90}{5592.36} = -0.045$$

It is apparent from the values of α_3 obtained from the three formulae, that the distribution of marks is slightly negatively skewed.

Now to calculate the measure of kurtosis α_4, we have to calculate μ_4.

$$\mu_4 = \left[\frac{1}{N}\Sigma_i f\hat{i}(d\hat{i} - \bar{d})^4\right]\times I^4$$

$$= \left[\frac{1}{N}\left\{\Sigma_i f_i d_1^{\,4} - 4\bar{d}\,\Sigma_i f_i d_i^{\,3} + 6\bar{d}^2\ \Sigma_i f_i d_i^{\,2} - 4\bar{d}^3\,\Sigma_i f_i d_i + \bar{d}^4\right\}\right]\times I^4$$

$$= \left[\frac{1}{60}\left\{1535 - 4\left(\frac{-11}{60}\right)(-119) + 6\times\left(\frac{-11}{60}\right)^2 \times 191 - 4\left(\frac{-11}{60}\right)^3(-11) + \left(\frac{-11}{60}\right)^4\right\}\right]\times 10^4$$

$$= \left[\frac{1}{60}\{1535 - 87.27 + 38.52 - 0.27 + 0.001\}\right]\times 10^4$$

$$= 24.7664 \times 10000 = 247664$$

Measures of Skewness and Kurtosis based on Moments Methods

In mechanics, the term moment is used to denote a measure of the tendency of a force to cause rotation of an object about a point. The strength of the tendency depends upon two things–the amount of the force and the distance from the point at which the force acts. Hence, a moment is the product of force times distance (M = F × D). There may be moments applying the force in one direction and others applying it in the other direction. When the sum of the moments tending to cause rotation in one direction is equal to the sum of the moments tending to cause rotation in the opposite direction, the object is in balance. In a statistical series, an item may be considered as a unit force acting at a distance *x* from the arithmetic mean, i.e. as a moment of force. Since the sum of negative deviations from the mean is equal to the sum of positive deviations, the mean is analogous to a point of balance. In statistics, the algebraic sum of the distance or deviations from the mean divided by N is called the first moment of the series.

The second moment of the series can be obtained, if deviations from the mean are squared, summed and divided by N. The third and fourth moments are based respectively upon the third and fourth powers of the deviations. Thus, the first four moments about the mean can be defined as follows:

$$\mu_1 = \frac{\Sigma x}{N} = 0 \quad ...(9.45)$$

$$\mu_2 = \frac{\Sigma x^2}{N} = \sigma^2 \quad ...(9.46)$$

$$\mu_3 = \frac{\Sigma x^3}{N} \quad ...(9.47)$$

$$\mu_4 = \frac{\Sigma x^4}{N} \quad ...(9.48)$$

where, 1, 2, 3, 4 are first, second, third and fourth moments respectively and x = X – M and the deviations are taken from the actual mean. When data are grouped in terms of class intervals of the constant size I and frequencies, the second, third and fourth moments about the mean can be calculated by using the following formulas:

$$\mu_2 = i^2\left[\left(\frac{\Sigma fd^2}{N}\right) - \left(\frac{\Sigma fd^2}{N}\right)\right] = \sigma^2 \quad ...(9.49)$$

$$\left[\left(\frac{\Sigma fd^4}{N}\right) - 4\left(\frac{\Sigma fd^3}{N}\right)\left(\frac{\Sigma fd}{N}\right) + 6\left(\frac{\Sigma fd^2}{N}\right)\left(\frac{\Sigma fd}{N}\right)^2 - 3\left(\frac{\Sigma fd}{N}\right)^4\right] \quad ...(9.50)$$

It may be noted that the calculation of 2 is exactly alike that of calculation of variance by the coded method. The initial steps in the calculation of other moments also follow the same method with the difference that these go up to Σfd^3 in case of μ_3 and up to Σfd^4 in case of 4. The value of Σfd^3 can be obtained by multiplying each fd^2 by corresponding d and summing over all such values thus obtained. The value of fd^4 is obtained by multiplying the entries in fd^3 further by d and obtaining the column sum. These values may then be divided by N separately and substituted in the formulas given above. There is hardly any need to substitute the value of i (class interval) and express the moments in the original units of measurements. When the moments are substituted in formulas 9.55 and 9.56, the i's cancel out. Necessary attention regarding the correct substitution and multiplication signs should be given to avoid errors in computing moments.

After the moments have been obtained, skewness and kurtosis can be computed by using the formulas given below:

$$\alpha_3 = \frac{\mu_3}{\mu_2\sqrt{\mu_2}} \quad ...(9.51)$$

$$\alpha_4 = \frac{\mu_4}{\mu_2^2} \quad ...(9.52)$$

in which, α_3 and α_4 = skewness and kurtosis, respectively,

μ_2, μ_3, μ_4 = second, third and fourth moments, respectively.

Interpretation: For the purpose of interpretation of α_3 and α_4, the following quick guide may be used.

Value		*Interpretation*
α_3=0		Normal
$\alpha_3 < 0$	(negative value)	Negative skewness
$\alpha_3 > 0$	(positive value)	Positive skewness
α_4=3		Normal
$\alpha_4 < 3$		Platykurtosis
$\alpha_4 > 3$		Leptokurtosis

In case of α_3, the greater the departure from 0, the greater the negative or positive skewness. In case of α_4, the greater the departure from 3, the greater the platykurtosis or leptokurtosis.

Significance of the Measures of Skewness and Kurtosis

The values of α_3 and α_4 obtained for any distribution are compared with the values of α_3 and α_4 found in normal distribution and significance of the difference determined. The questions precisely are: Does the obtained value of α_3 differ significantly from zero? If yes, at what level of confidence? Does the obtained value of α_4 differ significantly from 3? If yes, at what level of confidence?

Egon S Pearson has devised a table of 0.10 and 02 limits of α_3 when based on samples drawn from a normal population. Another table showing the upper and lower 0.01 and 0.05 limits of α_4 when based on random samples from a normal distribution has also been prepared. These tables are given in Appendix H and I.

Importance of Measures of Skewness and Kurtosis

The measures of skewness and kurtosis are of interest to the researchers and statisticians for a number of reasons and uses which these can be put to. Some more of them are discussed below in brief:

1. Measures of skewness and kurtosis together with measures of central tendency and variability, and the number of cases, N, convey all the information ordinarily needed to understand and interpret any distribution.
2. Measures of skewness and kurtosis indicate the extend of "non-normal" variation in a series of scores. Since a large number of parametric tests presuppose normality at some point of their application and to departure from normality, the measures of skewness and kurtosis can be helpful in ascertaining whether the assumption of normality had been fulfilled by the experimental data to warrant the use of a particular statistical test. The shape of the distribution is always of first concern to the statistician even in such simple descriptive measures as those of central tendency and variability.

   It can further be argued that those measures quantitatively indicate departure from normality and hence provide more precise and unambiguous meaning to such expressions as "slightly non-normal", "markedly non-normal", "approximately normal" and "severely skewed". The alphas are interpretable in a clear way. The more α_3 differs from 0, the more skewed the distribution; the more α_4 differs from 3, the greater the departure from normal peakedness.
3. Another important use to which the measures of skewness and kurtosis are generally put, relates to the comparison of the shape of two or more distribution. Thus, they furnish additional information to supplement that which is obtained from measures of central tendency and variability. These indicate the shape of the scatter of the items in a series about the average value.
4. In educational and psychological measurement, skewness assumes importance because it makes the central tendency difficult to interpret. Non-normal peakedness distorts the normal standard scores and area relationships and hence an important measure to compute.

Since the main purpose of calculating measures of skewness and kurtosis is to add to the adequacy of description of a distribution and to facilitate comparisons between two or more distributions, it would be worthwhile if the student takes certain precautions in the use of the same. The frequent occurrence of symmetrical distributions for psychological and educational variables may result from an artifact and the occurrence of a skewed distribution may also be artifactual. Most of the instruments in psychological and educational measurements involve unequal units decided upon arbitrarily and sometimes accidentally. Generally, the score a person gets on a test depends upon the number of items checked or done correctly. Since the number of items correct is an artifact of the difficulty level of the items the shape of the distribution is largely determined by the latter.

With items of medium difficulty, the scale is likely to yield a symmetrical distribution when applied to a group; if the items are very easy, the scores will pile up toward the top thus leading to negative skewness; if the items are very difficult, the concentration of scores toward the bottom will occur, thus generating a positive skewness.

Ordinarily, it is not necessary to compute measures of skewness and kurtosis unless there are indications to the same. However, the nature of the investigation, the size of the sample and the nature of the variable under study are important factors to be considered in determining whether these measures should be computed or not. If the size of the sample is less than 100, these measures may not give very reliable results.

Sampling Distributions

Sampling distribution describes the way in which a statistic or a function of statistics, which is/are the function(s) of the random variables $X_1, X_2, ..., X_n$, will vary from one sample to another sample of the same size. Such sampling distributions have given a fillip to the number of test statistics for hypotheses testing. Hence, some important sampling distributions are discussed in this chapter.

Student's *t*-Distribution

The '*t*' distribution also known as student's *t*-distribution is a sampling distribution derived from the parent normal distribution, introduced by WS Gosset and developed by RA Fisher. The statistics of small samples were revolutionized by this distribution.

Take a sample (of size for example) from the 500 Hb, values given in Appendix B and calculate the quantity '*t*' which is given by the equation.

$$t = \frac{!x - \mu!}{s\sqrt{n}} \quad ...(9.53)$$

where x is the mean of the sample; μ is the mean of the population; n is the size of the sample; s !√ is the estimate of the standard error of mean and s is given by the formula:

$$\sqrt{\frac{\text{Sum of squares of deviations of observations from mean (sample)}}{n-1}}$$

If many samples of the same size are taken from the normal population then the quantity t (both positive and negative values) will follow this distribution.

This t distribution is also a symmetric distribution about its' mean. Like in all symmetric distributions, mean, median and mode coincide. Unlike the normal distribution, the shape of *t*-distribution varies according to the size of the sample or according to the degrees of freedom. The size of the sample minus the number of parameters estimated is called degrees of freedom. In the present case only one quantity is used as an estimate. Therefore, the number of degrees of freedom is $n - 1$. The degrees of freedom is also defined as the number of independent members in the sample. When the size of the sample is large, the *t*-distribution closely approximates the normal distribution.

Under the heading 'Standard Error', that if a random sample $X_1, X_2, ..., X_n$ of size n, with observed values $x_1, x_2, ..., x_n$ is drawn from a normal population having mean μ and SD. σ, the mean $\bar{x}$ is distributed normally with mean μ and SD.

$\sigma/\sqrt{n}$, i.e. $\bar{x} \sim N(\mu, \sigma/\sqrt{n})$.

Also the variable Z, where

$$Z = \frac{x - \mu}{\sigma/\sqrt{n}} \quad ...(9.54)$$

is a normal variate with mean 0 and standard deviation 1, i.e. Z ~ N (0,1).

In practice, the standard deviation σ is not known and in such a situation the only alternative left is to, use s, the sample estimate of standard deviation σ. Thus the variate $\sqrt{n(\bar{x} - \mu)}/s$ is distributed as t and hence

$$t = \frac{\bar{x} - \mu}{s/\sqrt{n}} \quad ...(9.55)$$

where $$s^2 = \frac{1}{n-1}\Sigma_i (x_1 - \bar{x})^2$$

t is a widely used variable and the distribution of t is called student's t-distribution. This distribution was discovered by WS Gosset in 1908. The statistician Gosset is better known by the pseudonym 'student' and hence t-distribution is called student's t-distribution. He drived the distribution of $\overline{x}/s\,\overline{x}$ (where $s\,\overline{x}$ = s/ $\sqrt{n}$) to find an exact test of a mean by making use of estimated standard deviation s, based on a random sample of size n. RA Fisher in 1925, published that t-distribution can also be applied to the test of regression coefficient and other practical problems. Here, we give the density function and properties of t-distribution without derivation.The readers interested in the derivation should consult a book on mathematical statistics. The density function of variable t with $k = n - 1$ degrees of freedom$_2$ is,

$$f_k(t) = \frac{1}{\sqrt{k}B\left(\frac{1}{2},\frac{k}{2}\right)} \frac{1}{\left(1\frac{t^2}{k}\right)^{(k+1)/2}} - \infty < t < \infty \quad ...(9.56)$$

$$B\left(\frac{1}{2},\frac{k}{2}\right) = \frac{\sqrt{1/2}\sqrt{k/2}}{\sqrt{\frac{k+1}{2}}} = \frac{\sqrt{\pi}\sqrt{k/2}}{\sqrt{\frac{k+1}{2}}}$$

Therefore,

$$f_k(t) = \frac{\Gamma(k+1)/2}{\sqrt{k\pi}\Gamma\sqrt{\frac{k}{2}}}\left(1+\frac{t^2}{k}\right)^{\frac{-(k+1)}{2}} \quad ... (9.56.1)$$

Properties of *t*-Distribution

1. t-distribution is a unimodal distribution (Fig. 9.20).
2. The probability distribution curve is symmetrical about the line $t = 0$.
3. It is a bell-shaped curve just like a normal curve with its tails a little higher above the abscissa than the normal curve. Its spread increases as degrees of freedom 'k' decreases. This means that for the same value of t-variable and x, the normal variate, the area beyond t is larger than the area beyond x.

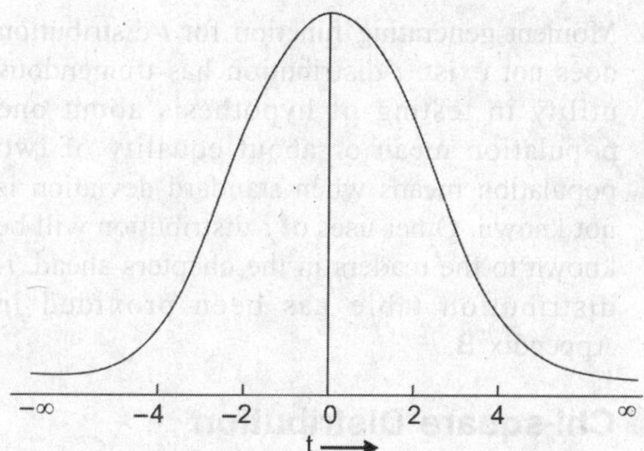

Fig. 9.20: *t*-distribution curve

4. t-distribution has only one parameter k, the degrees of freedom equal to $(n - 1)$.
5. The constants of t-distribution are as follows:
   (Mean) $\mu = 0$ for $k \geq 2$.

   (Variance) $\sigma^2 = \frac{k}{k-2}$ for $k \geq 3$

   (Skewness) $\alpha_3 = 0$ for $k \geq 4$

   (Kurtosis) $\alpha_4 = \frac{3(k-2)}{(k-4)}$ for ≥ 5
6. The area under t-distribution curve for $t < t'$ is determined by the equation,

$$Fk(t') = p(t < t') = \int_{-\infty}^{t'} f(t) \quad ...(9.57)$$

Students and other readers need not integrate actually for the area as the tables of area under the curve for different values of t are available and vice-versa.

Equation (9.57) is given to acquaint the reader with the know-how of getting the area if t is given and the value of t if area is given (Fig. 9.20).

7. t-distribution tends to normal distribution as k increases. For practical purposes, t is taken as equivalent to the normal distribution provided $k \geq 30$.

8. Moment generating function for t-distribution does not exist. t-distribution has tremendous utility in testing of hypothesis about one population mean or about equality of two population means when standard deviation is not known. Other uses of t-distribution will be known to the readers in the chapters ahead. t-distribution table has been provided in Appendix B.

Chi-square Distribution

So far, we have been discussing the distribution of mean obtained from all possible samples, or a large number of samples drawn from a normal population, distributed with mean μ and variance σ^2/n. Now we are interested in knowing the distribution, of sample variances s^2 of these samples. Consider a random sample $X_1, X_2, ..., X_n$ of size n. Let the observations of this sample be denoted by $x_1, x_2, ..., x_n$. We know that the variance,

$$s^2 = \frac{1}{n-1}\Sigma_i (x_i - \bar{x})^2 \text{ for } i = 1,2,...n.$$

or

$$\Sigma_i (x_i - \bar{x})^2 = (n-1)\, s^2 = ks^2 \quad ...(9.58)$$

where $k = (n - 1)$.

A quantity ks^2/σ^2, which is a pure number, is defined as χ^2_k. Now we will give the distribution of the random variable χ^2_k, which was first discovered by Helmert in 1876 and later independently given by Karl Pearson in 1900. Another way to understand chi-square is: if $X_1, X_2, ... X_n$ are n independent normal variates with mean zero and variance unity, the sum of squares of these variates is distributed as chi-square with n *df*. The chi-square distribution was discovered mainly as a measure of goodness of fit in case of frequency distribution, i.e. whether the observed frequencies follow a postulated distribution or not. The probability density function (pdf) of χ^2-variate is,

$$fk\,(\chi^2) = \frac{1}{2^{k/2}\Gamma(k/2)}(\chi^2)^{\frac{1}{2}k-1_e-\frac{1}{2}\chi^2} \quad ...(9.59)$$

Properties of Chi-square Distribution

1. The whole chi-square distribution curve lies in the first quadrant since the range of χ^2 is from 0 to ∞.
2. From the density function given by (9.59), it is evident that χ^2 distribution has only one parameter k, the degrees of freedom for χ^2. Thus, the shape of the probability density curve mainly depends on the parameter k. The shape of the curves for four different degrees of freedom say, $k = 2, k = 7, k = 12, k = 20$ are given below:
3. Chi-square distribution curve is highly positive skewed (Fig. 9.21).
4. It is an unimodal curve and its mode is at the point, $\chi^2 = (k - 1)$.
5. The shape of the curve varies immensely specially when k is small. For $k = 1$ and 2, it is just like an hyperbola.
6. Chi-square distribution is completely defined by one parameter 'k', which is known as the degrees of freedom of chi-square distribution.
7. The constants for chi-square distributions are as follows:

   (mean) $\mu = k$

   (variance) $\sigma^2 = 2k$

   (Skewness) $\alpha_1 = 2\left(\frac{2}{k}\right)^{\frac{1}{2}}$

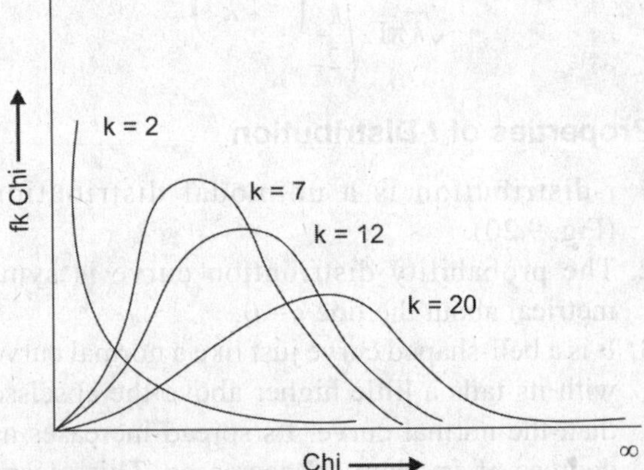

Fig. 9.21: Chi-square distribution curves

8. The moment generating function for chi-square distribution is,

$$\Phi_x^2(t) = (1-2t)^{-k/2}$$

9. μ_r the raw moment of chi-square distribution is,

$$\mu'_r = \frac{2^r \Gamma\left(\frac{k}{2}+r\right)}{\Gamma k/2}$$

Putting $r = 1$, $$\mu'_r = \frac{2\Gamma\left(\frac{k}{2}+1\right)}{\Gamma k/2} = k$$

$r = 2$, $$\mu'_2 = \frac{2^2\Gamma\left(\frac{k}{2}+2\right)}{\Gamma k/2}$$

$$= 4\left(\frac{k}{2}+1\right)\frac{k}{2} = k(k+2)$$

Again,

$$\mu_2 = \mu'_2 - (\mu'_1)^2$$
$$= k(k+2) - k^2 = 2k$$

and so on.

10. It can be shown that for large degrees of freedom say, $k \geq 100$, the variable $\left(\sqrt{2x^2} - \sqrt{2k-1}\right)$ is distributed normally with mean 0 and variance 1.

11. If χ_1^2 and χ_2^2 are two independent chi-squares with degrees of freedom k_1 and k_2 respectively, their sum ($\chi_1^2 + \chi_2^2$) will be distributed as chi-square with $(k_1 + k_2)$ *df*. This additive property of independent chi-squares, holds good for any number of chi-squares, i.e. if there are m independent chi-squares with $k_1, k_2, \ldots k_m$ *df* respectively, the sum $\Sigma_i \chi_i^2$ $(i = 1, 2, \ldots, m)$ will be distributed as chi-square with $\Sigma_i k_i$ *df*.

Fisher's Z-Distribution

Sir Ronald A. Fisher defined a statistic Z which is based upon the ratio of two-sample variances. Suppose s_1^2 and s_1^2 are two variances of random samples of sizes n_1 and n_2 respectively, drawn from two normal populations.

The statistic Z is defined as

$$Z = \frac{1}{2}\log\left(\frac{s_1^2}{s_2^2}\right) \quad \text{...(9.60)}$$

or $$Z = \log_e s_1 - \log_e s_2 \quad \text{...(9.60.1)}$$

or $$e^{2z} = \frac{s_1^2}{s_2^2} \quad \text{...(9.60.2)}$$

Putting

$$\frac{s_1^2}{s_2^2} = \text{F},$$

we get $$e^{2z} = \text{F} \quad \text{...(9.60.3)}$$

The letter F is the first letter of Fisher's name as a mark of respect. Z-distribution is of the form,

$$y = \frac{ce^{k_1 Z}}{(k_2 + k_1 e^{2Z})^{(k_1+k_2)/2}} \quad \text{...(9.61)}$$

where c is a constant, $k_1 = (n_1 - 1)$ and $k_2 = (n_2 - 1)$.

Properties of Z-Distribution

1. Z-distribution is symmetrical about the point Z = 0.
2. Z-distribution is a family of distributions in which each one exists for a pair of degrees of freedom k_1 and k_2.

Here the readers are acquainted with Fisher's Z-distribution as it is closely associated with F-distribution given below.

F-Distribution

From (9.61.3) it is evident that the ratio of two independent sample variances is denoted as F. Now we will consider the distribution of the ratio of two-sample variances in another manner and based on this new approach, the distribution of F is given. The distribution of F was worked out by GW Snedecor.

Consider two normal populations N (μ_1, σ_1^2) and N (μ_1, σ_2^2). An independent sample of size n_1 is drawn from a population N (μ_1, σ_1^2), and of size n_2 from a population N (μ_2, σ_2^2). Let the sample variances be s_1^2 and s_2^2 respectively. From the chi-square distribution theory we know $k_1 s_1^2 / \sigma_1^2$ is distributed as chi-square with k_1 d.f., i.e.

$$\frac{k_1 s_1^2}{\sigma_1^2} \sim \chi_1^2 \qquad ...(9.62)$$

where χ_1^2 has d.f. $k_1 = (n_1 - 1)$.

Similarly,

$$\frac{k_2 s_2^2}{\sigma_2^2} \sim \chi_2^2 \qquad ...(9.63)$$

where χ_2^2 has d.f. $k_2 = (n_2 - 1)$.

From (9.63), and (9.64) we can write that,

$$\frac{s_1^2 / \sigma_1^2}{s_2^2 / \sigma_2^2} = \frac{\chi_1^2 / k_1}{\chi_2^2 / k_2} \qquad ...(9.64)$$

$$= Fk_1,k_2 \qquad ...(9.64.1)$$

In (9.65.1), k_1 and k_2 are called the degrees of freedom of F. Dividing s_u^2 ($\mu = 1, 2$) by its corresponding population variance standardizes the sample variance, in the sense that on the average both the numerator and denominator approach 1. Now we may be interested in testing the hypothesis that both the normal populations have the same variance, i.e. $\sigma_1^2 = \sigma_2^2$. Under this hypothesis,

$$\frac{s_1^2}{s_2^2} = \text{F}k_1,k_2 \qquad ...(9.65)$$

As a norm, the greater sample variance is taken as the numerator.

From (9.65) it is apparent that the ratio of two independent chi-squares is distributed as F and (9.66) reveals that under the hypothesis $\sigma_1^2 = \sigma_2^2$, the ratio of two independent sample variances is distributed as F. The probability density function of F-distribution is,

$$fk_1,k_2\,(\text{F}) = \frac{(k_1/k_2)^{k_1/2}}{\text{B}\left(\frac{k_1}{2}, \frac{k_2}{2}\right)} \frac{\text{F}^{k_1/2-1}}{\left(1+\frac{k_1}{k_2}\text{F}\right)^{(k_1+k_2)/2}} \qquad ...(9.66)$$

Obviously, F is always a positive number and the F-distribution curve wholly lies in the first quadrant. There are two parameters of F-distribution namely, k_1 and k_2. Hence the shape of F-distribution curve depends on k_1 and k_2. For two pairs of degrees of freedom (k_1, k_2), the shape of the F-distribution are shown in Figure 9.22.

Properties of F-Distribution

1. F-distribution curve extends on abscissa from 0 to ∞
2. It is an unimodal curve and its mode lies on the point

$$\text{F} = \frac{k_2(k_1 - 2)}{k_1(k_2 + 2)}$$

which is always less than unity.

3. F-distribution curve is a positive skew curve. Generally the F-distribution curve is highly positive skewed when k_2 is small.

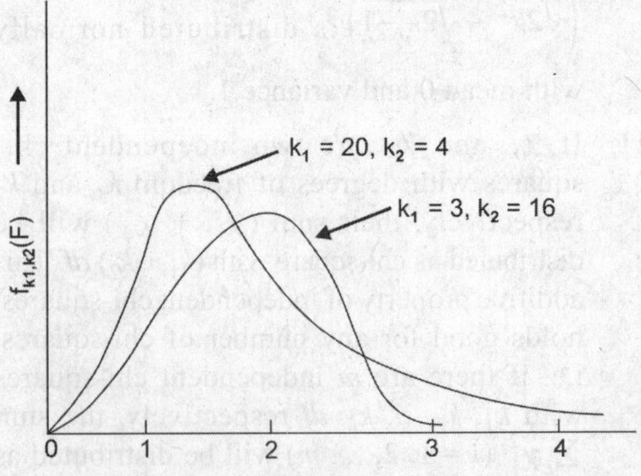

Fig. 9.22: F-distribution curves

4. The constants of F-distribution are,

(mean) $\mu = \frac{k_2}{k_2 - 2}$ for $k_2 \geq 3$

(variance) $\sigma^2 = \frac{2k_2^2(k_1 + k_2 - 2)}{k_1(k_2 - 2)(k_2 - 4)}$ for $k_2 \geq 5$

5. There exists a very useful relation for interchange of degrees of freedom k_1 and k_2, i.e.

$$F_1 - \alpha = (k_1 - k_2) = \frac{1}{F\alpha(k_2 - k_1)}$$

6. The moment generation function of F-distribution does not exist.

F-distribution is a very popular and useful distribution because of its utility in testing of hypothesis about the equality of several population means, two population variances and several regression coefficients in multiple regression, etc. As a matter of fact, F-test is the backbone of analysis of variance.

Wide use and application of the sampling distributions has been made in different chapters ahead while testing different null hypotheses about a variety of population parameters.

EXERCISES

1. In two throws of a coin what is the probability of throwing
   a. Both heads
   b. Both tails
   c. At least one head
   d. At least one tail
   e. One head or one tail?
2. If three coins are tossed, what is the possibility of obtaining
   a. At least two heads
   b. At least one head
   c. All three heads
   d. All three tails
   e. Exactly one head?
3. If the probability of answering a question correctly is 5 times the probability of answering it incorrectly, what is the probability of answering it correctly?
4. In a six-item test each item is scored right or wrong. If a student answers each item by guessing alone, (a) How many different outcomes are possible? (b) State the binomial. (c) Describe the different types of results. (d) What is the probability of getting (e) 4 or more items (f) All the 6 items correct (g) Exactly 3 items correct? (h) If 64 students attempted the test by guessing, how many students would obtain the situation d (i); d (ii), and d (iii) above?
5. If the probability of having a boy or a girl is equal, out of 64 families with four children each, how many would you expect to have (a) exactly one boy, (b) exactly three boys, (c) at least one boy, and (d) all girls?
6. If the probability of selecting an extrovert is 40. Out of a sample of 5 individuals selected independently, what is the exact probability that three of the individuals selected are extroverts and the remaining two are not?
7. Define a Normal Distribution? What are its principal properties?

8. In a group of 500 students based on normal distribution, M = 40; SD = 8, find out:
   a. Number of students between scores of 25 and 35.
   b. Values of P75 and P50
   c. If the group is divided into six subgroups on the basis of equal spread of ability, what will be the number in each subgroup?
9. Define the following:
   a. Skewness
   b. Kurtosis.
10. Explain why we call t, χ^2 and F as sampling distributions?
11. If $X_1, X_2, ..., X_k$ are k independent random variables distributed normally with mean 0 and variance 1, what is the distribution of $\Sigma_i X_i^2$ (i = 1, 2, ..., k)?
12. Write the parameters of the following distributions:
   a. Chi-square distribution
   b. t-distribution
   c. F-distribution
13. In what situation do the following distributions tend to normal distribution?
   a. t-distribution
   b. χ^2-distribution
14. Does moment generating function exist for the following distributions?
   a. t-distribution
   b. F-distribution
   c. x^2-distribution
15. Given $\alpha = 0.05$, $k_1 = 5$, $k_2 = 10$, find,
   i. $F_{\alpha'}(k_2, k_1)$
   ii. $F_{1-\alpha'}(k_1, k_2)$.
16. In what respects does t-distribution differ from a normal distribution?
17. For the same value of t-variate and a normal variate x, write whether the area to the left of t will be larger or smaller than area to the left of x.
18. Determine the values of the following:
   a. $t_{.01,18}$
   b. $t_{.05,12}$
   c. $t_{.10,15}$
   d. Find the ninetieth percentile of t-distribution with 10 *df*.

CHAPTER 10 Measures of Relative Position/Standards

Introduction

A raw score, taken by itself, rarely has meaning. A score may be given meaning by comparing it with a standard of performance. Absolute measurement in sciences are not so meaningful as they are the measures of relative standing with reference to a group. Relative position of a score means its distance from the mean expressed in terms of some deviational measures such as standard deviation. For example, knowledge that a nursing student has a score of 70 on a test of medical-surgical nursing does not tell us much. If the information that the mean of the group, to which the nursing student belongs, is 75 also is furnished, then we may infer that she is below average. This is also not sufficient. What is needed, in order to interpret a score of 70, is some measure of relative standing within the total distribution Percentiles and Standard scores to perform this function and that is the most commonly used measure of relative standing. In addition to these the agencies and grade norms are also popularly used.

Norms are the levels attained by a particular group of persons on a test. Norms may be defined as the average performance on a particular test made by a standardization sample. By standardization sample it is meant that a sample which is the true representative of the population takes the test for the express purposes of providing data comparison and subsequent interpretation of the test score. To be a standard sample, it must include a cross-section to compare raw score with the performance of the standardization sample. They are converted into "derived score" which denote the person's relative position in the standardization sample.

If the norms available for a different test are of the same kind and are based on comparable groups, all the tests can be expressed in comparable terms. The results can then be shown pictorially in the form of a profile. Profiles emphasize score differences within the individual. When profiles are used care must be taken not to over interpret their minor ups and downs.

Norms represent a descriptive framework for interpreting the score of an individual, a class group, or some large aggregation. However, before a judgment can be made as to whether an individual or group is doing well or poorly, allowance must be made for ability levels, cultural background and curricular emphasis. The norm is merely an average, not a strait jacket into which all can be forced to fit.

Methods of Interpreting Test Scores

An individual performance on some psychological, educational or other type is recorded in terms of the raw scores. Raw scores are expressed in terms of different units such as, number of correct responses made on a test. All these raw scores convey no meaning in themselves. In the absence of any interpretation of data, it is difficult to answer. Generally there are two methods which are used in interpreting the test scores, which include.

Normative Referencing and Criterion Referencing

i. *Criterion referencing* is defined as the way a test score is established. An external standard or criterion compares the examinees test score with it. For example, 90 percent of the items answered correctly. This method giving a raw score meaning is called, criterion referenced interpretations. Such an interpretation is appropriate for tests that are focused on a single objective and for which standards of performance can be either empirically or logically derived.

ii. *Normative referencing* is defined as the way to compare an examinee's test score with a score of a specific group of examinee's on that test. When raw scores are compared to the norms, a scientific meaning emerges. Since most tests are designed to appraise more than one objective and since meaningful absolute standards of performance are not available for most tests, a raw score is given meaning by comparison with some reference group or groups. This method of giving a raw score meaning is called normative referenced interpretation.

Developing Norms

The raw count of units or raw scores or even a crude percentage of the possible scores is not sufficient to allow comparison. The three main properties of units which can allow comparison and exhibit sound psychometric qualities one follows:

- Uniform measuring from test to test, so that a basis of comparison is provided through which we may compare different tests – for example, different arithmetic tests among scholastic aptitude test, or an achievement test with a scholastic aptitude test, etc.
- Units of uniform size, so that a gain of 5 points on one part of the scale signifies the something as a gain of 5 points on any part of the scale.
- A true zero point of "just none of" the quality in question, so that we can legitimately think of scores as representing 'twice as much as' or 'two-thirds as much as'.

The different types of norm that have been developed for the test represents marked progress towards the first two of the above objectives. The third can probably never be reached for the traits with which psychological and educational measurements are concerned. It is more or less impossible to arrive at "a total absence point" of intelligence or arithmetic ability or "sociability", although we may allot a student a zero score on any test. It would merely be an arbitrary zero. The fact of a general prevalence of inequality of units and absence of a real zero point brings us to the conclusion that a raw point score can be given meaning only by referring it to some type of group or groups. Hence, the need for norms.

The three important steps used in developing norms includes the following:

i. Defining the target population or the composition of population.
ii. Select the representative sample from each of the target population or group. Usually large sample in preferred.
iii. Standardized conditions should be implemented to secure standardized, valid and proper comparison of individual's test score to test norms.

Types of Norms

There are four main patterns for interpreting the score of an individual. The divided scores may be divided into four common types and depending upon each of these four scores, there are four types of norms. The four commonly derived scores are age score, grade score, percentile scores and standard scores. Accordingly, the main types of norms include the following:

- Age norms or age equivalent norms
- Grade norms or grade equivalent norms
- Percentile norms
- Standard score norms.

Age Norms

Age norms are defined as the average performance of representative sample of a certain age level on the measure of certain trait, ability or disease or treatment. Age norms are more suited to those traits or abilities which increases systematically with age. Most of the physical traits like weight, height and cognitive abilities are included.

The age norm for a particular age is the average value of the trait for persons of that particular age. Age norms can be established for a trait that shows a progressive change with age for example, weight, height, etc. we may take a representative sample of 8-year-old girls and measure their heights. The average value thus obtained will be the age norm for the 8-year-old girls. Similarly, age norms can be set-up for the 9-year-olds, 10-year-old and so on. Later on, each girl's height can be interpreted by comparing it with the average heights and identifying the age groups with whose height it was the closest. *If an 8-year-old girl has a height equal to the norm for the 12-year-old, we declare that she is as tall as an average girl of 12 years.*

The norms-based on age framework are relatively simple and familiar. They are convenient for a trait that shows continuous and relatively steady growth over a period of years. However, age norms suffer from certain disadvantages such as lack of standard and uniform units of growth in height from one year to another. Growth in a trait may slow down or even stop after a particular period. Moreover, these are less appropriate for the nonbiological framework of years of growth which may be based on training, schooling or amount of interaction with others.

There are some disadvantages of age norms, which include—

- Age norms lack standard and uniform unit throughout the period of growth of physical and psychological traits.
- Another problem in age norms arises from the fact that the growth rate of some traits are not comparable.
- Personality traits cannot be expressed in terms of age norms because these traits does not exhibit progressive change over the years.

Grade Norms/Grade Equivalent Norms

Grade equivalent norms defined as the average performance of a representative sample of a certain grade or class. The test whose norms are being prepared is given to a representative sample selected from each of the several grades or classes. After that the average performance of each grade on each given test is determined and then grade equivalent scores are obtained. These average performance is known as the grade equivalent norms.

A test is given to representative groups in each of a series of school grades (classes) and the average score determined for each grade (like 5th to 8th classes). Theses averages then represent the norms for various grades. Scores lying between the norm for two successive grades are assigned fractional credits by interpolation. Generally, the grade value of 5.0 is assigned to average performance at the beginning of the fifth grade, 5.5 to average performance at the middle of the grade, and so forth. If a child of 6th grade obtains a score equal to the norm for the 8th grade on a test of arithmetic, we say that the child though belonging to 6th grade is yet performing at a level equal to an average child of 8th grade.

Grade norms are relatively easy to determine as the administrative groups based on grades are easily available. They are easy to set-up and convenient to interpret. These are more useful for interpreting the academic accomplishments of children especially in primary schools. In the upper grades, slowing down of the progress makes the grade norms less meaningful and inappropriate. These should not be mistaken as the top achievement, neither more nor less.

Grade equivalent norms have certain limitations, which include:

- Grade equivalent norms of the same student in different subjects are not comparable.
- Grade equivalent norms assume that all students of a same class or grade will have similar curriculum experiences. This assumption may not be true in elementary classes and may not be true for higher classes.
- The grade norms are not suited to those students in which there occur a rapid growth in the elementary classes and a slow growth in higher classes.

Points to be remembered while using age norms and grade norms, include:

- Children learn and grow at different speed at different ages, so differences between second and third grade might be far different than the difference between 11th and 12th grade, though there is only one-year difference between each grade.
- Comparing grade norms and age norms is not equivalent as the advancement does not occur uniformly in all areas.

Percentile Norms

Percentile norms are the most popular and common type of norms. Such norms can be prepared for either adults or children and for any type of tests. A percentile norm indicates, for each raw score, percentage of standardization sample that falls below that raw score.

The nth percentile is that scale value or score point below which *n* percent of the cases in the distribution fall. The scale value of the variable is called *percentile point* or simply *percentile,* while its' corresponding percentage value is known as its' percentile rank.

While studying the concept and the method of calculation of the median, in the chapter on measures of central tendency, it was noted that median was another similar concept which stood for a score point below which 50 percent of the cases lie and hence equivalent to P_{50}. Q_1 and Q_3, introduced in yet another chapter stood for 25th percentile, and 75th percentile respectively indicating the score points below which 25 percent and 75 percent cases would lie. The method of calculation of percentiles is thus similar to that of calculating median, Q_1 or Q_3.

Centile or percentiles are values in a series of observation which is arranged in ascending order of magnitude which divides the distribution into 100 equal parts. They are values of variables such as height, weight, etc. which divide the total observation by an imaginary line into 2 parts expressed in percentages such as 25 percent and 75 percent. The median is 50th centile. The 50th centile will have 50 percent observation on either side.

Percentiles are used to divide a distribution in the convenient group. Those which are used widely are as follows:

1. **Quartiles:** They are three different points located on the entire range of variables.
2. **Quintiles:** They are four in number and divide the distribution into 5 equal parts.
3. **Deciles:** They are nine in number and divide the distribution into ten equal parts.

Calculation of Percentiles

There are basically two methods used to calculate percentiles.

1. Graphic method of presentation such as cumulative frequency table and Ogive curve
2. Arithmetic method such as, rank for group and ungroup data (Table 10.1)

(i) Calculation of percentiles from ungrouped data:

Table 10.1

Computation of percentile points from ungrouped data (scores of 40 students in nursing test)

Student	*Score*		*Student*	*Score*	
1	26		21	54	
2	28		22	55	
3	28		23	55	
4	29	$P_{10} = \frac{29+31}{2} = 302$	24	56	
5	31		25	58	
6	35		26	58	
7	35		27	58	
8	35		28	58	
9	35		29	59	
10	36		30	60	$P_{75} = \frac{60+62}{2} = 612$
11	38	$P_{25} = \frac{36+38}{2} = 372$	31	62	
12	39		32	63	
13	40	$P_{30} = \frac{39+40}{2} = 39.52$	33	64	$P_{80} = \frac{63+64}{2} = 63.52$
14	41		34	65	
15	45		35	65	
16	50		36	68	
17	51		37	71	
18	52		38	72	$P_{95} = \frac{72+73}{2} = 72.52$
19	52		39	73	
20	52		40	77	

(a) *When no duplication near percentile exists:* Suppose we desire to calculate P_{30} or the score value below which 30 percent of the 40 cases lie.

Thirty percent of 40 students $= 40 \times \frac{30}{100} = 12$ students must be below P_{30}. The scores in the table have been arranged in an ascending order. Counting up, we find that the 12th student scored 39 and the 13th student scored 40. The desired point must fall between these two score values. It is a convention that the average of such scores will be taken as the desired percentile. Hence,

$$P_{30} = \frac{39+40}{2} = 39.5$$

In the same manner, the values of the following percentile points have been calculated:

Percentile	*Number of cases required below Percentile*	*Percentile value*	
P_{10}	$40 \times \frac{10}{100} = 4$	$\frac{\text{4th score + 5th score}}{2}$	$= \frac{29 + 31}{2} = 30.2$
P_{25}	$40 \times \frac{25}{100} = 10$	$\frac{\text{10th score + 11th score}}{2}$	$= \frac{36 + 38}{2} = 37.2$
P_{30}	$40 \times \frac{30}{100} = 12$	$\frac{\text{12th score + 13th score}}{2}$	$= \frac{39 + 40}{2} = 39.52$
P_{75}	$40 \times \frac{75}{100} = 30$	$\frac{\text{30th score + 31st score}}{2}$	$= \frac{60 + 62}{2} = 61.2$
P_{80}	$40 \times \frac{80}{100} = 32$	$\frac{\text{32nd score + 33rd score}}{2}$	$= \frac{63 + 64}{2} = 63.52$
P_{95}	$40 \times \frac{95}{100} = 38$	$\frac{\text{38th score + 39th score}}{2}$	$= \frac{72 + 73}{2} = 72.52$

This student may try the calculation of other percentile points where no duplication of scores occur at the percentile.

(b) *Arithmetic method of calculating percentiles:* It is similar to that employed for the calculation of median.

The formula is

$$Pp = L + \frac{(P_N - F)}{fp} \times 1 \qquad ...(10.1)$$

Calculate P_{50} from the data given below:

Class interval	*f*	*Cum fq*	*X*
20-24	3	3	22
25-29	3	6	27
30-34	8	14	32
35-39	0	14	37
40-44	6	20	42
45-49	2	22	47
50-54	1	23	52
55-59	2	25	57
60-64	5	30	62
65-69	1	31	67
70-74	2	33	72
75-79	4	37	77
80-84	1	38	82
85-89	1	39	87
90-94	1	40	92

Pp = Percentage required or required percentage of the distribution, e.g. 30 percentage or 50 percentage

L = Exact lower limit of class interval where Pp lies.

P_N = Part of N to be counted off in reaching Pp

F = Sum of all frequencies upto intervals below *i*

i = Size of the CI

fp = Number of scores upon which Pp falls.

For example:

$P_N = P_{40}$ CI = 40 – 44

50% of 40 = 20 L = 39.5

Compute $P_N = P_{50}$ F = 14

$P_{50} = 20$ $fp = 6$

$i = 5$

$$Pp = L + \frac{(P_N - F)}{fp} \times i$$

$$P_{50} = 39.5 + \frac{20 - 14}{6} \times 5$$

$$= 39.5 + \frac{6}{6} \times 5$$

$$= 39.5 + 1 \times 5$$

$$= 39.5 + 5$$

$$P_{50} = 44.5$$

(ii) Calculation of percentile rank for grouped data: Sometimes the situation arises where the investigator wishes to calculate percentile rank (Pp) on the basis of given raw score in a grouped data.

It can be done with the help of the following formula.

Refer the previous table

$$P_R(X) = \frac{100}{N}\left\{F + \frac{(X-L)}{I} f\right\} \quad ...(10.2)$$

where X = score whose percentile rank is described

N = Number of scores

L = Lower limit of class interval

F = Cumulative frequency of CI below it

f = frequency of the CI containing X

I = Length of CI

Suppose in a group of 20 students. Neha gets the 10th rank calculate P_R

To calculate P_R the formula is as follows

$$P_R = 100 - \left(\frac{100R - 50}{N}\right)$$

$$= 100 - \left(\frac{100 \times 10 - 50}{20}\right)$$

$$= 100 - \left(\frac{1000 - 50}{20}\right)$$

$$= 100 - \frac{950}{20} = 47.5 = 52.5$$

R = Rank position

N = Number of persons

Take 52 as the P_R

$$P_R(X) = \frac{100}{N}\left\{F + \left(\frac{X-L}{I}\right) f\right\}$$

$$P_R(52) = \frac{100}{40}\left\{22 + \left(\frac{52-49.5}{5}\right) \times 1\right\}$$

$$= 2.5\left\{22 + \frac{2.5}{5} \times 1\right\}$$

$$= 2.5\{22 + 0.5 \times 1\}$$

$$= 2.5\{22 + 0.5\}$$

$$= 2.5\{22.5\} = 56.25$$

Thus, a score (X) of 52 has a P_R of 56 or P_{56}.

Thus, a percentile is a score below which a specified percentage falls where as percentile rank is the percentage below a specified score.

Despite such advantages of calculation with graphic and arithmetical method percentiles has two distinct limitations:

1. Layman as well as skilled persons sometimes fail to distinguish between percentile and the percentage score and this obviously results in confusion. But the two should not be confused because percentile is a derived score usually expressed in terms of percentages of persons whereas, the percentage score is a raw score expressed in terms of percentages of items carefully answered or solved.
2. The biggest limitations of the percentile norms is that of inequality of units throughout the percentile scale.

When duplication near percentile exists: The procedure of calculating the value of percentile points when the score value containing the percentile point has more than one frequency is different from the procedure mentioned above.

Example 1: For example, consider the score point corresponding to P_{20}. Twenty percent of 40 students is 8 students. However, the 8th and 9th, and also the 6th and 7th, students (Table 10.1) have a score of 35 each. The real lower limit of score of 35 is 34.5. Five cases are covered upto 34.5. To reach the target of 8 cases, 3 more cases are to be taken from the 4 cases which are within the score interval 34.5 – 35.5 (real lower and upper limits of the score 35) whose size is equal to one score unit. Hence, 3 out of 4 students scoring 35 fall below the 20th percentile. It would mean an addition of 3/4th of the class interval (i.e. 75) to the lower limit of 34.5.

Hence, $P_{20} = 34.5 + 0.75 = 35.25$.

This procedure is very much similar to the one already described in a previous chapter on the calculation of median. Similarly, the following percentile values can also be calculated.

Example 2: P_{65} = 26th score; the class interval of score 58 (exact limits 47.5–58.5) contains 4 students (serial 25 to 28). To reach the 26th student, two out of four cases are to be covered over and above the score of 57.5. These two cases span 2/4 or 0.5 or half of the CI size. Hence,

$$P_{65} = 57.5 + 0.5 = 58.00$$

The student may check the following values also

$$P_{15} = 34.75;\ P_{45} = 51.83;\ P_{85} = 65.00$$

(iii) Calculation of percentile ranks from ungrouped data

Percentile points answer the question What is the score point below a given percentage of cases?" In such cases, a score point was computed. However, if the question is reversed as follows, "What percentage of cases lie below a given score point"?, we have to find out Percentile Rank (PR) of the score of the person holding that score.

(a) *When no duplication near percentile exists:* From Table 10.1, one may ask "What is the percentile rank (PR) of a score of 63?" The score of 63 holds 32nd position in the descending order of the score distribution. This means that 31 persons or $\frac{31}{40} \times 100 = 77.5$ percent student scored less than the lower limit of 63 which is 62.5. By the same argument, 8 persons or $\frac{8}{40} \times 100 = 63.5$. The total percentage of cases below an above the score interval of 62.5 – 63.5 = 77.5 percent + 20 percent = 97.5. By subtraction, we may find the percentage of cases within the score interval of 62.5 – 63.5, which is 100.00 percent – 97.5 percent = 2.5 percent (This checks with the fact that only 1 case out of 40 or 2.5 percent cases are contained in this score interval). Since the midpoint of the class interval, is considered to be the most representative score, we need to divide the class interval into two equal halves to reach a score of 63.00 from 62.5. Hence, the percentage of cases contained in this interval is also to be divided into two equal halves; one half of this is then to be added to the percentage of 77.5 covered upto the score of 62.5.

Hence, P_R of score of 73 = 77.5 percent + 2.5 percent = 78.75 percent.

The percentile ranks are conventionally reported in whole percentages, the percentage of 78.75 is to be rounded off to the closest one, i.e. 79 percent. Hence the P_R of a score of 73 is equal to 79. The interpretation of this value is that a person holding a score of 73 has a rank of 79 on a 100-point scale. *In simple words 79 percent of the students lie below him in terms of scores.*

The above procedure can be diagrammatically shown in Figure 10.1 given below:

(b) *When duplication near percentile exists:* When more than one frequency exist at the given score value, the procedure adopted for the calculation of percentile ranks, in general, is the same as explained above.

For example, we wish to determine P_R of score 52. There are three persons holding a similar score of 52 leading to duplication (or triplication) of scores at the percentile. Seventeen $\left(\frac{17}{40} \times 100 \text{ or } 42.5 \text{ percent}\right)$ students scores are below the lower limit of 52 which is 51.5. There are three $\left(\frac{3}{40} \times 100 \text{ or } 7.5 \text{ percent}\right)$ frequencies within this score interval of 51.5 to 52.5. Hence, to reach from a score of 51.5 to 52.0, half of this percentage will be added to the percentage covered up to 51.5.

Hence, P_R of 52 = 42.5 percent + $\frac{7.5}{2}$ percent = 46.25 percent.

By rounding it off, we have 46 as the P_R of 52. The above procedure has been presented diagrammatically in Figure 10.2.

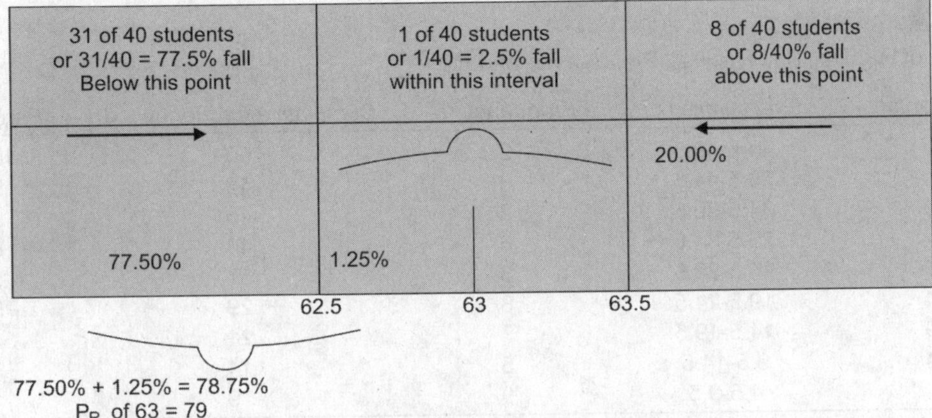

Fig. 10.1: Determination of percentile rank corresponding to the score value of 63

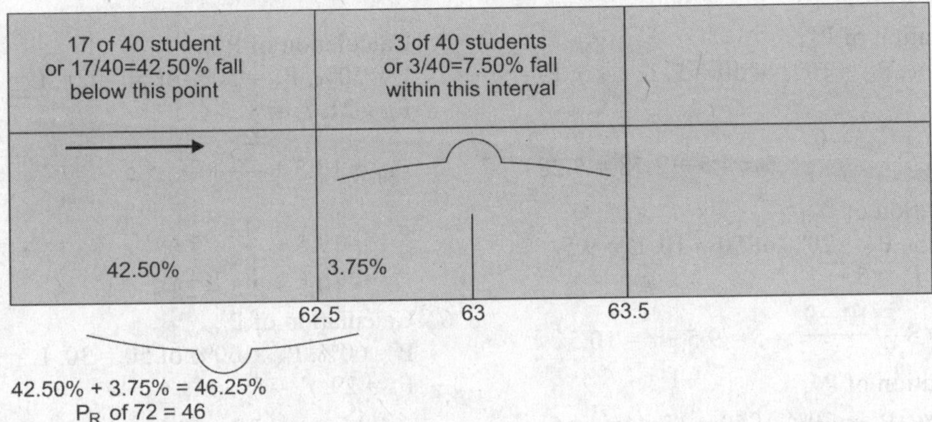

Fig. 10.2: Determination of percentile rank corresponding to a score value of 52

(iv) Calculation of percentile from the grouped data or frequency distribution

Calculation of percentile points from a frequency distribution of scores follows the same procedure as discussed in a previous chapter with reference to the calculation of median, Q_1 and Q_3. The same will be presented here and calculation of several percentile points will be done with reference to the data given below in Table 10.2.

$$\text{Formula} = P_p = L + \left(\frac{P_N - F_b}{fw}\right) \times i \quad ...(10.3)$$

where, Pp = the required percentile point

P = the proportion of the distribution wanted

N = Normal of cases

L = Exact lower limit of the class interval in which Pp falls

F_b = Cumulative frequency below the CI containing Pp

F_w = Frequency within the CI containing Pp

i = size of class interval

For the given data, N = 50, i = 5.

Table 10.2

Calculation of P_{10}, P_{20}, P_{30}, P_{40}, P_{50}, P_{60}, P_{70}, P_{80} and P_{90}

Class interval	*Exact limits (X)*	*Frequency (f)*	*Cumulative frequency (cf)*	*Percentage*
45-49	44.5-49.5	2	50	100.00
40-44	39.5-44.5	3	48	96.00
35-39	34.5-39.5	2	45	90.00
30-34	29.5-34.5	6	43	86.00
25-29	24.5-29.5	8	37	74.00
20-24	19.5-24.5	8	29	58.00
15-19	14.5-19.5	7	21	42.00
10-14	9.5-14.5	5	14	28.00
5-9	4.5-9.5	9	9	18.00
		N = 50		

1. Calculation of P_{10}

   P = 10%, P_N = 10% of 50 = 5, L = 4.5, $F_b = 0$, $f_w = 9$

   $$P_{10} = 4.5 + \frac{5-0}{9} \times 5 = 4.5 + 2.78 = 7.28$$

2. Calculation of P_{20}

   P = 20%, P_N = 20% of 50 = 10, L = 9.5, $F_b = 9, f_w = 5$

   $$P_{20} = 9.5 + \frac{10-9}{5} \times 5 = 9.5 + 1 = 10.5$$

3. Calculation of P_{30}

   P = 30%, P_N = 30% of 50 = 15, L = 14.5, $F_b = 14, f_w = 7$

   $$P_{30} = 14.5 + \frac{15-14}{7} \times 5$$

   $$= 14.5 + \frac{1}{7} \times 5$$

   $$= 14.5 + 0.71 = 15.21$$

4. Calculation of P_{40}

   P = 40%, P_N = 40% of 50 = 20, L = 14.5, $F_b = 14, f_w = 7$

   $$P_{40} = 14.5 + \frac{20-14}{7} \times 5$$

   $$= 14.5 + \frac{6}{7} \times 5$$

   $$= 14.5 + 4.29 = 18.79$$

5. Calculation of P_{50}

   P = 50%, P_N = 50% of 50 = 25, L = 19.5, $F_b = 21, f_w = 8$

   $$P_{50} = 19.5 + \frac{25-21}{8} \times 5$$

   $$= 19.5 + \frac{4}{8} \times 5$$

   $$= 19.5 + 2.5 = 22$$

6. Calculation of P_{60}

   P = 60%, P_N = 60% of 50 = 30, L = 24.5, $F_b = 29, f_w = 8$

   $$P_{60} = 24.5 + \frac{30-29}{8} \times 5$$

   $$= 24.5 + 0.62 = 25.12$$

7. Calculation of P_{70}

   P = 70%, P_N = 70% of 50 = 35, L = 29.5, $F_b = 29, f_w = 8$

   $$P_{70} = 24.5 + \frac{35-29}{8} \times 5$$

   $$= 24.5 + 3.75 = 28.25$$

8. Calculation of P_{80}

   P = 80%, P_N = 80% of 50 = 40, L = 29.5, $F_b = 37, f_w = 6$

   $$P_{80} = 29.5 + \frac{40-37}{6} \times 5$$

   $$= 29.5 + 2.5 = 32.0$$

9. Calculation of P_{90}

$P = 90\%$, $P_N = 90\%$ of $50 = 45$, $L = 34.5$, $F_b = 43, f_w = 2$

$$P_{90} = 34.5 + \frac{45 - 43}{2} \times 5$$

$$= 34.5 + 5 = 39.5$$

In Table 10.2, several percentile points have been calculated by using formula (10.1). The details of the calculations have also been presented in the latter half of the same table. However, for further clarification and understanding of the concept of percentile, the calculation of P_{40} is discussed here. Here $P_N = 20$ (40 percent of 50 = 20). From the frequency distribution Col. (4), it is evident that 14 cases are covered up to a score of 14.5, the exact upper limit of the class interval of 10–14 and also the exact lower limit of the class interval 15–29 in which P_{40} lies. Hence, to reach a score point below which 20 cases would die, we need 6 cases out of the 7 contained in the score interval of 15–29. The size of the class interval is 5. Now we need to add ($6/7 \times 5 = 40$) score units to the lower limit of 14.5 up to which 14 cases had been covered.

Hence $P_{40} = 14.50 + 4.29 = 18.79$

A similar value has been obtained by using Formula (10.1) as shown in Table 10.2.

P_0 is the exact lower limit of the lowest interval, and P_{100}, the exact upper limit of the top interval. These are called the limiting points. In Table 10.2, $P_0 = 4.5$ and $P_{100} = 49.5$. These values can be picked up simply by inspection.

The student, by slight understanding, can also pick up some values of percentile points by inspection only.

For example, in Table 10.2, $P_{28} = 14.5$ (upper limit of CI 10-14 upto which 14 cases or 28 percent cases are covered).

$P_{42} = 19.5$ (upper limit CI 15-29 upto which 21 cases or 42 percent cases are covered).

Similarly, $P_{58} = 24.5$; $P_{74} = 29$, $P_{56} = 34.5$; $P_{90} = 39.5$; $P_{96} = 44.5$. The student may check the correctness of these values of using Formula (10.1).

(v) Calculation of percentile ranks from the grouped data:

The calculation of percentile ranks requires the reverse of the procedure used for the calculation of percentile points. The cumulative percentages shown in column 5 of Table 10.2 are the percentile ranks corresponding to the exact top limits of the intervals. Thus, 18.0 are the PR corresponding to the percentile point of 9.5, the upper limit of the class interval 5–9. Similarly, 28.0 is the P_R corresponding to the percentile point of 14.5, the upper limit of the class interval. Other values are:

PR of score 19.5 = 42.0; PR of score 24.5 = 58.0; PR of score 29.5 = 74.0; PR of score 34.5=86.0; PR of score 39.5 = 90.0, etc.

These values of P_R's have been picked only by the inspection of Col. (5) of Table 10.2. Other values may require some further calculations.

PR of any score can be obtained by interpolation as illustrated below:

Suppose we wish to obtain P_R of a score of 22. The score 22 falls within the interval with exact limits 19.5 and 24.5. Hence, 22 is 2.5 score units above the lower limit of this class-interval. The lower limit has a percentile rank of 42.00 and the upper limit, 58.0 with a distance of 58.0 – 42.0 = 16 units on the percentile rank scale. The number of score units covered is 24.5 – 19.5 = 5. Hence the number of percentile rank units equal to score units of 2.5 are equal to (58.0 – 42.0) 2.5/5 = 8.0. We now take 42.0 + 8.0 = 50.0 as the percentile rank of the score 22. Fig. 10.3 given below will clarify the calculation. Percentile Ranks are reported in whole numbers and hence, be rounded to the nearest integer. In this example, the P_R has

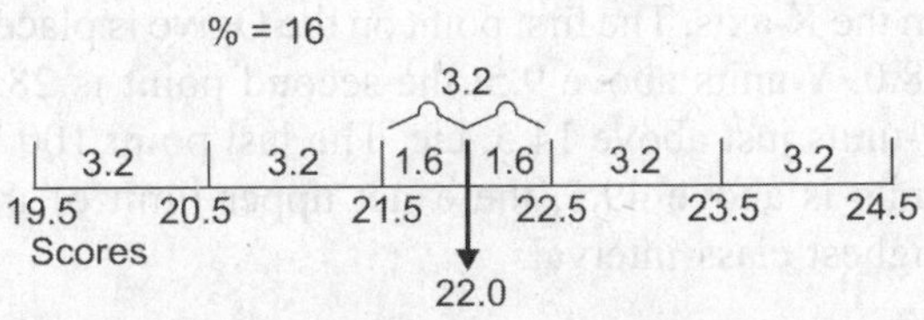

Fig. 10.3: Interpolation for the calculation of P_R

turned out to be an integer leaving no scope for rounding.

Note the steps required in the calculation of P_R's.

1. Find the class interval containing the score X whose percentile rank is required.
2. Find the exact lower limit of this class-interval.
3. Calculate the difference between X and this lower limit by subtracting the lower limit from X.
4. Divide this difference by the size of the class-interval and multiply by the percentage within the interval.
5. Add this to the percentile rank corresponding to the lower limit of the interval (or the percentage covered upto the lower limit of the interval).

The Cumulative Percentage Curve or Ogive

The cumulative percentage curve or Ogive is different from the cumulative frequency graph in one important aspect. In an Ogive, the frequencies are expressed as cumulative percents of N on the Y-axis instead of as cumulative frequencies. Table 10.2 shows the process of converting the cumulative frequencies (Col. 4) into cum. percentages (Col. 5). This conversion can be carried out by dividing each cum. frequency by N and multiplying it by 100. The multiplication can be performed simply by shifting the decimal points two spaces to the right.

The curve in Figure 10.4 is an Ogive plotted from the data in column (5) of Table 10.2. Exact interval limits have been laid off on the X-axis and a scale of 10 equal distances, each representing 10 percent of the distribution has been marked off on the X-axis. The first point on the Ogive is placed 18.0. Y-units above 9.5; the second point is 28.0 Y-units just above 14.5, etc. The last point 100 Y units is above 49.5, the exact upper limit of the highest class-interval.

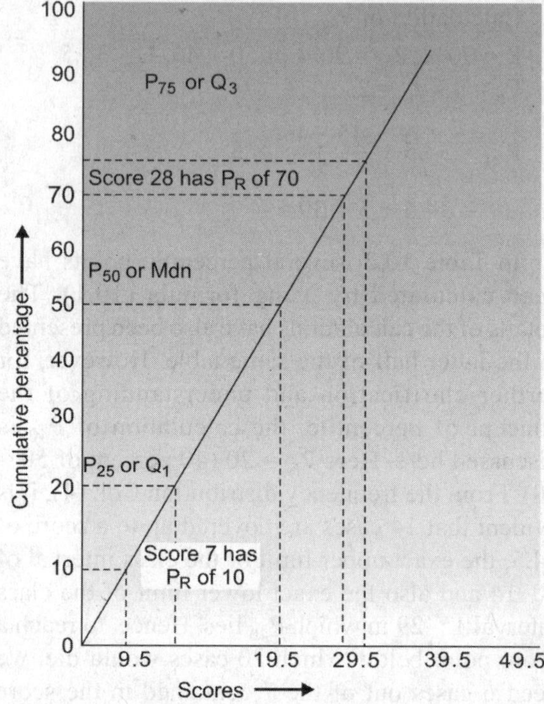

Fig. 10.4: Cumulative frequency curve for the calculation percentiles and P_R's

Percentiles and Percentile Ranks from Ogive

Percentiles and P_R's may be determined quickly and fairly accurately from an Ogive. In figure 10.4, an Ogive based on the data of Table 10.2 has been shown. The median or P_{50} Q_1 or P_{25}, Q_3 or P_{75} and a few other percentiles have been marked off on the Ogive. To obtain median or P_{50}, draw a line from 50 on the Y scale parallel to the X axis and from where this line cuts the curve, drop a perpendicular on the X-axis. Read this point of intersection on the X-axis. This value is 21.83 which is the median. Similarly, locate P_{26} and P_{75} on the Y scale and determine X values by drawing perpendiculars. These values are 12.83 and 30.00 respectively.

Determination of percentile ranks require a reversal of the above procedure. Here, we start off with a score on X-axis and draw a perpendicular on it. From the point where it meets the curve, we draw a line parallel to the X-axis. The point where it cuts the Y-axis is read as the required percentile rank. Percentiles and percentile ranks read from an Ogive will often be slightly in error, yet accurate enough to serve the practical purposes for which these are generally used. However, when the diagram is fairly large, the scale divisions precisely marked and the curve is carefully drawn, percentiles and P_R's can be read more accurately.

The Ogive has several other uses. It can be used to compare two or more groups on some variables of interest to the researcher. For this purpose, the scores of both the groups are plotted upon the same coordinate axes. Differences and similarities between the two distributions at all the points of the scale can then be studied.

The percentile points also serve as percentile norms for the comparison of a persons score with reference to his group. These are particularly useful in dealing with educational achievement examinations. Intra-student comparisons on more than one subject are also possible.

Standard Score (Z)

A standard score which is a kind of derived score is a method of expressing the distance of the score from the mean in terms of standard deviation. In other words it is a dimensionless quality derived by subtracting the sample mean from an individual (raw) and then dividing the difference by the same standard deviation.

Standard score can be classified into two types:

1. Linear standard score
2. Normalized standard score.

Linear Standard Score

The underlying purpose of transforming any original score into standard score is to make the scores on different tests comparable. A linear standard score is one where linear transformation of original score is made. When standard scores are based upon linear transformation, they retain all the characteristics of original raw scores because they are computed by subtracting a constant (such as mean) from each raw score and then dividing the obtained value by another constant (such as SD). Since all characteristics of original raw score are duplicated in linear standard scores, any statistical computation that can be done with original raw scores can also be done with such standard scores. The Z score is an example of linearly transformed standard score which has a mean of zero and a standard deviation of 1. It is computed by subtracting the mean from the individuals raw score and dividing the same by the standard deviation of the distribution. In terms of equitation, a Z score may be read as

$$Z = \frac{X - M}{SD} \qquad ...(10.4)$$

where Z = Z score/sigma score
X = Raw score
M = Mean
SD = Standard deviation

Or

A standard score is a deviation from the mean divided by the standard deviation. It is denoted by *Z* and the formula is

$$Z = \frac{X - M}{\sigma}$$

In which,
Z = Standard score
X = Raw score
M = Mean of raw scores
σ = Standard deviation of raw scores

Example: Suppose Lalitha has obtained a score of 60 on a test and the mean and SD are 30 and 15 respectively. Then,

$$Z = \frac{X - M}{SD} = \frac{60 - 30}{15}$$

$$= \frac{30}{15} = 2$$

This means that Lalitha's score is 2 sigma or standard deviation above the mean of the distribution.

There are some difficulties associated with the use of Z scores.

1. It may be obtained in plus or minus form. Z score in minus are cumbersome to handle.
2. Z score may be expressed in decimal points which tend to further complicate handling then.

Standard scores have a mean equal to zero, equal to unity or one. Thus, the mean serves the purpose of the origin and SD, the unit of measurement. Thus, a particular score value is Z standard deviation units above or below the mean (Table 10.3).

Transformation of raw scores into Z scores do not, in any way, change the other characteristics of the distribution like, skewness and kurtosis. The shape of the distribution remains absolutely unchanged. It does not, in any way, change the proportionality of the scale intervals. It means that the relative distances between the score values remain unchanged under a standard score transformation. The procedure of calculation of Z scores is shown in Table 10.4.

Thus, each nursing student's level of excellence is expressed as so many standard deviation units above or below the mean of the comparison group. Standard scores have essentially the same meanings from one test to another test.

Table 10.3

Computation of standard scores

Test	*Person* (σ)	*Raw score*	*Mean*	*Standard deviation*	*X – M*	$\frac{X-M}{\sigma}$ *or Z*
Child health nursing	Lalitha	62	56	8	62 – 56 = 6	6/8 = 0.67
	Anitha	42	56	8	42 – 56 = –14	–14/8 = –1.67
Community health nursing	Lalitha	68	70	6	68 – 70 = –2	– 2/6 = –0.33
	Anitha	58	70	6	58 – 70 = –12	–12/6 = –2.0

Table 10.4

Computation of standard scores with M = 50, SD = 10

	Formula $Z = 10\left(\frac{X-M}{\sigma}\right) + 50$
Child health nursing	Lalitha $Z = 10\left(\frac{62-56}{8}\right) + 50 = 57.7$ or 58
	Anitha $Z = 10\left(\frac{42-56}{8}\right) + 50 = 32.5$ or 33
Community health nursing	Lalitha $Z = 10\left(\frac{68-70}{8}\right) + 50 = 46.67$ or 47
	Anitha $Z = 10\left(\frac{58-70}{6}\right) + 50 = 30$

Interpretation: Lalitha is 0.67 SD units above the mean of the group on child health nursing while Anitha is 1.67 SD units below the group. On community health nursing test, both the persons are below the average by 0.33 and 2.0 standard deviation unit.

Intertest comparisons reveal that Lalitha though having a higher raw score on community health nursing test is yet 0.33 standard deviation units below the mean while with a smaller raw score, she is 0.67 units above the group mean on child health nursing test.

Standard scores in standard deviation units are quite satisfactory for several purposes but they involve two difficulties:

i. Plus and minus signs are used which can be miscopied, overlooked, or misunderstood, and
ii. Decimal points are involved which may be misplaced.

Hence, it has been suggested that a mean of 50 instead of zero and an SD of 10 instead of one, be used to avoid both the negative signs and the decimal points. For example, the raw scores given in Table 10.3 can be changed into standard scores with M = 50 and σ = 10, through the procedure shown in Table 10.4.

The values of mean and standard deviation can be set-up arbitrarily for the purpose of conversion. However, we may come across M = 50 and SD = 15; and M = 500 and SD =100 more often in the literature than any other values.

Stanine Scale

The stanine (abbreviated from standard nine) is a condensed or coarser form of the normalized T scale. Only nine score categories or groups are formed and the integer values 1 to 9 are assigned to each. The base line of the normal curve is divided into 9 equal divisions in terms of standard deviation units and thus the following percentages of areas obtained (Table 10.5).

Table 10.5

The stanine score system

Stanine scale	*% in each interval (rounded)*	*Cum. %'s*
9	4	100
8	7	96
7	12	89
6	17	77
5	20	60
4	17	40
3	12	23
2	7	11
1	4	4

If a set of scores is ordered from the lowest to the highest, the lowest 4 percent is assigned a score of 1, the next lowest 7 percent a score of 2; and the process continues till the top 4 percent get a score of 9, as shown in Table 10.5. The transformed scores are roughly normal and form a stanine scale.

The stanine scale has mean = 5, SD = 1.96.

A stanine of 5 covers the interval –0.25 to +0.25 in standard deviation units. The relationship of stanines with the s scores and area percent is given in Figure 10.5.

A stanine scale provides a quick method of converting scores to an approximate normal form. The grouping, although coarse, is sufficiently refined for many practical purposes.

Normalized standard score/non-linear standard score: Sometimes researchers wish to compare the scores obtained from distribution having dissimilar shapes. In such a situation they may employ some non-linear transformation so that the scores may conveniently fit into a specified type of distribution, preferably the normal distribution. Normal distribution facilitates further statistical computation. Thus, the normalized standard scores may be defined as those standard scores which have been expressed in the form of a distribution that has been transformed in a way that fits a normal curve. Like linear standard scores, normalized standard scores can be expressed in terms of the mean of zero as a normalized standard score, it indicates that the performance of that person lies exactly at the mean and he excels over 50 percent of the persons in the group.

T-Scale

Normalized standard scores are generally called T-scores. McCall (1939) devised T-scale for the first time which became very popular later on. In the standard scores or *Z* scores, the mean is at zero and the unit of measurement is 1. However, in T scores, a mean of 50 and σ of 10 are used. See Figure 10.6 for a comparison of various scales.

Only slight changes are needed to convert the *z* scale into a T-scale. The T-scale begins at –5 σ and ends at +5 σ. But σ is multiplied by 10 so that the mean is 50 and the other divisions are 0, 10, 20, 30, 40, 50, 60, 70, 80, 90 and 100. The T-scale thus ranges from 0 to 100; and its unit is 1 and mean, 50. Ability ranges beyond –3.5 σ to + 3.5 σ is rare to find, hence in actual practice t-scales range from about 15 to 85. Calculation of *t*-scores has been illustrated in Table 10.6.

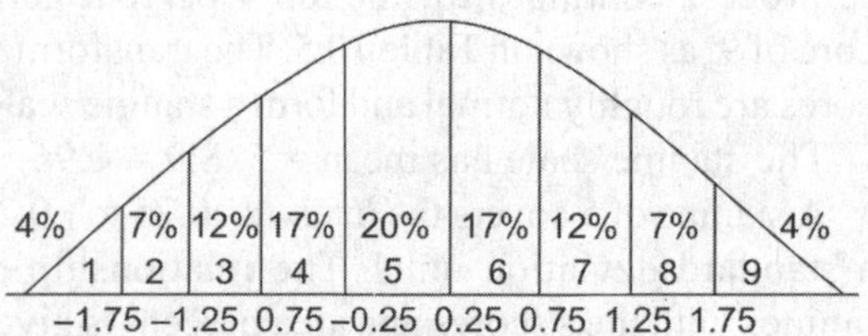

Fig. 10.5: Stanine scale showing standard deviation intervals and percents in each score from 1 to 9

Steps in the Calculation of T-Scores

1. List up the class intervals in Col. (1); mid-point of each CI in Col. (2) and *f* in Col. (3).
2. Calculate cum. frequencies (4)
3. Col. (5) shows the cum. F to the mid-points. These are frequencies below a particular CI plus 1-2 off for that CI. For example, CI 5-9 has 2 frequencies in it and zero frequencies below it. Hence cum. Frequency to mid-point for this CI = 0 + 2 × (1/2) = 1.0. Similarly, for CI 10-14 *two* frequencies below and 4 in it, leading to cum. *f* up to midpoint equal to 2 + 4 × (1/2) =4, and so on.
4. Calculate cum. percentage to midpoint (Col. 6) for each CI. These virtually are percentile ranks corresponding to each midpoint.

Table 10.6

Computation of T-scores

Test-scores	*Mid-point*	*F*	*Cum. f*	*Cum. f below score + 1/2 on given score (to mid-point)*	*Cum. % to mid-point*	*Normal standard deviation unit Z*	*T-Score* Z x 10	Z ×10 +50	*T-Scores from Appendix*
(1)	(2)	(3)	(4)	(5)	(6)	(7)	(8)	(9)	(10)
45-49	47	1	50	49.5	99.0	2.33	23.3	73.3	73
40-44	42	4	49	47	94.0	15.6	15.6	65.6	66
35-39	37	7	45	41.5	83.0	9.5	9.5	59.5	60
30-34	32	8	38	34	68.0	4.7	4.7	54.7	55
25-29	27	10	30	25	50.0	0.0	0.0	50.0	50
20-24	22	8	20	16	32.0	–4.7	–4.7	45.3	45
15-19	17	6	12	9	18.0	–9.2	–9.2	40.8	41
10-14	12	4	6	4	8.0	–14.0	–14.0	36.0	36
5-9	7	2	2	1.0	2.0	–20.5	–20.5	29.5	30

5. Col. (7) carries the values of normal deviate, Z, corresponding to each cum. percentage.
6. Z values have been multiplied by 10 and a constant of 50 added to each to arrive at the value of T scores (Col. 9). For example for CI 10–14, T = (–1.40 × 10) + 50 = 36; for CI 40-44, T = (1.56 × 10 + 50 = 65.6) and so on.
7. Col. (9) shows T scores corresponding to each cum. percent to midpoint, read from Appendix, Table L. It would eliminate the need of calculating Z values and further computational work. Values read from the Appendix are very close to those worked out by actual calculation. However, for a student, it is better to do all the calculations to understand the concept of T-scale (Fig. 10.6).

T-scale scores have general applicability, a very convenient unit and cover a wide range of ability. The minus and fractional values are eliminated. They are comparable from test to test and provide the same meaning. However, if suspicion about the normality of the trait in the population arises, T scores should not be used. However, it has been seen that when large samples are tested on mental abilities, normality is a reasonable assumption.

Chi-square (χ^2)

The chi-square test is one of the most important non-parametric test. It is also called as general-purpose statistics because it involves no assump-

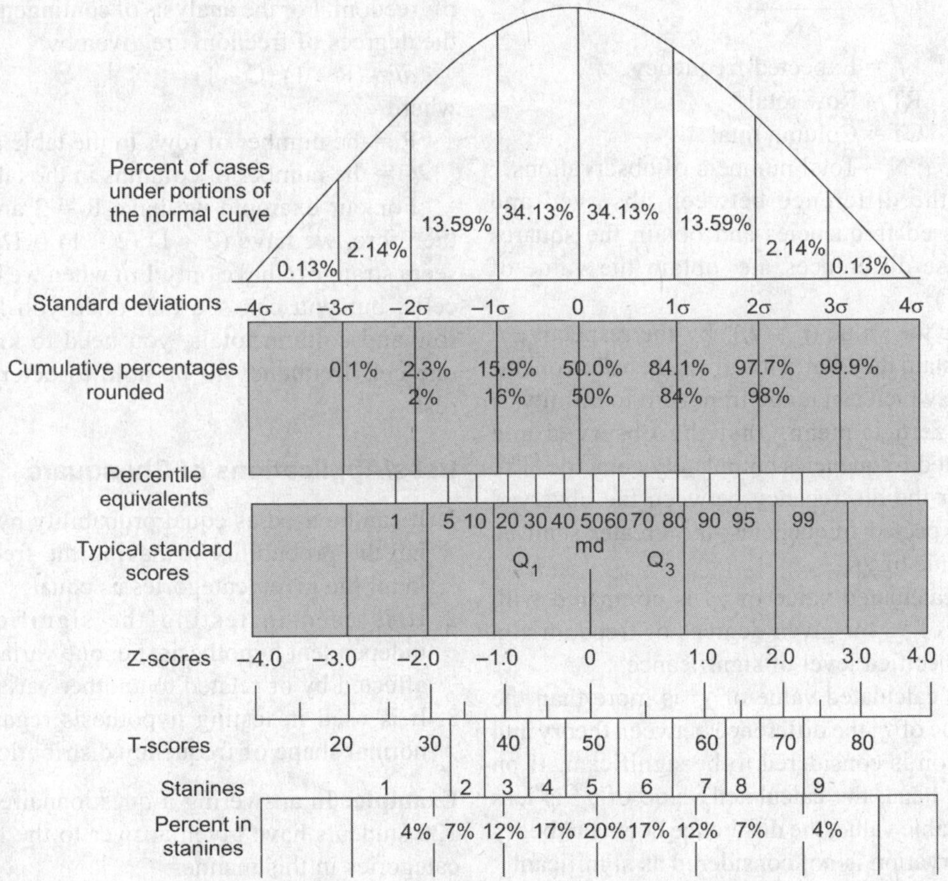

Fig. 10.6: Various types of standard score in relation to percentile and the normal curve

tion regarding the normalcy of distribution. The chi-square test (χ^2) is used when the data are expressed in terms of frequencies or proportions or percentages. It was first used by Karl Pearson in the year 1900. The formula for calculating χ^2 is as follows:

$$\chi^2 = \Sigma \frac{(f_0 - f_e)^2}{f_e} \qquad \text{...(10.5)}$$

where f_o = observed frequency
f_e = expressed frequency

Steps: To determine χ^2 the steps required are:

1. Calculate the expected frequency with the help of the following equation

$$f_e = \frac{\text{RT} \times \text{CT}}{\text{N}}$$

where f_e = Expected frequency
RT = Row total
CT = Column total
N = Total numbers of observations

2. Take the difference between observed and expressed frequencies and obtain the squares of these differences, i.e. obtain the value of $(f_o - f_e)^2$.
3. Divide the value $(f_o - f_e)^2$ by the respective f_e and obtain the total. This gives the value of chi-square which can range from zero to infinity. If χ^2 is zero it means that the observed and expected frequencies completely coincide. The greater the discrepancy between the observed and expected frequencies, the greater shall be the value of χ^2.

The calculated value of χ^2 is compared with the table of χ^2 for given degrees of freedom at a certain specified level of significance.

If the calculated value of χ^2 is more than the table value of χ^2 the difference between theory and observation is considered to be significant. If on the other hand, the calculated value of χ^2 is less than the table value, the difference between theory and observation is not considered as significant.

Degrees of Freedom

While comparing the calculated χ^2 with the table value we have to determine the degrees of freedom. Degrees of freedom refers to the number of classes to which the values can be assigned arbitrarily or at will without violating the restrictions or limitations placed.

In chi-square where we will prepare 2 × 2 table the degree of freedom can be calculated with the help of following formula:

$$df = (r - 1)(c - 1) \qquad \text{...(10.6)}$$

where r = row
c = column

Before we can compare our value of χ^2 to the value in Appendix χ^2, we must know the degrees of freedom. For the analysis of contingency tables, the degrees of freedom are given by:

$$df = (\text{R} - 1)(\text{C} - 1)$$

where

R = the number of rows in the table and
C = the number of columns in the table

For our example we have R = 2 and C = 2; therefore, we have (2 – 1) (2 – 1) = 1*df*. It may seem strange to have only 1 *df* when we have four cells, but you can see that once you know the row and column totals, you need to know only one cell frequency to be able to determine the rest.

Uses/Applications of Chi-square

1. It can be used as equal probability hypothesis, i.e. the probability of having the frequencies, in all the given categories as equal.
2. It is used in testing the significance of independent hypothesis, i.e. one variable is not affected by or related to another variable.
3. It is used in testing hypothesis regarding the normal shape of frequency distribution.

Example: In answering a questionnaire, a set of 120 students have given answer to the following categories in this manner:

Yes	Cannot say	No	Total
25	65	30	120

Answers	Yes	Cannot say	No	Total
f_o	25	65	30	120
f_e	40	40	40	120
f_o-f_e	–15	25	-10	
$(f_o-f_e)^2$	225	625	100	
$\frac{(f_0-f_e)^2}{f_e}$	5.625	15.625	2.5	23.75

$$\chi^2 = \sum\left[\frac{(f_0-f_e)^2}{f_e}\right]$$

$$\chi^2 = 23.75$$

$$df = (r-1)(c-1)$$

$$= (2-1)(3-1) = 1 \times 2$$

$$df = 2$$

Interpretation – referring to table distribution of χ^2 – the obtained value is significant beyond 0.001 level. Therefore the obtained value is significant.

Example: Take an example of 3 × 3 contingency table which shows data of 200 students who were into 3 classes on the basis of their educational qualification. Their educational attainment is measured in course of study by classifying them superior, average, inferior. Now the question is – Is educational achievement related to educational qualification?

	Superior	Average	Inferior	Total
Master	30	15	5	50
Bachelor	25	10	15	50
Intermediate	45	35	20	100
Total	100	60	40	200

Calculation of expected frequency (f_e)

Upper left	100 × 50/200 = 25
Upper middle	60 × 50/200 = 15
Upper right	40 × 50/200 = 10
Middle left	100 × 50/200 = 25
Middle middle	60 × 50/200 = 15
Middle right	40 × 50/200 = 10
Lower left	100 × 100/200= 50
Lower middle	60 × 100/200 = 30
Lower right	40 × 100/200 = 20
	200

The Chi-square may be calculated as follows:

f_0	f_e	f_0-f_e	$(f_0-f_e)^2$	$\frac{(f_0-f_e)^2}{f_e}$
30	25	5	25	1
15	15	0	0	0
5	10	–5	25	2.5
25	25	00	0	0
10	15	–5	25	1.67
15	10	5	25	2.5
45	50	–5	25	0.5
35	30	5	25	0.83
20	20	0	0	0
200	200	$(f_0-f_e) = 0$		$\sum\frac{(f_0-f_e)^2}{f_e}$

$$\chi^2 = \sum\left[\frac{(f_0-f_e)^2}{f_e}\right]$$

$$\chi^2 = 9.00$$

$$df = (r-1)(c-1)$$

$$= (3-1)(3-1) = 2 \times 2 = 4$$

Interpretation: p falls at 0.05 level indicating that there is no relationship between educational achievement and educational qualification.

Chi-square with 2 × 2 contingency table (where $df = 1$) we need not calculate expected frequency. Chi-square can be calculated with the help of following formula:

$$\chi^2 = \frac{N\,[(AD-BC)]^2}{(A+B)(C+D)(A+C)(B+D)}$$

- Suppose the researcher wants to know whether or not the given 2 items in the tests are independent. Both items have been answered in "Yes" or "No" form. The test was administered to a sample of 400 students and the obtained data were as follows:

	Yes	No	
No	180_A	120_B	300
Yes	90_C	10_D	100
	270	130	400

$$\chi^2 = \frac{N[(AD - BC)]^2}{(A+B)(C+D)(A+C)(B+D)}$$

$$= \frac{400\left[(180 \times 10) - 120 \times 90\right]^2}{(180+120)(90+10)(180+90)(120+10)}$$

$$= \frac{400\,[1800 - 10800]^2}{300 \times 100 \times 270 \times 130}$$

$$= \frac{400\,[-9000]^2}{1053000000} = \frac{400 \times 81000000}{1053000000}$$

$$= \frac{32400}{1053} = 30.76$$

$df = (r - 1)(c - 1)$
$= (2 - 1)(2 - 1)$
$= 1 \times 1 = 1$

$\therefore df = 1$

Interpretation: The two items on a test are related.

t-test

This is also called as test of significance. It is computed to compare performance of a group under two different conditions of the experiment. It indicates the extent to which the obtained difference is significant or not. As we usually compare the performance of the same group in a classroom situation, this test is very useful.

When the sample size is less than 30 we use the *t*-test or *t* for testing the significance of the difference between two means. The concept of small sample size test was developed in 1915, by William Seely Gosset, a statistician in Ireland.

When the sample size is more than 30, the ratio of the difference between two samples means the standard error of the difference is calculated by the Z-test, which is interpreted through the use of normal probability tables. As the sample size increases, the critical ratio or values of '*t*' necessary for rejecting the null hypothesis gradually reduce and approach the Z-values where the mean of the experimental group is equal to the mean of the control group. If it is rejected, we accept the alternative hypothesis.

Three types of situation arise while one is calculating the *t*-ratio

1. *t*-ratio from independent groups
2. *t*-ratio from correlated groups
3. *t*-ratio from matched groups

Regardless of the nature of group *t*-ratio is calculated by the following formula:

$$t = \frac{(M_1 - M_2) - 0}{SE_D} \qquad (10.7)$$

$$SE_D = \sqrt{SE_{M_1}{}^2 - SE_{M_2}{}^2}$$

$$SE_M = \frac{SD}{\sqrt{N}}$$

where

M_1 = Mean of first group
M_2 = Mean of second group
SE_D = Standard error of the difference between two sample means
SE_M = Standard error of the mean
SD = Standard deviation
N = Number.

Where Means are not Correlated (2 Groups)

Suppose one group of girls (22) and one group of boys (20) were administered a test, their data was summarized as under:

Girls	*Boys*
$N_1 = 22$	$N_2 = 20$
$M_1 = 30.56$	$M_2 = 34.56$
$SD_1 = 6.98$	$SD_2 = 5.68$

Solution.

In order to calculate *t* – ratio the following steps are used:

$$t = \frac{(M_1 - M_2) - 0}{SE_D}$$

Number of students	*Marks in 1st test*	*Marks in 5th test*	*D*	*D × D = D²*	*D – M = X*	*(X) × (X) = X²*
1	50	62	–12	144	2.84	8.06
2	42	40	2	4	7.16	51.26
3	51	61	–10	100	0.84	0.70
4	26	35	–9	81	0.16	0.02
5	35	30	5	25	4.16	17.30
6	42	52	–10	100	0.84	0.70
7	60	68	–8	81	1.16	1.34
8	41	51	–10	100	0.84	0.70
9	70	84	–14	196	4.84	23.42
10	55	63	–8	64	1.16	1.34
11	62	72	–10	100	0.84	0.70
12	38	50	–12	144	2.84	8.06
Total			110	1139		113.6

D = difference

$$SE_D = \sqrt{SEM_1{}^2 + SEM_2{}^2}$$

$$SE_M = \frac{SD}{\sqrt{N}}$$

$$SE_{M_1} = \frac{6.98}{\sqrt{22}} = \frac{6.98}{4.69}$$

$$SE_{M_1} = 1.489$$

$$SE_{M_2} = \frac{5.68}{\sqrt{20}} = \frac{5.68}{4.47}$$

$$SE_{M_2} = 1.270$$

$$SE_D = \sqrt{SEM_1{}^2 + SEM_2{}^2}$$

$$SE_D = \sqrt{1.489^2 + 1.270^2}$$

$$SE_D = \sqrt{2.217 + 1.612} = \sqrt{3.829}$$

$$= 1.956$$

$$t = \frac{(M_1 - M_2) - 0}{SE_D} = \frac{(30.56 - 34.56)}{1.956} - 0$$

$$= \frac{4 - 0}{1.956} = 2.04$$

$$df = (N_1 - 1) + (N_2 - 1)$$

$$= (22 - 1) + (20 - 1)$$

$$= 21 + 19 = 40$$

$$df = 40$$

Entering '*p*' table of *t*-ratio the obtained *t* of 2.04 and *df*(40) is significant at 0.05 level. Here true difference is found.

Where Means are Correlated (same Group under Two Conditions)

$$t = \frac{Mean_D}{SEM_D}$$

$$SEM_D = \frac{SD_D}{\sqrt{N}}$$

$$SD_D = \sqrt{\frac{\Sigma X^2}{N - 1}}$$

$$Mean = \frac{\Sigma D}{N}$$

$$df = N - 1$$

Marks of 12 students are given below under 1st test and 5th test. Calculate *t*-ratio

Note = Ignore minus signs

$$t = \frac{Mean_D}{SEM_D}$$

$$\text{Mean} = \frac{\sqrt{\Sigma x^2}}{N-1} = \frac{\sqrt{113.6}}{12-1}$$

$$= \frac{\sqrt{113.6}}{11} = \sqrt{10.327}$$

$$SD_D = 3.213$$

$$SEM_D = \frac{SD_D}{\sqrt{N}} = \frac{3.213}{\sqrt{12}}$$

$$= \frac{3.213}{3.464} = 0.927$$

$$t = \frac{\text{Mean D}}{SEM_D}$$

$$= \frac{9.16}{0.927} = 9.881$$

$$= 9.881$$

$$df = N - 1 = 12 - 1 = 11$$

Interpretation: The obtained *t*-value of 9.881 with the *df* of 11 is significant beyond 0.005 level.

EXERCISES

1. A researcher adopted different sampling techniques while investigating the same group of students to find the number of students falling in different intelligence levels. The results are as follows:

Researcher	*Below Average*	*Average*	*Above*	*Genius*	*Total*
X	86	60	44	10	200

2. For 3 × 3 contingency table:
Three samples are taken comprising 120 doctors, 140 advocates and 130 university teachers. Each person chosen is asked to select one of the three categories that best represents his feeling towards a certain national policy. The three categories are in favor of policy (F), against the policy (A) and indifferent towards the policy (I). The results of the interviews are given below:
Calculate χ^2 test

Occupation	*F*	*A*	*I*	*Total*
Doctors	80	30	10	120
Advocates	70	40	40	150
University Teachers	50	50	30	130
Total	200	120	80	400

3. For 2 × 2 contingency table
In a survey 200 boys, of which 75 were intelligent, 40 had skilled fathers while 85 of intelligent boys had unskilled fathers. Do these figures support the hypothesis that skilled fathers have intelligent boys?
Use χ^2 test and find out if there may be relation between having intelligent boys and skilled fathers. where $df = 1$.

	Skilled	*Unskilled*	*Total*
Intelligent	40	35	75
Unintelligent	40	85	125
Total	80	120	200

4. Calculate *t*-test for the following set of scores:

Subjects	T_1	T_2
A	16	14
B	14	11
C	17	16
D	16	15
E	15	16
F	12	14
G	13	17
H	14	15
I	18	16
J	16	16

5. Calculate percentile rank for the following set of data (Grouped data):

Class interval	*f*
31-35	3
36-40	4
41-45	7
46-50	9
51-55	13
56-60	16
61-65	12
66-70	8
71-75	4
76-80	4

6. Suppose Seema has obtained a score of 95 on a test and the mean and SD are 43.67 and 6.21 respectively. Calculate her Z-score.
7. In answering a questionnaire, a set of 150 students have given answer to the following categories in this manner:

Yes	*No*	*?*
92	32	26

Calculate χ^2.

CHAPTER

11 Statistical Correlation

Introduction

The relationships (or association) between two quantitatively measured (continuous) variable called 'correlation'.

Correlational designs allow the researcher to determine relationships between variables rather than drawing cause-and-effect conclusions, which can lead to spurious (incorrect) conclusions. Researchers who conclude that a high possitive or high negative correlations is necessarily a cause-and-effect relationship have failed to interpret correlations correctly.

Correlation means a possible connection or relationship or interdependence, between the value of two or more variables of the same phenomenon or individual series. It indicates the strength of relationship. For example, study the relationship of the type between height and weight or price and demand or wage and price index. For example, such a relationship is called 'statistical relationship'.

Regression technique provides the actual relationship between two or more variables. But the scientists are not always interested in this linear or curvilinear relationship. Often the interest lies only in knowing the extent of interdependence between two or more variables. In this situation, correlation methods serve our purpose. If the two variables, say X and Y, are linearly related, they are said to be correlated. The correlation between two variables is also known as simple correlation. It means that the change in one variable is accompanied by the proportionate change in the other variable. The change is likely to occur in both directions namely, (i) the increase in one variable is accompanied by the proportionate increase in the other variable, (ii) the increase in one variable causes the proportionate decrease in the other variable. In the first case the two variables are said to be positively interrelated, whereas in the second case, they are said to be negatively interrelated. For example, there exists a positive correlation between the age of a husband and age of his wife, the income and expenditure of families. On the other hand, the price of a commodity and its consumption, the soil temperature and germination period are the variables that are negatively correlated. The readers will come across many more correlation problems in numerical examples.

The mathematical measure of correlation was given by the statistician Karl Pearson in 1896 in the form of correlation coefficient. This was extensively used by Sir Francis Galton to explain many phenomena in biology and genetics. Its use in economics was emphasized by Professor Neiswanger as he wrote, "correlation analysis contributes to the understanding of economic behavior, aids in locating the critically important variable on which others depend, may reveal to the economist the connections by which disturbances spread and suggest to him the paths through which stabilising forces may become effective". Since its innovation the application of correlation methods has always been increasing. Besides Pearsonian correlation, many more types of correlations are being invented which are suitable for particular kinds of variables. To name a few are: rank correlation, biserial correlation, intraclass correlation, etc. Multiple correlation and partial correlation are associated with multivariate analysis. In this chapter we will confine to simple correlation and rank correlation.

When dealing with two sets of variables, it may so happen that one variable may be in a way related to the other. That is to say, with the change in one variable from one value to the other, the other variable will also change in its' value corresponding to the change in the first variable. Then, it is assumed that there is a correlation between the two variables. This correlation may be either due to some direct relationship between the two variables. To discover the existence or statistical relationship between the two variables from the bivariable data, some special methods have been developed in statistics.

When both variables in the bivariate data are quantitative, use the terms *correlation analysis* to describe the methods designed to find out whether the statistical relationship between the two variables exist or not. When the variables are of such a character, they may be measured and the results expressed in quantitative units and paired measurements for two variables and available for a group of individuals; it is possible under certain conditions to calculate a constant known as the *correlation coefficient*. This will express the degree of the relationship. Here the degree of this correlation is measured in terms of coefficient correlation. This measure takes into consideration the co-variation between two variables in relation to the variation within themselves.

Often two variables or attributes are simultaneously recorded (i.e., bivariate data) to know whether one influences the other, e.g. height and weight, age and blood pressure, weight or pregnant mother and weight of the newborn, temperature and pulse etc. The purpose of such study is to know whether change in one variable is associated with the change in the other variable. If there is a change like that, then it is assumed that there is a "correlation" between the two variables and the degree of this correlation is measured in terms of "Correlation Coefficient".

Correlation is the linear relationship or mutuality of association of two variables; it is independent of the units of measurements (where as x^2-test indicates the presence or absence of relationship between the qualitative data but not the degree of association).

Coxton and Cowden defined the correlation as the relationship of quantitative nature. The appropriate statistical tool for discovering and measuring the relationship and expressing it in a brief formula is known as *correlation.*

Before studying the correlation analysis, it is better to introduce the concept of *covariance* between two quantitative variables X and Y. Let the corresponding values of the two variables X and Y on the given set of n units of observations be given by the ordered pairs.

$$(x_1, y_1), (x_2, y_2), (x_3, y_3), \ldots, (x_n, y_n)$$

Then, the covariance between X and Y is denoted by covariance (X, Y). It is defined as

$$\text{Cov. (X, Y)} = \frac{(x_1-\bar{x})(y_1-\bar{y})+(x_2-\bar{x})(y_2-\bar{y}) + \cdots + (x_n-\bar{x})(y_n-\bar{y})}{n}$$

$$= \frac{1}{n}\sum_{i=1}^{n}(x_i-\bar{x})(y_i-\bar{y}) \quad \ldots(11.1)$$

where x and y are the means of X and Y respectively, i.e.

$$x = \frac{x_1+x_2+\cdots+x_n}{n},\ y = \frac{y_1+y_2+\cdots+y_n}{n}$$

Calculation of Covariance

The above formula for the calculation of covariance is complicated and may have more chances of the occurrence of an error. We now give below that which makes the calculations easier to carry out and which also reduce the chances of error.

The formula is

$$\text{Cov. (X,Y)} = \frac{1}{n}\left\{\sum_{i=1}^{n} x_i y_i - \frac{1}{n}\left(\sum_{i=1}^{n} x_i\right)\left(\sum_{i=1}^{n} y_i\right)\right\} \quad \ldots(11.2)$$

Cov. (X,Y) = E(XY) – E(X) E(Y), ...(11.3)

where E(X), E(XY) are the expectations of X, Y and XY respectively.

Determination of Correlation by Graphical Method

It has already been stated, while explaining the regression, that scatter diagram gives a fair idea of relationship between two variables, X and Y. Here too, we have paired observations of variables X and Y. These measurements for both the variables are taken either on the same unit or on paired units, e.g. the height and weight of a person form one pair, the age of husband and his wife form one pair, the income and expenditure of a family form one pair, the cost price and selling price of an article form one pair. When the paired observations are plotted on the graph paper for all the objects or units under consideration, their pattern of location gives a fair idea of correlation between two variables. Figures 11.1 to 11.6 of scatter diagrams are given here to show the extent of relationship between two variables. The population correlation coefficient is denoted by ρ (rho).

i. This scatter diagram shows the perfect positive correlation, as all the points lie on a straight line. As the variate value of X increases, Y also increases and vice-versa.

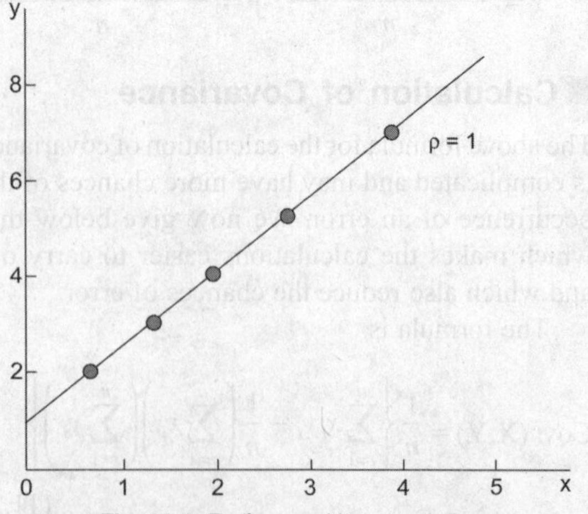

Fig. 11.1: Perfect positive correlation

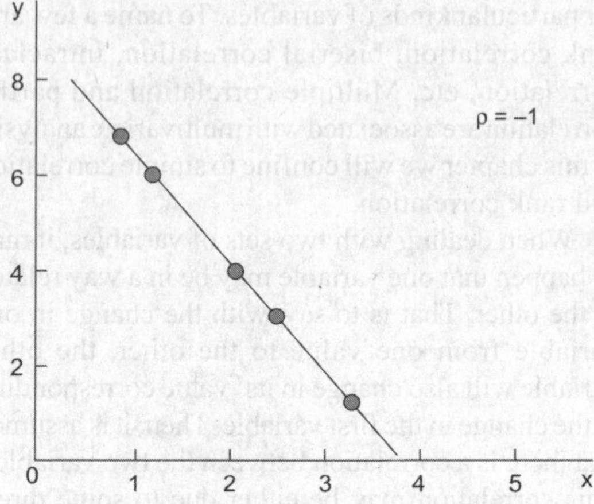

Fig. 11.2: Perfect negative correlation

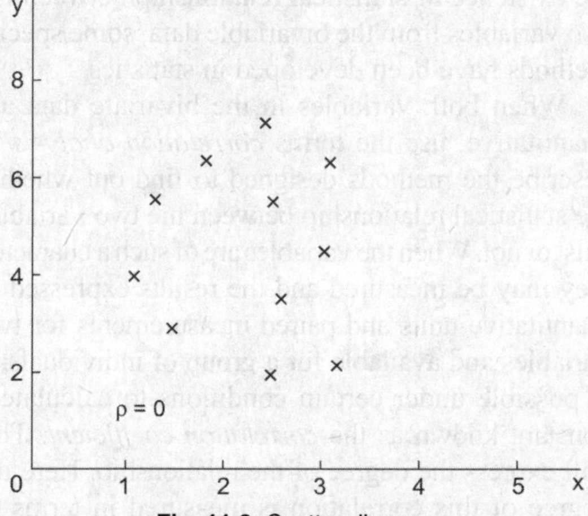

Fig. 11.3: Scatter diagram

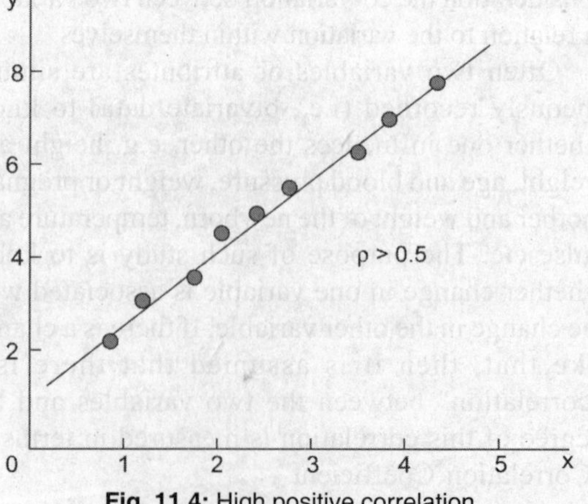

Fig. 11.4: High positive correlation

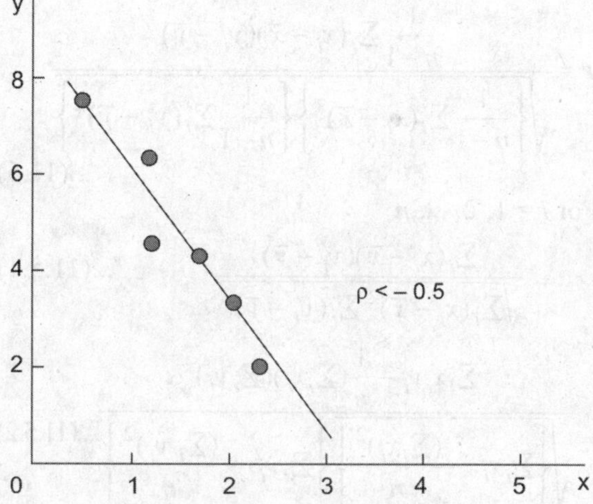

Fig. 11.5: High negative correlation

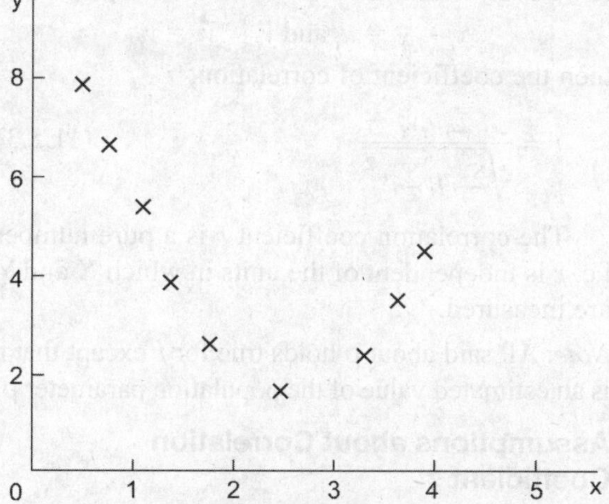

Fig. 11.6: Correlation not expressible

ii. This scatter diagram depicts a perfect negative correlation. All points lie on the straight line. The slope of the line is such that as X increases, Y decreases proportionately.

iii. No line can be drawn passing through most of the plotted points. The points are totally scattered. Hence it shows no correlation between the variables X and Y.

iv. Most of the plotted points lie on the line. Others are near to this line. Hence, the diagram shows a high positive correlation.

v. This scatter diagram shows a high negative correlation as the slope of the line is more than 90°. Most of the points either lie on the straight line or are in close vicinity.

vi. Points lie on a curve. Hence, there is no linear relationship between X and Y. Under the circumstances, the correlation is not expressible.

The above Figures 11.1 to 11.6 give a vague idea about the correlation between two variables. Still their importance cannot be ignored as they enable a person to know whether the data are suitable for finding out the correlation mathematically or not. From the Figures 11.1 and 11.4, it is apparent that in positive correlation, the points flow from lower left corner to the right top. Whereas the Figures 11.2 and 11.5 reveal that in negative correlation, the points flow from the upper left to the right bottom. Figure 11.3 shows that points do not follow any set pattern and hence the variables are independent. Figure 11.6 depicts a curvilinear trend and the simple correlation, which is a measure of linear association, is not expressible.

If only a few points lie on trend line and other points are away from this line, we consider that there is a low degree of linear relationship between the two variables.

Another way of judging the correlation between two variates is to plot both the variate values on the same axis corresponding to each paired number and see the trend of both the graphs. If both these trend lines or curves are parallel to each other, they are positively correlated.

Figure 11.7 shows that there is a high degree of positive correlation between the height of a Father and his Son.

Correlation Analysis

Correlation Coefficient (ρ)

The extent of relationship in measured by correlation-coefficient. In some situation, find that two variables are related because both are related to 3rd variable.

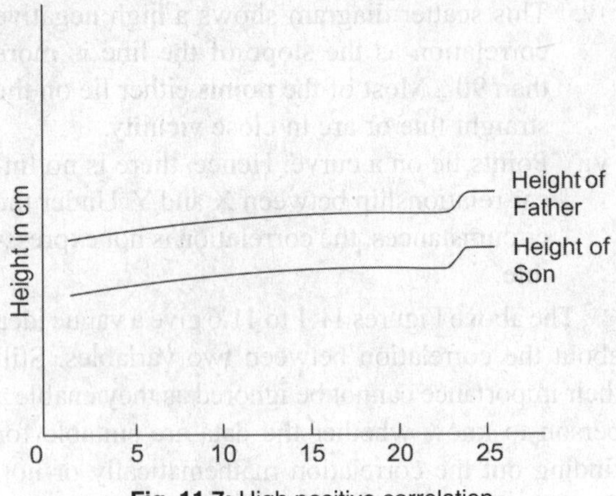

Fig. 11.7: High positive correlation

The correlation between two variables is termed as simple correlation and its general measure is Karl Pearson coefficient of correlation. The estimated value of population correlation coefficient ρ between two variables X and Y is denoted by ρ. Here we shall give all the formulae for r. If in some study all the units of the population are measured, we should use the formulae given for r over all the observations of the population and, instead of r, use the symbol ρ. But in rare cases we study the whole population. Therefore, we have given the formulae for sample observations. Sometimes, the suffix XY is added to r, i.e. r_{XY}, to connote that it is the correlation coefficient between the variables X and Y. Theoretically, the sample correlation coefficient is given as,

$$r_{XY} = \frac{\text{cov}(X, Y)}{\sqrt{u(X)u(Y)}} \quad ...(11.4)$$

$$= \frac{s_{xy}}{s_x s_y} \quad ...(11.4.1)$$

where s_x and s_y are the sample standard deviations of variables X and Y respectively, and s_{xy} is the estimated covariance between X and Y. If we have n pairs of sample observations, (x_1, y_1), (x_2, y_2), (x_3, y_3), ...(x_n, y_n), then the correlation coefficient,

$$r = \frac{\frac{1}{n-1}\Sigma_i(x_i - \bar{x})(y_i - \bar{y})}{\sqrt{\left\{\frac{1}{n-1}\Sigma_i(x_i - \bar{x})^2\right\}\left\{\frac{1}{n-1}\Sigma_i(y_i - \bar{y})^2\right\}}} \quad ...(11.5)$$

For $i = 1, 2, ..., n$

$$= \frac{\Sigma_i(x_i - \bar{x})(y_i - \bar{y})}{\sqrt{\Sigma_i(x_i - \bar{x})^2 \Sigma_i(y_i - \bar{y})^2}} \quad ...(11.5.1)$$

$$= \frac{\Sigma_i x_i y_i - \frac{1}{n}(\Sigma_i x_i)(\Sigma_i y_i)}{\sqrt{\left\{\Sigma_i x_i^2 - \frac{(\Sigma_i x_i)^2}{n}\right\}\left\{\Sigma_i y_i^2 - \frac{(\Sigma_i y_i)^2}{n}\right\}}} \quad ...(11.5.2)$$

For $i = 1, 2, ..., n$.

If we take the deviations from mean and denote

$$x_i - \bar{x} = u_i \text{ and } y_i - \bar{y} = v_i$$

then the coefficient of correlation,

$$r = \frac{\Sigma_i u_i v_i}{\sqrt{\Sigma_i u_i^2 \Sigma_i v_i^2}} \quad ...(11.5.3)$$

The correlation coefficient r is a pure number i.e. r is independent of the units in which X and Y are measured.

Note: All said about ρ holds true for r except that r is an estimated value of the population parameter ρ.

Assumptions about Correlation Coefficient

There are three assumptions made in giving the correlation coefficient by the above formulae. They are:

1. The random variables X and Y are distributed normally.
2. The variables X and Y are linearly related.
3. There is a cause and effect relationship between factors affecting the values of X and Y in the series of data.

Correlation and Coefficient of Correlation

Correlation: Correlation may be defined as a tendency towards interrelation variation.

Coefficient of correlation is a measure of such a tendency, i.e. the degree to which the two variables are interrelated is measured by a coefficient which is called the **Coefficient of correlation.** It gives the degree of correlation.

Definition: The relationship between two variables is such that, a change in one variable results in a positive or negative change in the other and also a greater change in one variable, results in a corresponding greater or smaller change in the other variable this is known as correlation.

The coefficient of correlation between the two variables x, y is generally denoted by r or r_{xy} or $p(x, y)$ or p.

Properties of Co-efficient of Correlation

1. It is a measure of the closeness of a fit in a relative sense.
2. Correlation coefficient lies between –1 and +1, i.e. $-1 \leq r \leq 1$.
3. The correlation is perfect and positive if $r = 1$ and it is perfect and negative if $r = -1$.
4. If $r = 0$, then there is no correlation between the two variables and thus the variables are said to be independent.

So far, we have looked into the distribution of a single variable at a time. Very often, however, there is interest in examining as to, how variations in one variable are associated with or related with the variations in another variable. This is called a bivariate situation. For this purpose, we need an index of association or relationship between the two variables. This is known as *coefficient of correlation. A coefficient of correlation is a single number that tells us to what extent two variables or things are related and to what extent variations in one variable go with variations, with the other.* Whenever, two measurements for the same individual can be paired for all the individuals in a group, the degree of relationship between the paired scores is called 'correlation'.

For example, a teacher finds that students having high IQ's have secured high marks and students having low IQ's have secured low marks on a test of academic achievement. It shows a definite trend of relationship in the variations of IQ's and marks. Let us examine the three sets of X and Y scores given in Table 11.1 for 10 children. Scores for the X variable have been ordered from the highest to the lowest and remain uniformally so in all the three A, B and C situations. Data for the Y variable are arranged in three different ways corresponding to the column headings, A, B and C.

The data in column A show that each person attains the same score on both variables. The child with the highest X score has also the highest Y score; conversely the child with the lowest score on X has the lowest score on Y. Each X score corresponds exactly with each Y scores. This leads to a perfect relationship. Since an increase in the value of X scores results in a corresponding increase in the Y scores, the direction of relationship is positive. The scatter plot for set A represents the placement of scores along a straight line which runs from the lower left hand corner to the upper right hand corner. The correlation coefficient, r, in this case = 1.00. The scores in Column B of Table 11.1 show a trend which is exactly opposite to the trend of set A. The person obtaining the highest score on the X variables has the lowest score on the Y variable. Conversely, the lowest score on the X variable corresponds to the highest score on the Y variable. The positions of other scores have also been reversed in a perfectly or maximal correlation but with a negative direction. The scatter plot for set B in Figure 11.8 represents the placement of scores along a straight line which runs from the lower right hand corner to the upper left hand corner. The correlation coefficient in this case = –1.00. Compare the direction of the straight lines of scatter plots A and B. What is the difference?

Table 11.1

Paired scores for three levels of correlation

Persons	*A*		*B*		*C*	
	X	*Y*	*X*	*Y*	*X*	*Y*
1	20	20	20	11	20	19
2	19	19	19	12	19	14
3	18	18	18	13	18	13
4	17	17	17	14	17	11
5	16	16	16	15	16	20
6	15	15	15	16	15	12
7	14	14	14	17	14	17
8	13	13	13	18	13	18
9	12	12	12	19	12	16
10	11	11	11	20	11	15
Interpretation	Perfect positive $r = +1.00$		Perfect negative $r = -1.00$		Zero correlation $r = 0$	

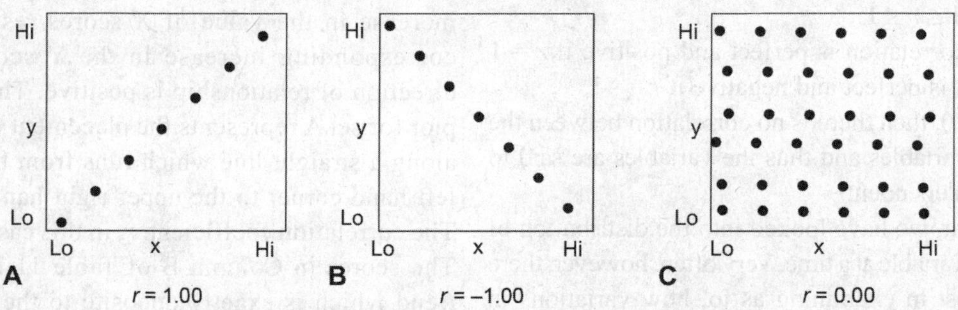

Figs 11.8A to C: Scatter plots for three levels of correlation

The scores in column C of Table 11.1 show that it was difficult to find any particular trend of association between the variations in the scores of X and Y. The correlation is essentially non-existent. The scatter plot for set C in Figures 11.8A to C shows that the scores fall all over the surface of the graph in such a way that change or variation in one variable is unrelated with the other variable. Hence value of $r = 0.00$.

There are four types of correlation, which includes perfect positive correlation; moderately positive correlation, perfect negative correlation, moderately negative correlation and absolutely, no correlation. This interpretation of correlation coefficient (r) as given below:

$r =$ 0.8 and above → High correlation coefficient

$r =$ 0.5 around → Moderate correlation coefficient (0.4 to 0.7)

$r =$ 0.3 (and above) → Low correlation coefficient

$r =$ 0 (zero) → Absolutely no correlation.

Example: The age in years of fourteen young couples is given below:

Husband (X)	21	25	26	24	22	30	19	24	28	32	31	29	21	18
Wife (Y)	19	20	24	21	21	24	18	22	19	30	27	26	19	18

To know the extent of relationship between the age of husbands and wives, we calculate the coefficient of correlation r from the given data. For the given variate values,

$$n = 14$$
$$\Sigma_i x_i = 350$$
$$\bar{x} = 25$$
$$\Sigma_i y_i = 308$$
$$\bar{y} = 22$$

Since means are whole numbers, it is convenient to make use of the formula (11.5.1). To do the calculations systematically, prepare the following Table:

From the Table we have,

$\Sigma(x_i - \bar{x})^2 = 264$

$\Sigma_i(y_i - \bar{y})^2 = 178$

$\Sigma_i(x_i - \bar{x})(y_i - \bar{y}) = 185$

Putting these values in the formula (11.5.1) we get,

$$r = \frac{185}{\sqrt{264 \times 178}} = \frac{185}{216.78} = 0.85$$

The coefficient of correlation between the age of husband and that of the wife is 0.85 which is close to 1. Hence it can be said that there is a high degree of positive relationship between the age of husbands and wives.

The Product Moment Correlation, r

The commonly used parametric statistic for correlation is the Pearson product-moment correlation coefficient, otherwise known as the **Pearson *r*,** or more simply as r. The Pearson r can be either descriptive or inferential. As a descriptive statistic, the correlation coefficient demonstrates the size and the direction of a stataistical relationship. As an inferential statistic, the Pearson r can be used to test

x	y	$x - \bar{x}$	$y - \bar{y}$	$(x - \bar{x})^2$	$(y - \bar{y})^2$	$(x - \bar{x})(y - \bar{y})$
21	19	– 4	– 3	16	9	12
25	20	0	– 2	0	4	0
26	24	1	2	1	4	2
24	21	– 1	–1	1	1	1
22	21	– 3	– 1	9	1	3
30	24	5	2	25	4	10
19	18	– 6	– 4	36	16	24
24	22	– 1	0	1	0	00
28	19	3	– 3	9	9	– 9
32	30	7	8	49	64	56
31	27	6	5	36	25	30
29	26	4	4	16	16	16
21	19	– 4	– 3	16	9	12
18	18	– 7	– 4	49	16	28
Total 350	308	0	0	264	178	185

hypotheses about relationships between data sets whithin and between populations. In this test, two different sets of interval or ratio data are compared to determine the degreee of relationship between them. Because r values range from –1 throught 0 to +1, pairs of items are related either positively or negatively. As the correlation coefficient approaches –1 or +1, the items become more hightly related. If the correlation coefficient approaches 0, the items have little or no relationship. The researcher can then determine whether the correlation coefficient is statistically significant by referring to the appropriate statistical table.

Based on information in Appendix D, it shows the correlation between pain quality and pain intensity and behavioural responses. Person r values have been computed. The number in parenthesis shows the degrees of freedom. The arteribs refers to the levels of significane.

The Pearson product-moment statistic was used by Clark (1997) "to determine associations between body composition and bone-mineral density.... between women with and without evidence of disordered eating behaviors". The investigator found a "moderate positive correlation between bone-mineral density of the femoral neck and body weight" ($r = 0.51, p = 0.01$).

Karl Pearson's product moment coefficient of correlation can be computed by using the definitional formula:

$$r = \frac{\Sigma z_x z_y}{N} \qquad \text{...(11.6)}$$

Table 11.2

Pearson product-moment correlation

	Pain intensity	Behavioral responses
Pain quality	$r(94) = 0.59^{**}$	$r(93) = 0.41^{**}$

**p <0.001

The student will recall that z or standard scores can be obtained by dividing the deviation scores by standard deviation. Hence, using the paired z scores, the product moment correlation can be defined as the average product of the paired z scores. It can be shown algebraically that the maximum value of the term $\Sigma z_x z_y$ is attained when, for each pair of z scores, $z_x = z_y$. It can also be shown that, when the z scores for each pair are identical, the sum of their products equal N. Using standard scores for the calculation of correlation coefficient, involves a tedious process. However, several formulas exist which have been derived from the basic definitional formula and involve less labor in the computation of r. The process of calculation of r is explained below:

Some Other Formulas

In Table 11.2, two different formulae have been used for the calculation of r. Both the formulae are mathematically equivalent and give the same results. The formula based on the raw scores is more convenient when a calculating machine is available or the analysis is to be done on a computer. The formula using deviation scores is more useful when N is small and means of X and Y scores are whole numbers. Another formula based on raw scores and mathematically equivalent to the two formulas mentioned in Table 11.2 is

Formula

$$r = \frac{N\Sigma XY - (\Sigma X)(\Sigma Y)}{\sqrt{[N\Sigma X^2 - (\Sigma X)^2][N\Sigma Y^2 - (\Sigma Y)^2]}} \qquad \text{...(11.7)}$$

$$r = \frac{5(210) - (30)(30)}{\sqrt{[5(220)^2 - (30)^2][5(226)^2 - (30)^2]}}$$

$$r = \frac{1050 - 900}{\sqrt{(1100 - 900)(1130 - 900)}}$$

$$r = \frac{150}{\sqrt{200 \times 230}} \qquad r = 0.7$$

Table 11.3

Calculation of product moment *r* by two different formulas. Raw score method

X	*Y*	X^2	Y^2	*XY*
10	11	100	121	110
8	7	64	49	56
6	2	36	4	12
4	6	16	36	24
2	4	4	16	8
$\Sigma X = 30$	$\Sigma Y = 30$	$\Sigma X^2 = 220$	$\Sigma Y^2 = 226$	$\Sigma XY = 210$

Steps

1. Calculate squares of each X and Y score as shown in Cols. (3) and (4)
2. Calculate products of X and Y by multiplying the value of Cols. (1) and (2)
3. Sum up all columns
4. Insert the values in the formula.

$$r = \frac{\Sigma XY - \dfrac{(\Sigma X)(\Sigma Y)}{N}}{\sqrt{\left[\Sigma X^2 - \dfrac{(\Sigma X)^2}{N}\right]\left[\Sigma X^2 - \dfrac{(\Sigma Y)^2}{N}\right]}} \quad ...(11.8)$$

(Coefficient of correlation from raw scores)

Formula

$$r = \frac{\Sigma XY}{\sqrt{\Sigma X^2\, \Sigma Y^2}} \quad ...(11.9)$$

$$r = \frac{30}{\sqrt{(40)(46)}}$$

$$r = \frac{30}{\sqrt{42.9}} \quad r = 0.7$$

Steps

1. Calculate means of X and Y scores
2. Obtain deviation scores *x* and *y* as follows: $x = X - M_x$; $y = Y - M_y$
3. Obtain squares of deviation scores
4. Multiply Cols. (1) and (2) to obtain *xy*
5. Sum up all columns
6. Insert the values in the formula.

Another formula using raw scores and mean is as follows:

$$r = \frac{\Sigma XY - NM_x M_y}{\sqrt{(\Sigma X^2 - NM_x{}^2)(\Sigma Y^2 - NM_y{}^2)}} \quad ...(11.10)$$

(Coefficient of correlation from raw scores and means).

Where M_x and M_y are means of X and Y scores, respectively. Difference formula may also be used for the calculation of *r*. The same is given below:

$$r = \frac{\Sigma x^2 + \Sigma y^2 - \Sigma d^2}{\sqrt[2]{\Sigma x^2 \times \Sigma y^2}} \quad ...(11.11)$$

(Coefficient of correlation using difference formula, deviations from the means of the distribution).

Where $\Sigma d^2 = \Sigma(x - y)^2$, symbols are the same as used above. The difference formula does not require the calculation of gross products (*xy*'*s*). The student may try the difference formula on scores given in Table 11.3. All values, except Σd^2, have already been presented there. Another variation of the difference formula which is often useful in machine calculation is also given here. This version uses raw or obtained scores instead of deviation scores.

$$r = \frac{N[\Sigma X^2 - \Sigma Y^2 - \Sigma(X - Y)^2 - (\Sigma X)(\Sigma Y)^2]}{\sqrt[2]{[N\Sigma X^2 - (\Sigma X)^2][N\Sigma Y^2 - (\Sigma Y)^2]}} \quad ...(11.12)$$

Table 11.4

Deviation score method

X	Y	X^2	Y^2	XY
4	5	16	25	20
2	1	4	1	2
0	–4	0	16	0
–2	0	4	0	0
–4	–2	16	4	8
$M_x = 0$	$M_y = 0$	$\Sigma X^2 = 40$	$\Sigma Y^2 = 46$	$\Sigma XY = 30$

(Coefficient of correlation by difference formula based on raw or obtained scores). In which $\Sigma(X - Y)^2$ is the sum of the squared difference between X and Y sets of scores.

The student may use this formula on data given in Table 11.3. All calculations, except $\Sigma(X - Y)^2$, are already available (Table 11.4).

Correlation Coefficient Calculated from Ungrouped Data

A constant known as the correlation coefficient (r) may be used to measure the degree of this relationship. This is calculated from the following formula:

$$r = \frac{\left(\frac{x-\bar{x}}{\sigma_x}\right)\left(\frac{y-\bar{y}}{\sigma_y}\right)}{n} \quad ...(11.13)$$

where x and y represent measurements for the two variables taken at the same time. X and Y means of the two distributions of measurements and standard deviations of the measurements. For the series of the five patients given below, if x represents the temperature and y the pulse for individual patients:

$$\bar{x} = \frac{500}{5} = 100 \qquad \sigma_x = \sqrt{2}$$

$$\bar{y} = \frac{400}{5} = 80 \qquad \sigma_x = \sqrt{200}$$

$$r = \frac{+100/\sqrt{400}}{5} = \frac{5}{5} = +1$$

The correlation is +1. This indicates first that, there is positive correlation; that is, the variables change in the same direction; second, that the correlation is perfect.

Suppose the measurements on the five individuals had been:

Individual	*Temperature*	*Pulse*
A	102	60
B	101	70
C	100	80
D	99	90
E	98	100

Plotting these data on a scatter diagram gives the picture in Figure 11.9A. Again all the points fall on a straight line, except that now the line has a downward or negative slope. This indicates an inverse relationship, that is, as one variable increases the other decreases. In this instance, as temperature increases, the pulse rate decrease. The change again is uniform; for an increase of one degree of temperature the pulse decrease 10 beats.

What would be the correlation coefficient for these data? Using the same method, the calculations are:

$$\bar{x} = \frac{500}{5} = 100 \qquad \sigma_x = \sqrt{2}$$

$$\bar{y} = \frac{400}{5} = 80 \qquad \sigma_x = \sqrt{200}$$

$$r = \frac{-100/\sqrt{400}}{5} = \frac{-5}{5} = -1$$

Patient	Temperature x	Pulse y	$\left(\frac{x-\bar{x}}{\sigma_x}\right)$	$\left(\frac{x-\bar{x}}{\sigma_y}\right)$	$\left(\frac{x-\bar{x}}{\sigma_x}\right)\left(\frac{x-\bar{y}}{\sigma_y}\right)$
A	102	100	$2/\sqrt{2}$	$20/\sqrt{200}$	$40/\sqrt{400}$
B	101	90	$1/\sqrt{2}$	$10/\sqrt{200}$	$10/\sqrt{400}$
C	100	80	$0/\sqrt{2}$	$0/\sqrt{200}$	$0/\sqrt{400}$
D	99	70	$-1/\sqrt{2}$	$-10/\sqrt{200}$	$10/\sqrt{400}$
E	98	60	$-2/\sqrt{2}$	$-20/\sqrt{200}$	$40/\sqrt{400}$
Total	500	400	0		$+100/\sqrt{400}$

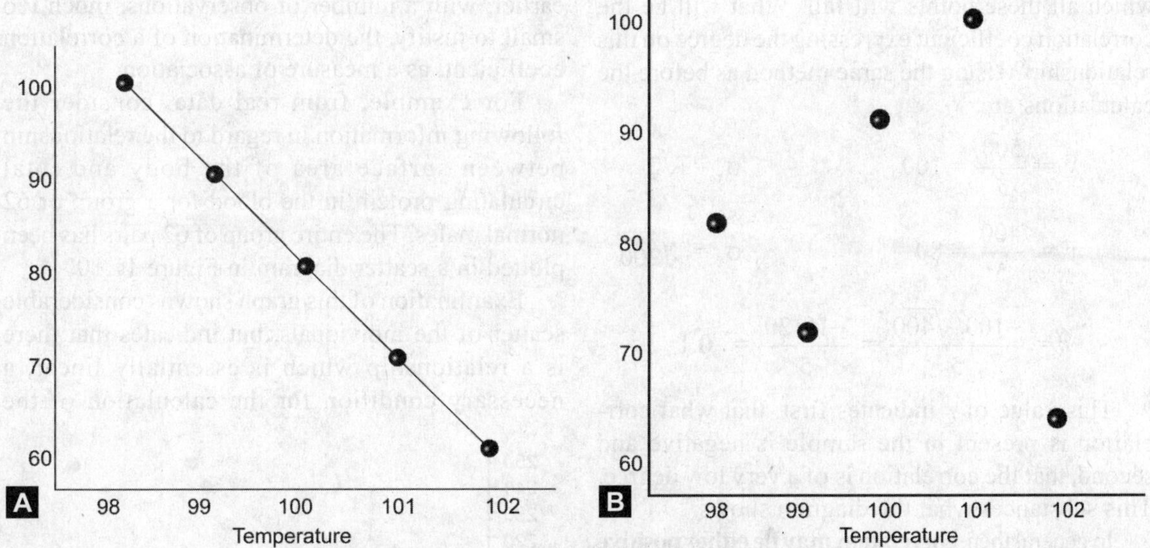

Figs 11.9A and B: Relationship between pulse and temperature for five individuals

Note that the only difference here is that the product terms $\left(\frac{x-\bar{x}}{\sigma_x}\right)\left(\frac{y-\bar{x}}{\sigma_x}\right)$ are all negative. This indicates that for these data there is perfect negative correlation, shown by the fact that $r = -1$.

Now suppose the paired values had been:

Individual	Temperature	Pulse
A	102	60
B	101	100
C	100	90
D	99	70
E	98	80

These data are plotted in Figure 11.9B. It can easily be seen that no straight line can be drawn on

Patient	*Temperature* x	*Pulse* y	$\left(\frac{x-\bar{x}}{\sigma_x}\right)$	$\left(\frac{x-\bar{y}}{\sigma_y}\right)$	$\left(\frac{x-\bar{x}}{\sigma_x}\right)\left(\frac{x-\bar{y}}{\sigma_y}\right)$
A	102	100	$2/\sqrt{2}$	$-20/\sqrt{200}$	$-40/\sqrt{400}$
B	101	90	$1/\sqrt{2}$	$-10/\sqrt{200}$	$-10/\sqrt{400}$
C	100	80	$0/\sqrt{2}$	$0/\sqrt{200}$	$0/\sqrt{400}$
D	99	70	$-1/\sqrt{2}$	$10/\sqrt{200}$	$-10/\sqrt{400}$
E	98	60	$-2/\sqrt{2}$	$20/\sqrt{200}$	$-40/\sqrt{400}$
Total	500	400	0	0	$+100/\sqrt{400}$

which all these points will fall. What will be the correlation coefficient expressing the degree on this relationship? Using the same method as before the calculations are:

$$\bar{x} = \frac{500}{5} = 100 \qquad \sigma_x = \sqrt{2}$$

$$\bar{y} = \frac{400}{5} = 80 \qquad \sigma_x = \sqrt{200}$$

$$r = \frac{-100/\sqrt{400}}{5} = \frac{-10/20}{5} = -0.1$$

This value of r indicates first, that what correlation is present in the sample is negative and second, that the correlation is of a very low degree. This substances what the diagram shows.

In general then, **correlation may be either positive or negative or zero. Positive correlation indicates that the change in two variables is in the same direction, that is, as one increases the other increases; or if one decreases the other decreases. Negative correlation indicates that the variables change in opposite direction, that is, as one increases the other decreases. The value of the correlation coefficient must lie between 0 and +1 or 0 and –1. A coefficient of 0 indicates no correlation; a coefficient of 1 (either positive or negative) indicates perfect correlation.** Obviously, the closer the value of the coefficient is to one, the greater is the degree of intensity of association.

For sake of simplicity, the concept of correlation was presented from fictitious data and as stated earlier, with a number of observations, much too small to justify, the determination of a correlation coefficient, as a measure of association.

For example, from real data, consider the following information in regard to the relationship between surface area of the body and total circulating protein in the blood for a group of 62 normal males. The entire group of 62 pairs has been plotted in a scatter diagram in Figure 11.10.

Examination of this graph showns considerable scatter of the individuals, but indicates that there is a relationship which is essentially linear, a necessary condition for the calculation of the

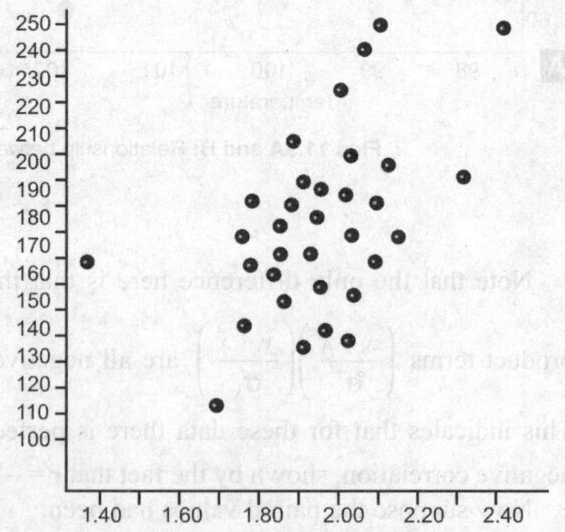

Fig. 11.10: Relationship between total circulating protein and surface area

Patient	Temperature x	Pulse y	$\left(\frac{x-\bar{x}}{\sigma_x}\right)$	$\left(\frac{x-\bar{y}}{\sigma_y}\right)$	$\left(\frac{x-\bar{x}}{\sigma_x}\right)\left(\frac{x-\bar{y}}{\sigma_y}\right)$
A	102	60	$2/\sqrt{2}$	$-20/\sqrt{200}$	$-40/\sqrt{400}$
B	101	100	$1/\sqrt{2}$	$+10/\sqrt{200}$	$+10/\sqrt{400}$
C	100	90	$0/\sqrt{2}$	$0/\sqrt{200}$	0
D	99	70	$-1/\sqrt{2}$	$-10/\sqrt{200}$	$10/\sqrt{400}$
E	98	80	$-2/\sqrt{2}$	$0/\sqrt{200}$	0
Total	500	400	0	0	$+100/\sqrt{400}$

correlation coefficient. A few representative pairs of values are given below:

Individual no.	Surface area (sq. meter) (x)	Total circulating protein (gm) (y)
1	1.75	170
2	2.18	182
3	1.74	160
4	1.77	174
60	2.00	188
61	2.12	199
62	1.67	144

The method used in the three previous examples could be used in this instance, but the calculations would be very laborious.

The formula for the calculations of r originally given: can be written also in the following form which is easier to use for computation:

$$r = \frac{\sum\left(\frac{x-\bar{x}}{\sigma_x}\right)\left(\frac{y-\bar{y}}{\sigma_y}\right)}{n} \quad ...(11.14)$$

can be written also in the following form which is easier to use for computation:

$$r = \frac{\frac{\Sigma xy}{n} - \frac{\Sigma x}{n}\frac{\Sigma y}{n}}{\sqrt{\frac{\Sigma x^2}{n} - \frac{(\Sigma x)^2}{n}} \cdots \sqrt{\frac{\Sigma y^2}{n} - \frac{(\Sigma y)^2}{n}}} \quad ...(11.15)$$

or simplifying,

$$r = \frac{n\Sigma xy - \Sigma x \Sigma y}{\sqrt{n\Sigma x^2 - (\Sigma x)^2}\sqrt{n\Sigma y^2 - (\Sigma y)^2}} \quad ...(11.16)$$

For the above 62 observations the following sums have been computed:

$$\Sigma x = 117.76 \qquad \Sigma x^2 = 225.4290$$
$$\Sigma y = 11016 \qquad \Sigma y^2 = 2000748$$
$$\Sigma xy = 21050.38$$
$$n = 62$$

Substituting the appropriate values in the last formula gives:

$$r = \frac{62\,(21050.38) - 117.76 \times 11016}{\sqrt{62 \times 225.4290 - (117.76)^2} \times \sqrt{62 \times 2000748 - (11016)^2}}$$

The above example shows that the computation is not simple.

We give the following direct method:

Direct Method. If X and Y, two variates having their means $\bar{x}$ and $\bar{y}$ respectively, then

$$\rho(X, Y) = \frac{\Sigma dx\, dy}{\sqrt{\Sigma dx^2 \times \Sigma dy^2}}$$

where $dx = x_i - x$, $dy = y_i - y$, $dx^2 = (x_i - x)^2$, $dy^2 = (y_i - y)^2$.

It can also be written as $r_{xy} = \dfrac{\Sigma dx\, dy}{n\sigma_x \times \sigma_y}$ ...(11.17)

where n is the number of observations in X or Y series, σ_x, σ_y are standard deviation of X and Y respectively.

The following formula can also be deduced from above:

$$\rho(X, Y) = \frac{\Sigma dxdy - \left(\dfrac{\Sigma dx\, \Sigma dy}{n}\right)}{\left(\sqrt{\Sigma dx^2 - \dfrac{(\Sigma dx)^2}{n}} \times \sqrt{\Sigma dy^2 - \dfrac{(\Sigma dy)^2}{n}}\right)} \quad ...(11.18)$$

where n is the number of observations

Working Rule: The coefficient of correlation is calculated by the following steps:

Step I. Denote one series by x and the other series by y.

Step II. Calculate x and y of the x and y series respectively

Step III. Take the deviations of the observations in x series from x and write it under the column headed by $dx = x - \overline{x}$. Take the deviations in y series from $\overline{y}$ and write it in a column headed $dy = y - \overline{y}$.

Step IV. Square these deviations and write them under the columns headed by dx^2 and dy^2.

Step V. Multiply the respective dx and dy and write it under the column headed by $dxdy$.

Step VI. Apply the following formula to calculate r or r_{xy}, the coefficient or correlation.

$$r = \frac{\Sigma dxdy}{\sqrt{\Sigma dx^2 \times \Sigma dy^2}}, \quad (11.19)$$

or

$$r = \frac{\Sigma dxdy}{n\sigma_x \times \sigma_y} \quad ...(11.20)$$

where n is the number of observation in x or y series, σ_x and σ_y are the standard deviations of x and y. The above method is illustrated by the following example:

Example: Find the coefficient of correlation between the heights of fathers and sons from the following data:

Heights of fathers (in inches) (x)	65	66	67	68	69	70	71
Heights of sons (in inches) (y)	67	68	66	69	72	72	69

Let the heights of fathers be denoted by x and that of sons be y, then

$$x = \frac{65 + 66 + 67 + 68 + 69 + 70 + 71}{7} = 68$$

$$y = \frac{67 + 68 + 66 + 69 + 72 + 72 + 69}{7} = 69$$

x	*dx* (*x* – 68)	*dx*² (*x* – 68)²	*y*	*dy* (*y* – 69)	*dy*² (*y* – 69)²	*dxdy*
65	–3	9	67	–2	4	6
66	–2	4	68	–1	1	2
67	–1	1	66	–3	9	3
68	0	0	69	0	0	0
69	1	1	72	3	9	3
70	2	4	72	3	9	6
71	3	9	69	0	0	0
	$\Sigma dx = 0$	$\Sigma dx^2 = 28$		$\Sigma dy = 0$	$\Sigma dy^2 = 32$	$\Sigma dxdy = 20$

X	dX (X – 13)	dX² (X – 13)²	Y	dY (Y – 25)	dY² (Y – 25)²	dXdY
5	–8	64	12	–13	169	104
9	–4	16	20	–5	25	20
13	0	0	25	0	0	0
17	4	16	33	8	64	32
21	8	64	35	10	100	80
	ΣdX = 0	ΣdX² = 160		ΣdY = 0	ΣdY² = 160	ΣdXdY = 236

Let us prepare the above Table:

Now $r = \dfrac{\Sigma dxdy}{\sqrt{\Sigma dx^2 \times \Sigma dy^2}} = \dfrac{20}{\sqrt{(28 \times 32)}}$

$= \dfrac{5}{7.5} = 0.67$ (approximately)

Example 1: Calculate the correlation coefficient between X and Y from the following data.

X	5	9	13	17	21
Y	12	20	25	33	35

Solution. Here $\bar{X} = \dfrac{65}{5} = 13,\ \bar{Y} = \dfrac{125}{5} = 25.$

$$r = \frac{\Sigma dxdy}{\sqrt{\Sigma dx^2 + \Sigma dy^2}} = \frac{236}{\sqrt{160 \times 358}}$$

$$= \frac{236}{239.33} = 0.986$$

Short-cut Method: The above direct method for calculating r is not convenient when (*i*) the terms of the series x and y are big and the calculation x and y becomes difficult or (*ii*) the means $\bar{x}$ and $\bar{y}$ are not integers. In these cases we apply the following formula of assumed mean:

$$r = \frac{\Sigma dxdy - \dfrac{(\Sigma dxdy)}{n}}{\sqrt{\Sigma dX^2 - \dfrac{(\Sigma dx)^2}{n}} \times \sqrt{\Sigma dX^2 - \dfrac{(\Sigma dx)^2}{n}}} \quad ...(11.21)$$

where $dx = x - a$, a is the assumed mean of x series, $dy = y - b$, b is the assumed mean of y series and n is the number of observations of x or y.

Working Rule

Step I. Take any term a (perfectly the middle one) of x series as assumed mean and any term b (preferable middle one) as assumed mean for y series.

Step II. Take deviations of the observations in x series from a, i.e. $dx = x - a$. Take deviations of the observations in y series from b, i.e. $dy = y - b$ and write it under columns dx and dy.

Step III. Find dx^2 and dy^2 and write it under columns dx^2 and dy^2.

Step IV. Find $dxdy$ and write it under the column $dxdy$.

Step V. Apply the formula

$$r = \frac{\Sigma dxdy - \dfrac{(\Sigma dxdy)}{n}}{\sqrt{\Sigma dx^2 - \dfrac{(\Sigma dx)^2}{n}} \times \sqrt{\Sigma dx^2 - \dfrac{(\Sigma dx)^2}{n}}} \quad ...(11.22)$$

The method is illustrated by the following example

Example 2: Calculate the coefficient of correlation between x and y for the following data:

x	1	3	4	5	7	8	10
y	2	6	8	10	14	16	20

x	y	dx	dy	dx^2	dy^2	dxdy
1	2	–4	–12	16	144	48
3	6	–2	–8	4	64	16
4	8	–1	–6	1	36	6
5	10	0	–4	0	16	0
7	14	2	0	4	0	0
8	16	3	2	9	4	6
10	20	5	6	25	36	30
n = 7	n = 7	$\Sigma dx = 3$	$\Sigma dy = 22$	$\Sigma dx^2 = 59$	$\Sigma dy^2 = 300$	$\Sigma dxdy = 106$

Let 5 be the assumed mean for the values of x and 14 be assumed mean for the values of y.

Let $dx = x - 5$, $dx^2 = (x - 5)^2$, $dy = (y - 14)$, $dy^2 = (y - 14)^2$. We have the below Table:

Since we have taken the deviations from assumed means, so we shall apply the following formula of correlation for assumed mean:

$$r = \frac{\Sigma dxdy - \dfrac{(\Sigma dxdy)}{n}}{\sqrt{\Sigma dx^2 - \dfrac{(\Sigma dx)^2}{n}} \times \sqrt{\Sigma dx^2 - \dfrac{(\Sigma dx)^2}{n}}}$$

$$r = \frac{106 + \dfrac{66}{7}}{\sqrt{\left(59 - \dfrac{(9)^2}{7}\right)} \times \sqrt{\left(300 - \dfrac{484}{7}\right)}}$$

$$r = \frac{808}{\sqrt{404} \times \sqrt{1616}}$$

$$= \frac{808}{\sqrt{652864}} = \frac{808}{808} = 1$$

Thus, the coefficient of correlation between x and y is positive and perfect.

Spearman's Rank Correlation Coefficient

It was seen that for the calculation of correlation coefficient, at least one of the variables is distributed normally. In cases where it is not so or when measurements are in terms of certain ranks and not in exact quantitative terms, then Spearman's rank correlation coefficient is applied to determine whether there is a monotonic relation between the two variables, whether an increase in one is associated with an increase or decrease in the other.

In this case, one of the series is arranged in the order of magnitude and ranked from 1 to n and the other variable also is ranked. Thus the test ignores the actual values. The correlation coefficient [i.e., Spearman's rank order correlation (Rho)] of these two rankings is calculated, using the formula Rho

$$= 1 - \frac{6 \times \Sigma D^2}{n(n^2 - 1)}$$

Where D is the difference in the ranks of each pair of data, n is the number of pairs or observations.

Note:

- Whenever there is a tie in the ranks, then for each of the tied pairs average of the ranks is assigned.
- The range for rank correlation coefficient is also between –1 and +1.
- One of the applications of this test is in determining whether the pairs formed for conducting a randomized controlled trial are really matched.

The coefficient of rank correlation is based on the various values of the variates and is also denoted by R. It is applied in the problems in which data cannot be measured quantitatively but, qualitative assessment is possible such as beauty, honesty, etc. In this case, the best individual is given rank number 1, next rank 2 and so on. The coefficient of rank correlation is given by the formula.

$$R = 1 - \frac{6\Sigma D^2}{n(n^2-1)} \quad ...(11.23)$$

Where D^2 in the square of the difference of corresponding ranks, and n is the number of pairs of observations.

Working Rule

Step I. Assign ranks to each item of both the series

Step II. Calculate the difference of ranks of x from. the ranks of y and write it under the column headed by D.

Step III. Square the difference D and write it under the column D^2.

Step IV. Apply the formula

$$R = 1 - \frac{6\Sigma D^2}{n(n^2-1)}$$

The above method is explained with the help of the following example.

Example 1: Ten students got the following percentage of marks in Medical Surgical (MSN) and Reproduction Health Nursing (RHN):

MSN (X)	8	36	98	25	75	82	92	62	65	35
RHN (Y)	84	51	91	60	68	62	86	58	35	49

Find the coefficient of rank correlation (below in Table).

X	*Y*	x_i = *Rank in X*	y_i = *Rank in Y*	$D = x_i - y_i$	D^2
8	84	10	3	7	49
36	51	7	8	–1	1
98	91	1	1	0	0
25	60	9	6	3	9
75	68	4	4	0	0
82	62	3	5	–2	4
92	86	2	2	0	0
62	58	6	7	–1	1
65	35	5	10	–5	25
35	49	8	9	–1	1
				$\Sigma D = 0$	$\Sigma D^2 = 90$

$$R = 1 - \frac{6\Sigma D^2}{n(n^2-1)} = 1 - \frac{6 \times 90}{10(100-1)}$$

$$= 1 - \frac{6}{11} = 1 - 0.545$$

$$= 0.455$$

Example 2: The average age-wise systolic blood-pressure in a community were as follows:

Age (yrs)	*Blood pressure (mm of Hg)*
15	120
25	125
30	130
40	130
50	130
60	150

Does age significantly influence blood pressure?

Step 1: The variables are arranged in the rank. Number 1 is awareded to the lowest numerical figure, 2 to the next higher one and so on. If there are two or more measurements of same value, each of them is given the average of the next two or more numbers.

The above data is ranked as follows.

Step 2: In the next step, the difference (D) in the ranks, for age and corresponding blood pressure is calculated and its square (D^2) is worked out as follows.

Age	Age rank	BP	BP rank	D	D^2
15	1	120	1	0	0
25	2	125	2	0	0
30	3	130	4	1	1
40	4	130	4	0	0
50	5	130	4	1	1
60	6	150	6	0	0

Step 3:

$$\text{Rho} = 1 - \frac{6 \times \Sigma D^2}{n(n^2 - 1)}$$

$$= 1 - \frac{6 \times 2}{6(6 \times 6 - 1)}$$

$$= 1 - \frac{12}{6(36 - 1)}$$

$$= 1 - \frac{12}{210}$$

$$= 1 - 0.05$$

$$= 0.95$$

The significance of rank correlation coefficient is assessed by referring to Kendall table (Annexure V). According to that table, the value for a sample size of 6 at 5 percent level (p = 0.05) is 0.88. Since the calculated value is more than the table value, age and BP are significantly correlated.

Scatter or Dot Diagram—Graphical Method

Scatter diagram is a graphical method of showing the correlation between the two variables. Let (x_i, y_i), $i = 1, 2, 3 \ldots n$ be a bivariate distribution. The values of the variables x and y be plotted along the x-axis and y-axis in a coordinate plane by choosing a suitable scale, so that it measures the range of the data of both the variates (series) under consideration. Then, corresponding to every ordered pair (x_i, y_i), there corresponds a point or a dot in the coordinate plane.

The diagram of dots or points so obtained is called a **scatter diagram or a dot diagram.**

The scatter diagram may indicate both degree and the type of correlation.

In many problems, it is more important to know the exact mathematical relationship between two variables than, to have a measure of it expressed in terms of the *correlation coefficient*. Also such measure can be determined only when the relationship between the two variables is linear. It is necessary, therefore, to know the pattern of the relationship.

As a first step in determining the pattern of the relationship between two quantitatively measured variables, data are plotted on a scatter diagram. Examination of the arrangement of the dots representing the individual pairs of values gives certain information as to the possible relationship. The dots may or may not form a distinct pattern. If, as in Figure 11.11, they scatter all over the diagram, this is the evidence that, little relationship between the two variables is present. The dots may however, form a distinct pattern. If, as in Figure 11.11, they scatter all over the diagram, this is also evidence that, little relationship between the two variables present. The dots may, however, form a distinct pattern, which may be of a linear nature as in Figure 11.12 or they may form a pattern which is in the form of a curve as in Figure 11.13. The relationship represented in the Figure is linear in nature; that of Figure 11.13 is curvilinear. If the red blood count and the white blood count are determined the same time for a group of normal individuals and plotted in a scatter diagram, the resulting graph will in all probability resemble that of Figure 11.11.

Nor, is there reason to expect any relationship between blood sugar and the weight of an individual. However, if the body temperature and pulse rate of normal persons are compared, linear relationship is usually found. This is also true of surface area of the body and blood plasma volume. The urinary nitrogen of pregnant women goes down in a linear relationship as the stage of pregnancy increases. Growth curves by contrast represent a curvilinear relationship; for example, growth of the embryo and

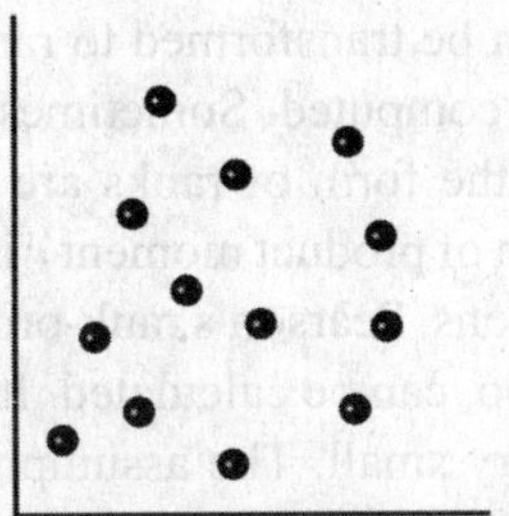

Fig. 11.11: No relationship

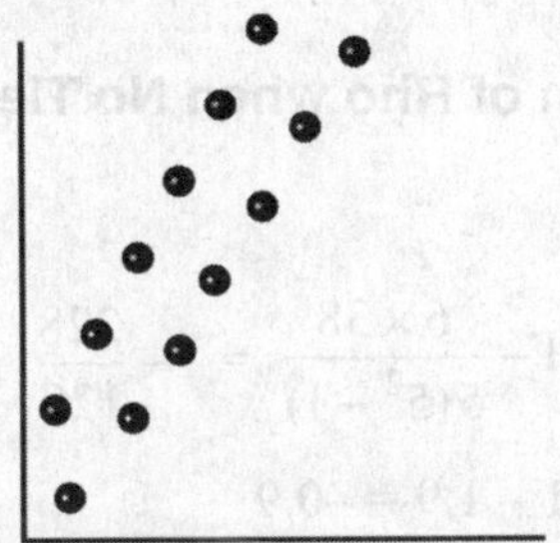

Fig. 11.12: Linear relationship

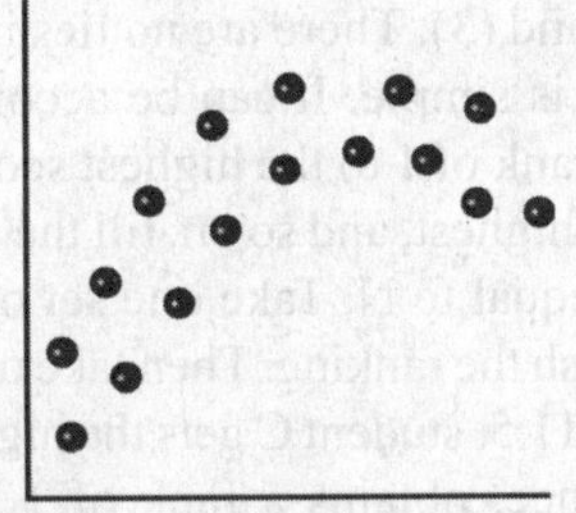

Fig. 11.13: Curvilinear relationship

length of pregnancy and growth of the individual represented either by height or weight when compared with age or growth of bacteria with time. In the first examples, growth precedes rapidly at first and then gradually shows up with, duration of time. In the latter example bacteria go through a lag phase immediately after inoculation that is followed by a period of rapid growth, then a gradual showing up, ending by a decrease in growth. All these patterns are curvilinear in nature.

Spearman's Rho Calculation

There are many nonparametric correlation techniques. One of the most common is the Spearman's Rho Correlation. Researchers using this statistic rank their observations of the two variables under consideration and then determine the level of relationship between them. For example, a researcher might want to test the relationship between patients' perceived level of comfort and their perception of the quality of care provided by the nursing staff in a hospital. In this instance, the patients would be given two attitude-evaluation scales (one to measure each variable), and then the two scores would be ranked and a Spearman's rho computed.

An examples of the use of the Spearman's rho is the study conducted by Walker and Sofaer (1998) in their attempt to identify sources of psychological distress in patients attending pain clinics. Among other statistical measures, the investigators used the Spearman's rho to correlate ordinal scores between five measures of pain and six measures of psychological distress. The data analyses demonstrated that all the measures of psychological distress. The data analyses demonstrated that all the measures of psychological distress, except age, had statistically significant relationships with the measures of pain at the 0.01 level or below. The researchers concluded that the findings of this study might be used in developing an easily used nursing assessment instrument that might be used to improve the psychological well-being of patients with chronic pain.

Partial and Multiple Correlation

Occasionally, the researcher needs to analyze a number of variables that might be interrelated. In this instance, partial correlations can be computed. The intent of this method is to eliminate the confounding effects of one or more variables when measuring the relationshps between a number of variables. This is shown as $r_{1,2,3}$ where variables 1 and 2 are correlated and variable 3 is eliminated mathematically. Conversely, if a researcher wants to combine the varibales, this can be done by a technique called multiple correlation (symbolized by the letter R).

Correlations can be used for prediction by using a technique called regression analysis. This technique allows the researcher to predict the score an individual will make on a third assessment by correlating the scores obtained by that individual on two assessments.

The researcher whose study is reprinted in Appendix D used a multiple correlation technique known as canonical correlation that measured the relationship between a set of independent variables (age, medical fears, distractibility, threshold of pain) and a set of dependent varibales (pain quality, behavioral responses, magnitude of heart rate change). Although canonical correlations can be used to determine regression scores, and thus can be used as predictors, the researcher chose not to do this.

Stein and colleagues (1998) used both partial and multiple correltions to determine whether self-reported risky behaviors (sexual intercourse, tobacco use, alcohol used, and poor school performance) by students in the eighth grade predicted risky behaviors by the same students in the ninth grade. They found that risky behaviors are intercorrelated and that adolescent self-concept, especially as being socially popular, was a predictor of engagement in risky behaviors, which then "contributed to the conceptualization of the self as currently deviant and expectation that one will be deviant in the future". The researchers concluded that interventions to limit risky behaviors may help prevent the development and continuation of risky pattern of behavior.

Spearman's Rank—Difference Correlation Coefficient (Rho)

In case when distributions of scores are markedly skewed, measurements made with an interval or ratio scale can be transformed to ranks before the correlation is computed. Sometimes, only ordinal scale data in the form of ranks are available and the calculation of product moment *r* is not possible. In such situations, Pearson's rank-order correlation coefficient, rho, can be calculated. It is also useful when N is very small. The assumption of normal distribution of the characteristic in the population is not required. The procedure of calculation of rho is shown in Table 11.5.

Calculation of Rho when No Ties Exist

Formula

$$R = 1 - \frac{6 \times 38}{5(5^2 - 1)} = 1 - \frac{228}{120}$$

$$= 1 - 1.9 = -0.9$$

Interpretation: Relationship between X and Y is very high and inverse in Table 11.5, students have been listed in Col. (1); scores on test I and test II, in Cols. (2) and (3). There are no ties in the scores, and ranking is simple. It can be accomplished by assigning a rank of 1 to the highest score, a rank of 2 to the next highest, and so on, till the lowest score gets a rank equal to N. Take one set of scores at a time and finish the ranking. Then take up the second set. In Table 11.5, student C gets the highest X score of 9 and hence, obtains a rank of 1 (see Col.4); Student A with the next highest X score of 8 gets the next rank of 2; student B, a rank of 3; student D, a rank of 4; and student E, with the lowest score, gets the last rank of 5 which is equal to N. The same procedure is repeated for ranking the students on test II and the ranks written in Col. (5). In column (6), differences of ranks for each student are mentioned. For example, for student A; $D = R_1 - R_2$ or $2 - 5 = -3$. Col. (7) shows each rank difference squared. Col. (7) is summed up to obtain ΣD^2 which is 38 in our example. The number of students in this example is five, hence N = 5. The numerical values 1 and 6 in the formulae are constants and

Table 11.5

Rank—difference coefficient of correlation (Case of no ties)

Student	*Score test I* *X*	*Score on test II* *Y*	*Rank on test I* R_1	*Rank on test II* R_2	*Difference between ranks* *D*	*Difference squared* D_2
A	8	4	2	5	–3	9
B	7	7	3	3	0	0
C	9	6	1	4	–3	9
D	5	8	4	2	2	4
E	1	10	5	1	4	16
	N = 5					$\Sigma D^2 = 38$

Table 11.6

Rank—difference coefficient of correlation

Student	*Score test I* *X*	*Score on test II* *Y*	*Rank on test I* R_1	*Rank on test II* R_2	*Difference between ranks* *D*	*Difference squared* D_2
A	10	16	6.5	5.5	1.0	1.0
B	15	16	3	5.5	–2.5	6.25
C	11	24	5	1.5	3.5	12.25
D	14	18	4	4	0	0
E	16	22	2	3	–1.0	1.00
F	20	24	1	1.5	–0.5	0.25
G	10	14	6.5	7.5	–1.0	1.00
H	8	10	9	10	–1.0	1.00
I	7	12	10	9	1.0	1.00
J	9	14	8	7.5	0.5	0.25
	N = 10					$\Sigma D^2 = 24.00$

remain the same in all cases. The values of ΣD^2 and N are inserted in the formula and the value of rho obtained. Necessary precaution should be taken regarding the sign of the value of rho when it is negative least it is omitted inadvertently. In our example, rho = –0.9 a value which is quite high and shows an inverse relationship between X and Y.

Calculation of Rho when Tied Ranks Exist

Sometimes, two or more persons obtain the same score or have the same age, years of service or some other numerical value. This introduces ties in the scores which are then reflected in their ranks also. The procedure of assigning ranks in such situations will be described with reference to the example solved in Table 11.6. Column (1) shows student serial number in terms of letters. In Cols. (2) and (3) each student's scores on test I and test II have been given. For ranking, one set of scores say X, is taken at a time. Ranks assigned to scores on test I have been shown in Col. (4). Student F with the highest score of 20 has been given a rank of 1; and student E whose scores is the next highest, a rank of 2. In this way, the ranking has been completed till student I got a rank of 10. Students A and G have similar scores of 10 each and they possess 6th and 7th positions. Instead of assigning either 6 or 7 to both of them, the average or the two positions, i.e. (6 + 7)1/2 = 6.5 has been assigned to each of them.

The same procedure has been followed in respect of scores on test II. In this case, ties occur at three places. Students C and F have the same score and hence, obtain the average rank of (1+2)1/2 = 1.5. Students A and B have rank positions of 5 and 6 hence are assigned (5 + 6)1/2 = 5.5 each. Similarly, students G and J have been assigned (7 + 8)1/2 = 7.5 each. The same procedure is to be adopted when more than two persons tie up for the same position.

The rest of the procedure follows the same steps as have been used in the calculation of rho without ties. Difference of the ranks D, i.e. Col. (4) – Col. (5), has been calculated and summed to obtain SD^2, in Col. (6). This value has been inserted in the formula and the sum solved for the value of rho which is 0.855.

When ranks are treated as scores and there are no ties, the value of the product moment coefficient of correlation equals the value of rho. In case of tied positions, a correction may be used to make rho equal to *r*. However, in case of a small number of ties, the correction can be ignored and rho accepted as an approximation to *r*. Rank—difference correlation is a quick and convenient method of estimating the correlation when N is small. In case only ranks are available, rho is the only answer. With larger N's, rho may be useful as an exploratory measure. However, it must be amply evident to the student that *r* is based on both the sizes of the measures and also their relative positions in the series while rho takes account of the positions only.

Formula

$$(\rho) = 1 - \frac{6\Sigma D^2}{N(N^2 - 1)}$$

$$= 1 - \frac{6 \times 24}{10\,(10^2 - 1)}$$

$$= 1 - \frac{144}{10 \times 99}$$

$$= \frac{990 - 144}{990} = 0.855$$

Interpretation: The correlation between X and Y is very high and positive.

Properties of the Correlation Coefficient

The Range of r

The correlation coefficient may assume values from – 1 through zero to +1. This is inherent in the very formula propounded by Pearson for the calculation of *r*. The values of $r = -1$ and $r = +1$ present a case of perfect relationship, though the direction of relationship is negative in the first case and positive in the latter. The value of *r* can never be greater than +1 and less than –1. These are the limits of *r*.

The Coefficient of Determination, r^2

The correlation coefficient, *r*, can be interpreted in terms of r^2 which is called the *coefficient of determination.* This may be called as the variance interpretation of r^2. When multiplied by 100 the coefficient r^2 gives us the percentage of variance in Y that is associated with, determined by, or accounted for by variance in X. When $r = 0.60$, the value of $r^2 = (0.60)^2 = 0.36$. Expressed in terms of percentage, it means that 36 percent, ($0.36 \times 100 = 36$) of the variance in Y scores has been accounted for by the variance in X scores. The proportion of the variance in Y, not determined by or not associated with the variance in X is given by k^2. which is called *the coefficient of non-determination.* Hence, $k^2 = 1 - r^2$. Another index derived from the same is the *coefficient of alienation, k.*

$$k = \sqrt{1 - r^2} \qquad \text{...(11.24)}$$

Table 11.7

Values of coefficient of determination and coefficient of alienation for some selected values of *r*

Correlation coefficient (r_{xy})	*Coefficient of determination* (r^2_{xy} x 100)	*Coefficient of alienation* (*k*)
0.00	0.00	1.000
0.05	0.00	1.000
0.10	1.00	0.999
0.15	2.25	0.989
0.20	4.00	0.980
0.30	9.00	0.954
0.40	16.00	0.917
0.50	25.00	0.866
0.60	36.00	0.800
0.70	49.00	0.714
0.80	64.00	0.600
0.90	81.00	0.436
0.95	90.25	0.312
0.98	96.00	0.199
0.99	98.00	0.141
0.995	99.00	0.100
0.999	99.80	0.045

while *r* indicates the degree of relationship between two variables, the coefficient of alienation, *k* indicates the degree of lack of relationship. Table 11.7 shows the three indices in relation to each other:

An inspection of the above Table 11.7 reveals that the coefficients of determination for small *r*'s emphasize the very slight degree of association which these *r*'s disclose. An *r* of 0.10, 0.20 or even 0.30 between two tests X and Y indicates only 1 percent, 4 percent and 9 percent, respectively, of the variance of Y accounted for by X. At the other extreme, *r*'s equal to 0.90 and 0.99 indicate 81 percent and 98 percent, respectively, of the variance in Y accounted for by X.

The value of *r* is invariant under transformations of unit and/or origin. *The correlation coefficient does not change if every score in either or both distributions is increased or multiplied by a constant.* The result has important implications for the use of correlation coefficient. It leads us to conclude that it does not matter if the measurements is in feet or inches, minutes or seconds, units or dozens. The correlation between the variables will be the same. This quality of *r* gives it a large range of applications. While working with large values in the calculation of *r* by raw score method, it would always be advisable to subtract a constant from all the scores. It would help avoid working with large numbers.

The correlation is sometimes misunderstood as indicating a casual relationship between the two variables and at times to the extent that the first was the cause and the other, effect. However, such inferences are not legitimately possible. Although, having a running nose correlates with having a cold, one would hardly believe that the running nose causes the cold. The fact the sun rises when we wake up in the morning does not suggest that our getting up causes the sun to rise.

If X correlates with Y, these casual relationships are possible:

X causes Y,
Y causes X, or
Z causes both X and Y.

Z may be very remote with long casual chain interposed before X and Y actually occur but the point serves the purpose of indicating a third source of causation. Hence, causality cannot be inferred solely on the basis of a correlation between two variables. It can be inferred only after conducting controlled experiments.

Factors Influence the Size of the Correlation Coefficient

The student should be aware of the following factors which influence the size of the correlation coefficient and can lead to misinterpretation.

1. The size of *r* is very much dependent upon the variability of measured values in the correlated sample. The greater the variability, the higher will be the correlation, everything else being equal.
2. The size of *r* is altered when researchers select extreme groups of subjects in order to compare these groups with respect to certain behaviors. Selecting extreme groups on one

variable increases the size of r over what would be obtained with more random sampling.

3. Combining two groups which offer in their mean values on one of the variables is not likely to faithfully represent the true situation as far as the correlation is concerned.
4. Addition of an extreme case (and conversely dropping of an extreme case) can lead to changes in the amount of correlation. Dropping of such a case leads to reduction in the correlation while the converse is also true.

Assumptions Underlying the Product Moment Correlation

Pearson's product moment r is based on some assumptions which must be filled before its use is made. These assumptions include linearity of regression. It means that the trend of relationship between the two variables be rectilinear. This can be determined, as a rule, by inspection of the scatter diagram. If the distribution of the cases within the correlation diagram appears to be elliptical, without any indication of a definite bending of the ellipse, the chances are that the relationship is rectilinear. In case of curvature, of regression, *correlation ratio* instead of product moment r as a measure of relationship would be more appropriate. Curvilinearity of regression can be eliminated by transformations to binomial or to an approximately normal form.

Pearson's does not assume that the distribution of the two variables should be normal. The forms of distribution may vary, so long as they are fairly symmetrical and unimodal. Even rectangular distributions can be used.

Many other circumstances affect the correlation coefficient. Among these may be mentioned sampling errors and errors of measurement.

The Interpretation of *r* in Terms of Verbal Description

The correlation coefficient is generally interpreted in different ways by different statisticians. However, there is a fairly good agreement among them that the following verbal descriptions may be assigned to different values of correlations.

Value of r	*Verbal description*
0.00 to ± 0.20	indifferent or negligible relationship
± 0.20 to ± 40	low correlation; present but slight
± 0.40 to ± 0.70	substantial or marked
± 0.70 to ± 1.00	high to very high (Garrett, 1966)

The above categorization is broad and tentative and may be used with advantage as a general guide by less sophisticated students. However, a correlation coefficient must as a rule be judged with regard to

i. The nature of variables under study
ii. The statistical significance of the coefficient
iii. The degree of reliability of the tests used
iv. The purposes for which r has been computed, and
v. The extent of variability of the group.

Biserial Correlation

Some experiments require an estimate of the relationship between a continuous variable and a dichotomous variable. The term 'dichotomous' means 'cut into two parts'. The variable of social adjustment can be dichotomized as "socially adjusted subjects: and "socially maladjusted subjects". The two-fold classification may appear in the following example—Passes and failures; drop-outs and stay-ins; and successful and unsuccessful, etc. However, the essential assumption is that the variable underlying the dichotomy should be continuous and normal. It means that it should be based on artificial dichotomy and not on a natural dichotomy.

The formula for biserial correlation is

$$r_{\text{bis}} = \frac{M_p - M_q}{\sigma} \times \frac{pq}{y}$$

(calculation of r_{bis})

In which, r_{bis} = biserial r

$M_p–M_q$ = mean test scores respectively for those who pass and fail the item

p and q = proportions who pass and fail the item

y = height of the ordinate of the normal curve at the point of division between p and q proportions of cases

s = SD of the entire group

Example: A rehearsal group and a non-rehearsal group obtained the following Table 11.8 scores on their performance. Find out the correlation between rehearsal and performance in dramatization.

Table 11.8

Worksheet for the calculation of r_{bis}

Scores	*Rehearsal group*	*Nonrehearsal group*
90–99	3	9
80–89	6	15
70–79	5	18
60–69	12	36
50–59	10	18
40–49	8	30
30–39	6	24
Sum	50	150

Steps

1. Calculate means for the two groups separately and combined. Also calculate SD for the total.

Group	*Mean*	*SD*
Rehearsal	60.9	(Mean and SD have been calculated using the standard procedures)
Non-Rehearsal	59.5	
Total	59.85	17.63

2. Obtain p = N1/N = 50/200 = 0.25; $q = 1 - p$ $= 1 - 0.25 = 0.75$
3. From Table M, ordinates of normal curve, pick up the height of y ordinate corresponding to the point of dichotomy of 0.25 and 0.75. In our example, it is 0.318.
4. Substitute the values in Formula

$$r_{bis} = \frac{60.0 - 59.5}{17.63} \times \frac{0.25 \times 0.75}{0.318} = 0.047$$

The correlation is negligible

An alternative formula for r_{bis} is

$$r_{bis} = \frac{M_p - M_q}{\sigma} \times \frac{pq}{y} \qquad ...(11.25)$$

(Alternative formula for r_{bis}) in which, M is the mean for the whole sample.

Values of r_{bis} may not always range between –1 and +1. In case of gross departure from normality, values of r_{bis} greater than unity may occur.

Point Biserial Correlation

In cases, when test items are scored simply as 1 if correct and 0 if incorrect, that is right or wrong, the assumption of normality in the distribution of right/wrong responses is generally not met. Other examples of genuine or natural dichotomies are, male-female, rural-urban, living-dead, convicted-not convicted, loyal-disloyal. In such cases, the point biserial correlation, r_{pbis} instead of r_{bis} can be used.

Example: Scores obtained by 11 students on the total test and item No. 12 of the test are given in Table 11.9. Calculate item total correlation.

Step 1

Calculate the following:

Proportion of students who passed the item,

$$p = \frac{6}{11} = 0.55$$

Proportion of students who failed, $q = \frac{5}{11} = 0.45$

Table 11.9

Worksheet for the calculation of point biserial correlation r_{bis}

Score of test (Criterion) X	*Item number 12 Y*	X^2
15	1	225
14	0	196
13	0	169
15	1	225
10	1	100
15	1	225
13	0	169
12	1	144
15	1	225
10	0	100
11	0	121
Σ143	6	1899

M_x of students who passed the item,

$$M_p = \frac{15+15+10+15+12+15}{6} = 13.67$$

M_x of students who failed the item,

$$M_p = \frac{14+13+13+10+11}{5} = 12.20$$

$$M_i = \frac{\Sigma X}{N} = \frac{143}{11} = 13.30$$

Step 2

Calculate σ_x for the total group:

$$\sigma_x = \frac{1}{N}\sqrt{N\Sigma X^2 - (\Sigma X)^2}$$

$$= \frac{1}{11}\sqrt{11(1899) - (143)^2} = 1.91$$

Step 3

Use the following formula to find out r_{pbis}:

$$r_{pbis} = M_p - M_q \sqrt{pq}$$

$$= \frac{13.67 - 12.20}{1.91}\sqrt{5.5 \times 0.45}$$

$$= 0.38$$

The point biserial correlation is a product-moment correlation. If we assign *a* 1 to individuals in one category and *a* 0 to individuals in the other category and calculate product moment *r* the result is a point biserial *r*. In the above example, those who did item No. 12 correctly were assigned *a* Y score of 1 and those who did it incorrectly, *a* Y score of 0. Weights other than 1 and 0 can also be assigned. The point biserial *r* is specially useful in the analysis of the items of a test. The relation between biserial and point biserial correlation is given by the expression.

$$r_{bis} = r_{pbis}\frac{\sqrt{pq}}{y} \quad ...(11.26)$$

The factor $\sqrt{pq/y}$ varies from 1.25 when $p = q = 0.5$, to 3.73 when $p = 0.99$ and $q = 0.01$. Thus r_{bis} is always greater than r_{pbis} and the difference increases with extremeness of the dichotomies.

Tetrachoric Correlation

The biserial and point biserial correlations were used when one variable was continuous and expressed as test scores and the other variable was dichotomous or in a two fold classification. However, when both the variables are dichotomous, we cannot calculate biserial or point biserial correlation. For such situations, tetrachoric correlation, *rt* can be calculated. Tetrachoric correlation is suitable for situations in which neither of the two variables can be measured in terms of scores but both the two variables can be separated in terms of two categories. For example if we wish to find out correlation between residence and punishment for indiscipline at school, we may dichotomize the variables as rural residence and urban residence; and punished and not-punished. Some other examples are:

1. Intelligence (Above average and below average); and social maturity (socially mature and socially immature).

2. School attendance (graduated from high school and those who did not); and employment (presently employed and not employed).

Tetrachoric correlation assumes that the two variables under study are essentially *continuous* and would be normally distributed if it were possible to obtain scores or exact measures on them.

Example: In the 2 × 2 Table below the two-fold distribution of students on training and success is given. Calculate tetrachoric correlation.

Table 11.10

Worksheet for the calculation of tetrachoric correlation

Given	*Pass*	*Fail*		
Trained	20 (A)	40 (B)	60	AD = 20 x 22 = 440
Untrained	15 (C)	22 (D)	37	BC = 40 x 15 = 600
	35	62	97	

Step 1: Both the variables are classified into two categories, marked + and –. Entries in cell A are + +, entries in D, – –, so that concentration of frequencies into these two cells means close agreement and positive correlation. The other two cells are designated as B and C which would be + – and – +, or in our example trained-failed and untrained-passed. A generalized model of designating the cells is given on the next page:

Y \ X	+	–
+	A + +	B – +
–	C + –	D – –

Or

Y \ X	–	+
+	B – +	A + +
–	D – –	C + –

Step 2: The full equation for tetrachoric r is *algebraically* very complex and hence a simplified formula which gives good approximation to r_t is used:

$$r_t = \cos \frac{(180° \times \sqrt{BC})}{\sqrt{AD} + \sqrt{BC}} \quad ...(11.27)$$

(An approximate formula for tetrachoric r)

AD and BC are the products of the cells designated in the 2 × 2 table above and cos is a trigonometric function whose value is available from Tables.

In our example BC *is greater than AD, hence AD is to be put in the numerator.*

Substituting the values in formula we get,

$$r_t = \cos \frac{(180° \times \sqrt{440})}{\sqrt{440} + \sqrt{600}}$$

$$= \cos \frac{(3775.71)}{45.47} = \cos 83°$$

Step 3: Convert cos 83° into r_t, consulting Table N in appendix.

$$r_t = -0.122$$

(Minus sign has been fixed to r_t because BC is greater than AD).

When the value of AD entries (agreement) is larger than the value of BC entries (disagreement), the correlation is positive. In the reverse situation, the experiment should fix a minus sign to the value of r_t.

The Phi Coefficient (ø)

When we have to find out correlation between two items of a test and the items are restricted to a scoring of 1 and 0, we can calculate phi coefficient instead of product moment r. The data is arranged in a 2 × 2 table and the cells are marked as below:

And then the following formulae are used: Phi coefficient,

$$= \frac{AD - BC}{\sqrt{(A+B)(C+D)(A+C)(B+D)}} \quad ...(11.28)$$

(Phi coefficient from frequencies)

$$\text{Phi coefficient} = \frac{p_{ij} - p_i p_j}{\sqrt{p_i p_j q_i q_j}}$$

(Phi coefficient from proportions)

In which, p_i = proportion passing item i

p_j = proportion padding item j

q_i = proportion failing item i

q_j = proportion failing item j

p_{ij} = proportion passing both items i and j

Example: The number of candidates passing and failing two items are given below. Calculate a Phi coefficient between the two items.

Solution:

		Item I		
		Fail	Pass	
Item II	Pass	65 (B)	90 (A)	155 (A + B)
	Fail	80 (D)	30 (C)	110 (C + D)
		145 (B + D)	120 (A + C)	265

Substituting the values in formula we get Phi coefficient

$$= \frac{90 \times 80 - 65 \times 30}{\sqrt{155 \times 110 \times 145 \times 120}}$$

$$= \frac{7200 - 1950}{17224.11} = 0.30$$

The phi coefficient has been widely used in statistical work associated with psychological tests. Usually when researchers speak of the correlation between dichotomously scored test items, the reference is to the phi coefficient. The Phi coefficient is a particular case of product moment correlation when the integers 1 and 0 are assigned to represent the two categories of each variable. The values of phi coefficient range between –1 and +1 and are influenced by the marginal totals. Negative and positive perfect correlation is obtained when the two variables are evenly divided, i.e. $p_i = p_j = q_i = q_j$.

Rank Correlation

It is not always possible to take measurements on units or objects. Many characters are expressed in comparative terms such as beauty, smartness, temperament, etc. In such cases the subjects are ranked pertaining to that particular character instead of taking measurements on them. Sometimes, the units are also ranked according to their quantitative measure. In these types of studies, two situations arise, (i) the same set of units is ranked according to two characters A and B, (ii) two judges give ranks to the same set of units independently, pertaining to one character only. In both these situations, we get paired ranks for a set of units. For example, two judges rank the girls independently in a beauty competition. The students are ranked according to their marks in Mathematics and Statistics. In all these situations, the usual Pearsonian correlation coefficient cannot be obtained. Hence, the psychologist, Charles Edward Spearman (1906) developed a formula for correlation coefficient, which is known as rank correlation or Spearman's correlation. It is denoted by r_s. Suffix s to r is a connotation for Spearman, the name of the inventor.

Frequencies				*Proportions*			
	Item 1				*Item 2*		
	Fail	*Pass*	*A + B*		*Fail*	*Pass*	
Pass	B	A		Pass	(b)	(a)	p_1
Item II				Item I			
Fail	D	C	C + D	Fail	(d)	(c)	q_2

The formula for r_s is derived as the ratio of covariance to the product of standard deviation of two series of ranks. Here the derivation is omitted and thus the formula for rank correlation is,

$$r_s = 1 - \frac{6\Sigma_i d_i^2}{n(n^2-1)} \qquad ...(11.29)$$

where $i = 1, 2, ..., n$

d_i is the difference between the ranks of the i-th units and n is the total number of units.

The value of r_s also lies between – 1 and 1.

Example: Two judges gave the following ranks (from the highest to the lowest) to eleven girls who contested in a beauty competition. Whether or not, there is an agreement between the independent rankings of the two judges, can be ascertained only by finding out the rank correlation between the ranks awarded by two judges.

Here $\Sigma_i d_i^2 = 66$ and $n = 11$

From (11.29),

$$r_s = 1 - \frac{6 \times 66}{11 \times 120} = 1 - 0.30 = 0.70$$

The value of rank correlation $r_s = 0.70$, which is quite high. Hence, it can be concluded that there is an agreement between judges with regard to the beauty of the girls.

Problem of Tied Observations

Formula (11.29) is based on the assumption that n units received n sets of paired ranks from 1 to n independently assigned in each set. As a matter of fact no ties should occur in case of samples from continuous populations. But ties seldom occur due to rounding of measurements. Hence, the problem of ties comes in while calculating Spearman's rank correlation.

If ties occur between measurements across sets x and y, it creates no problem. But if ties occur within a set of sample values, the problem of ties cannot be ignored. In this situation, of course, the ranks are assigned by mid rank method. Under this process, the sum of ranks remains the same as $n(n + 1)/2$, but there is a decrease in the sum of squares of ranks. Hence, adjustment has to be made in the formula of Spearman's rank correlation. It is given here without proof.

Suppose m_h is the number of tied measurements in the ith group of tied values ($h = 1, 2, ..., k$) for the set x. It means there are k groups of tied values in the set x. Then the correction factor u_x for ties for the set x is given as,

$$u_x = \sum_{h=1}^{k} m_h(m_h^2 - 1)$$

A similar expression u_y, i.e., the correction factor for groups of tied measurements within the set y can be given as

Girl no.	1	2	3	4	5	6	7	8	9	10	11
	Ranks										
Judge A	3	4	1	2	5	10	11	7	9	8	6
Judge B	2	4	3	1	7	9	6	11	10	5	8

Following the usual procedure, the rank correlation is calculated.

d	1	0	–2	1	–2	1	5	–4	–1	3	–2	Total
*d*²	1	0	4	1	4	1	25	16	1	9	4	66

$$u_y = \sum_{j=1}^{l} g_j(g_j^2 - 1)$$

where g_j is the number of tied measurements in the jth group of tied values for $j = 1, 2, ..., l$. In case of ties in both the sets, the amended formula for Spearman's rank correlation is

$$r = \frac{n(n^2-1) - 6\sum_{i=1}^{n} d_i^2 - (u_x + v_y)/2}{\sqrt{(n^2(n^2-1)^2 + (u_x + v_y)(n^3 - n) + u_x v_y}} \quad ...(11.29.1)$$

$$= \frac{(n^3-n) - 6\sum_{i=1}^{n} d_i^2 - (u_x + v_y)/2}{\sqrt{(n^3-n)^2 - (n^3-n)(u_x + v_y) + u_x v_y}} \quad ...(11.29.2)$$

In the above formula, if no ties occur in the set x, $u_x = 0$ and if no ties occur in the set y, $u_y = 0$. If no ties occur in both the sets, $u_x = 0$, $v_y = 0$ and thus formula (11.29.2) reduces to formula (11.29).

Spearman's rank correlation between percentage of marks in ICWA and CA examinations by eleven students is calculated in the manner explained in theory.

From percentage of marks it is apparent that the ties occur in both the sets. Further there are two groups of tied percentages in each set.

Using mid rank method, the ranks of percentages for ICWA (x) and CA (y) and their differences $d_i (i = 1, 2, ..., 11)$ are displayed in the given Table.

Calculation of correction factors

For the set x,

$$m_1 = 2, m_2 = 3 \text{ and } h = 1, 2.$$

Hence, $u_x = (2^3 - 2) + (3^3 - 3)$

$= 6 + 24 = 30$

Similarly for the set y,

$$g_1 = 2, g_2 = 2 \text{ and } l = 1, 2$$

$v_y = (2^3 - 2) + (2^3 - 2)$

$= 6 + 6 = 12$

$$\Sigma d_i^2 = (-1)^2 + 2^2 + (-2.5)^2 + 3.5^2 + 2^2 + 1.5^2 + (-1)^2 + 0^2 + 2.5^2 + (-3)^2 + (-4)^2$$

$$= 1 + 4 + 6.25 + 12.25 + 4 + 2.25 + 1 + 0 + 6.25 + 9 + 16 = 62.00$$

Also, $n^3 - n = (11^3 - 11) = 1320$

Thus, from the formula (11.29.2), Spearman's correlation is,

$$r_s = \frac{1320 - 6\times 62 - (30+12)/2}{\sqrt{(1320)^2 - 1320(30+12) + 30\times 12}}$$

$$= \frac{1320 - 372 - 21}{\sqrt{1687320}} = \frac{927}{1298.97} = 0.714$$

Since, the value of r_s is high, it shows that a high positive correlation exists between percentage of marks in ICWA and CA earned by the eleven students.

Example: The percentage marks secured by eleven students in ICWA and CA examinations are as follows:

Student	1	2	3	4	5	6	7	8	9	10	11
ICWA marks (*x*)%	40	55	40	60	62	78	58	96	85	60	60
CA marks (*y*)%	65	45	68	65	70	75	69	88	75	72	82

Students	1	2	3	4	5	6	7	8	9	10	11
Ranks for *x*	1.5	3	1.5	6	8	9	4	11	10	6	6
Ranks for *y*	2.5	1	4	2.5	6	7.5	5	11	7.5	9	10
Difference d_i	–1	2	–2.5	3.5	2	1.5	– 1	0	2.5	– 3	– 4

Coefficient of Determination

The coefficient of determination, which is given as r^2, explains to what extent the variation of dependent variable y is being expressed by the independent variable x.

$$r^2 = \frac{\text{Variance explained}}{\text{Total variance}} \quad \text{...(11.30)}$$

More the value of r^2, better it is. A high value clearly shows that a good linear relation exists between the two variables. Obviously, if $r = 1$, then $r^2 = 1$, which is an indicator of perfect relationship between the two variables. Also the quantity $(1 - r^2)$ is called the coefficient of non-determination or coefficient of alienation. $(1 - r^2)$ is thus a measure of deviation from perfect linear relationship. For example, if $r = 0.08$, it means high degree of correlation. But $r^2 = 0.64$, which means that only 64 percen of variations in the dependent variable are due to the independent variable, remaining 36 percent variations are due to other independent variables yet to be located.

Spurious Correlation

If we have paired observations on two variables and the assumptions hold good, it is always possible to calculate the correlation coefficient between the two variables. But correlation coefficient is not always meaningful unless the two variables are properly chosen. For example, if we find out the correlation between the total imports and the number of shoes produced per year, it would not lead to any conclusion. Because there is no cause and effect relationship between the total imports and number of shoes produced per year. Such a correlation is known as *spurious* or *nonsense* correlation between two variables. Another example of spurious correlation is the correlation between the number of tourists who visited Taj Mahal and the number of TV sets produced. From this discussion, we come more important to see the nature of the variables. If they have a cause and effect relationship, and if one variable can be explained with the help of the other, then the correlation has sense, otherwise it is spurious.

The description of correlation coefficient, in this chapter, does not cover all types of correlation coefficients. Those not covered in this chapter are correlation ratio, intraclass correlation, biserial correlation, etc. Whatever has been embodied in this chapter is in accordance to the requirement of the syllabi.

EXERCISES

1. What do you understand by a regression model? What are it uses?
2. What is a scatter diagram and what role does it play in regression theory?
3. Explain the method of estimating parameters of a regression equation.
4. Can a regression equation be used for projections? If so, what are the assumptions underlying it? Also give some examples.
5. Explain the regression of Y on X and X on Y. At what point do the two regression lines intersect? Also derive the relation of two regression coefficients with correlation coefficient.
6. Answer the following questions with reasoning in a one line or two.
   a. Can regression coefficient be negative?
   b. Can correlation coefficient be negative?

c. If the regression coefficient is negative, then correlation coefficient will also be negative.
d. It the regression coefficient of Y on X is negative, does it mean that regression coefficient of X on Y will also be negative?
e. What inference would you draw by a negative value of regression coefficient?
f. If the two coefficients of regression are negative, does it mean that the correlation would be positive?

CHAPTER 12 Statistical Regression

Introduction

It was observed that the degree of correlation between the two variables could be measured using the correlation coefficient.

In some cases, one variable (known, called independent variable) causes the change in the other variable (unknown, called dependent variable). For example, change in height (independent) of the child causes change in weight (dependent variable) of the child.

This change of dependent variable with respect to change in independent variable is known as "Regression".

Sometimes, it may happen that the dependent variable increases for each change of the independent variable upto a certain value and then it may start decreasing with the change in the independent variable. The reverse process may also happen. In such cases, the regression is said to be "Non-linear". For example, the prevalence rate of tuberculosis in a community rises with the age upto a certain age and then starts decreasing with the increase in the age after reaching a maximum at certain age group. This may be due to immunity attained by the community by the time they reach a certain age.

In such a case, the relationship is said to be quadratic.

In simple correlation, it is observed that there is one dependent variable and only one independent variable. But it may so happen that there may be more than one independent variable for the causation of the dependent variable. For example, wt of the newborn baby (dependent variable) is related to more than one independent variable such as age of the mother, period of gestation at the time of birth, parity of delivery, health condition of the mother and so on. If the overall correlation of all these independent factors with the dependent factor is considered, then it is known as "multiple correlation".

If an equation is fitted to estimate the dependent variable (e.g. weight of the baby at birth) in terms of other independent variables (as in above factors), then the equation is called as the "multiple regression equation".

The concept of regression was first given by Sir Francis Galton (1822-1911) in a study of inheritance of stature in the human being. To prove this biometrical fact, Karl Pearson found the regression of son's height on father's height. But soon the use of regression technique became too common for a variety of problems. The relationship between variables, if it exists, may be linear or curvilinear. In this chapter a detailed discussion of linear regression and a brief discussion of curvilinear regression have been given.

Linear relationship between two variables is represented by a straight line which is known as a *regression line*. *The line of average relationship* is another name for a regression line. In the study of linear relationships between two variables Y and X, suppose the variable Y is such that it depends on X, then we call it the regression line of Y on X. If X depends on Y, it is called the regression of X on Y. To find out the regression line, the observations

(x_i, y_i) on the variables X and Y are necessarily taken in pairs, on the units which may be people, animals, plots, spare parts, plants or any other thing. For example, if the height of Rama is measured, only the weight of Rama has to be taken to form a pair for establishing the relationship between height and weight. Not that we form a pair of Rama's height and Krishna's weight. If a pair is formed of a father's height and eldest son's height at a particular age, in all cases this has to be maintained and not a combination of different sons with the father to form a pair of observations. Generally the studies are based on samples of size *n*, and hence *n* pairs of sample observations can be written as (x_1, y_1), (x_2, y_2), ..., (x_n, y_n). Before entering into the method of estimation or fitting of regression line, it will be appropriate to explain first the scatter diagram.

Scientific studies usually aim at one or more of the three important things—explanation, pre-diction and control. One of the most important tests of any scientific hypothesis is its ability to make predictions or estimations. Statistical reasoning has helped the researcher in framing statement of a predictive nature. The related problem of prediction or estimation of the value of the variable, from a known value of variable to which it is related, can be discussed by means of regression. Here the amount of error in the predictions can also be statistically measured.

Regression means to 'return' or 'to go back'. So it implies the act of returning or going back. Normal phenomena usually has a tendency to return to normal. In statistics, "regression" is used to denote backward tendency, which is going back to *average* or *normal*. The term regression was first used by Sir Francis Galton in study of heredity. Where he found tall fathers have tall sons. The concept of regression is now extended to other spheres of phenomena, which have a tendency to regress or set back to the normal.

The concept of regression is very helpful in the study of correlation. It shows a relationship between the average values of two variables. It is very helpful in estimating and predicting the average value of one variable for given value of the other variable. The estimate or prediction may be made with the help of regression line which shows the average value of one variable 'X' for a given value of the other variable 'Y'. The best average value of one variable associated with the given value of the other variable may also be estimated or predicted by means of an equation and the equation is known as 'Regression Equation'.

In the case of correlation, it was seen that the degree of correlation between the two variables could be measured using the correlation coefficient. In some cases this correlation is due to a latest factor associated with both the variables or in some others, it may be that one of the variable directly causes the change in the other variable as already explained. In the latter case the variable which causes the change is known as the independent variable and variables which change in the same pattern with the change in the independent variable is known as dependent variable. This change of dependent variable with respect to change in the independent variable is known as 'Regression' (Fig. 12.1).

For example, the height and weight of children given in the case charge, in the independent variable height of the child will cause a charge in the dependent variable weight of the child.

The relationship between the two variables can be represented by a mathematical equation known as "Regression Equation" when the relationship is linear, i.e. the dependent variable either increases or decreases throughout with the change in the independent variable, not in a linear manner, the equation will be the type $Y = a + bx$.

Scatter Diagram

Suppose, the correlation of height and weight of 100 children has to be studied and correlation coefficient is to be calculated, the extent and type of the relation between the two variables has to be known by plotting the variables into a scatter diagram, wherein one variable (X_1) is represented on X-axis and another variables (X_2) on the Y-axis. Each pair of observation is plotted as a dot. The diagram will be a scatter of dots. [each dot represents height on one axis and weight on another axis].

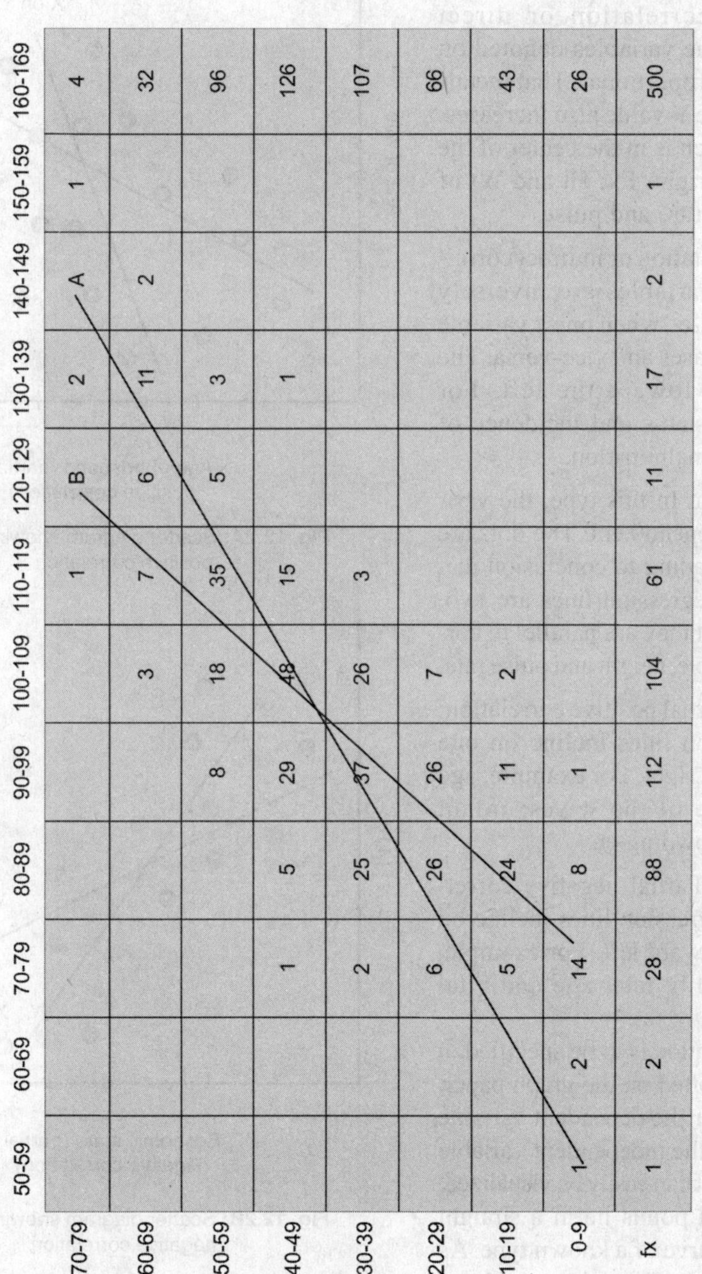

	50-59	60-69	70-79	80-89	90-99	100-109	110-119	120-129	130-139	140-149	150-159	160-169
70-79							1	B	2	A	1	4
60-69						3	7	6	11	2		32
50-59					8	18	35	5	3			96
40-49			1	5	29	48	15		1			126
30-39			2	25	37	26	3					107
20-29			6	26	26	7						66
10-19			5	24	11	2						43
0-9	1	2	14	8	1							26
fx	1	2	28	88	112	104	61	11	17	2	1	500

Line A: Regression of Y on X, $Y' = 0.70X - 33.14$

Line B: Regression of X on Y, $X' = 0.85Y + 70.25$

Fig. 12.1: Bi-variate frequency distribution showing regression lines of Y on X, and X on Y

There are 5 types of scatter diagram (Figs 12.2A to B).

Diagram 1: Positive correlation or direct correlation: In this type, the variables denoted on X and Y-axis are directly proportional. That means as the *x*-value increases, the Y-value also increases. The "regression line", which is in the center of the plots, ascends toward the right. Ex: Ht and Wt of growing children, temperature and pulse.

Diagram 2: Negative correlation or indirect correlation: In this type, the variables are inversely proportional to each other i.e., when one *x* variable increases, the other y decreases and vice-versa. The regression line ascends toward the left. For example, socioeconomic status and incidence of tuberculosis; income and malnutrition.

Diagram 3: No correlation: In this type, the variables are different and independ0.ent. The dots are haphazardly distributed, leading to conclusion that there is no relation. The regression lines are two, inclined on one another, but they are parallel to corresponding axes. For example, height and pulse rate.

Diagram 4: (Fig. 12.2a) Partial positive correlation: In this type, the regression lines incline on one another and ascend toward right. For example, age of the husbands and age of the wives; infant mortality rate and over-crowding etc.

Diagram 5: (Fig. 12.2b) Partial negative correlation: In this type, the regression lines incline on one another and ascend toward left. For example, income and infant mortality rate; age and vital capacity among adults.

When a regression equation is to be specified, *n* paired observations are plotted on the graph paper, setting the vertical scale for the dependent variable Y and horizontal scale for the independent variable X. From the plotted points, it can easily be visualized, whether or not the plotted points lie in a straight line or appear to lie on a curve of a known type. As a matter of fact, scatter diagram may be considered as a basis of deciding the type of regression equation, suited for the relationship, between the two variables, Y and X. In case, the plotted points are scattered in a haphazard manner, i.e. no pattern is observed, then it can be inferred that the variables are not related. Now we discuss the scatter diagram with special

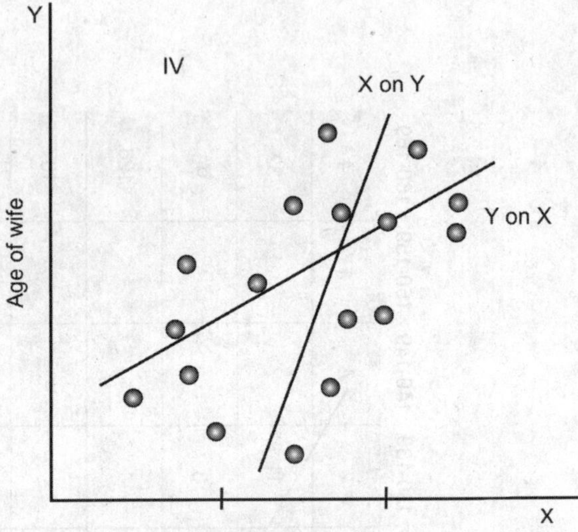

Fig. 12.2A: Scatter diagram showing partial positive correlation

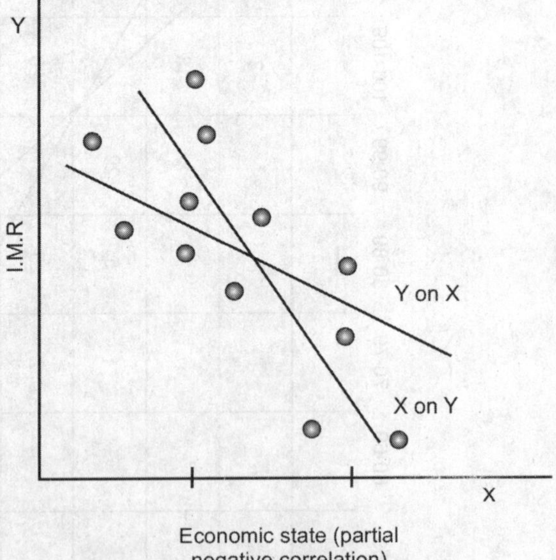

Fig. 12.2B: Scatter diagram showing partial negative correlation

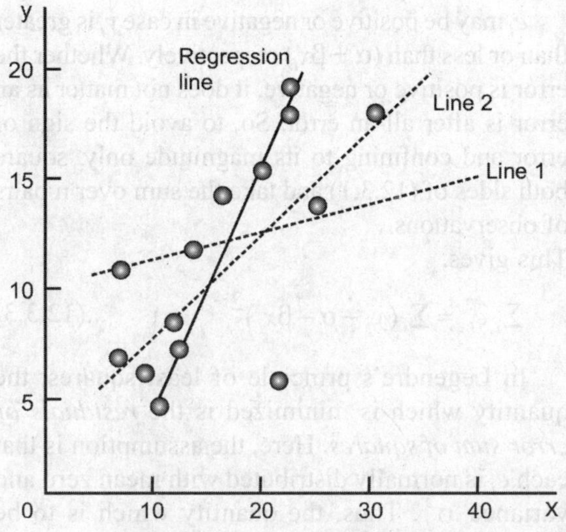

Fig. 12.2C: Fitting of a regression line

reference to the regression line. In practice, when we plot various paired observations, one would hardly come across a situation in which all the points are lying exactly in a line. But if a line is drawn suitably, some points will be lying on the line and others will be lying in the close vicinity of this line as depicted in Figure 12.2c.

It is observed that a few points are lying away from all the fitted lines. These extreme points may sometimes be considered outliers. As evident from the figure, a number of lines may be drawn and considered suitable. But the best line will be one for which the algebraic sum of the perpendicular distances of all the points from the line is zero. Hence, dotted lines in the figure are not such a good fit as the smooth straight line. In short, the scatter diagram can be thought of as a device to know how closely the two variables are related and in what form, i.e. linear or curvilinear. If no path is discernable, it means that the two variables are independent. Independence of two variables means that the change in one variable does not cause any change in the other variable, according to any rule. Scatter diagram pertaining to independent variables is shown in Figure 12.3.

From Figure 12.3, it is easily verifiable that if any line is drawn through the plotted points, not more than two points will be lying on the line and most of the other points will be at a considerable distance from this line.

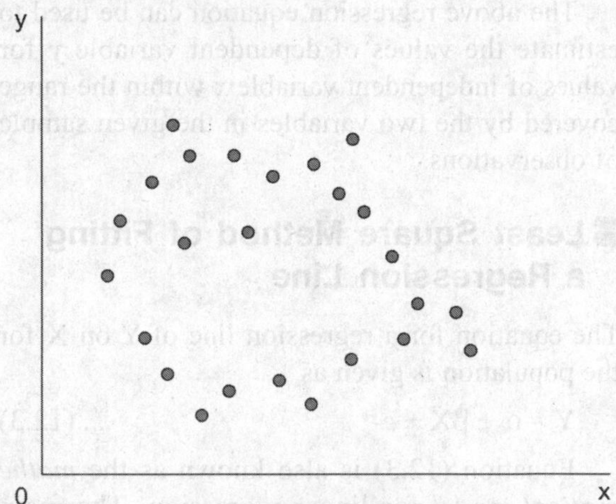

Fig. 12.3: Scatter diagram

Once it is decided on the basis of prior information or scatter diagram that the two variables are linearly related, the problem arises on deciding which of the many possible lines is the best fitted line. To cope with this problem, mathematical basis leads to the most logical and accurate solution. The least square method is the most widely accepted method of fitting a straight line and is discussed here adequately,

where y is the dependent variable
x is the independent variable
b is the regression coefficient
a represents the value of 'Y' for 'x' = 0

In the above linear equation, the regression coefficient b is calculated from the formula,

$$b = \frac{\Sigma xy - \left[(\Sigma x \, \Sigma y)/n\right]}{\left[\Sigma x^2 - (\Sigma x)^2/n\right]} \quad ...(12.1)$$

Where b is the regression coefficient of independent variable x, upon dependent variable y and usually represented as b.

After testing for the significance of regression coefficient, the linear regression line of y upon x can be fitted in the form Y = $a + bx$ by substituting the various calculated, in the formula

$$y = y + (x - \bar{x})\, b \quad ...(12.2)$$

where $\bar{y}$ and $\bar{x}$ are the means of the variable y and x and b is the calculated regression coefficient.

The above regression equation can be used to estimate the values of dependent variable y for values of independent variable x within the range covered by the two variables in the given sample of observations.

Least Square Method of Fitting a Regression Line

The equation for a regression line of Y on X for the population is given as

$$Y = \alpha + \beta X + e \qquad ....(12.3)$$

Equation (12.3) is also known as the *mathe matical model* for linear regression. The main difference between the cartesian equation of a line and a regression line is that a regression line is a probabilistic model which enables one to develop procedures for making inferences about the parameters a and b of the model. In this model, the expected value of Y is a linear function of X, but for fixed X, the variable Y differs from its expected value by *a* random amount. As a special case, the form $y = a + bx$ is called the *deterministic model.* In this model, the actual observed value of y is a linear function of x. In equation (12.1) a is the intercept which the line cuts on the axis of Y and b is the slope of the line b is also called the *regression coefficient* and is defined as, "b is the measure of change in the dependent variable (Y) corresponding to a unit change in the independent variable (X)". b is often written as b_{yx} to indicate that it is the regression coefficient of Y on X. In case no suffix is attached to b, it is considered by itself. b can take any real value within the range $-\infty$ to ∞.

Suppose the regression line given by (12.1) is to be fitted on the basis of n pairs of sample observations, $(x_1, y_1), (x_2, y_2), ..., (x_n, y_n)$. Each pair (x_i, y_i) for $i = 1, 2, ..., n$ will satisfy the regression line (12.1).

Thus, $$y_i = \alpha + \beta x_i + e_i \qquad ...(12.3.1)$$

or $$e_i = (y_i - \alpha - \beta x_i) \qquad ...(12.3.2)$$

e_i may be positive or negative in case y_i is greater than or less than $(\alpha + \beta x_i)$ respectively. Whether the error is positive or negative, it does not matter as an error is after all an error. So, to avoid the sign of error and confining to its magnitude only, square both sides of (12.3.1) and take the sum over n pairs of observations.

This gives,

$$\Sigma_i e_i^2 = \Sigma_i (y_i - \alpha - \beta x_i)^2 \qquad ...(12.3.3)$$

In Legendre's principle of least squares, the quantity which is minimized is the *residuals or error sum of squares*. Here, the assumption is that each e_i is normally distributed with mean zero and variance σ_e^2. Thus, the quantity which is to be minimized here $\Sigma_i e_i^2$. Let us denote this quantity by Q. Hence,

$$Q = \Sigma_i (y_i - \alpha - \beta x_i)^2 \qquad ...(12.3.4)$$

Interpretation of Regression

i. Linear regression equation should be used for estimating the values of the dependant variable, only when a straight line fully answers the relationship
ii. The regression line should not be extended beyond the values of the variable for which they are plotted
iii. Whenever there is correlation it does not mean that there is also a regression. The correlation may be due to an inherent factor acting on both variables and so, there may not be any regression
iv. The regression coefficient should be tested for significance
v. The standard error of regression coefficient is given by

$$S_b = \frac{S_{yx}}{\sqrt{(\Sigma x - x)^2}}$$

$$S_b = S_{y \cdot x} \sqrt{\left(\Sigma x^2 - (\Sigma x)^2 / n\right)} \qquad ...(12.4)$$

$S_{y \cdot x} =$

$$\sqrt{\frac{1}{(n-2)}\left(\Sigma y^2 - (\Sigma y)^2 / n\right) - \frac{\left(\Sigma xy - (\Sigma x)(\Sigma y)/n\right)}{\Sigma x^2 - (\Sigma x)^2 / n}} \quad \text{... (12.4)}$$

vi. The regression coefficient is to be tested for null hypothesis using t distribution where

$$t = \frac{b}{S_b} \text{ with } n\text{–}2 \; df \quad \text{...(12.5)}$$

vii. The standard error of the estimated value of y from the regression equation is given by the quantity $S_{y \cdot x / \sqrt{n}}$ where $S_{y \cdot x}$ is obtained as above.

In linear regression, the relationship between the two variables x and y is linear. In order to estimate the best average values of the two variables, two regression equations are required and they are used separately. One equation is used for estimating the value of X variable for a given value of Y variable and the second equation is used for estimating the value of Y variable for a given value of X variable. In both cases, the assumption is that one is an independent variable and the other is a dependent variable and vice versa.

The two lines of regression are:

1. Regression Equation of X on Y is

$$X - \overline{X} = r\frac{\sigma_x}{\sigma_y}(Y - \overline{Y}) \quad \text{...(12.6)}$$

[It estimates X for a given value of Y]

2. Regression Equation Y on X is

$$Y - \overline{Y} = r\frac{\sigma_y}{\sigma_x}(X - \overline{X}) \quad \text{...(12.7)}$$

[It estimates Y for a given value of X]

Where X = Value of X, Y = Value of Y

Y = Arithmetic Mean of X series,

X = Arithmetic Mean of Y series

σ_x = Standard Deviation X series

σ_y = Standard Deviation Y series

r = Correlation Coefficient between X and Y

It is important to note that the regression equation of X on Y should be used for predicting or timing the value of X for a given value of Y and the regression equation of Y on X should be used for predicting or estimating the value of Y for a given value of X.

Regression Coefficients

Regression means change in the measurements of a variable, on the positive or negative side, beyond the mean. This regression is measured through "Regression coefficient", a constant, which gives the amount of increase in the dependent variable (e.g. wt) for an unit increase in the independent (e.g. height) variable. This quantity is represented by "b", when these variables are plotted on a graph, gives "Regression-line", depicting that the relationship is linear.

The regression coefficient of y on x is

$$b_{yx} = r\frac{\sigma_y}{\sigma_x} \text{ and that of } x \text{ on } y$$

$$b_{xy} = r\frac{\sigma_x}{\sigma_y} \quad \text{...(12.8)}$$

Properties of Regression Coefficient

1. It can take any value between $-\infty$ and ∞.
2. Its sign is same as that of σ_{xy}, i.e. cov (X, Y). Further, if the whole population has been studied, i will vary from 1 to N for all the N units of the population. In this situation we get population regression coefficient β_{yx} directly, for which the formula is

$$\beta_{yx} = \frac{\sigma_{xy}}{\sigma_x^2} \quad \text{...(12.9)}$$

In case of population regression coefficient β of Y on X, which can elaborately be specified as β_{yx} we can express it as

$$\beta_{yx} = \rho\frac{\sigma_y}{\sigma_x} \quad \text{...(12.9.1)}$$

where ρ is the population correlation coefficient between X and Y.

As a and b are the estimated values of α and β respectively, the equation of the estimated regression line is

$$\hat{Y} = a + bX \quad ...(12.10)$$

where, the hat (^) over Y indicates that Y is an estimated value. Substituting the value of α, the line of best fit is

$$\hat{Y} = (\bar{y} - b\bar{x}) + bX \quad ...(12.10.1)$$

$$(\hat{Y} - \bar{y}) = b(X - \bar{x}) \quad ...(12.10.2)$$

Properties of Correlation Coefficients

a. The coefficients of correlation is the geometric mean of the coefficients of regression, i.e., $r = \sqrt{b_{yx} \times b_{xy}}$
b. If one of the regression coefficients is greater than unity, then the other is less than unity
c. Arithmetic mean of the regression coefficient is greater than the correlation coefficient
d. Regression coefficients are independent of change of origin but not of scale.

Linear Regression Line or Equation

A method, which expresses in the form of a mathematical equation the relationship between the two variables x and y, is relatively simple when the *relationship is linear in character*. This equation is known as the *regression equation*. Methods are also available for determining the regression equation when the relationship is not linear but are beyond the scope of this presentation. An understanding of the method used in determining the linear regression equation will aid the student in understanding curvilinear relationship, when they are encountered by the student.

The relationship between the two variables can be represented by a mathematical equation, known as "Regression Equation". When the relationship is linear, the equation will be of the type $y = a + bx$

Where,

y, is the dependent variable,

x, is the independent variable,

b is the regression coefficient,

a represents the value of y for $x = 0$.

The regression coefficient is calculated by using the formula,

$$b_{xy} = \frac{\Sigma xy - (\Sigma x \, \Sigma y)/n}{\Sigma x^2 - (\Sigma x)^2/n}$$

Where b_{xy} is regression coefficient of independent variable x, upon dependent variable y and usually represented as b.

Since, in most instances of linear regression the dots representing the individual pairs of values for the two variables will not all fall in such a way that every dot will fit on a straight line (perfect correlation), the problem resolves itself into determining the equation of the straight line that best fits the dots or in other words, the line around which the dots have the least scatter. This line is called a regression line and its equation can be found by a method known as least squares. This involves finding the line for which the sum of the squares of the distances of each observed point from the line shall be as small as possible. Consider Figure 12.4 where for simplicity only three points, W, S and T have been plotted. If the distance from point W to the line be measured by w, that from S by s, and that from T by t, the problem is to find the equation of the line which will make $w^2 + s^2 + t^2$ a minimum. Let the equation of this line be, in general terms, $y = a + bx$, where y and x represent the two variables, a the y-intercept or the distance between the x axis and the point where the line crosses the y axis and b the slope or the increase in the y value per unit change in the x value (Fig.12.5).

Using mathematical principles developed in calculus, the value of $w^2 + s^2 + t^2$ will be a minimum if the value of a and b are such that they satisfy two simultaneous linear equations known as the normal equations. These are:

1. $\Sigma y = na + b\Sigma x$ ...(12.11)
2. $\Sigma xy = a\Sigma x + b\Sigma x^2$ ....(12.12)

Solving the two equations by the ordinary methods of algebra gives the value of b in general terms:

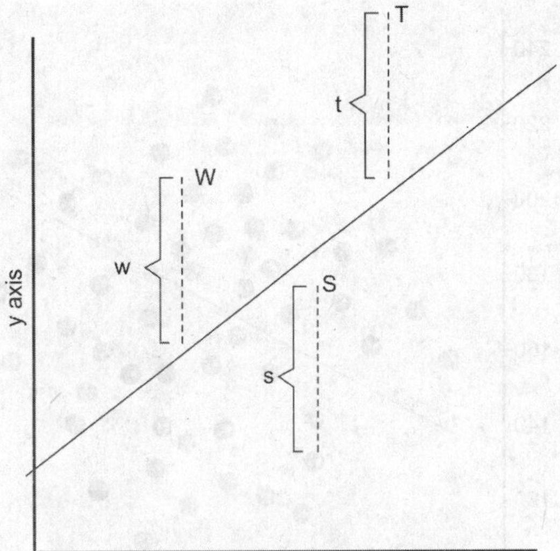

Fig. 12.4: Illustration of deviations from the line in the *y* direction

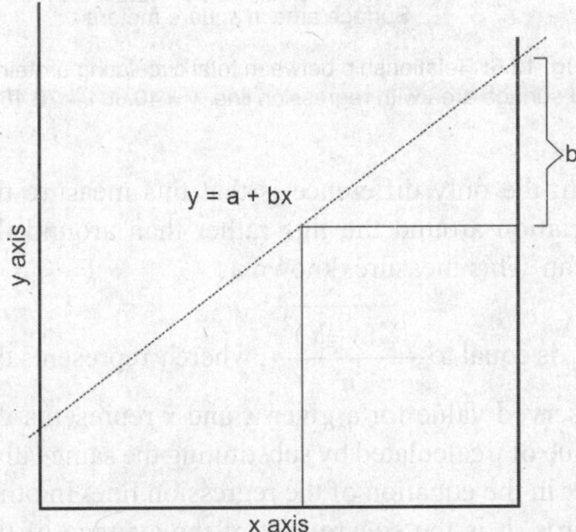

Fig. 12.5: Illustration of interpret and slope for the regression line

$$b_{yx} = \frac{n\Sigma xy - \Sigma x \Sigma y}{n\Sigma x^2 - (\Sigma y)^2} \quad ...(12.13)$$

After the value of b_{yx} is found, this value together with the values of Σy, n, Σx can be substituted in equation (12.11) and the value of a calculated. The accuracy of the computations can be checked by substituting the values a and b in Equation (12.12).

For the data previously used showing the correlation between surface area of the body (designated as the x variable) and circulating protein of the blood (designated as the y variable), the following sums were given as:

$\Sigma x = 117.76 \qquad \Sigma x^2 = 225.4290$
$\Sigma y = 11016 \qquad \Sigma y^2 = 20007.48$
$\Sigma xy = 21050.38$
$n = 62$

To determine the equation of the regression line that minimizes the squares of the y deviations (i.e. the difference between the observed y for any given value of x and the y value calculated from the equation for the same value of x) these values may be substituted in the above formula for b:

$$b_{yx} = \frac{62(21050.380) - (11016)(117.76)}{62(225.4290) - (117.76)^2}$$

$$= \frac{7879}{109.1804} = 72.1686$$

Substituting this value for b together with the other necessary values in equation (12.11) gives:

$11016 = 62a + (72.1686)(117.76)$
$11016 = 62a + 8498.5743$
$62a = 2517.4257$
$a = 40.6036$

Checking by substituting the necessary values in equation (12.12) gives:

$$21050.38 = (40.6036)(117.76) + (72.1686)(225.42\,90) = 21050.38$$

These values of a and b can now be substituted in the equation of the line $y = a + bx$, giving for the regression line the equation:

$$y = 40.604 + 72.169x$$

To plot the regression line on the scatter diagram, it is necessary to find two paired values of x and y. First, one value of x such as 1.6 is substituted for x in the equation $y = 40.604 + 72.169x$ and the corresponding value of y is obtained. Then, a second value of x such as 2.0 is substituted for x

and the value of y obtained. These two paired values for x and y (1.6,156.1) and 2.0,184.9) are now plotted on the diagram and the line connecting them is the regression line.

What do the values of a and b indicate? The value of b indicates the for each unit change in surface area of the body, the circulating protein increases (because b is positive) by 72.169 gm. The a value tells simply what the value of y is when x is 0 or tells where the regression line crosses the y axis.

The second alternate formula for calculation of x is especially useful when dealing with grouped data. This is

$$b_{yx} = r\frac{\sigma_y}{\sigma_x} \quad ...(12.14)$$

The subscript yx is used to show that the value of by x being calculated is that which is to be substituted in the line $y = a + bx$. The value of A can then be calculated, as before, by substituting the appropriate figure in the equation:

$$\Sigma y = a + b\Sigma x \quad ...(12.15)$$

This equation can also be written as:

$$\frac{\Sigma y}{n} = a + b\frac{\Sigma x}{n} \quad ...(12.16)$$

$$\text{or} \quad \bar{y} = a + b\bar{x} \quad ...(12.17)$$

Therefore, knowing b, x and y, it becomes easy to find the value of a. Use of this formula gives the same line as did the first method.

This last formula emphasizes the fact that the regression line will always pass through the mean of the x values and the mean of the y values. This, is a further check on the accuracy of computations.

This line has been plotted on the scatter diagram (Fig. 12.6). Inspection shows that there is considerable scatter of the dots about the line. This is to be expected because of the low correlation coefficient previously found for these data.

A measure of the variation of these points around the line can be determined. This measure is comparable to the standard deviation of a distribution; the only difference is that this measure the variation around the line rather than around the mean. This measure, known as

σ_{yx}, is equal to $\frac{\sqrt{\Sigma(y-Y)^2}}{n}$, where y represents the observed value for a given x and y represents the value of y calculated by substituting the same value of x in the equation of the regression line. In other words, it is the square root of the average of the squares of the y deviations from the regression line. It can be shown algebraically that:

$$\frac{\sqrt{\Sigma(y-Y)^2}}{n} = \sigma_y\sqrt{1-r^2} \quad ...(12.18)$$

when n, or the number of observations is large, the value of yx may be calculated more easily from the alternate formula. If the first formula is used, the value of Y must be calculated for every value of x, n differences must be calculated, squared and

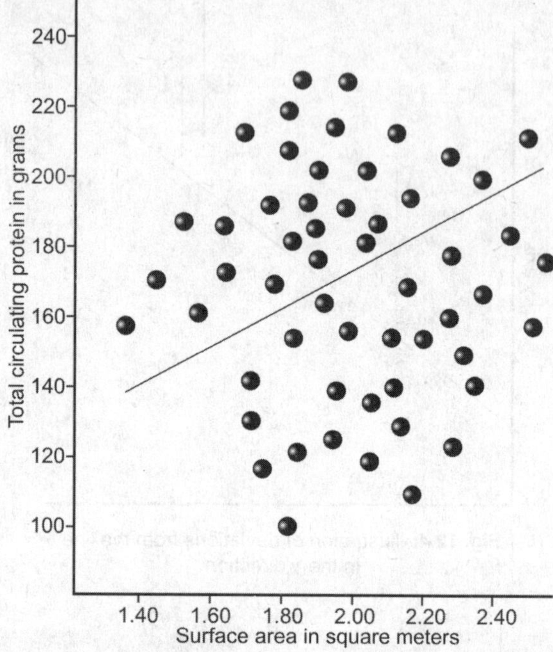

Fig. 12.6: Relationship between total circulating protein and surface area with regression line, $y = 40.604 + 72.169x$

summed. All the added calculations necessary for the second formula are the summation of the squares of the y values and the determination of y and r from the appropriate formulas.

For these particular data, the alternate formula is much simpler. Substituting in the alternate formula.

$$\sigma_{yx=} 26.47\sqrt{1-(0.46)^2} = 23.48\,\text{gm}$$

This standard error of estimate, as it is often called, is a measure of the residual variation about the line. It measures the agreement between the y values observed and those predicated from the observed values of x. If there is correlation between the two variables, yx, will always be smaller than y, the standard deviation of the y values from the mean, all the y observations. In this particular example, the variation around the line is not much less than the variation of the y values from y since the correlation coefficient is small.

This standard error of estimate is also useful in determining confidence intervals for the prediction of the y value for any given value of x. For details of this method a good textbook at the more advanced level should be consulted.

It would be possible to minimize the x deviations as well as the y deviations. The distances of the points W, S and T, which were shown as distances in the y direction in Figure 12.7, have been measured now as distances from the line in the x directions. To do this, involves the same method as before except that the x and y values are interchanged. The equation of the line is $x = \text{A} + \text{B}y$. The equations which must be solved to determine A and B are:

$$\Sigma x = n\text{A} + \text{B}\Sigma y \qquad ...(12.19)$$

$$\Sigma xy = \text{A}\Sigma y + \text{B}\Sigma y^2 \qquad ...(12.20)$$

In this equation, B is the increase in the average value of x per unit increase in y and A is the value of x when y is zero or it tells when the regression line crosses the x-axis.

The variation around this line is measured as before except that the differences are those between the x values for a given y value and the X calculated from the regression line for the same y value. The

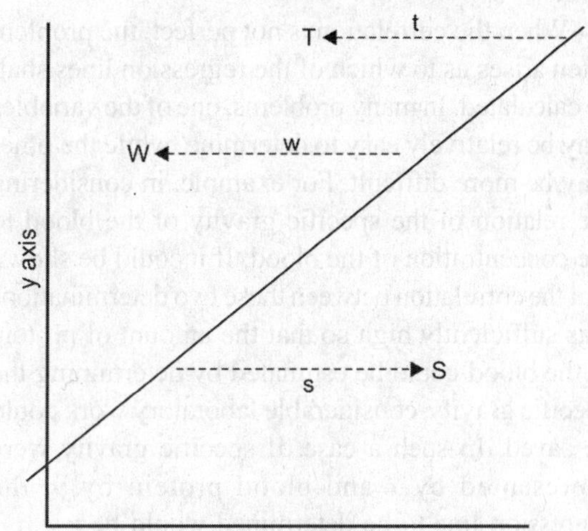

Fig. 12.7: Illustration of deviations from the line in the x direction

formula written in the two forms used before is:

$$\sqrt{\Sigma(x-\text{X})^2} \text{ or } \sigma_x\sqrt{1-r^2} \qquad ...(12.21)$$

Fundamentally, what is the difference in these two regression lines and under what circumstances will there be only one line? The first line ($y = a + bx$) is known as the regression line of y on x. That is, it is the line that would be used for the prediction of value of y, from given values of x. It was calculated in such a way that the sum of the squares differences between the observed y and the predicted Y (determined by substitution in the equation of the regression line) would be the smallest possible.

The second line ($x = \text{A} + \text{B}y$) is known as the regression line of x on y. It is the line that would be used for the prediction of x values for given y values. It was calculated in such a way that the sum of the squares of the differences between the observed x value and the predicted x should be minimum.

When there is perfect correlation, the two lines will be identical. The higher the degree of relationship or the higher the value of r, the smaller will be the residual variation. The two lines will always intersect at the point that represents the mean of the x values and the mean of the y values, since both must pass through the point $\bar{x}$, $\bar{y}$.

When the correlation is not perfect, the problem often arises as to which of the regression lines shall be calculated. In many problems, one of the variables may be relatively easy to determine, while the other may be more difficult. For example, in considering the relation of the specific gravity of the blood to the concentration of the blood. If it could be shown that the correlation between these two determinations was sufficiently high so that the amount of protein in the blood could be estimated by determining the specific gravity, considerable laboratory work could be saved. In such a case, if specific gravity were represented by x and blood protein by y, the regression line to be determined would be $y = a + bx$ what is the line so calculated that the y deviations are minimized. When only one line is to be fitted it is customary, although not necessary, to designate the variable to the estimated (sometimes called the dependent variable) as the y variable and the variable from which the other is to be estimated as the x variable (called the independent variable).

If estimations of both y from x and x from y are to be made, which is very uncommon, both regression lines must be calculated. To be useful in estimations, the correlation between the two variables must be high and the variability about the line must be low. It should also be stated that in most instances, prediction of values beyond the range of those used in determining the equation of the regression line should not be made. Regression lines are used also in certain problems is calibration in which only one variable is measured at fixed points on a scale of time, temperature, dilution, etc. Such a problem would be measurement of optical density for solutions of varying but predefined dilution. Here, only the regression of optical density on dilution has any meaning.

Example 1: From the data given below estimate the most likely height of a father whose son's height is 70".

Father's: Mean height is 67" and a sd of 3.5"

Son's: Mean height is 65" with a sd of 2.5"

The coefficient of correlation between the heights of fathers and sons is +0.8.

Solution: Let x, y be the variables corresponding to the heights of sons and fathers.

$\therefore$ Then, $\bar{x} = 65, \bar{y} = 67, \sigma_x = 2.5, r_{xy} = 0.8$

Now, $b_{yx} = \dfrac{r\sigma_y}{\sigma_x} = \dfrac{(0.8)(3.5)}{2.5} = 1.12$

$\therefore$ The equation of line of regression of y on x is

$$y - \bar{y} = b_{yx}(x - \bar{x})$$

$\Rightarrow y - 67 = 1.12\,(x - 65)$

$\Rightarrow y = 1.12x - 5.8$ ...(i)

Height of a father whose son's height is 70" is = Estimate of y for $x = 70$.

Putting $x = 70$ in (i), we get

$$Y = (1.12) \times 70 - 5.8 = 78.4 - 5.8 = 72.6"$$

Example 2: Given the following results of the height and weight of 1,000 students: $\bar{Y} = 68$ inches, $\bar{X} = 150$ lbs, $r = 0.60$, $\sigma_y = 2.50$ inches, $\sigma_x = 10$ lbs. Amit weighs 100 lbs. Sumit is 5 feet tall. Estimate the height of Amit from his weight and the weight of Sumit from his height.

Solution: Here,

Height = Y Weight = X

$\bar{Y} = 68$ inches $\bar{X} = 150$ lbs

$\sigma_y = 2.50$ inches, $\sigma_x = 10$ lbs

a. The regression equation of Y on X is

$$Y - \bar{Y} = r\frac{\sigma_y}{\sigma_x}(X - \bar{X})$$

Or $Y - 68 = 0.60 \times \dfrac{2.50}{10}(X - 150)$

$\Rightarrow Y - 68 = 0.15X - 9$

$\Rightarrow Y = 0.15X - 9 + 68$

$\therefore Y = 0.15X + 59$

When Amit's weight X = 100 lbs, his height

$Y = 0.15 \times 100 + 59$

$= 15 + 59 = 74$ inches

$\therefore$ Required height of Amit = 74 inches.

b. The regression equation of X on $\overline{Y}$ is

$$X - \overline{X} = r\frac{\sigma_x}{\sigma_y}(Y - \overline{Y})$$

or $X - 150 = 0.60 \times \frac{10}{2.5}(Y - 68)$

or $X - 150 = 2.4(Y - 68)$

or $X - 150 = 2.4Y - 163.2$

or $X = 2.4Y - 163.2 + 150$

$\therefore$ $X = 2.4Y - 13.2$

When Sumit's height Y = 5 feet = 60 inches,

His weight $X = 2.4 \times 60 - 13.2 = 144 - 13.2$

$= 130.8$ lbs.

$\therefore$ Required weight of Sumit = 130.8 lbs.

Example 3: Find the regression of x on y from the following data:

$\Sigma x = 24$, $\Sigma y = 44$, $\Sigma xy = 306$, $N = 4$

Find the value of x, when y = 6.

Solution: Here,

$$\overline{X} = \frac{\Sigma x}{N} = \frac{24}{4} = 6$$

$$\overline{Y} = \frac{\Sigma y}{N} = \frac{44}{4} = 11$$

Regression coefficient $(b_{xy}) = r\frac{\sigma_x}{\sigma_y}$

$$\frac{N\Sigma xy - \Sigma x\Sigma y}{N\Sigma y^2} = \frac{4 \times 306 - 24 \times 44}{4 \times 576 - (44)^2}$$

$$= \frac{1224 - 1056}{2304 - 1936} = \frac{168}{368} = 0.46$$

The regression equation of x on y is

$$x - \bar{x} = r\frac{\sigma_x}{\sigma_y}(y - \bar{y})$$

Or $x - 6 = 0.46(y - 11)$

Or $x - 6 = 0.46y - 5.17$

Or $x = 0.46y - 5.06 + 6$

Or $x = 0.46y + 0.94$

When $y = 6$, $x = 0.46 \times 6 + 0.94 = 3.70$

Required value of $x = 3.70$

Simple Regression

As mentioned earlier, for predicting a variable from another, it is essential to set up a regression equation or equation of the regression line. Furthermore, it has also been mentioned that the equation of a straight line is based upon two constants, *a* and *b*. Hence, it is necessary to calculate the values of these constants before predictions can be made. The procedure of setting up regression equations will be demonstrated on raw data as well as on the information about coefficient of correlation, standard deviations and means.

Regression Equations from Raw Scores

Five subjects have been given two tests, X and Y. Their scores are given in Table 12.1 under the

Table 12.1

Simple regression from raw scores

X	Y	X^2	Y^2	XY
10	12	100	144	120
11	18	121	324	198
12	20	144	400	240
9	10	81	100	90
8	10	64	100	80
X = 50	**Y = 70**	**$\Sigma X^2 = 510$**	**$\Sigma Y^2 = 1068$**	**XY = 728; $M_x = 10$; $M_y = 14$**

columns X and Y. Set up regression equations for predicting Y from X and also X from Y.

Prediction Equation

The regression line is also known as *prediction equation*. Once the constants *a* and *b* are calculated, there remains two unknown variables in the regression equation viz., Y and X. Moreover, we know Y depends on X in the case of regression equation of Y on X. Under the presumption that the trend of change in Y corresponding to X remains the same, the value of Y can be estimated for any value of X. But such a presumption rarely holds good for a very wide range of X values. Hence, the fitted regression line gives a better estimate of Y for a given value of X, which is within the range of X values, taken into consideration at the time of calculation of *a* and *b* or not much beyond the values of X involved in the calculations. For example, we know that the crop yield increases with the increases in the quantity of fertilizers applied in the field. But beyond certain fertilizer-dose, the increase in yield is negligible. Hence, the estimation of the yield of a crop for a fertilizer dose should be restricted only for doses within certain limits. In industry, the production of a product depends on the consumption of electricity. But it does not mean that if we go on increasing the consumption of electricity, the production of a product will keep on increasing in the same proportion. It holds true only up to a certain limit because many other factors besides consumption of electricity affect the production. The fitting of a regression line through actual data is given below.

Predicting Y from X Scores

Step I: Find the Value of b Coefficient for Predicting Y from X

$$b_{yx} = \frac{N\Sigma XY - (\Sigma X)(\Sigma Y)}{N\Sigma X^2 - (\Sigma X)^2} \quad ...(12.22)$$

Substituting the values

$$b_{yx} = \frac{(5)(728) - (50)(70)}{(5)(510) - (50)(50)} = 2.8$$

Step II: Find the Value of a Coefficient for Predicting Y from X

The formula for calculating the value of *a* is as follows:

$$a_{yx} = M_y - b_{yx} M_x$$

Substituting the values, we obtain

$$a_{yx} = 14 - (2.8)(10)$$
$$= 14 - 28$$
$$= -14$$

Due care should be taken about the sign of this value, especially when it is negative.

Step III: Step up the Full Regression Equation

The full regression equation for predicting Y scores from X scores would be

$$Y' = bX + a$$

In which *y'* is the predicted y score and *b* and *a* are regression constants.
Substituting the values, we obtain

$$Y' = 2.8X + (-14)$$
$$= 2.8X - 14$$

It means that a Y score can be viewed as 2.8 times the X score with a constant of 14 subtracted.

Predicted X from Y Scores

In this situation, Y is the independent variable and X is the criterion variable. The steps are the same as shown above for predicting Y from X. The formulas will, no doubt, undergo some change which may be noted carefully.

$$b_{xy} = \frac{N\Sigma XY - (\Sigma X)(\Sigma Y)}{N\Sigma Y^2 - (\Sigma Y)^2} \quad ...(12.23)$$

There is a change in the denominator only.

Substituting the values, we obtain

$$b_{yx} = \frac{(5)(728) - (50)(70)}{(5)(1068) - (70)(70)} = 0.318$$

$a_{xy} = \text{Mx} - b_{xy}\, \text{M}_y$

Substituting the value, we obtain

$a_{xy} = 10 - (0.318)\,(14)$
$= 10 - 4.452$
$= 5.548$

The regression equation for predicting X from Y will be:

$X' = bY + a$
$= 0.318Y - 5.548$

It means that an X score can be viewed as 0.318 times the Y score plus a constant of 5.548 added.

Values of regression coefficient *a* and *b* both the situations can also be obtained by using and solving the simultaneous normal equations given below:

Predicting Y from X

$\Sigma Y = Na + b\Sigma X$ and
$\Sigma XY = a\Sigma X + b\Sigma X^2$

Predicting X from Y

$\Sigma X = Na + b\Sigma Y$ and
$\Sigma XY = a\Sigma Y + b\Sigma Y^2$

The student may try the above simultaneous normal equations to check the solution by the other method given earlier. The notation is the same as shown in Table 12.1.

Regression Equations from SD's, r and M's

In situations when standard deviations, coefficient of correlation and means are given it is advisable to use this information to set up regression equations for predicting Y from X and X from Y.

Example: On the basis of the following information, set up the two regression equations:

	M	σ	
X	65	6	0.80
Y	75	8	

Predict values of Y for X = 70, 72, 48 and 60.

Predicting Y from X

The values of the two regression coefficients *a* and *b* can be calculated as below:

$$b_{yx} = r_{yx} \frac{\sigma_y}{\sigma_x} \qquad ...(12.24)$$

b_{yx}, with the subscripts in this order implies that we are predicting Y from X.

$b_{yx} = 0.8\frac{8}{6} = 1.064$

$a_{yx} = M_y - (M_x)\, b_{yx}$
$= 75 - (65)\,(1.064)$
$= 5.84$

The complete prediction equation will now is

$Y = b_{yx}X + a_{yx}$

$Y = 1.064x + 5.84$

The entire regression equation can also be obtained by using the composite formula given below

$$Y' = r\left(\frac{\sigma_y}{\sigma_x}\right)(X - M_x) + M_y \qquad ...(12.25)$$

Substituting the values, we obtain

$Y' = 0.8\,(8/6)\,(X\text{-}65) + 75$
$= 1.064\,((X\text{-}65) + 75$
$= 1.064X + 5.84$ (checks with the previous result).

Predicting X from Y

$b_{xy} = r_{xy} \frac{\sigma_x}{\sigma_y}$

$= 0.8\,(6/8)$
$= 0.6$

$a_{xy} = M_x - (M_y)\, b_{xy}$
$= 65 - (75)\,(0.6)$
$= 20$

The regression equation then will be X = 0.6Y + 20.

By Using Composite Formula

$Y' = r\frac{\sigma_x}{\sigma_y}(Y - M_y) + M_x$
$= (0.8)(6/8)\,(Y - 75) - 65$
$= (0.6)(Y - 75) - 65$
$= 0.6Y + 20$ (checks with previous result).

On the basis of the regression equations set up by the process shown above, prediction of Y scores from X scores and X scores from Y scores can be made simply by substituting the given values of a variable.

Predicting Y Values from X = 70, 72, 48 and 60

∴ Y' = 1.064X + 5.84 (set up earlier)

∴ X = 70; Y' = (1.064) (70) + 5.84 = 80.32

X = 72; Y' = (1.064) (72) + 5.84 = 82.45

X = 48; Y' = (1.064) (48) + 5.84 = 56.85

X = 60; Y' = (1.064) (60) + 5.84 = 69.68

Predicting X values from Y = 75, 65, 82, and 72

X' = 0.6Y + 20 (Already set up)

Then

For Y = 75; X' = (0.6) (75) + 20 = 65.00

Y = 65; X' = (0.6) (65) + 20 = 59.00

Y = 82; X' = (0.6) (82) + 20 = 69.2

Y = 72; X' = (0.6) (72) + 20 = 67.2

The student may try some other values of one variable and predict the values of the other variable.

Relationship between b coefficients and r

One important check of the accuracy of the two regression equations is that

$b_{yx} b_{xy} = r^2$ (Relation of *b's* to r^2) ...(12.26)

or $r = \sqrt{b_{xy}\, b_{xy}}$

In other words the coefficient of correlation is equal to the square root of the product of the two *b* coefficients. In our example, $b_{yx} = 1.064$, $b_{xy} = 0.6$

Hence, $r^2 = 1.064 \times 0.6$

$= 0.64$ (rounded)

$r = \sqrt{0.64}$

$= 0.8$ (checks with our *r* above)

Another check of the accuracy of the prediction equations is that the Y' for the M_x will be equal to M*y*; and X' for M_y will be equal to M*x*.

Standard Error of the Estimates

The deviations between the predicted scores and the actual scores introduce an error. These deviations (Y – Y' and X – X') can be squared, summed, averaged and then the square root extracted. This index of the discrepancies between the observed and the predicted values is called the standard error of the estimates. When we predict on the basis of the regression equations, we need not calculate Y – Y' or X – X'. The SE of the estimate can be calculated from the correlation coefficient and the standard deviation. The formulas are:

SE of estimate for predicting Y from X,

$$\sigma_{yx} = \sigma_y \sqrt{1 - r^2_{xy}} \quad \text{...(12.27)}$$

SE of estimate for predicting X from Y,

$$\sigma_{yx} = \sigma_x \sqrt{1 - r^2_{xy}} \quad \text{...(12.28)}$$

$$\sigma_{yx} = 8\sqrt{1 - 0.64} = 8 \times 0.6 = 4.8 \text{ and}$$

$$\sigma_{yx} = 6\sqrt{1 - 0.64} = 6 \times 0.6 = 3.6$$

The interpretation of SE of the estimate is like that of SE of measurement. We assume normality and interpret the results by setting up probability or odds. In our example above, an X score of 60 has a Y' score of 69.68. Hence, the confidence interval for various odds can be set up as follows:

68% or 2 to 1 odds: Y' ± $1\sigma_{xy}$

: 69.68 ± 4.80

: 64.88 to 74.48

Hence, the odds are two to one that any individual whose X score is equal to 60 will not fall below 64.88 or go above 74.48, these scores being one *xy* below and above the predicted Y.

For 95% : Y' ± 1.96 *xy*

For 99% : Y' ± 2.58 *xy*

The values of 1.96 and 2.58 have been taken from the normal curve area tables.

The student may try the interpretation of other scores at these levels.

Assumptions

The setting up of regression equation, making predictions and calculation of the SE of the estimate involve certain assumptions which need to be made explicit.

Firstly, we assume that the relationship between the two variables is linear. It means that a straight line is the best way to describe the relationship. Linearity can be gauged by taking a look at the scatter plot. Statistical tests of linearity also exist.

Secondly, we assume homoscedasticity which means that Y scores in any 6 single column have essentially the same standard deviation. Homoscedasticity can be translated as "similar variability" in each column.

Thirdly, we assume that Y scores within any one column are normally distributed. This assumption is essential when we interpret scores by using normal distribution.

Multiple Prediction

We have already discussed the correlation and regression based on two variables – one independent and the other dependent or criterion. It was a situation involving simple regression. However, actual relationships in social sciences are not always as simple as that. There could be two or more variables affecting or jointly related to a dependent variable. School marks may be a joint function of intelligence and the number of hours at study or a rural and urban setting. Hence, in such situations one has to keep in view multiple dependence instead of the idea of dependence of one variable on another single variable. Multiple dependence means the dependence of one variable on two or more independent variables. Success in sports may be related both to aptitude and training. Multiple dependence can be indicated by the statistic, the coefficient of multiple correlation, R.

The Coefficient of Multiple Correlation, R

Multiple correlation indicates the strength of relationship between dependent variable and two or more independent variables taken together. It is related to the inter-correlations among independent variable as well as to their correlations with the dependent variable. The process of calculation of the coefficient of multiple correlation. R is illustrated below by taking hypothetical data.

Table 12.2

Inter-correlation among four variables

Variables	X_2	X_3	X_4	X_1
X_2		0.50	0.60	0.70
X_3	0.50	-	0.20	0.80
X_4	0.60	0.20	-	0.90
X_1	0.70	0.80	0.90	-
M_x	73	55	60	78
σ_x	12	10	15	16

X_1 = Criterion or dependent variable

X_2, X_3, X_4 = Means and SD's respectively of the four variables

Three-Variable Solution

We take a three-variable problem and demonstrate the process of calculation of R and setting up the regression equation. The formula for the calculation of coefficient of multiple correlation is:

$$R^2_{1\text{-}23} = \frac{r^2_{12} + r^2_{13} - 2r_{12}r_{13}r_{23}}{1 - r^2_{23}} \quad ...(12.29)$$

$R_{1\text{-}23}$ is the square root of $R^2_{1\text{-}23}$

r_{12}, r_{23}, r_{34}, are correlations between pairs of variables as indicated by their subscripts

$R_{1\text{-}23}$ = Coefficient of multiple correlation between X_1 and a combination or X_2 and X_3

Substituting the values of correlation coefficients in formula (12.29), we obtain

$$R^2_{1\text{-}23} = \frac{(0.70)^2 + (0.80)^2 - 2 \times 0.70 \times 0.80 \times 0.50}{1 - (0.50)^2}$$

$$= \frac{0.49 + 0.64 - 0.56}{1 - 0.25} = 0.76$$

$$= R_{1\text{-}23} = \sqrt{0.76} = 0.87$$

Formula 12.29 can be easily modified to obtain multiple correlation among other combinations of variables. For example

$$R^2_{1\text{-}34} = \frac{r^2_{13} + r^2_{14} - 2r_{13} 2r_{14} r_{34}}{1 - r^2_{34}}$$

The student may try to write the formula for $R^2_{1\text{-}24}$ himself. We should remember two important principles regarding multiple correlation. These are based on extent of correlation between the independent variables and each independent variable with dependent variable.

1. An increase in the correlation between the dependent variable and independent variable leads to an increase in the value of R.
2. A decrease in the correlations between independent variables leads to an increase in the value of R.

From these principles, it is implied that a maximum R will be obtained when correlations with X_1 (criterion) are large and intercorrelations of X_2, X_3 ….. , X_m are small.

If intercorrelation of independent variables is zero, formula (12.29) will be reduced to:

$$R^2_{1\text{-}23} = r^2_{12} + r^2_{13}$$

Therefore, the last term in the numerator to 0: and the denominator to 1.

The Multiple-Regression Equation

In the preceding section, a multiple correlation has been calculated by taking a three variable problem. The same will be extended for the purpose of setting up the multiple regression equation for prediction of values of X_1 from knowledge of the values of X_2 and X_3. The equation for multiple prediction for our problem will be:

$$X_1 = a + b_{12\text{-}3} X_2 + b_{13\text{-}2} X_3 \qquad ...(12.30)$$

In which, X_1 = the predicted or dependent variable

b coefficients = the multiplying constant or weights

a coefficients = a constant to be added.

B coefficients are the optimal weights which ensure maximization of correlation between predicted and observed X values. These are based on the principle of least squares.

To set up the prediction, we must solve for the value of *b* coefficients. The various formulas are:

$$b_{12\text{-}3} = \frac{\sigma_1}{\sigma_2} \beta_{12-3} \qquad ...(12.31)$$

(Partial regression coefficient, keeping X_3 variable constant)

$$b_{13\text{-}2} = \frac{\sigma_1}{\sigma_3} \beta_{12-3} \qquad ...(12.32)$$

(Partial regression coefficient, keeping X_2 variable constant) in which σ_1, σ_2 and σ_3 are standard deviations of variables X_1, X_2, and X_3. $b_{12\text{-}3}$ and $b_{13\text{-}2}$ are standard partial regression coefficients. The first partials out or keeps constant the effect of X_3, while the second, that of X_2, as is done in partial correlation. The beats, $b_{12\text{-}3}$ and $b_{13\text{-}2}$ are found as below:

$$\beta_{12\text{-}3} = \frac{r_{12} - r_{13} r_{23}}{1 - r^2_{23}}$$

$$\beta_{13\text{-}2} = \frac{r_{13} - r_{12} r_{23}}{1 - r^2_{23}}$$

(Standard partial regression coefficient or weights) in which correlation coefficients, for various combinations of variables have been indicated by the subscripts.

Substituting the values from Table 12.2, we solve the formulas from 12.31 to 12.32. We first calculate the values of β weights:

$$\beta_{12-3} = \frac{0.70 - (0.80)(0.50)}{1 - (0.50)^2}$$

$$= \frac{0.80 - 0.40}{1 - 0.25} = 0.4$$

$$\beta_{13-2} = \frac{0.80-(0.70)(0.50)}{1-(0.50)^2}$$

$$= \frac{0.80-0.35}{1-0.25} = 0.6$$

We may now solve for the b coefficients by means of Formulas 12.31 and 12.32.

$$b_{12\text{-}3} = \frac{16}{12}(0.4) = 1.333 \times 0.4 = 0.533$$

$$b_{13\text{-}2} = \frac{16}{10}(0.6) = 1.6 \times 0.6 = 0.96$$

Now, let us calculate the value of a constant

$$a_{1\text{-}23} = M_1 - b_{12.3}\, M_2 - b_{13\text{-}2}\, M_3$$

In which M_1, M_2 and M_3 are the means of the variables X_1, X_2, and X_3 respectively.

Substituting the values, we obtain

$$a_{1\text{-}23} = 78 - (0.4)(72) - (0.6)(55)$$
$$= 78 - 28.8 - 33 = 16.2$$

Now, substituting these values in equation (12.30)

$$X'_1 = a + b_{12\text{-}3} \times 2 + b_{13\text{-}2} \times 3$$
$$= 16.2 + 0.533 \times 2 + 0.96 \times 3$$

Now we can predict the values of X_1 from the knowledge of the values of X_2 and X_3.

For example, if X_2=60 and X_3 = 40, the predicted X_1 score will be:

$$X'_1 = 16.2 + 0.533\, X_2 + 0.96\, X_3$$
$$= 16.2 + 31.98 + 38.40$$
$$= 86.58$$

Calculation of R from Betas

Beta coefficients can also be used to calculate multiple R as follows:

$$R^2_{1\text{-}23} = \beta_{12\text{-}3}\, R_{12} + \beta_{13\text{-}2}\, r_{13}$$

(R from Beta weights)

Substituting the values

$$R^2_{1\text{-}23} = (0.4)(0.7) + (0.6)(0.8)$$
$$= 0.28 + 0.48$$
$$= 0.76$$
$$R^2_{1\text{-}23} = 0.76 = 0.87$$

(Checks with our value calculated earlier by formula 12.29).

Standard Error of Estimate from Multiple Prediction

Standard error of estimate from multiple prediction can be calculated to know as to how far the predicted values would deviate from the obtained ones. The formula for the purpose is:

$$\sigma_{1-23} = \sigma_1 \sqrt{1 - R^2_{1-23}} \qquad ...(12.33)$$

In which, σ_1 is the SD of the X_1 variable and R^2 is the multiple R squared.

In our example,

$$\sigma_{1-23} = 16\sqrt{1-(0.87)^2}$$
$$= 16 \times 0.24 = 3.84$$

The interpretation of SE of estimate is similar to that in the case of simple regression. Here, it can be said that two-thirds of the obtained X_1 values will lie between 3.84 points of the predicted X_1 values.

Other Methods

Multiple correlation with more than three variables can be calculated and prediction equations set up, by using the Doolittle-solution and other methods which are given in texts on advanced statistics. Statisticians have devised methods to find out a correlation between a combination of dependent variables and a combination of independent variables. It is called Canonial correlation and requires the help of a computer as the computation work involved is enormous. Multiple regression equations are used in the preparations of tests on the basis of the weights allotted to various sub-tests. The contribution of various components can also be calculated.

EXERCISES

1. Briefly explain the concept and uses of regression.
2. What is scatter diagram and its role in regression?
3. Explain the method of estimating parameters of a regression equation.

CHAPTER 13 Standard Estimates

Introduction

Estimation is concerned with making inference and generalization about the values of the parameter. An estimator as a rule, is a method or a formula, for estimating a parameter. Thus, a sample mean is frequently used as a estimator or estimate, of a population mean μ. Instead of estimating a parameter with a single number a point estimate, it is often desirable to use an internal called a class interval. A (1 – X) percent confidence internal for a parameter (P) is given by a pair of statistics 'P' and '*p*' which are such that one can assert with a probability of (1 – X) that the interval from P to P contain P and is usually chosen 0.05, 0.01 or 0.001. Standard deviations and standard errors are utilized for measuring the reliability of an estimate of population values or parameters. Confidence limits are fixed for mean values or proportions or percentages or variances are based on small sample.

Standard estimation is a method by which population parameters are estimated from sample information. Statistical helps in estimating the mean, standard deviation, etc., of population quantities. It is possible to draw valid conclusions about the population parameters from the sampling distribution. We have a sample from a population involving all unknown parameter, such as the mean. The problem is *to construct a sample quantity* that will serve *to estimate the unknown parameter*, viz. population mean μ. Such a sample quantity is called the *estimator* and the actual numerical value obtained by evaluating an estimator in a given instance is the estimate. For example, the sample mean is an estimator of population mean μ. If for a specific sample, the sample mean is 7.85, then 7.85 is our estimator for the population mean. It is important to note that an estimator must be a statistic and it must depend only on the sample and not on the parameter to be estimated. In other words, an estimator is a statistic which for all practical purposes, can be used in place of unknown parameter of the population. Estimation of population parameters like mean, standard deviation, variance, correlation, etc., from the corresponding sample statistic is one of the important problems of statistical inference.

There are many ways of estimating a parameter from the data of the sample and the knowledge of the form of sampling distribution. Some of these ways are better than others. The theory of estimation deals with these and related matters. Obviously, estimated are bound to differ from the true value of the population parameters. But the tolerable divergence between the estimates and the true value of the population parameter may be specified before hand. The theory of sampling helps in determining the probability of such divergence.

Types of Estimation

When estimating parameters of population, the following two types of estimate are possible:

i. Point estimation
ii. Interval estimation.

Point Estimation

In **point estimation** a single statistic is used to provide an estimate of the population parameter. In other words, **the estimate of a population given by a single number is called the point estimation of the parameter.** In point estimation, we find a statistic which may be used for or replace an unknown parameter of the population for all practical purposes. A good estimator is one which may be used for or replace an unknown parameter of the population for all practical purposes. A good estimator is one which is as close to the true value of the parameter as possible. A good estimator must possess the following characteristics:

- Unbiasedness
- Consistency
- Efficiency
- Sufficiency.

Unbiasedness

A static $t = r(x_1, x_2, x_3 \ldots\ldots, x_n)$ is said to be an unbiased estimate of the corresponding population parameter θ, if

$$E(x) = \mu$$

Consistency

A statistics $t = t_n = t(x_1, x_2, x_3 \ldots\ldots, x_n)$ based on the sample size n is said to be consistent estimator of the parameter θ, if $t_n \to \theta$ and $n \to \infty$ Symbolically,

$$\lim_{n \to \infty} P(t_n \to \theta)$$

Efficiency

If t_1 and t_2 are two consistent estimators of a parameter 0 such that **Var** $(t_1) <$ **Var** (t_2) for all sample size n, then t_1 is said to be more efficient than t_2. In other words, **an estimator with lesser variability is said to be more efficient and consequently more reliable than the other.**

Sufficiency

A statistic $t = t(x_1, x_2, x_3 \ldots\ldots x_n)$ is said to be a sufficient estimator of parameter if it contains all the information in the sample regarding the parameter. In other words, if $t = t(x_1, x_2, x_3 \ldots\ldots x_n)$ is a statistic based on a random sample $(x_1, x_2, \ldots x_n)$ of size n from a population with probability density function PĐf = P(x, θ), then it is a sufficient estimator of, if the conditional probability $P[(x_1 \cap x_2 \cap x_3 \ldots\ldots \cap x_n)/t = k]$ does not depend on, i.e. $P(x, \theta) = p(x)$.

Estimation of Population Parameters

Let $X_1, X_2, \ldots, X_n$ be a random sample of size n from a population of N units and $x_1, x_2, \ldots, x_n$ be the corresponding observed values. The values of the known parameter(s) should be estimated from the set of these sample observations. These estimates are often single valued which are known as point estimates. Also, many times an interval is to be estimated in which the parameter is expected to lie with a certain level of confidence. Here we will not pursue the estimation theory and hence the formulae for sample mean, sample variance, etc. are given directly.

Some properties of estimates are also discussed in this chapter. Formulae are presented in terms of x_i ($i = 1, 2, \ldots n$), the actual observed value corresponding to X_i.

Formulae for Mean and Variance

Let $U_1, U_2, \ldots, U_N$ be N population units. A random sample of n units is selected. Suppose the observations on the sampled units are $x_1, x_2, \ldots, x_n$. The sample mean,

$$\bar{x} = \frac{x_1 + x_2 + \ldots + x_n}{n} \qquad \ldots(13.1)$$

$$= \frac{1}{n} \sum_i x_i \qquad \ldots(13.1.1)$$

for $i = 1, 2, ..., n$.

The sample variance,

$$s^2 = \frac{1}{(n-1)}\sum_i (x_i - \bar{x})^2 \qquad ...(13.2)$$

$$= \frac{1}{(n-1)}\{\sum x_i^2 - n\bar{x}^2\} \qquad ...(13.2.1)$$

$$= \frac{1}{(n-1)}\left\{\sum_i x_i^2 - (\sum_i x_i)^2/n\right\} \qquad ...(13.2.2)$$

Let the population mean be μ and variance σ^2. $\bar{x}$ is an estimated value of μ and s^2 is an estimated value σ^2.

Now, we define a special term s^2, which is slightly different from σ^2 and is given as,

$$s^2 = \frac{1}{(n-1)}\sum_i (x_i - \mu)^2 \qquad ...(13.3)$$

$$= \frac{1}{(n-1)}\left\{\sum_i X^2 - n\mu^2\right\} \qquad ...(13.3.1)$$

where $i = 1, 2, ..., n$.

Properties of Estimates

Unbiasedness

An estimate is said to be unbiased if its expected value is equal to its parameter value. For example, if $\bar{x}$ is an estimate of μ, $\bar{x}$ will be an unbiased estimate if and only if:

$$E(\bar{x}) = \mu \qquad ...(13.4)$$

The expectation may well be understood with this example. If from a population, we take all possible samples of size n and take the mean of all samples, the mean of the estimates is known as the expected value. It can theoretically be proved that $\bar{x}$ is an unbiased estimate of μ. In formula (13.2) for s^2, the divisor is $(n-1)$ instead of n. The reason for this is that using the divisor $(n-1)$ makes σ^2 an unbiased estimate of s^2, i.e.,

$$E(s^2) = s^2 \qquad ...(13.5)$$

Hence, the above conjecture of unbiasedness will be shown through an example.

Example: A population of five units has the observations:

7, 6, 8, 4, 10

Random samples of three units are drawn such that no unit is repeated in a sample and the order of selection does not matter. Out of the 5 units, there can be 10 samples each consisting of 3 units.

Possible samples, their means and variances are given in the following Table 13.1:

Table 13.1

Means and variance of sample

Sample Nos.	1	2	3	4	5
Observations	7, 6, 8	7, 6, 4	7, 6, 10	7, 8, 4	7, 8, 10
$\bar{x}$	7	17/3	23/3	19/3	25/3
s^2	1	7/3	13/3	13/3	7/3
	6	7	8	9	10
	7, 4, 10	6, 8, 4	6, 8, 10	6, 4, 10	8, 4, 10
	7	6	8	20/3	22/3
	9	4	4	28/3	28/3

Mean of

$$\bar{x}' = \frac{1}{10}\left(7+\frac{17}{3}+\frac{23}{3}+\frac{19}{3}+\frac{25}{3}+7+6+8+\frac{20}{3}+\frac{22}{3}\right)$$

$$= \frac{210}{30} = 7$$

Similarly, mean of $s^2 = \frac{50}{10} = 5.0$

Population mean $\mu = \frac{35}{5} = 7$

and variance

$$S^2 = \frac{1}{4}\{(7-7)^2+(6-7)^2+(8-7)^2+(4-7)^2+(10-7)^2\}$$

$$= \frac{20}{4} = 5.0$$

The above calculations verify the statement that the sample mean is an unbiased estimate of population mean whereas, s^2 is an unbiased estimate of s^2.

Simple Consistency

The notion of consistency is mainly concerned with infinite population. If T_n is an estimator of a parameter θ where T_n is based on a random samplex $X_1, X_2, ..., X_n$ such that $T_n = t_n(X_1, X_2, ... X_n)$ then the sequence $\{T_n\}$ is said to be a consistent estimator of θ if for every $\varepsilon > 0$, the following condition holds:

$$\lim_{n\to\infty} P\{\theta - \varepsilon < T_n < \theta + \varepsilon\} = 1 \quad ...(13.6)$$

or $$\lim_{n\to\infty} P\{|T_n - \theta| > \varepsilon\} = 0 \quad ...(13.6.1)$$

Mean Squared Error

If $T_n = t_n(X_1, X_2, ..., X_n)$ be an estimator of a parameter θ, then $E\{(T_n - \theta)^2\}$ is said to be the mean-squared error of the estimator T_n. The sequence of estimators $\{T_n\}$ is said to be a mean squared error consistent if the following condition holds:

$$\lim_{n\to\infty} E\{(T_n - ,)^2\} = 0 \quad ...(13.7)$$

Note: When the observed values $x_1, x_2, ..., x_n$ for $X_1, X_2, ..., X_n$ are substituted in the estimator, we get the estimated value.

Interval Estimation

There are situations where the point estimation is not desirable and we are interested in finding such limits within a known probability or to a known degree of reliance, the value of the population **parameter** is expected to lie. Such a process of estimation is called the **interval estimation.** In other words, an interval estimation is the range of values used in making estimation of a population parameter. Thus, the interval estimation of the **population parameter is the estimation of the population parameter by an interval around the point.** The interval estimation of a population **parameter** θ is the estimation of the parameter θ with the help of the interval $[t-s, t+s]$ where it is the sample statistic i.e., $t - s \leq \theta\ t + s$.

Confidence Interval and Level of Confidence

Both point and interval estimation are ways of drawing inductive references and therefore involve an element of uncertainty. But the interval estimation has advantage over the point estimation as it provides a measure of degree of uncertainty in terms of probability attached to the conclusion. In the interval estimation, the estimate for the parameter lies between two limits. The two limits within which the estimate for the parameter lies are known as **Confidence Limits or Fiducial Limits** and the interval bounded by these two limits are **Confidence Interval or Fiducial Interval.** The confidence interval depends upon the confidence that is required to set it up. **The probability that we associate with an interval is called the confidence level.** It shows the confidently we can say that the interval estimate will include the population parameter. The higher the probability, the more is the confidence. Although any **confidence levels are** 90 percent, 95 percent, 98 percent and 99 percent. In the light of above discussion the interval estimation is defined as:

The interval $[\bar{x} - \delta, \bar{x} + \delta]$, is the interval estimation of the population mean and is called the **confidence interval** for a given value of $\bar{x}$. The end points x–δ are called **confidence or fiducial limits** for the parameter.

$P[C_1 < \theta < C_2]$ for given value of statistic t] $= 1 - \alpha$ where a is the level of significance, the interval $[C_1, C_2]$ within which the unknown parameter is expected to lie is known as Confidence Interval or Fiducial Interval and 1-α is called the confidence coefficient or level of confidence depending upon the desired precision of the estimate [For example $\alpha = 0.01$ gives 99 percent confidence limits], C_1, C_2 are respectively known as lower limit and upper limit of the confidence interval.

The probability with which the confidence interval is attained is called the **level of confidence or confidence coefficient.**

The term 95 percent confidence interval for μ for a normal distribution is

$$\left(\bar{x} - 1.96\frac{\sigma}{\sqrt{n}}, \bar{x} + 1.96\frac{\sigma}{\sqrt{n}}\right) \quad ...(13.8)$$

and it means that we are 95 percent confident of finding the population mean μ lying in the interval

$$\left(\bar{x} - 1.96\frac{\sigma}{\sqrt{n}}, \bar{x} + 1.96\frac{\sigma}{\sqrt{n}}\right)$$

Where x is the sample mean, σ is the variance of population and n is the size of the sample.

In other words, it means that the probability of μ lying in the interval

$$\left(\bar{x} - 1.96\frac{\sigma}{\sqrt{n}}, \bar{x} + 1.96\frac{\sigma}{\sqrt{n}}\right) \quad ...(13.9)$$

is 0.95. Below we give some intervals for a certain level of confidence, when the sampling distribution is taken as normal.

Level of confidence	*Confidence interval around $\bar{x}$*
i. 68.27%	$\left[\bar{x} - \frac{\sigma}{\sqrt{n}}, \bar{x} + \frac{\sigma}{\sqrt{n}}\right]$
ii. 95%	$\left[\bar{x} - 1.96\frac{\sigma}{\sqrt{n}}, \bar{x} + 1.96\frac{\sigma}{\sqrt{n}}\right]$
iii. 95.45%	$\left[\bar{x} - \frac{2\sigma}{\sqrt{n}}, \bar{x} + \frac{2\sigma}{\sqrt{n}}\right]$
iv. 98%	$\left[\bar{x} - \frac{2.33\sigma}{\sqrt{n}}, \bar{x} + \frac{2.33\sigma}{\sqrt{n}}\right]$
v. 99%	$\left[\bar{x} - \frac{2.58\sigma}{\sqrt{n}}, \bar{x} + \frac{2.58\sigma}{\sqrt{n}}\right]$
vi. 99.73%	$\left[\bar{x} - \frac{3\sigma}{\sqrt{n}}, \bar{x} + \frac{3\sigma}{\sqrt{n}}\right]$

If 't' is the sample statistic used to estimate the corresponding population parameter θ, then $(1 - \alpha)$% confidence limits for $\theta = t \pm \text{S.E.}(t) \times t_\alpha$, where S.E. (t) is the standard error t, and α the significant or critical value at significant level α, $t + \text{S.E.}(t) \times t_\alpha$, is the upper limit and $t - \text{S.E.}(t) \times t_\alpha$, is the lower limit of confidence interval

$$[t - \text{S.E.}(t) \times t_\alpha, t + \text{S.E.}(t) \times t_\alpha] \quad ...(13.10)$$

Method to Compute Confidence Limits for a Population Parameter

The following steps enable to compute the confidence limits for the population **parameter** θ in terms of the sample **statistic** t.

1. Compute or select the appropriate sample **statistic** t.
2. Obtain **S.E. (t),** the standard error of the sampling distribution for the sample t.
3. Select the confidence level and corresponding to that **"specific level of confidence"** note down the critical value t_α.

Interval Estimation for Large Samples

As per the central limit theorem for large samples, the underlying distribution of the standardized variate corresponding to the sampling distribution of the sample statistic t will be asymptotically normal, i.e.,

$$Z = \frac{t - E(t)}{\text{S.E.}(t)} \sim N(0,1) \quad ...(13.11)$$

Is a standardized normal variate with mean zero and variance one as $n \to \infty$.

Confidence Interval Estimate of the Mean

Let μ be the population mean and x be the sample mean of the sampling distributions of means. It is also assumed that the sample mean is normal or the sample is large. Then the interval estimate or population mean μ by the sample mean of the sampling distribution of means is given by the following rule:

Working Rule

Step I

Compute $\bar{x}$

Step II

Select the confidence level and the corresponding to that specific level of confidence and note the value of confidence coefficient Z_α or t_α.

Step III

Compute S.E. $(\bar{x})$ with the help of the following results:

Case I

When σ, the standard deviation of the normal population σ is known:

$$\textbf{S.E. }(\bar{x}) = \frac{\sigma}{x} = \frac{\sigma}{\sqrt{n}} \quad ...(13.12)$$

where n is the sample size.

Case II

When σ, the standard deviation of population is not known.

$$\textbf{S.E. }(\bar{x}) = \frac{s}{\sqrt{n-1}} \quad ...(13.13)$$

Where n = Sample size and n is large

s = Standard deviation of the sampling distribution of sample.

Step IV

Construct a confidence level as follows:

Case I

Where s is known and population is normal or any population with large n.

$$\text{Confidence Interval} = [\bar{x} - \text{S.E.}(\bar{x}) \times Z_\alpha, \bar{x} + \text{S.E.}(\bar{x}) \times Z_\alpha] \quad ...(13.14)$$

$$\text{Or} \left[(\bar{x}) - \frac{\sigma}{\sqrt{n}} \times Z_\alpha \le \mu \le \bar{x} + \frac{\sigma}{\sqrt{n}} \times Z_\alpha\right] \quad ...(13.15)$$

$$\left(\text{S.E.}(\bar{x}) = \frac{\sigma}{\sqrt{n}}\right)$$

Case II

When σ is unknown and n is large.

In this case Coefficient Interval

$$= [\bar{x} - \text{S.E.}(\bar{x}) \times Z_\alpha, \bar{x} + \text{S.E.}(\bar{x}) \times Z_\alpha] \quad ...(13.16)$$

$$= \left[(\bar{x}) - \frac{s}{\sqrt{n-1}} \times Z_\alpha, \bar{x} + \frac{s}{\sqrt{n-1}} \times Z_\alpha\right]$$

$$\left[\text{S.E.}(\bar{x}) = \frac{s}{\sqrt{n-1}}\right]$$

Step V

Select the value of Z_α from the following Table:

Confidence level $(1-\alpha)\%$	*Value of confidence coefficient* Z_α *or* t_α
90%	1.64
95%	1.96
98%	2.33
99%	2.57
Without any reference to the confidence level	3.00

Note: Where no reference to the confidence level is given, then always take t_α or $Z_\alpha = 3$

The above method is illustrated by the following examples:

i. Construction of a 95 percent Confidence Interval

It is reasonable to use x as the basis for an interval estimator of μ. It is a good point estimator. If mean is based on a random sample of size n from a normally distributed population with unknown mean μ and known variance σ^2, then its sampling distribution is normal with mean μ and variance σ^2/n. The standard normal variable related to mean is obtained by subtracting μ and variance $\sigma\sqrt{n}$, the standard deviation or standard error of mean. This gives

$$Z = \frac{\bar{x}-\mu}{\sigma/\sqrt{n}} \qquad \text{...(13.17)}$$

In constructing an interval estimator of μ we want limits between which μ will lie with high probability, say 0.95. These limits will be random variables, and in order to determine them we use Z.

We use from Table

$$P(-1.96 < Z > 1.96) = 0.95$$

And we examine the event $-1.96 < Z > 1.9$. This really the event $-1.96 < (x-\mu)/(\sigma/\sqrt{n})$ 1.96, if we use the definition of Z. We seek to recast the form of this event and construct a completely equivalent event of the form $a < \mu < b$. This event will then also have probability 0.95. To do this we will make use of the properties of inequalities. Notice that mean is the only component of the event which is a random variable.

Whenever $-1.96 < (\bar{x} - \mu)/(\sigma/\sqrt{n}) < 1.96$, then multiplying through by $\sigma/\sqrt{n}$, we obtain

$$-1.96\,\frac{\sigma}{\sqrt{n}} < x - \mu < 1.96\,\frac{\sigma}{\sqrt{n}}$$

That is, in exactly those random samples for which $(\bar{x} - \mu)/(\sigma/\sqrt{n})$ is between plus and minus 1.96, $\bar{x} - \mu$ is between plus an minus $1.96\sigma/\sqrt{n}$. Recall that multiplying both sides of an inequality by the same positive quantity, $\sigma/\sqrt{n}$ in this case, does not change the sense or direction of the inequality. Now, subtracting mean from the three parts of our chain inequality, we have a completely equivalent event:

$$-\bar{x} - 1.96\frac{\sigma}{\sqrt{n}} < -\mu < -\bar{x} + 1.96\frac{\sigma}{\sqrt{n}}$$

Recall that subtracting the same quantity from both sides of an inequality does not change its sense. Now, multiplying through by -1, we obtain the equivalent event.

$$-\bar{x} + 1.96\frac{\sigma}{\sqrt{n}} < -\mu < -\bar{x} - 1.96\frac{\sigma}{\sqrt{n}}$$

Multiplication of both sides of an inequality by a negative quantity reverses the inequality. But now reversing the order the terms of this chain inequality and writing the smallest quantity on the left instead of the right, we have the equivalent event

$$-\bar{x} - 1.96\frac{\sigma}{\sqrt{n}} < -\mu < -\bar{x} + 1.96\frac{\sigma}{\sqrt{n}}$$

an event of the form we are seeking. Note well that this is the same event as

$$-1.96 < Z < 1.96$$

That is, for the same random samples in which $Z = (x - \bar{\mu})/(\sigma/\sqrt{n})$ is between plus and minus 1.96, will be between $(x - 1.96\,\sigma/\sqrt{n}$ and $x + 1.96\sigma/\sqrt{n})$. Notice, however, that in the original form of the event, the middle expression in the chain inequality was the random variable, since it involved mean, whereas in the revised form the outside expressions are the random variables. Because, we have changed only the form of the original event and have not changed its probability, we can write:

$$\left(\bar{x} - 1.96\frac{\sigma}{\sqrt{n}} < \mu < \bar{x} + 1.96\frac{\sigma}{\sqrt{n}}\right) \quad ...(13.18)$$

This statement takes into account the fact that mean is a random variable with a sampling distribution. All we need to do is select a random sample, calculate the numerical value of mean, and substitute this value into the expressions ($\bar{x} - 1.96\sigma/\sqrt{n}$ and $\bar{x} + 1.96\sigma/\sqrt{n}$) along with the known numerical values of σ and *n*. In a specific numerical case this will produce two numbers, such as 1.7 and 4.9, for the limits. But here we run into a snag. We cannot assert that the probability that μ lies between 1.7 and 4.9 is 0.95. The quantities 1.7, 4.9 and μ lie between these numbers or it does not, and it is not sensible to assign a probability of 0.95 to the statement that it is between them.

The difficulty here arises at the point of substitutions of the observed numerical value for mean. The random sample in mean is variation from random sample to random sample and it is this variation to which the probability refers. However, if we denote the observed numerical value of $\bar{x}$ by $\bar{x}_0$, we know that this value arose from a process that could have produced infinitely many different values of mean and hence infinitely many different intervals of the form $x \pm 1.96\sigma/\sqrt{n}$. The probability statement says that 95 percent percent of these intervals would actually include or trap μ between their limits. Since, we have only one random sample, one value x_0 of *x* and one interval $x_0 \pm 1.96\sigma/\sqrt{n}$, we say we are 95 percent confident that μ lies between these limits. We might write:

$$P\left(\bar{x} - 1.96\frac{\sigma}{\sqrt{n}} < \mu < \bar{x}_0 + 1.96\frac{\sigma}{\sqrt{n}}\right) = 0.95 \quad ...(13.19)$$

This indicates that the confidence is 0.95, not the probability. The interval $x_0 \pm 1.96\sigma/\sqrt{n}$ is called a 95 percent confidence for μ and is the interval estimator. The figure 0.95 is called the confidence level.

Subscript Notation for Percentages

We shall use the notation Z or *t* for 100 percentile of the standard normal distribution. In other words, $Z_{0.95}$ is the 95th percentile, $Z_{0.975}$, the 97.5th percentile and so on. The subscript is a probability, it is multiplied by 100, when one is speaking of a percentile. In this notation the quantity 1.96, which arose in the 95 percent, confidence interval is $Z_{0.975}$. The 0.975 comes from the fact that the original event $-1.96 < Z < 1.96$ allowed Z to fall outside the limits 1.96 with probability 0.025 in either side. That is the balance between a probability of 1.00 and 0.95 was divided equally between two sides of the distribution. In general, if we want confidence level 1, we must use the quantity $Z_{1-(\alpha/2)}$ in forming the interval. For example, the confidence level 1 – 0.99, we have = 0.01. Then $Z_{1-(\alpha/2)} = Z_{0.975} = 2.57$. The general form of a 1–α level confidence interval for population mean becomes

$$\bar{x} \pm Z_{1-(\alpha/2)}\left(\frac{\alpha}{\sqrt{n}}\right) \text{ or } x \pm Z_{1-(\alpha/2)}\, x\, [\text{S.E. } (\bar{x})] \quad ...(13.20)$$

Summary of Formulae of Confidence

We state below the most useful and important formulae of confidence intervals for the some important parameters (Table 13.2).

Example 1: The quality control manager of a tyre company has sampled 100 years and has found the mean life time to be 30.214 kms. The population s.d. is 860. Construct a 95 percent interval for the mean life time for this particular brand of tyres.

Solution: Here $n = 100$, $\bar{x} = 30214$, $\sigma = 860$. Also $(1 - \alpha)\% = 95\%$ so that $Z_\alpha = 1.96$ [From table]

Table 13.2

Summary of formulae of confidence

Parameter	*Confidence Interval*
Mean of a normal distribution with known variance:	$x \pm Z_{1-(\alpha/2)}\left(\dfrac{\sigma}{\sqrt{n}}\right)$
Mean of a normal distribution with unknown normal:	$x \pm Z_{1-(\alpha/2)}\left(\dfrac{\sigma}{\sqrt{n}}\right)$
Variance of a normal distribution:	$\dfrac{(n-1)s^2}{X^2_{1-(\alpha/2)}} \dfrac{(n-1)s^2}{X^2_{(\alpha/2)}}$
Standard deviation of a normal distribution:	$\sqrt{\dfrac{(n-1)s^2}{X^2_{1-(\alpha/2)}}} \sqrt{\dfrac{(n-1)s^2}{X^2_{(\alpha/2)}}}$
Difference between means of two normal distributions, with known variances:	$\bar{x}_1 - \bar{x}_2 + t_{1-(\alpha/2)}\sqrt{\dfrac{\sigma_1^2}{n_1} + \dfrac{\sigma_2^2}{n_2}}$
Difference between means of two normal distributions, unknown but equal variances:	$\bar{x}_1 - \bar{x}_2 \pm t_{1-(\alpha/2)} S_P \sqrt{\dfrac{1}{n_1} + \dfrac{1}{n_2}}$
Confidence interval for the mean difference:	$\bar{d} \pm t_{1-(\alpha/2)} \dfrac{S_d}{\sqrt{n}}$
Ratio of variances of two normal distribution:	$\dfrac{s_1^2 \sqrt{s_2^2}\; s_1^2 \sqrt{s_2^2}}{Ft_{1-(\alpha/2)} Ft_{(\alpha/2)}}$
p, the parameter of the binominal distribution, normal approximation:	$p \pm Z_{1-(\alpha/2)}\sqrt{\dfrac{p(1-p)}{n}}$
$p_1 - p_2$, the difference between the parameters of two binomial distributions:	$p_1 - p_2 \pm z_{1-(\alpha/2)}\sqrt{\dfrac{p_1(1-p)}{n_1} + \dfrac{p_2(1-p_2)}{n_2}}$
Pooled variance:	$s^2{}_p = \dfrac{(n_1-1)\,s_1^2 + (n_2-1)s_2^2}{n_1 + n_2 - 2}$

$$\therefore \quad \text{S.E.}(\bar{x}) = \left(\frac{\sigma}{\sqrt{n}}\right) = \frac{860}{\sqrt{100}} = \frac{860}{10} = 86$$

$$\therefore \text{Confidence Interval} = \left[\bar{x} - \frac{\sigma}{\sqrt{n}} \times Z_\alpha, \bar{x} + \frac{\sigma}{\sqrt{n}} \times Z_\alpha\right]$$

$$= [30214 - 86 \times 1.96, 30214 + 86 \times 1.96]$$
$$= [30214 - 168.56, 30214 + 168.56]$$
$$= [30046.56, 30382.56]$$

Example 2: A sample random sample of size 100 has mean 15, the population variance being 25. Find the interval estimate of the population mean with a confidence level of (i) 99 percent and (ii) 95 percent.

Solution: Here $n = 100$, $\sigma^2 = 25$, $\bar{x} = 15$.

$$\text{S.E. }(x) = \frac{\sigma}{\sqrt{n}} = \frac{5}{\sqrt{100}} = \frac{5}{10} = 0.5.$$

(i) 99 percent confidence level = $Z_\alpha = 2.58$

$\therefore$ Confidence Interval $= x \pm \text{S.E. }(x) \times Z_\alpha$
$= 15 \pm 0.5 \times 2.58$
$= 15 \pm 1.29$

i.e. 13.71 to 16.29

(ii) 95 percent confidence level = $Z_\alpha = 1.96$

$\therefore$ Confidence Interval $= x \pm \text{S.E. }(x) \times Z_\alpha$
$= 15 \pm (0.5) \times 1.96$
$= 15 \pm 0.98$

i.e. 14.02 to 15.98

Example 3: The data given below are the specimens obtained from 10 individuals for the determination of percent calcium content of sound teeth.

36.39, 34.20, 36.19, 35.15, 35.22, 35.47, 36.19, 36.63, 35.63, 35.59.

(a) Calculate 95 percent and 99 percent confidence intervals for the mean percentage of calcium in the population

(b) Find 95 percent and 99 percent confidence interval for the variance and standard deviation of the population.

Solution. Here,

$$\sum_{i=1}^{10} x_i = [36.39 + 34.20 + 36.19 + 35.15 + 35.22 + 35.47 + 36.11 + 36.33 + 35.63 + 35.59] = 356.58$$

$$\therefore \quad \bar{x}_0 = \frac{356.58}{10} = 35.658$$

Also $\sum_{i=1}^{10} x_i^2 = 12{,}719.5140$

$$\sigma_0^2 = 0.5094 \; \sigma_0^2 = 0.7137$$

$$\therefore \quad \text{S.E.} = \frac{\sigma_0}{\sqrt{n}} = \frac{0.7137}{\sqrt{10}} = 0.2257$$

$$\therefore \quad (n-1)\sigma_0^2 = 4.5846.$$

$$\therefore \quad \psi^2_{0.025} = \mathbf{2.70},\ \psi^2_{0.975} = \mathbf{19.02},$$
$$\psi^2_{0.005} = \mathbf{1.73},\ \psi^2_{0.995} = \mathbf{23.59}$$

Number of degrees of freedom $v = n - 1 = 10 - 1 = 9$

Also $t_{0.975} = \mathbf{2.262},\ t_{0.975} \times \dfrac{\sigma_0}{\sqrt{n}} = \mathbf{0.5105}$

$t_{0.995} = \mathbf{3.250},\ t_{0.995} \times \dfrac{\sigma_0}{\sqrt{n}} = \mathbf{0.7335}$

$\therefore$ **95 percent interval for $\mu = x_0 \pm t_{0.975}\dfrac{\sigma_0}{\sqrt{n}}$**
$= 35.66 \pm 0.51$

$\therefore$ **Lower limit = 35.15; Upper limit = 36.17**

99 percent interval for $\mu = x_0 \pm t_{0.995}\dfrac{\sigma_0}{\sqrt{n}}$
$= 35.66 \pm 0.73$

$\therefore$ **Lower limit = 34.93; Upper limit = 36.39**

95 percent confidence interval for σ^2

$\therefore$ Lower limit $= \dfrac{4.5846}{19.02} = 0.241$

Upper limit $= \dfrac{4.5846}{2.70} = 1.698$

99 percent confidence interval for σ^2:

$\therefore$ Lower limit $= \dfrac{4.5846}{23.59} = 0.194$

Upper limit $= \dfrac{4.5846}{1.73} = 2.650$

95 percent confidence interval for σ:

$\therefore$ Lower limit $= \sqrt{0.241} = 0.491$

Upper limit $= \sqrt{1.628} = 1.303$

99 percent confidence interval for σ:

∴ Lower limit = $\sqrt{0.194} = 0.440$

Upper limit = $\sqrt{2.650} = 1.628$

Confidence Interval Estimate of the Proportion

Population Proportion

The population proportion P is the ratio of the number of elements possessing a characteristic to the total number of elements in the population, i.e.,

$$P = \frac{\text{Number of elements possessing the characteristic}}{\text{Total number of elements in the population}} \quad ...(13.21)$$

If we multiply the population by 100, then we get the percentage and we may take use of percentage for the proportion and vice-versa.

Sample Proportion

The sample proportion P is the ratio of the number of elements possessing a characteristic to the total number of elements 'n' in the sample.

$$p = \frac{\text{Number of elements possessing a characteristic}}{n = \text{Total number of elements in the sample}} \quad ...(13.22)$$

It is important to note that the mean of sampling distribution of P equals the population proportion, i.e., $E(p) = P$.

Standard Error (or Standard Deviation) of Sample Proportion

Case I

When the population size is infinitely large or the sample is drawn with replacement

(i) **Standard Error of Sample Proportion is**

$$\textbf{S.E. }(p) = \sqrt{\frac{PQ}{n}}$$, if P is known, where $Q = 1 - P$, n = the sample size.

(ii) **Standard Error of Sample Proportion** = $\sqrt{\frac{PQ}{n}}$, if P is not known, where $Q = 1 - p$, n = the sample size.

It is then estimated value.

Case II

When the population size is finite and the sample is drawn without replacement.

(i) Standard Error of Sample Proportion

$$\textbf{S.E.(p)} = \sqrt{\frac{PQ}{N}} \times \sqrt{\frac{N-n}{N-1}}, \textbf{ if P is known}$$

where $Q = 1 - p$, N = Size of population, n = size of sample.

Confidence Interval Estimate of the population proportion P is given by the following results:

Case I

When P is known. In this case the **confidence interval** of the sample proportion is given [$p - Zx$ S.E.(p), $p + Z \times$ S.E.(p)] where Z is the confidence coefficient and (S.E. p) is the standard Error of p.

Case II

When P is not known. In this the confidence interval of the sample proportion is given by [$p -$ S.E.(p) × Z, S.E.(p) × Z] where Z is the confidence coefficient, and standard error of p = S.E.(p).

Example 1: A random sample of 800 units from a large consignment showed that 200 were damaged. Find 95 percent confidence limits for the population proportion of damaged units in the consignment.

Solution: Here $n = 800$,

Sample proportion, $p = \frac{200}{800} = 0.25$,

$$q = 1 - 0.25 = 0.75.$$

$$\text{S.E. }(p) = \sqrt{\frac{pq}{n}} = \sqrt{\frac{0.25 \times 0.75}{800}} = 0.031$$

Also $(1 - \alpha)\% = 95\%$ so that $Z_{\alpha/z} = 1.96$

Confidence limits for the population proportion are $p \pm Z_{\alpha/z} \times \text{S.E.(p)}$

Lower limit $= p - Z \times \text{S.E. }(p) = 0.25 - 1.96 \times 0.0031$

$= 0.25 - 0.06 = 0.19$

Upper limit $= p + Z \times \text{S.E. }(p) = 0.25 + 1.96 \times 0.0031$

$= 0.25 + 0.06 = 0.31.$

Hence 95 percent confidence limits for the population proportion of damaged units in the consignment are 0.19 and 0.31.

Example 2: Out of 300 households in a town 123 have refrigerator. Find 95 percent confidence limits to the true value of the proportion of the households with refrigerators in the whole town.

Solution: Here $n = 300$, Sample proportion,

$$p = \frac{123}{300} = 0.41$$

$$\therefore \quad q = 1 - \frac{123}{300} = \frac{177}{300} = 0.59$$

$$\text{S.E. }(p) = \sqrt{\frac{pq}{n}} = \sqrt{\frac{0.41 \times 0.59}{300}} = 0.0283$$

Also $(1 - \alpha)\% = 95\%$ so that $Z = 1.96$

Confidence limits $= p \pm Z \times \text{S.E. }(p)$

$= 0.41 \pm 1.96 \times 0.0283$

$= 0.41 \pm 0.055$

Lower limit $= 0.41 - 0.055 = 0.355$

Upper limit $= 0.41 + 0.055 = 0.465$

Hence 95 percent confidence limits for the proportion of the households with Refrigerators in the whole town are 0.355 and 0.465.

Example 3: A factory is producing 50,000 pairs of Gloves daily. From a sample of 500 pairs, 2 percent were found to be of substained quality. Estimate the number of pairs that can be reasonably expected to be spoiled in the daily production and assign limits at 95 percent level of confidence.

Solution. Here $n = 500$, Sample percentage $p = 2\%$

$$\text{S.E.}(p) = \sqrt{\frac{p(100 - p)}{n}} = \sqrt{\frac{2(100 - 2)}{500}}$$

$$= \sqrt{\frac{2 \times 98}{500}} = 0.63$$

Also $(1 - \alpha)\% = 95\%$ so that $Z = 1.96$

$\therefore$ 95 percent confidence limits for the percentage of substained quality are

$p \pm \text{S.E.}(p)\ Z = 2 \pm (1.96 \times 0.63) = 2 \pm 1.23$

$= 2 - 1.23$ and $2 + 1.23$

$= 0.77$ and 3.23.

Number of pairs of gloves that can be expected to be spoiled in daily production lies between $\frac{0.77}{100} \times 50{,}000 = 385$ and $\frac{3.23}{100} \times 50{,}000 = 1615$.

Estimation: Examples for Large Samples

Example 1: In a Health Survey of 856 school boys it is found that the mean hemoglobin level is 10.4 g. per 100 mL with a standard deviation of 1.5. Estimate the *mean* hemoglobin level of the population of such school boys.

Solution: It is theoretically proven that the mean of the sample is the best estimate of the mean of the population. Therefore, the estimate of the population mean is 10.4 g per 100 mL. This is a point estimate it specifies one value (one point) as the estimated hemoglobin level. We can also get confidence interval as an interval estimate. The confidence interval of mean is given by

$\bar{x} - z_p$ (S.E. of mean) to $\bar{x} + z_p$ (S. E. of mean) or $\bar{x} \pm z_p$ (S. E. of mean).

Where Z_p is the value in the normal distribution corresponding to the confidence probability *p*.

To get 95 percent confidence interval, look at the last two columns of Appendix D, and note that from Z = – 1.96 to Z = 1.96, 95 percent of the observations of the Normal Distributions lie. Z_p = 1.96. Therefore the 95 percent confidence interval is 10.4 – 1.96 (0.05) to 10.4 + 1.96 (0.05) or 10.30 to 10.50.

This indicates that population mean will lie in the interval 10.30 to 10.50 with 95 percent probability.

To determine 99 percent confidence interval, again, find from Appendix D that from Z = – 2.576 to Z = 2.576, 99 percent of the observations of Normal Distribution lie. So Z_p = 2.576. Therefore that 99 percent confidence interval is 10.4 – 2.576 (0.05) to 10.4 + 2.576 (0.05) or 10.27 to 10.53

This means the population mean will lie in the interval 10.27 to 10.53 with 99 percent probability.

Example 2: Using the data from the problem 1, find the 95 percent confidence interval for the *difference in means*.

Solution: Following the procedure used in the previous problem, for 95 percent confidence interval Z_p is obtained as 1.96. The confidence interval for *difference in means* is

Difference in means ± 1.96 (S.E. of difference in means) using data from problem 1, the 95 percent confidence interval is

4.5 – 1.96 (0.2756) to 4.5 + 1.96 (0.2756) or 3.96 to 5.04

Hence, the population difference in means will lie between 3.96 and 5.04 with 95 percent probability.

Example 3: Find the 99 percent confidence interval for the *proportion* of children with otological abnormalities, using data from problem 1.

Solution: The Z_p for 99 percent confidence interval is given by 2.576. The 99 percent confidence interval of the proportion is

P ± 2.576 (S.E. of proportion)

Where P = proportion with otological abnormalities, and

$$\text{S.E. of proportion is } \sqrt{\frac{18.3 \times 81.7}{246}} = 2.4653$$

i.e. 18.3 percent ± 2.576 (2.4653) or 11.95 to 24.47 This means, with 99 percent probability, the population proportion will lie between 11.95 percent and 24.47 percent.

Estimation: Examples for Small Samples

Example 1: For the data given in problem 1 estimate the mean of the population and the 95 percent confidence interval of mean.

Solution: The best estimate of the population mean is the sample mean which is 7.2 g%.

The 95 percent confidence interval is given by $x \pm t_{0.05}$ S.E. of *x* where $t_{0.05}$ is obtained from the *t* distribution given in Appendix E for n_1 (=15) degrees of freedom. Here $t_{0.05}$ = 2.131 and the confidence interval is thus

7.2 ± 2.131 (0.1298) or 6.92 to 7.48

Example 2: Find the 95 percent confidence interval of the *difference in means* for the data of above problem.

Solution: The 95 percent confidence interval of difference in means is given by

Difference in means ± $t_{0.05}$ (S.E. of difference in means)

The $t_{0.05}$ with $n_1 + n_2 - 2$ (=30) degrees of freedom is 2.042 which is obtained from the *t* distribution given in Appendix E. Since the difference in means is:

$$\bar{x} - \bar{x}_2 = 1.6387,$$

The 95 percent confidence interval is:

1.6387 ± 2.042 (0.5607) or 0.49 to 2.78.

CHAPTER 14

The Significance of Mean and Other Statistics

Introduction

Inferential statistics is that branch of statistics which primarily deals with inferences from a sample to a larger population from which the sample has been taken. By implication, then, it is concerned also with the comparison of two of the sample estimates with a view to find out if they did not differ significantly from each other on a given characteristic or property. A significant difference means a difference larger than expected by chance or due to sampling fluctuations. Means and other measures computed from samples are called *statistics* and are subject to chance difference due to sampling fluctuations. Measures descriptive of a population, on the other hand, are called *parameters* and are to be thought of as fixed reference values. We do not know the parameters, but they do exist. Under specified statistics with known degrees of accuracy. The degree to which a sample mean represents its parameter is an index of the *significance* or trustworthiness of the computed sample mean. When a statistic has been calculated, the question which is generally asked is: How good an estimate is this statistic of the parameter based upon the entire population from which this sample was drawn? This question applies to all statistics but, only a few more important ones will be discussed in this chapter.

If two or more samples are drawn from the same universe (population), their means (m_1, m_2, m_3.......) may not be equal but will-show variation, even-though they are from the same universe. Such a difference between the means of the samples, is known as "sampling variation".

The mean of the sample-means (i.e., grand mean however will be approximately equal to the mean (M) of the universe).

The variation between the sample mean and the universal mean (m_1 and M; m_2 and M and m_3 and M) is known as "Inherent Sampling Variation".

The sampling variation, from one sample to another, may be by chance, when it is called "Natural or Biological variability" or due to play of certain factors, when it is called "real variability", (e.g. effect of nutrition, vaccine, smoking etc. Hts and Wts in England is more than that in India because of good nutrition; attacks among vaccinated is lesser than that among unvaccinated; incidence of cancer is more among smokers than among non-smokers etc.).

Sampling Distribution and the Standard Error of the Mean, SE_M

Standard Error

Standard deviation has been discussed in earlier chapter as a measure of variability. Another measure is standard error (SE), which is the standard deviation of the sampling distribution of an estimator. The idea is that if we draw a number of repeated samples of fixed size *n* from a population having a mean μ and variance σ_2, each sample mean, say $\bar{x}$, will have a different value. Here $\bar{x}$ itself is a random variable and hence it has a distribution. The standard deviation of $\bar{x}$ is called *standard error*. It has been proved that the standard error '$\sigma\bar{x}$' of the mean $\bar{x}$ based on a sample of size n is,

$$\sigma_{\bar{x}} = \frac{\sigma}{\sqrt{n}} \qquad ...(14.1)$$

From formula (14.1), it is obvious that the larger the sample size, the smaller the standard error and vice-versa. The advantage of considering standard error instead of a standard deviation is that this measure is not influenced by the extreme values present in a population under consideration. Moreover, it upholds all the virtues of standard deviation.

In practice we avoid studying or surveying the whole population. The process of drawing repeated samples is still more cumbersome. Hence, in reality neither we use σ to calculate the standard error of $\bar{x}$ nor we take more than one sample. As a matter of fact, what we do is, that we select only one sample, find its standard deviation s and use the following formula to find out the standard error of $\bar{x}$, i.e.,

$$SE(\bar{x}) = \frac{s}{\sqrt{n}} \qquad ...(14.2)$$

Standard error is commonly used in testing of hypothesis and interval estimation. Many distributions, which are originally not normally distributed, have been taken as normal by considering the distribution of mean $\bar{x}$ for a large n. This result follows from a most celebrated theorem known as *central limit theorem*. This theorem has been stated below:

- If $X_1, X_2, ..., X_n$ are n identically and independently distributed random variables with mean $\bar{X}_n$ and variance σ_x^2, the standardized variable$\{\bar{X}_n - E(\bar{X}_n)\}/\frac{\sigma_x}{\sqrt{n}}$ approaches a standard normal distribution as n approaches infinity.

Remark. The standard error may be considered as the key to the sampling theory.

Standard Error of Mean

The means of the samples (m_1, m_2, m_3 etc.) show dispersion around the population mean (M) (or universe mean) symmetrically as in normal distribution with a central tendency and with a definite standard deviation. The variation in the sample means is measured in terms of a parameter called "Standard error", which in fact is not an error but is a standard deviation of sample means (or proportions) from that of the universe or population (M). This standard deviation of the sample mean with that of the population mean, is called the "Standard error of the mean", denoted as SE $\bar{x}$ or simply the standard error (SE).

SE defines the limits of variation that occurs mainly due to chance. Variation beyond these limits is significant and is probably due to play of some external factors.

Similarly, the standard error of a proportion gives the standard deviation of proportions of several samples of a qualitative data taken from the same population and is denoted as SEP.

The standard error can be reduced by increasing the size of the sample. To illustrate, if the average number of attacks of diarrhea per child per year is 4 in a particular area, we will not necessarily get an average of 4 a sample of children from an hygiene area, where it may be only 2 per child or from an unhygienic area where it may be 6 per child. These variations in samples are inherent. If we take a very large sample of children from the three areas, included almost equally, the average attacks per child will be more or less 4 per year. Thus by increasing the size of the sample, the variations can be reduced and vice-versa.

On the other-hand, if the variations in means is large, such as 10 attacks in one example and 30 and 40 in others, the standard error will be increased. Thus the SE depends upon 2 factors.

- Standard deviation of the sample, which measures the variability of the observations (i.e. SD of the means)
- Size of the sample.

Thus standard error can be calculated by the formula

$$SE = \frac{SD}{\sqrt{n}}$$

Thus it is clear that SE varies inversely with the root of the sample size (n) and directly proportional to the SD of the means.

Since the distribution of the means, follows the pattern of normal distribution, (Fig. 35.16) it is not difficult to visualize that 95 percent of the sample means will lie within the limits of two standard error [Population mean M ± 2SE or M ± 2 $\frac{SD}{\sqrt{n}}$] on either side of the population mean (M).

Therefore, the chance that the population mean (M) lies between the limits defined by sample mean ± 2SE is also 95 percent. This is referred to as 95 percent "Confidence limits" (or Confidence interval) (Fig. 35.19). The confidence of the limits is increased to 99 percent by increasing the number of standard errors to ± 3SE.

In otherwords 95 percent confidence limits or interval which cover the range, mean ± 2SE, includes 95 percent of sample values in normal distribution. Any value lying outside this range will be rare. Its probability of occurrence (p-value) by chance will be only 5 percent i.e. 0.05 or 1 in 20.

Similarly, 99 percent confidence limits or interval cover the range mean ± 3SE, include 99 percent of sample values. The probability (chance) of any value falling outside the range is 1 percent or 0.01.

The standard error (of the mean) is a value which is smaller than the standard deviation and does not give a measure of the scatter of individual results but only the likely accuracy of the *mean* value. This point is important when constructing curves from a limited number of observations since the use of the standard error may give a false picture of the reliability of the curve. If one took repeated samples of ten people and measured height, the means would differ and would also be seen to be distributed around an average mean, or population mean if the number of samples was large enough. Ninety-five percent of all sample means lie within two standard errors of the population mean. Hence a set of results may be expressed as mean ± 2SE. The standard error can be calculated by dividing the standard deviation of a set of results by the square root of the number of observations if the numbers are more than 30, i.e. SE = $\frac{SD}{\sqrt{n}}$

Suppose a simple random sample of size n is drawn from a normal population of N units. The variance of the sample mean is

$$V(\bar{x}) = \left(\frac{1}{n} - \frac{1}{N}\right)s^2 \qquad ...(14.3)$$

$$= \frac{N-n}{N} \cdot \frac{s^2}{n} \qquad ...(14.3.1)$$

An unbiased estimate of $V(\bar{x})$ is

$$s_{\bar{x}}^2 = \left(\frac{1}{n} - \frac{1}{N}\right)s^2 \qquad ...(14.4)$$

where s^2 is given by (14.2). If 1/N is negligible, we obtain

$$s_{\bar{x}}^2 = \frac{s^2}{n} \qquad ...(14.5)$$

$$s_{\bar{x}} = \frac{s}{\sqrt{n}} \qquad ...(14.5.1)$$

Finite Population Correction

The quantity $\left(\frac{N-n}{N}\right)$ appears in (14.3.1) and other formulae only if N is finite. In case N is large (tending to infinity), the quantity $\left(\frac{N-n}{N}\right) = \left(1 - \frac{n}{N}\right)$ reduces to 1 in the limiting case since n/N becomes negligible. The quantity n/N is known as the *sampling fraction*. Though there is no rule governing the value n/N to be taken as small, even then as a tradition, n/N is taken as negligible if its value is equal to or less than 0.05 $\left(\frac{n}{N} \le 0.05\right)$.

In this situation, the factor $\left(\frac{N-n}{N}\right)$ disappears from the formulae.

Often we estimate population total instead of population mean. Let $\overline{X}$ be the estimate of population total $\overline{X} = \sum_{i=1}^{N} x_i$. The formula for $\hat{X}$ is,

$$\hat{X} = N\bar{x} \quad ...(14.6)$$

The variance of $\overline{X}$ is given by the formula,

$$V(\hat{X}) = N^2 V(\bar{x}) \quad ...(14.7)$$

$$= N^2\left(\frac{1}{n} - \frac{1}{N}\right)S^2 \quad ...(14.8)$$

$$= N\left(\frac{N-n}{n}\right)S^2 \quad ...(14.8.1)$$

The estimate of $V(\hat{X})$ is obtained when we replace s^2 by its unbiased estimate s^2.

Thus the estimated variance of $\hat{X}$ is.

$$S_{\bar{x}}^2 = N\left(\frac{N-n}{n}\right)S^2 \quad ...(14.9)$$

Means and Variance for Proportions

In many studies, the investigators want to know the proportions of units belonging to either of the two categories. For example, the number of people in favor of a plan and the number against it, the proportion of people in a specified area suffering from leprosy or the proportion of defective items produced in a factory, etc. In such type of studies, observations are not based on measurements but on the number in the two categories, classes or groups. Let the classes be c_1 and c_2. Let the units falling in class c_1 be N_1 and in class c_2 be N_2, out of the total number of units N. Also assume that P denotes the proportion of units in class c_1, i.e. $P = N_1/N$ and the proportion of units in class c_2 denoted by Q will be N_2/N. Since there are only two classes, any unit will belong to either of the classes and hence $P + Q = 1$. Instead of studying the whole population, let a simple random sample of size n be drawn and the study be made. Out of n, suppose n_1 units fall in c_1 and $n_2 = (n - n_1)$ units fall in c_2. Let the sample proportion in c_1 be denoted by p and in c_2 by q. Also suppose our observations are coded in the manner in which if a unit belongs to c_1, it is given the value 1 and if a unit belongs to c_2 it is given the value 0. The mean and variance for proportions in the case of population and in the case of sample are as given below.

It is trivial to prove that p is an unbiased estimate of P.

If a large number of samples are taken from the same population and the same test administered to them under identical conditions, the average scores or means of these samples can be calculated. If the means so obtained are arranged in the form of a frequency distribution and also plotted on a graph as a frequency polygon, we obtain *the distribution of means,* which is called the sampling distributions of mean. The difference between a distribution of

Population	Sample
$\mu = \frac{1}{N}\sum_{i=1}^{N} x_i = \frac{N_1}{N} = P \quad ...(14.10)$	$\bar{x} = \frac{1}{n}\sum_{i=1}^{n} x_i = \frac{n_1}{n} = p \quad ...(14.12)$
Since $x_i = 1$ if $x_i \in c_1$ $= 0$ if $x_i \in c_2$ or $N_i = NP \quad ...(14.11)$	Since $x_i = 1$ if $x_i \in c_1$ $= 0$ if $x_i \in c_2$ $n_i = np \quad ...(14.12.1)$
$\sum_{i=1}^{N} x_i^2 = N_i = NP$	$\sum_{i=1}^{n} x_i^2 = n_i = np$

Contd...

Contd...

Hence, $S_p^2 = \frac{1}{N-1}\left\{\sum_{i-1}^{n} x_i^2 - N\bar{x}^2\right\}$	Hence, $s_p^2 = \frac{1}{n-1}\left\{\sum_{i=1}^{n} X_i^2 - n\bar{x}^2\right\}$
$= \frac{1}{N-1}(NP - NP^2)$	$= \frac{1}{n-1}(np - np^2)$
$= \frac{N}{N-1}P(1-P)$	$= \frac{n}{n-1}p(1-p)$
$= \frac{N}{N-1}PQ$ ...(14.11)	$= \frac{n}{n-1}pq$ ...(14.13)

scores and a sampling distribution lies in the fact that the former is based on an arrangement of scores while the latter of means or any other statistic. It has been found that even if the distribution of scores is skewed, the sampling distribution tends to reach a normal shape.

However, it may not be true in the case of very small samples. The smaller the sample, the more the form of distribution of the population affects the form of distribution of the means. It is important to have a knowledge of the form of sampling distribution of a statistic before we can draw any inferences from it about the parameters. It warrants the use of the theoretical models or theoretical mathematical distributions like binomial, normal, poisson and hyper-geometric. However, in educational and psychological data, the normal distribution generally provides a good fit and hence is most popularly used. *The Standard Error (SE) is the standard deviation of the sampling distribution* and is to be interpreted in the same manner. The sampling distributions, though, are not calculated, yet they exist. The SE is also not calculated direct from the sampling distribution, but it is estimated from the sample standard deviation which is the only value available to us.

Computation of the Standard Error of the Mean, SE_M. For the computation of SE_M, we need to know the population standard deviation and then to use the following formula:

$$\sigma_M = \frac{\sigma}{\sqrt{N}} \qquad ...(14.14)$$

(SE of a Mean computed from a known population parameter) in which s = SD of the population; N = number of cases in the sample.

However, the population parameter, s, is generally unknown and cannot be directly obtained experimentally. It may involve a huge expense in terms of money and time to test the whole population and may defeat the very purpose of the experiment itself. Hence, statisticians have devised methods of estimating s_M from the sample statistics available to the experimenter. The formula for the purpose is

$$\text{SE of the Mean, } SE_M, \sigma_M = \frac{\sigma}{\sqrt{N}} \qquad ...(14.15)$$

(SE of the Mean estimated from sample standard deviation) in which, s is the sample SD; and N is the number of cases in the sample.

Some authors suggest the use of N in the denominator of formula (14.15) for large samples ($\geq$30) and of N–1 for small samples (N<30). The plea is, that in very large samples generally used in social sciences, no appreciable difference takes place in the value of σ_M by N–1 instead of N. The use of N or N–1 thus remains a matter of arbitrary decision. However, if N–1 instead of N has not been used in calculating the sample SD, then it becomes imperative to use N–1 instead of N in the denominator of the formula (14.15) for obtaining an unbiased estimate of the population standard deviation, *s*. It has been shown that SD of a random sample underestimates (is smaller than) the corresponding population σ. Hence for the correction of this underestimation, the SD of a sample should be computed by the formula

$SD=\frac{\sqrt{\Sigma x^2}}{N-1}$ instead of the usual formula $\frac{\sqrt{\Sigma x^2}}{N}$

The student will easily understand that sample *s* is the only estimate of the *s* available to us and hence, the former be used in the calculation of the SE of the mean.

Formula (14.15) above makes it clear that the size of the SE_M, varies directly with the size of the sample SD and inversely with the size of N.

Application and Interpretation of SE_M in Large Samples

Standard error of mean measures the degree to which the mean is affected by the errors of measurement as well as by the errors of sampling or sampling fluctuations from one random sample to the other. The interpretation of the SE of the mean is done to answer the question – how dependable is the mean? Further, it may be asked, as to how good an estimate is the sample mean, of the population mean. The answer to these questions is provided by setting up the *confidence limits* or the *Fiduciary limits* of the mean. These limits, for a particular level of confidence, are supposed to embrace the population mean. Thus, the interpretation of the SE_M is done in terms of the *confidence intervals* for the population mean.

Example: The mean achievement score of a random sample of 400 students on a test of statistics is 57 and SD is 15. How dependable is the mean? How good an estimate is it of the population mean?

Solution

Step 1: Calculate SE_M

$$SE_M = \frac{\sigma}{\sqrt{N}} = \frac{15}{\sqrt{400}} = \frac{15}{20} = 0.75$$

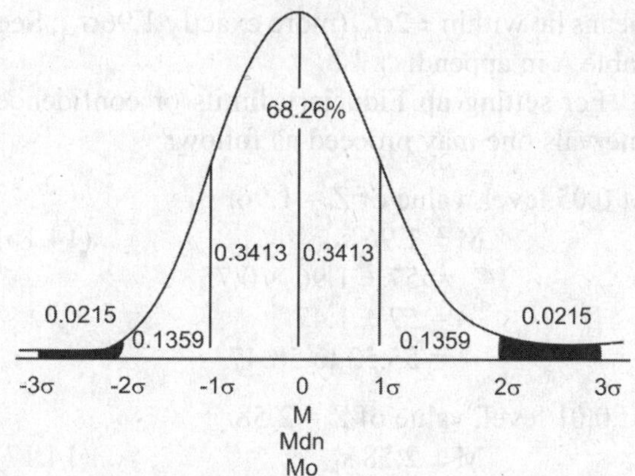

Fig. 14.1: Properties of the normal curve

We have used SD of the sample as our estimate of the population *s*. SE_M is the standard deviation of a distribution of sample mean around the fixed population mean (population mean is a constant value).

Assuming normal distribution the position of the SE_M is shown is Figure 14.1.

Step 2: Set up Confidence Intervals

In Figure 14.1, the population mean which is unknown is at the center of the curve. Normal curve, being symmetrical, sample means fall equally often on + (upper) side and –(lower) side of the M_{pop}. Looking at the divisions of area, 68.26 percent or about 2/3 of the sample means fall between $\pm \sigma 1_M$ of M_{pop} i.e. within a range of $\pm 1 \times 0.75$ units. Proceeding further out towards the two tails of the curve, one may notice that 95 percent sample means lie within $\pm 2\sigma_M$ (More exactly 1.96 σ_M; See Table A in appendix).

For setting up Fiduciary limits or confidence intervals one may proceed as follows:

At 0.05 level, value of Z = 1.96.

$$\begin{aligned} M &\pm 1.96\, s_M \\ &= 57 \pm 1.96 \times 0.75 \\ &= 57 \pm 1.47 \\ &= 55.53 \text{ to } 58.47 \end{aligned}$$

$\pm 1\sigma_M$ of M_{Pop}, i.e., within a range of $\pm 1 \times 0.75$ units. Proceeding further out towards the two tails of the curve, one may notice that 95 percent sample means lie within $\pm 2\sigma_M$ (more exactly $1.96\sigma_M$; See Table A in appendix).

For setting up Fiduciary limits or confidence intervals one may proceed as follows:

At 0.05 level, value of Z = 1.96.

$$M \pm 1.96\, s_M \quad ...(14.16)$$
$$= 57 \pm 1.96 \times 0.75$$
$$= 57 \pm 1.47$$
$$= 55.53 \text{ to } 58.47$$

At 0.01 level, value of Z = 2.58

$$M \pm 2.58\, s_M \quad ...(14.17)$$
$$= 57 \pm 2.58 \times 0.75$$
$$= 57 \pm 1.94$$
$$= 55.06 \text{ to } 58.94$$

The above confidence intervals, i.e. at 0.05 and at 0.01 levels, are in general use accepted as standard by most of the statisticians. However, confidence intervals with lesser degrees of assurance can also be set up.

Step 3: Interpret the Results

The confidence intervals represent a range within which the parameter, M_{Pop} is likely to fall. *Hence, with respect to our data above, there are 95 chances out of 100, that the M_{Pop} would fall between the score values 55.53 to 58.47; and there are 99 chances out of 100, that the M_{Pop} would fall between the score limits 55.06 to 58.94. Our confidence that these intervals contain M_{Pop} is 95 percent or P of 0.95; and 99 per cent or P of 0.99 respectively.*

The Distribution of *t*

The *t* distribution is a theoretical distribution discovered by an English, statistician, WS Gossett in 1908 writing under the pen name 'Student' in respect of his teacher RA Fisher. The distribution is therefore known as 'Student's distribution. The *t* ratio is obtained by the formula

$$t = \frac{M - \mu}{S_M} \quad ...(14.18)$$

(Basic formula of *t* ratio)

in which m is the population mean; M, mean of the sample; and S_M, an estimate of the σ_M obtained from SD of the sample. Gossett had shown that for random samples drawn from normal populations, the sampling distribution of *t* is given by

$$y = \frac{y_o}{\left(1 + \frac{t^2}{n-1}\right)^{n/2}} \quad ...(14.19)$$

(Equation for sampling distribution of *t*)

in which *n* is the number of cases in the sample and *y* stands for length of the ordinate. The denominator of the equation will be minimum if $t = 0$, and hence, the height of the ordinate the maximum at this point. Since the squared value of *t* is used, the ordinate *y* will be the same for positive and negative values and will generate a symmetrical distribution. Finally, as *t* increases, the ordinate *y*, or the height of the curve decreases. The curve is asymptotic to the base line. The curve is much like the normal curve except that it is more peaked for small *n*'s. As the *n*'s grow in size, the *t* distribution approaches normality.

As depicted in Figure 14.1, the *t* distribution is not a single distribution but a family of distributions depending on *df*. Like binomial and normal distributions already discussed in a previous chapter, *t* distribution is another theoretical model having wide applications to several sampling problems. Tables of values of *t* have been devised by statisticians. Table B in appendix shows these values for different levels of confidence and is very simple to use. The value of *t* at the intersection of a given *df* and level of confidence is to be picked up as the critical value.

Degrees of Freedom, *df*

The concept of degrees of freedom is of key importance in inferential statistics. Almost all tests of significance require the calculations of degrees of freedom. It is a mathematical concept. The geometric interpretations of the concept relates to the movement of a point in relation to the number of dimensions it is attached with. A point on a line is free to move in on dimension only and thus has 1 degree of freedom. A point on a plane has freedom of movement in two dimensions and has 2 degrees of freedom. A point in space of three dimensions has 3 *df*.

The expression degrees of freedom is abbreviated form of the full expression "degrees of freedom to vary". When a sample statistic is used to estimate a parameter, the number of degrees of freedom depends upon the number of restrictions placed upon the scores, each restriction reducing one *df*. To a less mathematically oriented student, the idea of *df* can be presented through two sets of scores given below.

Sl. No.	*Set I Given scores*	*Set II Altered scores*	
1.	8	10	
2.	7	6	Can vary in any way
3.	6	12	
4.	10	13	
5.	19	9	Its value gets fixed or automatically determined
ΣX	50	50	
Mx	10	10	

In set I original scores have been presented. We can vary the first four scores, 1-4, in any way we like. But the value of the 5th score gets fixed due to the restriction that ΣX in each must be 50. Hence, in this situation the four scores out of five are free to vary and hence the *df* = 5 – 1 = 4. Thus, in this case, the number of df depended upon the number of scores minus the number of restrictions (The idea of *df* has, also been explained in a chapter on chi-square).

Significance

"Significance" is opposite of "chance". If the (*m*) mean of one sample differs from that of another sample or of the universe (M) by more than two times the SE (2SE), i.e. lying outside the 95 percent confidence limits, the difference is said to be "Statistically Significant" at 5 percent level (probably due to play of some external factors and not due to chance), (i.e. *p* value lesser than 0.05) (Fig. 14.2).

A value lying outside 3SE or 99 percent confidence limits is very rare and the difference is considered to be "highly significant". (P value lesser than 0.01) at 1 percent level.

This level of significance is expressed as "*p*" value (i.e. probability value). If the *p*-value is less than 0.05 (or 5%) it is said to be significant and if less than 0.01 (1%) it is highly significant. 5 percent level of significance is also called as "critical level of significance".

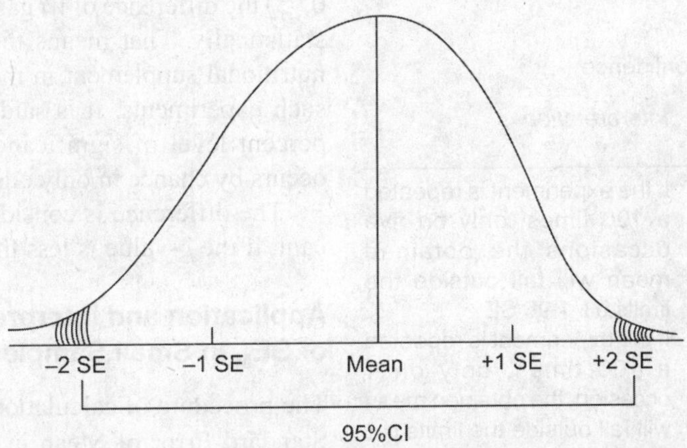

Fig.14.2: Normal curve showing 95% confidence limits. The shaded areas indicate values that fall beyond these limits on either side

Thus the "*p*" value denotes whether the difference in the sample estimates (sampling variation) is due to chance or due to an external (reality) factor.

To illustrate, suppose on weighing 100 mangoes individually and found that 95 percent of them weigh between 435 gms and 565 gms, we can say that 101st mango has 5 percent chance of weighing either lesser than 435 gms or more than 565 gms, in either case it means that the mango has lost or achieved a "significance weight", because that weight is lying beyond 95 percent confidence limits (beyond 2SE). If it is beyond 99 percent confidence limits (beyond 3SE) it is considered "highly significant".

Levels of Significance

Experimenters and researchers have selected some arbitrary standards – called *levels of significance to serve as the cut-off points or critical points along the probability scale, to separate the significant difference from the non-significant difference* between the two statistics, like means or SD's. Generally, the 0.05 and the 0.01 levels of significance are the most popular in social sciences research. The confidence with which an experimenter rejects – or retains – a null hypothesis depends upon the level of significance adopted. These may, hence, sometimes be termed as *levels of confidence.* Their meaning may be clear from the following Table 14.1.

Table 14.1

Meaning of Levels of Confidence

Level	*Amount of confidence*	*Interpretation*
0.05	95%	If the experiment is repeated a 100 times, only on five occasions the obtained mean will fall outside the limits $\mu \pm$ 1.96 SE
0.01	99%	If the experiment is repeated a 100 times, only on 1 occasion, the obtained mean will fall outside the limits $\mu \pm$ 2.58 SE

The values 1.96 and 2.58 have been taken from the *t* tables keeping large samples in view. The 0.01 level is more rigorous and higher a standard as compared to the 0.05 level and would require a larger value of the critical ratio for the rejection of the H_0. Hence, if an obtained value of *t* is significant at 0.01 level, it is automatically significant at 0.05 level but the reverse is not always true.

Tests of Significance

These are the statistical tests or mathematical methods employed to measure the probability or chance of occurrence of biological variation, in samples by standard error. It defines the limits of variation by chance and determines the probability of the factor playing the role.

For example, suppose the mean weight gain in 100 children receiving a nutritional supplement was 2 kg after 9 months (increase in mean weight of 15 to 17 kgs) while the gain in the control group was 1 kg (increase of mean weight of 15 to 16 kgs). Whether this difference of 1 kg in weight gain is a chance occurrence of no significance or whether it is attributable to supplementary feeding has to be decided to establish the value of latter.

The test of significance will measure the probability (*p* value) of increase in weight by chance. If the *p*-value is less than 5 times out of 100 ($p < 0.05$) the difference of *wt* gain of 1 kg, is significant statistically. That means the difference is due to nutritional supplement in more than 95 percent of such experiments. It is said to be significant at 5 percent level of significance, i.e., the difference occurs by chance in only one in twenty such trials.

The difference is considered as highly significant, if the *p*-value is less than 0.01.

Application and Interpretation of SE_M in Small Samples

The procedure of calculation and interpretation of Standard Error of Mean in small samples differs from that for large samples, in two respects.

1. The denominator N-1 instead of N is used in the formula for calculation of the SD of the sample.
2. The appropriate distribution to be used for small samples is *t* distribution instead of normal distributions.

The rest of the line of reasoning used in determining and interpreting SE_M in small samples is similar to that for the large samples.

Simply denoted as SE, is a parameter, used to measure the variation among the sample means (m_1, m_2, m_3 etc.) (i.e., sampling variation). SE is not an error, but it is the standard deviation of the sample means from the population mean (M) explained already). It helps to measure the chance variation or biological variation.

Uses of SE $\bar{x}$

- To find the confidence limits of population mean if standard deviation of the sample is known. Population mean (M) = Sample mean (*m*) ± 2 SE of mean (for 95% confidence limits).
- To tell whether a particular sample is drawn from the known population or not, if the population mean (M) is known. Here the characteristics of the normal curve are used. If the sample mean (*m*) ($\bar{x}$) lies within the range of M ± 2 SE$\bar{x}$. It is considered as belonging to the known population because 95 percent of the sample means lie within M ± 2 SE$\bar{x}$. If the sample mean is outside this range (beyond 95% confidence limits) then the sample is considered to be from some other population or it is under the influence of some other factor.
- To find the SE of difference between two means to know if the observed difference between the means of two samples is real and statistical significant or it is apparent and insignificant due to chance (i.e., to test the significant difference between two sample means).
- To calculate the size of the sample in order to have desired confidence limits, SD of the population is known, by the formula SE $\bar{x}$ = $\frac{SD}{\sqrt{n}}$

Example: A randomly selected group of 16 students was administered a test of verbal ability. The mean and SD obtained by the group are 52 and 8. Determine the 95 percent and 99 percent confidence intervals for the M_{pop}.

Solution

Step I: Calculate SE_M

$$SE_M = \frac{\sigma}{\sqrt{N}} = \frac{8}{\sqrt{16}} = 2.00$$

Step II: From Table B Pick up the Values of t

For *df* = N–1 = 16–1 = 15:

t at 0.05 level = 2.13

And *t* at 0.01 level = 2.95

Step III: Set up Confidence Intervals

at 0.05; M ±1.96 SE_M

= 52±2.13 × 2.00

= 47.74 and 56.26

at 0.01; M ± 2.95 SE_M

= 52 ± 2.95 × 2.00

= 46.10 and 57.90

Step IV: Interpret the Results

There is a probability of 0.95 that the M_{pop} will be within the score range 47.74 to 56.26; and 0.99 probability that M_{pop} will be within the score range 46.10 – 57.90.

The placement of the limits of the two confidence intervals in terms of SE_M and scores. The width of the 0.99 confidence interval (i.e. 46.10 – 57.90) is larger than the 0.95 confidence interval (i.e. 47.74 – 56.26). If the experiment or observation is repeated over a large number of times, chances are that the M_{pop} will be within 46.10 – 57.90 with our chances of being correct 99 percent times and being wrong only once in 100 times. Small n's do not necessarily generate stability of the results because smalln ess of the sample may not lead to an accurate representation of the parent population. Randomness in such cases may prove ineffective to guarantee this condition.

Calculation of SE of the Mean

First the SD of means of samples is calculated, by squaring the summation of the difference between sample mean and population mean, by using the formula

$$SD = \sqrt{\frac{\Sigma(m - M)^2}{n}}$$

But in practice, the SD of means of all samples is not known because only one sample is drawn of which SD and mean are calculated, by the formula $\frac{SD}{\sqrt{n}}$ i.e., SD is divided by the square root of the number of observations.

Example: Mean and SD for the height of 50 boys were 150 cm and 7 cm respectively. Find SE of mean and 95 percent confidence limits of heights in nature. Could this sample be from the universe with a population mean (M) of 154 cms?

Mean height = 150 cms
SD = 7 cms
n = 50 boys

$$SE\bar{x} = \frac{SD}{\sqrt{n}} = \frac{7}{\sqrt{50}} = \frac{7}{7.07} = 0.98$$

95 percent confidence limits (or 2 SE range) in nature will be

Mean height ± 2 SE
150 ± 2 × 0.98
= 150 + 1.96 = 151.96
and 150 – 1.96 = 148.04

This sample of 50 boys with a mean height of 150 cms is not drawn from the universe with a population mean if 154 cm, because 154 is much more than 95 percent of confidence limit of 151.96 cm.

$$\text{Relative deviate, } Z = \frac{\text{Observation} - \text{mean}}{SE\ \bar{x}}$$

$$= \frac{154 - 1504}{0.98} = \frac{}{0.98} = 4.08$$

4.08 is more than 4 times the SE.

Since this ratio is more than 3 (i.e. beyond 3 SD), it is considered to be highly significant, i.e. beyond 99 percent confidence limits. So the probability of this sample (with a mean *ht* of 150 cms) being drawn from the specified universe (with a mean height of 154 cm) is less than 1 percent ($p < 0.01$).

The Standard Error of a Median, σ_{Mdn}

It has been established that the variability of the sample medians is about 25 percent greater than the variability of means in a normally distributed population. Hence the standard error of a median can be estimated by using the formulas:

$$SE_{Mdn}, \sigma_{Mdn} = \frac{1.253\sigma}{\sqrt{N}} \quad \text{...(14.20)}$$

$$\sigma_{Mdn} = \frac{1.858Q}{\sqrt{N}} \quad \text{...(14.21)}$$

(Standard Error of the Median in terms of s and Q)

It is clear from formula (14.20) above the SE_{Mdn} is roughly times the SE_M. Hence s_{Mdn}, is less dependable and more subject to sampling fluctuations as compared to s_M.

Example: On a test of mechanical aptitude 225 randomly selected students of an engineering course secure a Mdn = 25.50 and Q = 5.00. How well does this median represent the median of the population from which this sample was drawn?

Solution

By formula 14.21, the $s_{Mdn} = \frac{1.858 \times 5.00}{\sqrt{225}} = 0.62$

Since N is large, we can use normal curve tables to set up the confidence intervals.

Z for 99 percent = 2.58 The same values we used in large sample SE_M cases.

Z for 95 percent = 1.96

Hence the confidences intervals are:

0.99 confidence: Mdn ± 2.58 s_{Mdn}
= 25.50 ± 2.58 × 0.62

$= 25.50 \pm 1.60$
$= 23.90 \text{ to } 27.10$

0.95 confidence: $\text{Mdn} \pm 1.96\, s_{\text{Mdn}}$
$= 25.50 \pm 1.96 \times 0.62$
$= 25.50 \pm 1.22$
$= 24.38 \text{ to } 26.72$

The interpretation of the confidence intervals follow the same pattern as that of the mean. Here we can place 99 percent and 95 percent confidence respectively that the Population mdn. Will be within these ranges.

The Standard Error of a Standard Deviation, SEσ

Since standard deviation also records fluctuations from sample to sample, the SE of the standard deviation can also be estimated and used to find the limits within which population SD will fall. The formula for the purpose is

$$\text{SE}\sigma,\ \sigma_\sigma = \frac{\sigma}{\sqrt{2}} \qquad \text{...(14.22)}$$

(Standard error of a standard deviation)

For small samples with $N < 100$, the sampling distribution of SD is somewhat skewed but approaches normality as N increases. Hence inferences, based on normal distribution can be drawn. A comparison of the denominators of Formula (14.22) and (14.15) will reveal that the SE_M is about 40 percent greater than SEs and hence less stable than the SE.

After calculating SEs we can set up the confidence intervals as explained earlier.

The Standard Error of Percentage and Proportions

At times it is not possible to measure some traits. The only information available is the percentage of the group that possesses that trait. The SE of the percentage would then be required to estimate the degree of confidence we can place in our information. How reliable was the percentage as an index of the incidence of the behavior in which we are interested? The formula for the SE of the percentage is

$$\text{SE}_{\%}\ \sigma_{\%} = \frac{\sqrt{PO}}{2N} \qquad \text{...(14.23)}$$

(Standard error of percentage)

in which P = percentage of the group possessing the trait

Q = (1 – P)

N = Number of cases

Suppose, 80 or 40 percent of the 200 children were found to have shown signs of tiredness after a strenuous physical exercise. Assuming that the sample was randomly drawn from a specified population, how well do our results represent the population percentage.

Applying formula (14.23), we get

$$\text{SE\%} = \frac{\sqrt{40\% \times 60\%}}{200} = 3.46\%$$

The 0.99 confidence interval will be:

$40\% \pm 2.58 \times 3.46\%$
$= 40\% \pm 8.93\%$
$= 31.07\% \text{ to } 48.93\%$

The 0.95 confidence interval will be:

$40\% \pm 1.96 \times 3.46\%$
$= 40\% \pm 6.78\%$
$= 33.22\% \text{ to } 46.78\%$

We may feel sure with 99 percent confidence that the percentage of children in the population who are likely to be tired after the physical exercise will not be less than 31 percent and more than 48.93 percent.

The Standard Error of a Correlation Coefficient, SE$_r$

We may draw a large number of samples randomly from a population, compute a correlation for each sample and prepare a frequency distribution of correlation coefficients. The shape of this distribution depends upon r_{pop}. As r_{pop} departs from zero, the sampling distribution of r's becomes increasingly skewed. A high positive value of r_{pop} generates an extremely negative skewness, while a high negative value of r_{pop} produces an extremely positive skewness. The SE of r is given by the formula:

$$SE_r, \sigma_r = \frac{1-r^2}{\sqrt{N}} \quad ...(14.24)$$

(SE of a correlation coefficient)

For example, the value of r in a set of 100 scores is 0.6. How dependable is this value?
By formula (14.24) we have,

$$\sigma_r = \frac{1-6^2}{\sqrt{100}} = \frac{0.64}{10} = 0.064$$

Using normal distribution, we set up the confidence intervals as below:
The 0.99 confidence interval will be:

$$r \pm 2.58\ \sigma_r$$
$$= 0.6 \pm 2.58 \times 0.064$$
$$= 0.6 \text{ to } 0.165$$
$$= 0.435 - 0.765$$

The 0.95 confidence interval will be:

$$r \pm 1.96\ s_r$$
$$= 0.6 \pm 1.96 \times 0.064$$
$$= 0.6 \text{ to } 0.125$$
$$= 0.475 - 0.725$$

The interpretation is that the Pop. r will be within these limits.

This formula has a fundamental defect that the theoretical model of normal distribution is not a good fit to the sampling distribution of r's as explained earlier. Hence Z transformation of r is recommended.

Conversion of r's into Fisher's Z Function

Difficulties resulting from the non-normality of the sampling distribution of r were resolved by RA Fisher who suggested the conversion of r's into Z function by using the formula

$$Z_r = \frac{1}{2}\log_e(1-r) - \log_e(1-r) \quad ...(14.25)$$

(Conversion of r's into Fisher's Z function)

However, conversion tables are readily available and there is no need of using formula. See Table C in Appendix. The given r's are converted into Z's. The test of significance is then applied to Z and not to r's. The sampling distribution of Z is approximately normal and the values of Z's can be interpreted in this manner. The SE formula for Z, as given below is independent of the value of r's.

$$SE_z = \frac{1}{\sqrt{N-3}} \quad ...(14.26)$$

(SE for Fisher's Z Function)

For illustration, the problem mentioned above is taken in which $r = 0.6$ and $N = 100$.

1. Convert r of 0.6 into Z which = 0.69
2. By formula 14.26, $SE_z = \frac{1}{\sqrt{N-3}} = \frac{1}{9.85} = 0.1$
3. Set up the confidence intervals as below:
   The 0.99 confidence interval will be:

$$Z \pm 2.58\ \sigma_z$$
$$= 0.69 \pm 2.58 \times 0.1$$
$$= 0.69 \pm 0.26$$
$$= 0.43 \text{ to } 0.95$$
$$= 0.435 - 0.765$$

Convert back into r's = 0.405 to 0.740

The 0.95 confidence interval will be:

$$Z \pm 1.96\ s_z$$
$$= 0.69 \pm 1.96 \times 0.1$$
$$= 0.69 \pm 1.96$$
$$= 0.494 \text{ to } .786$$
$$= 0.49 \text{ to } 79 \text{ (rounded)}$$

Convert back into r's = 0.455 to 0.660

A comparison of these values with those obtained by formula (14.24) would reveal some differences but not very appreciable.

In addition of the above, SE formulas for some other statistics and in some special situations have also been suggested. Only formula for SE of the quartile deviation is given:

$$SE_Q, \sigma_Q = \frac{0.786\sigma}{\sqrt{N}} \quad ...(14.27)$$

Based on Q

$$SE_Q, \sigma_Q = \frac{1.17Q}{\sqrt{N}} \quad ...(14.28)$$

EXERCISES

1. On a test of nursing aptitude, a randomly selected group of 400 candidates obtains a mean = 25.6 and s = 5.00. Use 0.95 and 0.99 confidence, and set up the two confidence intervals.
2. A randomly selected group of 25, VI year BSc Nursing students have a mean height of 135 cm, and SD = 10 cm. How well does this value estimate the population mean? Use 0.99 and 0.95 confidence intervals.

CHAPTER 15 The Significance of Difference between Means and Other Statistics

Introduction

Generally, a hypothesis is established before hand. By hypothesis, we mean to give postulated or stipulated value(s) of a parameter. Also, instead of giving values, some relationship between parameters is postulated in the case of two or more populations. On the basis of observational data, a test is performed to decide whether the postulated hypothesis be accepted or not. This involves certain amount of risk. This amount of risk is termed as a level of significance. When the hypothesis is accepted, we consider it a nonsignificant result and if the reverse situation occurs, it is called a significant result. The tests, which are dealt within this chapter pertain to parametric tests. A test is defined as, "A statistical test is a procedure governed by certain rules, which leads to take a decision about the hypothesis for its acceptance or rejection on the basis of sample values."

Descriptive statistics give us a quantitative way of viewing the world. They enable a researcher to describe certain factual aspects of a population. Most researchers, however, are concerned with other kinds of judgments as well. This leads to the use of inferential statistics. Inferential statistics do not examine a whole population. A sample (or samples) is drawn from the population, and the characteristics of the population are deduced or inferred from the responses of this sample or samples.

In addition to this type of inference, the quantitative researcher uses inferential statistics to test hypothesis and to determine whether certain experimental treatments or techniques are better, worse, or not significantly different from other types of treatments or techniques. Hypothesis testing is based on probability. When reading research, the statement "$H_0 = p < 0.05$" often occurs. (Remember that H_0 is called the null hypothesis. Here, $p < 0.05$ is called the level of significance or level of confidence—that is, the researcher states that the results of the experimental treatment will probably not be significantly different from the stantdard or common treatment. Most researchers really want to reject the null hypothesis, but research convention has cast this as the most common type of research hypothesis. The symbol p stands for probability. The probability in the statement $p < 0.05$ means that there will be no conclusion of a significant difference between treatments unless 5 or fewer treatments out of 100 have the same results as the original or standard treatments. Probability is determined by connecting the appropriate statistics and then reading the statistical table that gives the probability for that statistics.

When a level of significance is selected, the experimenter is telling the world that chance has little to do with the results of the experiment. Medically related experiments may set extremely high levels of significance, usually, one chance in a thousand or less ($p < 0.001$). In cause of life and death, the chance of error must be diminished as much as possible.

Statistical tests of hypotheses play an important role in industry, biological sciences, behavioral sciences and economics, etc. The use of tests has been made clear through a number of practical problems.

1. A food manufacturer announces that his food contains forty per cent protein. Now to make sure whether his claim is correct or not, one has to take a random sample of the product and by chemical analysis, find the protein percentages in the samples. From these observed values, he would decide about the manufacturer's claim for his product. This is done by performing a test of significance.
2. There is a process A, which produces certain items. It is considered that a new process B is better than process A. Both the processes are put under operation and then the items produced by them are sampled and observations are taken on them. A statistical test is performed based on these observations which enables us to decide whether process B is better than A or not.
3. Often we are interested to know what is the best dose of a chemical treatment? Two or more doses of the chemical are applied or administered on a number of subjects and response is observed. Now it is tested statistically whether the doses differ significantly or not.
4. Psychologists are often interested in knowing whether the level of IQ of a group of school boys is up to a certain standard or not. In this case, some boys are selected and an intelligence test is conducted. The scores obtained by them pass through a statistical test and a decision is made whether their IQ is up to the standard or not.

There is no end to such types of practical problems where statistical tests can be applied. These are only a few examples. Here, one very important point is to be noted. Whatever conclusions are drawn about the populations(s), they are always subjected to some error. Hence, there is always some risks involved in these decisions. Thus, a level of significance is always associated with these decisions. Now, we will discuss various terms involved in testing of hypothesis in an exact way before describing the statistical tests.

In experimental and other research work, the determination of whether an observed difference is of such magnitude that it cannot be attributed to chance factors or sampling variations is often our major interest. For example, we may observe that a group of subjects tested under one set of experimental conditions have a higher mean than a comparable group tested under a different set of experimental conditions. Is the observed difference between the means one that might occur frequently by chance, that is, as a result of sampling variations? If not, then we might infer that the difference is a product of the experimental conditions. For this purpose, we need a statistical test of significance of difference between the means. The critical ratio or the *t* is the one generally used in such circumstances.

Statistical Significance

Statistical significance is a comment on the degree of probability that observed associations of whatever kind may have arisen through chance. Tossing a coin is a good example. If ten tosses are tried, heads may occur eight times, which may be held to prove that pennies come up heads 80 percent of the time; this is, of course, nonsense, for a different result may occur on the next trial. If however, anyone had the patience to do a thousand tosses, the results would very likely come out as half heads and half tails—which represents the real probability. Only when there is a substantial number of tests is the law of averages a useful description or prediction. Probability varies widely (Fig. 15.1). By convention a probability (P) of findings occurring by chance not more than one time in 20 ($P < 0.05$) or "significant at the 5 percent level" is normally accepted as being statistically significant. A probability of findings occurring not more than one time in 100, "significant at the 1 percent level", or ($P<0.01$) indicates that the findings are highly significant. Statistical significance is, of course, not the same as clinical importance.

Types of Hypothesis

"A hypothesis is an assertion or conjecture about the parameter(s) of population distribution(s)".

In case, we are considering more than one population, it may be about the relationship between

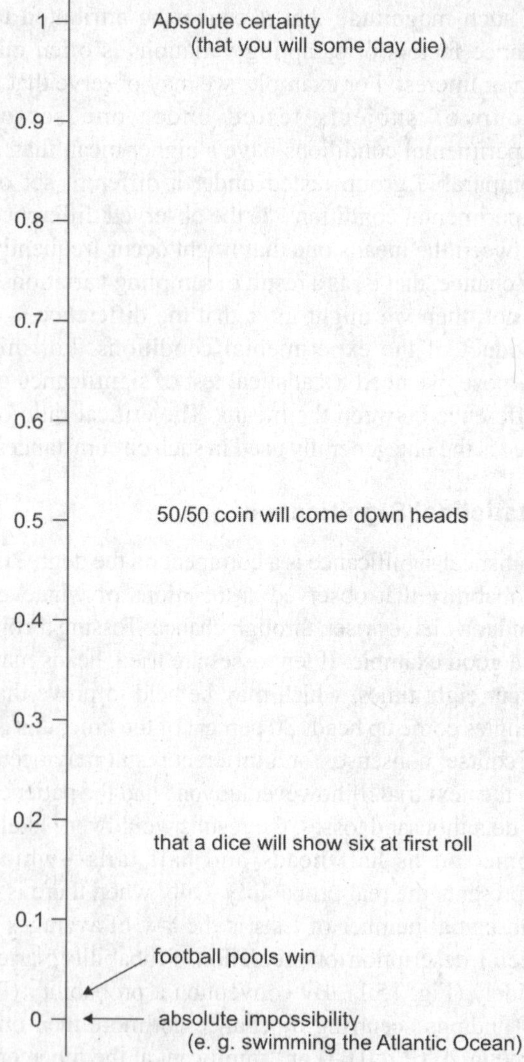

Fig. 15.1: Probability scale

the similar parameters of the distributions. For example, the mean μ of a distribution is fifty, i.e. H: $\mu = 50$. The variance σ^2 of a distribution is 36, i.e. H: $\sigma^2 = 36$. For two populations, the hypothesis may be that the means μ_1 and μ_2 or variances $\sigma_1{}^2$ and $\sigma_2{}^2$ are equal, i.e. H: $\mu_1 = \mu_2$ or H: $\sigma_1{}^2 = \sigma_2{}^2$. Many times, the statement in the notational form can be given in the following manner as well.

H: $\mu > 0$, H: $\mu < 0$, H: $\mu = 0$, H: $\mu = c$,
H: $\mu_1 > \mu_2$, H: $\mu_1 < \mu_2$, etc.

where, c is a known constant value. Similarly for variances(s), the hypotheses may be given as,

H: $\sigma^2 = \sigma_0^2$, H: $\sigma^2 > \sigma_0^2$, H: $\sigma_1^2 = \sigma_2^2$, H: $\sigma_1^2 < \sigma_2^2$,

etc. where $\sigma_0{}^2$ is a known fixed value. A hypothesis is further classified according to its nature and usage.

Alternative Hypothesis

It is a statement about the population parameter or parameters, which gives an alternative to the null hypothesis (H_0), within the range of pertinent values of the parameter, i.e. if H_0 is accepted, what hypothesis is to be rejected and vice-versa. An alternative hypothesis is denoted by H_1 or H_A. The idea of alternative hypothesis was originated by Neyman. For instance,

If H_0: $\mu = 0$, the alternatives are, H_1: $\mu \neq 0$, H_1: $\mu > 0$ or H_1: $\mu < 0$
if H_0: $\mu_1 = \mu_2$, the alternatives are, H_1: $\mu_1 \neq \mu_2$, H_1: $\mu_1 > \mu_2$ or H_1: $\mu_1 < \mu_2$.

if $H_0: \sigma^2 = \sigma_0^2$, the alternatives are,
$H_1: \sigma^2 \neq \sigma_0^2, H_1: \sigma^2 < \sigma_0^2$ or $H_1: \sigma^2 > \sigma_0^2$

if $H_1: \sigma_1^2 = \sigma_2^2$, the alternatives are,
$H_1: \sigma_1^2 \neq \sigma_2^2, H_1: \sigma_1^2 > \sigma_2^2$ or $H_1: \sigma_1^2 < \sigma_2^2$

Simple and Composite Hypothesis

If the statistical hypothesis completely specifies the distribution, it is called a simple hypothesis, otherwise it is called a composite hypothesis. For instance, we consider a normal population N (μ, σ^2), where σ^2 is known and we want to test the hypothesis, H_0: $\mu = 25$ against H_1: $\mu = 30$. From these hypotheses we know that μ can take either of the two values, 25 or 30. In this case, H_0 and H_1 are both simple. But generally H_1 is composite, i.e. of the form, H_1: $\mu \neq 25$, H_1: $M \neq 25$ or H_1: $\mu > 25$. Likewise, simple and composite hypothesis for any other parameter(s) can be stated.

Null Hypothesis

A hypothesis which is to be actually tested for acceptance or rejection is termed as null hypothesis. It is denoted by H_0.

The techniques to know how far the differences between the estimates of different samples are due to sampling variation is known as the "testing of hypothesis". This can be worked out by several methods.

The first step in testing of hypothesis (e.g. smoking resulting in cancer, drug resulting in cure of a disease or a vaccine resulting in protection etc.) is "Null hypothesis" (H_0) i.e. to study the effect of an external factor (smoking, drug, vaccine) on man in health and disease.

Assumption is made that the external factor plays no rule. Such an assumption is called "Null hypothesis". Smoking has no relation with lung cancer. Similarly, there is no difference between two drugs or vaccines. Then proceeded to test the hypothesis (e.g. Smoking results in lung cancer) in quantitative terms. In such studies 2 groups or samples called experimental group (smokers) and control group (non-smokers, taken for comparison) are taken. After the period of observation, or at the end of the experiment, the values (proportions or means) of the two samples or groups, are noted. If the difference between the samples is more than twice the standard error so that the probability of chance occurrence is less than 5 times in 100 experiments, the null hypothesis (of no difference between two drugs or no relation between smoking and lung cancer) is rejected and the hypothesis that "smoking results in lung cancer" is accepted. That means if the '*p* value' is less than 0.05, that means the difference is real (and not due to chance) and the factor under trial is considered to have definitive action on the experimental group. If the probability is more than 5 percent (*p* value more than 0.05) the null hypothesis is accepted. That means the diffence is by chance. Usually the level of significance (*p*-value) is stated while accepting or rejecting the hypothesis.

In certain conditions the null hypothesis (H_0) is rejected though it should be accepted, when there is no significant difference, i.e. when the observation lies within 95 percent confidence limits. This is stated as "Type 1 error".

Similarly, in certain other conditions, the null hypothesis is accepted, though it should be rejected, when there is significant difference, i.e. when the observation lies beyond 95 percent confidence limits. This is stated as "Type 2 error".

By increasing the limit or level of significance to 99 percent, type 1 error is increased.

The *null hypothesis* is a proposition of zero differences. Fisher has emphasized that every experiment may be said to exist only in order to give the facts a chance of disproving the null hypothesis. Thus, a hypothesis which is set-up with the possibility of it being rejected at some defined probability value is called a null hypothesis, the term "null" is referring to our interest in the possible rejection of the hypothesis. In statistical term, a null hypothesis may be stated as

$$H_0: \mu_1 = \mu_2$$

where μ_1 and μ_2 are population means.

It states that there is no significant difference in the means of the two populations. If facts lead to the rejection or non-retention of the H_0, then the alternative hypothesis (H_1) as stated below, stands accepted.

H_0: $\mu_1 \neq \mu_2$; in which $\neq$ means" not equal to"; and μ_1 and μ_2 are population means.

It means that the two populations differ significantly.

The term *null hypothesis* is used when the assumption is made, before statistical tests are applied, that there is no difference between two treatments. The statistical test used depends, largely, on the number of observations recorded and the distribution of the results. If the results have a Gaussian (or normal) distribution, familiar parametric tests such as Student's *t*-test can be used. If the distribution is skewed (non-Gaussian), then transformation will be needed or other statistical methods must be used. Non-parametric tests such as the χ^2 test can be used with any distribution (Fig. 15.2).

The Process of Testing Hypothesis

The process of testing for the significance of the difference between the two means include the following steps:

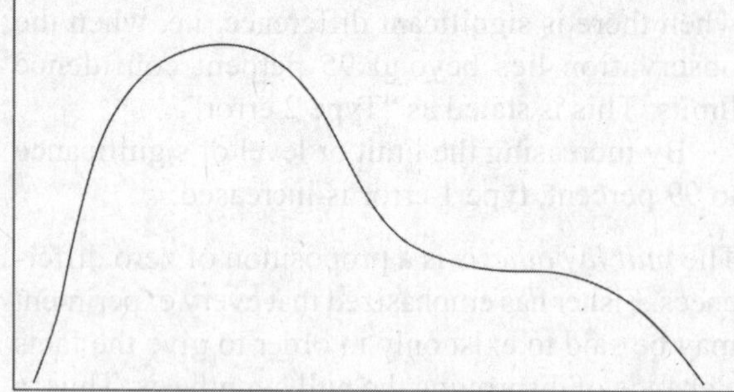

Fig. 15.2: Non-parametric skew distribution

i. Set up H_0 and H_1 according to the requirements of the problem
ii. Decide about the level of significance for the test. Customarily 0.05 and 0.01 levels are selected
iii. Decide whether one-tailed or two-tailed test of significance was needed
iv. Decide whether the data warranted a test of significance for the independent or the correlated means
v. Decide whether the large sample or the small sample was involved
vi. Use one of the following formulas appropriate to (iv) and (v) above, for the calculation of SE of Mean Difference, SE_D.
vii. Calculate the value of the critical ratio or t by using the formula $\frac{M_1 - M_2}{SE - SE_D}$, in which M_1 and M_2 are the means to be compared and SE_D is the SE of Mean Difference calculated under step (vi) above
viii. Calculate Degrees of Freedom (*df*) as below:
ix. Look up the tables of t values (See Appendix, Table B) with *df* (as decided in step VIII above) and the level of significance (step ii).
x. Decision Rule: Compare the calculated value of t.
   a. If the calculated value of t is larger than the table value of t, reject H_0 and accept H_1.
   b. If the calculated value of t is less than the table value of t, accept H_0.
xi. Interpret the results as below:
   a. H_0 rejected: There is a significant difference between the two means
   b. H_0 accepted: There is no significant difference between the two means. Whatever the difference, it has arisen due to sampling fluctuations and chance factors only
xii. The procedural steps in the use of the t test of significance of difference between two means will now be explained with the help of some numerical examples. For the purpose of convenience, the examples have been arranged in two sections. The first section is concerned with the comparison of independent or uncorrelated means. The second section is on comparison of correlated means.

General Procedures for Testing a Hypothesis

i. A "Null hypothesis" (H_0), suitable to the problem is set up.
ii. An alternate hypothesis is defined if necessary.
iii. A suitable statistical test, using a relevant formula, is calculated.
iv. The degree of freedom is determined.
v. Then the probability level (p-value) is found out, corresponding to the calculated value of the test and its degree of freedom. This can be found out from the tables.
vi. If the p-value is less than 0.05, the Null hypothesis is rejected and if the p-value is more than 0.05, null hypothesis is accepted.

The different tests employed are:

- Standard error of the mean
- Standard error of the difference between two means
- Standard error of proportion
- Standard error of difference between two proportions 't' test
- Chi-square test.

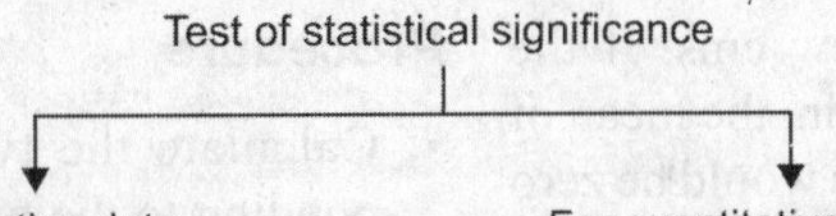

For quantitative data
a. For sample size more than 30
• Standard error of proportion
• Standard error of difference between two proportions
• Chi-square test

For quantitative data
a. Sample size more than 30
• Standard error of mean
• Standard error of difference between two mean
b. Sample size less than 30
• Paired *t*-test
• Unpaired *t*-test

Independent or Uncorrelated Means

Large Samples

$$\sigma_D = \sqrt{\frac{\sigma^2_1}{N_1} + \frac{\sigma^2_2}{N_2}} \quad ...(15.1)$$

Or $$\sigma_D = \sqrt{\sigma m_1^2 + \sigma m_2^2} \quad ...(15.2)$$

Small Samples

$$SE_D = SD$$

$$\text{where, } SD = \sqrt{\frac{\Sigma(X_1 - M_1)^2 + \Sigma(X_2 - M_2)^2}{(N_1 - 1) + (N_2 - 1)}} \quad ...(15.3)$$

Correlated Means

Large Samples

$$SE_D = \sqrt{\sigma^2_{M_1} + \sigma^2_{M_2} - 2r_{12}\sigma_{M_1}\sigma_{M_2}}$$

Small Samples

$$SE_D = \frac{SD}{\sqrt{N}} \quad ...(15.4)$$

Description of Symbols of Above Formulas

σ_{M_1} and σ_{M_2} = SE's of the Means of the two groups
σ_1 and σ_2 = SD's of the two groups
N_1 and N_2 = Number of cases in the two groups
SD = Pooled standard deviation of the two groups.

Other Symbols as Above

M_1 and M_2 = Means of two groups
X_1 and X_2 = Individual raw scores in the two groups
r_{12} = Correlation coefficient between scores of groups I and II.

Other Symbols as Above

SD = The standard deviation of the difference scores
N = Number of differences or Number of persons in the group.

Standard Error of the Difference of Two Independent Means (Large Sample) Standard Error of Difference between Two Means

Standard error (SE) is denoted as SE $(\bar{x}_1 - \bar{x}_2)$. Unlike the SE$\bar{x}$, which measures the chance difference between the sample mean and the population mean (*m* – *m*), standard error of difference in means (SEDM) measures the chance difference between the means of the two samples (a pair of samples) drawn from the same population.

Two samples (s_1 and s_2) are simultaneously drawn from the universe and their mean heights are recorded. The difference in these two means is noted $(\bar{x}_1 - \bar{x}_2)$. It will be plus or minus few cms.

The samples are returned to the universe and two fresh samples (s_3 and s_4) are obtained, their means are calculated, the difference in their means will be $(\bar{x}_3 - \bar{x}_4)$ plus or minus few cms. If the procedure is repeated again and again, the mean of the differences in the paired samples would be zero or nearly so.

Moreover, the differences in means of the different sets of twin samples will follow normal frequency distribution. The SD of these differences therefore will define the range within which 95 percent of differences in the means would lie. Such a SD is actually called "Standard Error of Difference in Means (SEDM), (unlike SE$\bar{x}$ which is the SD of sample means).

In practice it is not possible to find differences of large number of samples and then find SE of these differences. The test is applied to one pair directly if standard deviations of two means are known.

If the observed difference between the two means is more than twice the SE of difference, it is significant at 95 percent confidence limits.

If the observed differences between the two means is greater than three times the SE of difference, it is significant at 99 percent confidence limits. It is real variability in more than 99 percent cases and the chance factor is less than 1 percent.

Apply relative deviate (Z) test for large samples and '*t*' test, for small samples, for correct estimation of chance limits, because WS Gosset observed that the normal distribution gives biased results in case of small samples.

SE of difference between two means is denoted as SE $(\bar{x}_1 - \bar{x}_2)$. Mathematically it is the root of the sum of the squares of the standard error of two samples means.

It is already seen that the SE of a sample mean is equal to $\frac{SD}{\sqrt{n}}$

$\therefore$ SEDM denoted as $S\bar{d} = \sqrt{(SE_1)^2 + (SE_2)^2}$

Substituting $SE = \frac{SD}{\sqrt{n}} = \frac{SD^2}{n}$

$$= \sqrt{\left(\frac{SE_1}{n_1}\right)^2 + \left(\frac{SE_2}{n_2}\right)^2}$$

Procedure

- Calculate the two means $\bar{x}_1$ and $\bar{x}_2$, corresponding to the two samples with samples sizes n_1 and n_2 respectively.
- Set up the null hypothesis that the two samples are from the same population and that the difference between the two sample estimates is due to sampling variation.
- Calculate the standard deviation of the two samples and their standard errors (SE_1) and (SE_2) respectively.
- Calculate the SEDM as $\sqrt{(SE_1)^2 + (SE_2)^2}$
- Calculate the quantity

$$Z = \frac{\text{Difference between sample estimates}}{\text{SE of difference}}$$

- Refer to normal distribution table and corresponding to this calculated value of Z, find the value of probability '*p*'.
- If the *p*-value is less than 0.05 (or Z value is > 2 SE) reject the null hypothesis and conclude that the difference between two sample estimates as significant. If the Z value is > 3 SE ($p < 0.01$) it is highly significant.

If the *p*-value is greater than 0.05, accept the null hypothesis and conclude that the difference between the two sample estimates as insignificant.

When two distinct groups of subjects are involved, the groups may be termed as independent. These groups are drawn at random from totally different and unrelated populations. No attempt is made to equate the groups by using pair-comparison or any other method.

Example 1: Thirty boys and forty girls selected randomly from the first year of BSc Nursing Studying in a Nursing College were given a standard test of Nursing Skill. Their means and SD's are reported in Table 15.1.

	N	M	SD
Boys	30	20.5	4.0
Girls	40	16.2	5.0

Is the mean difference in the Nursing Skill significant?

Table 15.1

Summary of the test of difference of means of independent groups (Nursing Skill example)

Hypothesis

$H_0: \mu_1 = \mu_2$

$H_0: \mu_1 \neq \mu_2$

Decision rules

Given: 0.05 significance level; and $df = N_1 + N_2 - 2 = 68$; table value of $t = 2.00$:

If t obt. < 2.00 accept H_0.

If t obt. ≥ 2.00 reject H_0.

Computation

$$\text{Formula, } SE_D = \sqrt{\frac{\sigma_1^{\,2}}{N_1} + \frac{\sigma_2^{\,2}}{N_2}}$$

Substituting the numerical values.

$$SE_D = \sqrt{\frac{4^2}{30} + \frac{5^2}{40}} = 1.07$$

$$t = \frac{M_1 - M_2}{SE_D}$$

$$= \frac{20.5 - 16.2}{1.07} = \frac{4.3}{1.07} = 4.02$$

Interpretation: Reject H_0

Example 2: In a study on growth of children, one group of 100 children had a mean height of 60 cms and SD of 2.5 cm, while another group of 150 children had a mean height of 62 cm and SD of 3 cm. Is the difference between the means statistically significant?

$$\text{SEDM} = \sqrt{(\text{SE}_1)^2 + (\text{SE}_2)^2}$$

$$= \sqrt{\frac{(\text{SD}_1)^2}{n_1} + \frac{(\text{SD}_2)^2}{n_2}}$$

$$= \sqrt{\frac{(2.5)^2}{100} + \frac{(3)^2}{150}}$$

$$= \sqrt{\frac{6.25}{100} + \frac{9}{150}}$$

$$= \sqrt{0.06 + 0.06}$$

$$= \sqrt{0.12}$$

$$= 0.35$$

$$Z = \frac{\bar{x}_1 - \bar{x}_2}{\text{SE}(\bar{x}_1 - \bar{x}_2)} = \frac{60 - 62}{0.35} = \frac{2}{0.35} = 5.71$$

Since the observed difference is more than 3 times the SE, it is highly significant ($p < 0.01$). The growth is more in the second group than in the first.

Example 3: Pregnant women attending an *anganwadi* and receiving nutritional supplementation numbering 49 were matched with 64 pregnant women not attending *anganwadi* and not getting the supplementation. Both groups were followed-up. The mean birth-weight of babies born to the former was 3.5 kg with SD 1.4 kg and that of those born to the latter, 3.0 kg with SD 1.6 kg. Is the higher birth weight in the former due to the nutrition supplementation?

First, the SE of mean for each of the group is calculated as follows.

$$\text{SEDM} = \sqrt{(\text{SE}_1)^2 + (\text{SE}_2)^2}$$

$$= \sqrt{\frac{(\text{SD}_1)^2}{n_1} + \frac{(\text{SD}_2)^2}{n_2}}$$

$$= \sqrt{\frac{(1.4)^2}{49} + \frac{(1.6)^2}{64}}$$

$$= \sqrt{\frac{1.96}{49} + \frac{2.56}{64}}$$

$$= \sqrt{0.04 + 0.04}$$

$$= \sqrt{0.08}$$

$$= 0.28$$

$$Z = \frac{\bar{x}_1 - \bar{x}_2}{\text{SE}(\bar{x}_1 - \bar{x}_2)} = \frac{3.5 - 3.0}{0.28} = \frac{0.5}{0.28} = 1.78$$

Since the observed difference is less than 2 times the SE, (within 95% confidence limits) it is not significant. That means the difference in mean birth weight is due to chance and not due to nutritional supplementation.

Standard Error of the Difference between Two Correlated Means

Correlation between the two means is introduced in the following situations:

a. *The Single Group Situation:* This is, when a single group is tested twice on the same test or an equivalent form of the test is used on the second occasion.
b. *The Equivalent Group Situation:* When equivalent groups are formed by using "matching by pairs" or "matching by Means and SD's".

If the same group of students take the arithmetic ability test twice instead of two different groups taking it, we have the same individual's score on the first testing, to pair off with his score in the second testing. If, in a comparison of males and females, the two groups are standardized better by taking a brother or a sister from each family or if the boys and girls are paired with respect to age, IQ or social status and if these factors of common family, age, IQ or social status have any relation to arithmetic ability, they will automatically introduce correlation between the two samples.

A correlation coefficient is computed and introduced in the relevant formula. A numerical example using the single group situation is given below:

Difference Method (Small Samples)

When groups are small, the procedure called, the *difference method* is often to be preferred. It is quicker and easier to apply than the long method of calculating SE's for each mean and the SE of the difference. It is to be preferred if the value of the correlation coefficient between the two sets of scores is not required for any other purpose.

Example: Ten patients were given three successive trials on a stress test. The scores for the first and the last trials are shown below. Is the mean gain from the first to the third trial significant (Table 15.2)?

In the above example nondirectional hypothesis was put forward. The H_1 did not mention any direction of the difference. The difference could be in favor of the first trial also. However, if our hypothesis had been that practice increases test scores and there would be gain on successive trials, a one-tailed test would have been used. In that case the critical value of t from the table would have been read as follows:

i. For 9 *df*, the 0.1 level is read from the 0.02 col. ($p/2 = 0.01$); t value = 2.82.
ii. For 9 *df*, the 0.05 level is read from the 0.10 col. ($p/2 = 0.05$); t value = 1.83.

The calculated value of t in this example is much larger than the value of t required for significance at both the levels with the directional hypothesis. Hence, the mean gain from the first to the third on the test is significantly larger.

The Significance of Difference between Standard Deviations

Independent Samples

When samples are independent, i.e., different groups have been studied or there is evidence that the two tests given to the same group are uncorrelated, the significance of the difference between the two may be found by the formula:

$$SE_{\sigma_1-\sigma_2}, \sigma_{\sigma_1-\sigma_2} = \sqrt{\sigma^2_{\sigma_1} + \sigma^2_{\sigma_2}} \quad ...(15.5)$$

(SE of the difference in two independent samples).

At times, the psychologists and the educational researchers are interested more in the variability than in the means of the groups. Experimental treatments may be tried out which affect variability. Hence, the need for testing the difference in the standard deviations (Table 15.3).

Example: Suppose, on a test of communication skill, two groups of 32 students of Nursing School and 50 students of Nursing College obtain standard deviations equal to 8 and 6 respectively. Is the difference in the two standard deviations significant?

Table 15.2

Summary of the test of the difference between means for correlated groups (Non-sense syllable test example) Difference Method

Hypothesis

$$H_0: \mu_1 = \mu_2$$
$$H_0: \mu_1 \neq \mu_2$$

Decision rules

Given: 0.01 significance level; and $df = N_1 - 1 = 9$; table value of $t = 3.25$:

If t obt. < 3.25 accept H_0.
If t obt. ≥ 3.25 reject H_0.

Computation:

Trial-I	Trial-III	Difference (T-III – T-I)	x	x^2
12	16	4	1	1
14	18	4	1	1
10	17	7	4	16
8	10	2	–1	1
16	18	2	–1	1
17	25	8	5	25
18	18	0	–3	9
20	21	1	–2	4
16	17	1	–2	4
19	20	1	–2	4
ΣI = 150	ΣII = 180	ΣD = 30		$\Sigma x^2 = 66$

$$\text{Mean, D} = \frac{\Sigma D}{N} = \frac{30}{10} = 3.0$$

$$SD_D = \sqrt{\frac{\Sigma x^2}{N-1}} = \sqrt{\frac{66}{9}} = 2.71$$

$$SE_D = \frac{SD}{\sqrt{N}} = \frac{2.71}{\sqrt{10}} = 0.86$$

$$t = \frac{M_D - 0}{SE_D} = \frac{3-0}{0.86} = 3.49$$

Interpretation:

Reject H_0
Hence, there is a significant difference between the means on the two trials.

Table 15.3

Summary of the test of difference between means in small independent samples (attitude test example)

Hypothesis

$$H_0: \mu_1 = \mu_2$$
$$H_0: \mu_1 \neq \mu_2$$

Decision Rules

Given: 0.05 significance level; and $df = N_1 + N_2 - 2 = 13$; table value of $t = 2.16$:

If t obt. < 2.16 accept H_0.
If t obt. ≥ 2.16 reject H_0.

Computation

Maternity ward			*Medical ward*		
X	*x*	x^2	X	*x*	x^2
6	–4	16	4	1	1
7	–3	9	3	0	0
8	–2	4	2	–1	1
10	0	0	1	–2	4
15	+5	25	5	2	4
16	+6	36	$\Sigma X_2 = 15$		$\Sigma x_2^2 = 10$
9	–1	1	M = 15/5 = 3		
10	0	0	$N_1 - 1 = 9$, $N_2 - 1 = 4$.		
10	0	0			
9	–1	1			
$\Sigma X_1 = 100$		$\Sigma x_1^2 = 92$			
M = 10					

$$\text{Formula: SD} = \sqrt{\frac{\Sigma x_1^2}{N_1 - 1} + \frac{\Sigma x_2^2}{N_1 - 1}}$$

$$SE_D = 1.56$$

$$t = \frac{M_1 - M_2}{SE_D} = \frac{7}{1.56} = 4.46$$

Interpretation:

Reject H_0: It shows that the two groups differed significantly in their mean attitude scores.

Solution. First calculate the values of σ_1 and σ_2 by formula.

$$\sigma_{\sigma 1} = \frac{\sigma_1}{\sqrt{2N_1}} = \frac{8}{\sqrt{2 \times 32}} = 1.00$$

(SE for students of nursing school group)

$$\sigma_{\sigma 2} = \frac{\sigma_2}{\sqrt{2N_2}} = \frac{6}{\sqrt{2 \times 50}} = 0.6$$

(SE for students of nursing college group)

σ_1 and σ_2 are SD's for students of nursing school and college respectively and so are N_1 and N_2

$$\sigma_{\sigma_1-\sigma_2} = \sqrt{(1.00)^2 + (0.6)^2}$$
$$= 1.17$$
$$t = \frac{\sigma_1 - \sigma_2}{\sigma_{\sigma 1-\sigma 2}} = \frac{8-6}{1.17} = \frac{2}{1.17} = 1.71$$

Interpretation

The null hypothesis, $H_0 = \sigma_1 = \sigma_2$, could not be rejected because the observed value of t, 1.71, is less than the critical value of t with $df = 32 + 50 - 2 = 80$, at 0.05 level. Hence, the students of Nursing School and College do not differ significantly on variability on the test of verbal ability.

Correlated Samples

Situations arise when the same group of subjects is to be tested before and after a particular experimental treatment. The two groups, to be compared may be matched or correlation may be introduced due to some other factors. In these situations, formulas for the comparison of SD's for independent samples do not apply. However, the formula given below can be used for the purpose:

$$SE\sigma_1\_\sigma_2, \sigma_{\sigma_1-\sigma_2} = \sqrt{\sigma^2_{\sigma_1} + \sigma^2_{\sigma_2} - 2r_{12}^2\sigma_{\sigma 1}\sigma_{\sigma 2}} \quad ...(15.6)$$

(SE of the difference between two correlated SD's with large N). In which σ_1 and σ_2 are the SE's of the individual SD's calculated by formula and r_{12} is the value of correlation between the two sets of scores. The other procedure of calculation and interpretation remains the same as for independent samples above (Table 15.4).

The Significance of the Difference between Two Independent Proportions

Experimental results sometimes require a test of significance of the difference between two independent proportions taken from two randomly drawn samples. Of the N_1, members of the first group f_1, have the attribute A of the N_2 subjects of the second group, f_2 have this attribute. The question arises, do the two proportions, $f_1/N_1 = p_1$ and $f_2/N_2 = p_2$, differ significantly. Can the two samples be regarded random samples from the same population? This requires the computation of SE of the difference of the proportions. The SE of a single proportion is given by formula reproduced below:

$\sigma_p = \sqrt{pq/N}$ in which p = sample value of a proportion $q = 1 - p$
N = N_0 of cases in the sample

When a comparison of two sample proportions is involved, the SE of the difference is given by

$$\sigma_{p_1-p_2} = \sqrt{pq\left(\frac{1}{N_1} + \frac{1}{N_2}\right)} \quad ...(15.7)$$

In which p is an estimate based on the two samples combined and $q = 1 - p$. The value of p is obtained by adding up the frequencies of occurrence in the two samples and dividing it by the sum of the two N's.

$$p = \frac{f_1 + f_2}{N_1 + N_2} \quad ...(15.8)$$

A t value is then obtained by dividing the difference of the two proportions by $SE_{p_1-p_2}$.

Example: In Nursing College A, 350 students out of 500 and in Nursing College B, 250 students out of 300, passed in a University. If the two Nursing colleges have been selected randomly from a large number of colleges in a district, do the two colleges differ significantly in terms of their performance in the university examination?

Solution:

$$p_1 = \frac{350}{500} = 0.7$$

$$p_1 = \frac{250}{500} = 0.83$$

$$\text{Combined proportion, } p = \frac{350 + 250}{500 + 300} = \frac{600}{800} = 0.75$$

$$q = 1 - p = 1 - 0.75 = 0.25$$

Table 15.4

Summary of the test of the difference between means for correlated large samples (single group method)

Example: A group of 35 randomly selected nursing students was tested before and after an experimental treatment. The data so obtained is given below:

	Pre-test	Post-test	
M	15.5	21.6	$r = 0.70$
SD	5.2	4.8	N = 35

Find out if the groups differed significantly on the two testing.

Hypothesis

$$H_0: \mu_1 = \mu_2$$
$$H_0: \mu_1 \neq \mu_2$$

Decision rules

Given: 0.01 significance level; and $df = N_1 - 1 = 34$; table value of $t = 2.72$:

If t obt. < 2.72 accept H_0.
If t obt. ≥ 2.72 reject H_0.

Computation

$$SE_D = \sqrt{\sigma^2 m_1 + \sigma^2 m_1 - 2r_{12}\sigma m_1\, \sigma m_2}$$

$$\sigma_{M_1} = \frac{\sigma_1}{\sqrt{N}} = \frac{\sigma_2}{\sqrt{N}} = 0.88 \quad (\sigma_1 \text{ is the SD of pre-test})$$

$$\sigma_{M_2} = \frac{\sigma_2}{\sqrt{N}} = \frac{4.8}{\sqrt{35}} = 0.81 \quad (\sigma_2 \text{ is the SD of pre-test})$$

$$SE_D = (0.88)^2 + (0.81)^2 - 2 \times 0.70 \times 0.88 \times 0.81 = 0.658$$

$$t = \frac{M_1 - M_2}{SE_D} = \frac{6.1}{658} = 9.27$$

Interpretation:

Reject H_0:

There is a significant difference between the mean scores of the group on pre-test and post-test.

SE of the difference by formula (15.7)

$$\sigma_{p_1 - p_2} = \sqrt{0.75 \times 0.25\left[\frac{1}{500} + \frac{1}{300}\right]}$$

$$= \sqrt{0.19 \times 0.005}$$

$$= \sqrt{0.00095} = 0.031$$

$$t = \frac{0.70 - 0.83}{0.031} = \frac{0.13}{0.031} = 4.19$$

The value of t from Table B with $df = (500 + 300) - 2 = 798$, at 0.05 level = 1.96; and at 0.01 level = 2.58.

Interpretation

The calculated value of t is larger than the critical value of t at 0.01 levels. Hence, it is significant and thus the null hypothesis (H_0: $p_1 = p_2$) cannot be retained. The two Nursing colleges differ significantly in their performance in the University examination.

Standard Error of Proportion

The SEM and SEDM are the tests of significance of variation in means of samples (more than 30) of quantitative data. The SEP and the SEDP (Standard Error of Difference between two proportions) are the tests of significance of variation in proportions of samples of qualitative data (more than 30).

In qualitative data, the character remains the same while the frequency variations are dealt with.

If a sample consist of characters of two attributes (positive and negative) only, such as male and female, rich and poor, vaccinated and non-vaccinated, died and survived, successes and failures etc. it is a sample of binomial classification and if the division of the sample is made into more than two classes such as blood groups A, B, AB and O or WBCs into polymorphs, lymphocytes, eosinophils etc. the sample is of multinomial classification.

The proportion of individuals, having a specific character or attribute, in a binomial distribution, is expressed as "p", either as a fraction of 1 or as percentage.

$$p = \frac{\text{Number of individuals having a specific character}}{\text{Total number in the sample}}$$

The remaining proportion of individuals having the other (negative) character, is represented as "q". Arithmatically "q" = $1 - p$ in terms of fraction of 1 or $100 - p$ in percentage.

Thus 'p' is the probability of occurrence of a positive attribute and 'q' is the probability of occurrence of the negative attribute (or non-occurrence of the same positive attribute).

To illustrate, suppose there are 80 girls in a class of 200 strength, the proportion of girls and boys, is estimated as follows:

Proportion of girls (p) = $\frac{80}{200}$ 0.4 out of 1 in the sample

Proportion of boys (q) = $\frac{200-80}{200} = \frac{120}{200} = 0.6$ out of 1

or

$$q = 1 - p$$
$$= 1 - 0.4$$
$$= 0.6$$

For statistical analysis, the proportion of girls (p) and boys (q) are expressed in percentage as below.

$$p = \frac{80 \times 100}{200} = 40\% \text{ girls}$$

$q = 100 - p = 100 - 40 = 60\%$ boys in the example.

The Significance of the Difference between Two Correlated Proportions

When the two proportions have been obtained on the same sample of individuals or on matched samples, the paired observations may exhibit a correlation between the two proportions and must be taken care of while using a test of significance of difference in them.

Example: If 400 patients of Victoria Hospital, Bengaluru city answer the two questions as below, is the difference between the two proportions of persons saying 'Yes' to both the questions significant?

	Yes	No
1. Are you getting good treatment?	180	220
2. Are you getting good nursing care?	200	200

The data is arranged below in the shape of a 2 × 2 contingency table. This arrangment is, of course, based on detailed information about paired observations for each individual. One individual may say 'Yes' to both the questions; the second, 'No' to both the questions; the third 'Yes' to question one, and 'No' to question two and so on. This data can be tabulated as below in 2 × 2 contingency tables; showing frequencies and proportions based on frequencies. The cells in tables of frequencies have been marked by capital letters and those for proportions, by small letters whose arrangement may be noted carefully.

Frequencies

	Question 1 No	Question 1 Yes	
Question 2 Yes	220 (A)	180 (B)	400
No	200 (C)	200 (D)	400
	420	380	800

Proportions

	Question 1 No	Question 1 Yes	
Question 2 Yes	0.15 (a)	0.35 (b)	0.50
No	0.40 (c)	0.10 (d)	0.50
	0.45	0.45	1.00

The null hypothesis is that the proportions of 'Yes' responses to question 1 and question 2 do not differ, except beyond chance. The standard error of the difference between two correlated proportions is given by the formula

$$SEp_1 - p_2 = \frac{\sqrt{a+d}}{N} \qquad ...(15.9)$$

$$= \frac{\sqrt{0.15+0.1}}{400} = 0.0125$$

The value of $Z = \dfrac{p_1 - p_2}{SEp_1 - p_2}$

According to the problem, $p_1 - p_2$ are

$180/400 = 0.45$ and $200/400 = 0.50$

Hence, $$Z = \frac{0.45 - 0.50}{0.0125} = \frac{0.50}{0.125} = 4.00$$

The critical value of Z at 0.05 and 0.01 levels are 1.96 and 2.58 respectively (Consult Table A in Appendix). Hence, the calculated value of Z is significant at 0.01 level.

In case frequencies are to be used, the following formula will apply:

$$Z = \frac{D - A}{\sqrt{A + D}} \qquad ...(15.10)$$

(Formula for comparison of frequencies)

Another general formula for the calculation of $SEp_1 - p_2$ is

$$\sigma_{p_1} - {}_{p_2} = \sqrt{\sigma^2_{p_1} + \sigma^2_{p_2} - 2r_{p_1 p_2}\sigma_{p_1}\sigma_{p_2}} \qquad ...(15.11)$$

(SE of difference between two correlated proportions, based on calculation of r).

For this purpose, r between the two percents is given by the phi coefficient, a ratio equivalent to the correlation coefficient in 2 × 2 tables. Calculation of phi coefficient will be shown in chapter on correlational techniques. σ_{p_1} and σ_{p_2} are SE's of σ_{p_1} and σ_{p_2} computed according to formula (15.10).

Suppose from the universe (population), multiple samples are drawn, the value of the particular characteristic (otherwise called as proportion) in each sample is represented as "p" (just like the sample mean, $\bar{x}$), the proportion of the samples (p_1, p_2, p_3 .... etc.) have a tendency to concentrate around the proportion of the universe or population, represented as "P" (just like the sample means m_1, m_2, m_3, i.e., $\bar{x}_1$, $\bar{x}_2$, $\bar{x}_3$, ... etc. have central tendency around population mean M).

The sample proportions are symmetrically distributed around the population proportion, from which the samples are drawn, i.e. it gains the shape of a normal curve.

This distribution of the sample values (proportions) around the population proportion (P), is expressed arithmetically interms "Standard error of proportions" (SEP). In otherwords, SEP is the standard deviation of the sample proportions (just like SEM in the SD of the sample means).

The binomial confidence limits are as follows.

- 68 percent of sample proportions will lie within the range P ± 1SE of proportion.
- 95 percent of values lie within the range of P ± 2SEp. (95 percent confidence limits).
- 99 percent of values lie within the range of P ± 3SEp. (99 percent confidence limits).

Standard error of proportion is defined as a measure of variation occurring by chance between the sample proportion (p) and the population proportion (P) in a qualitative data.

This test of significance is employed to find the efficacy of a drug or a vaccine or a surgical procedure etc. To illustrate, if 35 percent cases died in previous epidemic and 30 percent in the present epidemic, whether this reduction of 5 percent is due to better treatment or increased immunity or decrease virulence of the pathogen or by chance is determined by calculation of SE of proportion.

Formula:

$$\text{SEP} = \frac{p \times q}{n}$$

Where,

p = % of positive character (proportion)

q = % of negative character $(100 - p)$

n = number of observations (size of the sample)

The significance of difference is found by relative deviate (Z) test.

$$Z = \frac{\text{Observed difference}}{\text{SEP}}$$

Example 1: The proportion of blood group A among Indians is 30 percent. Find SEP and the 95 percent confidence limits. Could this sample be from an universe, in which the prevalence of blood group A is 40 percent?

$$p = 30;\ q = 100 - 30;\ n = 100$$

$$\text{SEP} = \sqrt{\frac{p \times q}{n}} = \sqrt{\frac{30 \times 70}{100}} = \sqrt{21} = 4.58$$

95% confidence limits = $p \pm 2\text{SE}$

$$= 30 + 2 \times 4.58 \qquad 30 - 2 \times 4.58$$

$$= 30 + 9.16 \qquad = 30 - 9.16$$

$$= 39.16 \qquad = 20.84$$

Since the proportion 40 is outside the 95 percent confidence limits, we can say with 95 percent confidence that the sample is not drawn from the universe having 40 percent prevalence of blood group A.

Uses of SEP

- SEP is used to find the confidence limits of population proportion (ρ) if sample proportion (β) is given.
- To tell whether the sample drawn from the known population or not.
- To find the standard error of difference between two proportions, to know if the observed difference between proportions of two samples is real and statistically significant or due to chance and insignificant.
- To find the size of the sample if SEP and the proportions are known.

The Significance of the Difference between Two *r*'s

Situations arise in which two correlation coefficients are to be compared. There could be correlations between attitude towards a particular course and achievement in that course for two different groups, say, male and female students. The null hypothesis, $H_0: p_1 = p_2$ or $H_0: p_1 - p_2 = 0$. The procedure of calculating an SE of the r has already been explained in a section in the preceding chapter. The comparison of the r's involves the following steps.

1. Convert the two r's into Fisher's Z funtion.
2. The $\text{SE}z_1 - z_2 = \sqrt{\sigma_{z1}^2 + \sigma_{z2}^2}$

$$= \sqrt{\left(\frac{1}{N_1 - 3} + \frac{1}{N_2 - 3}\right)} \qquad \text{... (15.12)}$$

(Comparison of two r's through Z conversion)

N_1 and N_2 are number of cases in two groups.

$$\text{Value of } t = \frac{Z_1 - Z_2}{\text{SE}_{z_1 - z_2}} \qquad \text{...(15.13)}$$

The above steps will be demonstrated through an example.

Example: The two correlation coefficients in the illustration given above are 0.64 and $N_1 = 103$ and $N_2 = 63$. Is there a significant difference in the two r's.

$$\text{SE}_{z_1 - z_2} = \sqrt{\frac{1}{103 - 3} + \frac{1}{63 - 3}} = 0.164$$

$$t = \frac{1.05 - 0.76}{0.164} = \frac{0.29}{0.164} = 1.77$$

The $df = N_1 + N_2 - 3 = 103 + 63 - 3 = 163$, and critical value of t at 0.05 level is 1.97. The observed value of t is smaller than the critical value of t. Hence, the H_0 cannot be rejected. There is no significant difference between the two correlations.

In case where the same sample has been tested on more than one variables and the correlations between the variables have been computed, the situation involves an SE of the correlated samples. Suppose a group of 10 randomly selected students have been tested on their attitude towards Mathematics, their achievement in Mathematics and general mental ability. The three pairs of correlations are: r_{12}, r_{13} and r_{23} with their values, 0.8, 0.7 and 0.2 respectively. If we wish to compare r_{12} and r_{13}; or r_{12} and r_{23}; or r_{13} and r_{23} the procedure mentioned above does not apply because it is based on correlated samples.

Hence, to test the difference between r_{12} and r_{13}, we use

$$t = \frac{(r_{12} - r_{13})\sqrt{(N-3)(1+r_{23})}}{\sqrt{2(1 - r_{12}^2 - r_{13}^2 - r_{23}^2 + 2r_{12}r_{13}r_{23})}} \qquad ...(15.14)$$

(Difference in two r's in correlated samples)

Inserting the values, we obtained

$$t = \frac{(0.8-0.7)\sqrt{(103-3)(1+0.2)}}{\sqrt{2(1-0.8^2-0.7^2-2^2+2\times 0.8\times 0.7\times 0.2)}}$$

$$= \frac{0.1\times 10.06}{0.33} = 3.21$$

Interpretation

With $df = 103 - 3 = 100$, a t of 2.63 is required for significance. Since the observed value is higher than 2.63, it is significant at 0.01 level. Hence, there are significant differences in the two's and the H_0 cannot be retained.

Critical Region

A statistic is used to test the hypothesis H_0. The test statistic follows some known distribution. In a test, the area under the probability density curve is divided into two regions, viz., the region of acceptance and the region of rejection. The region of rejection is the region in which H_0 is rejected. It means that if the value of test statistics lies in this region, H_0 will be rejected. The region of rejection is called a critical region. Moreover, the area of the critical region is equal to the level of significance α. The critical region is always on the tail of the distribution curve. It may be on both the tails or on one tail, depending upon the alternative hypothesis.

One- and Two-tailed Tests

If the alternative hypothesis, H_1 is of the type $\mu > \mu_0$; $\mu_1 <$ or $> \mu_2$; $\sigma^2 > \sigma_0^2$ or $\sigma_1^2 < \sigma_2^2$; etc., the critical region lies on only one tail of the probability density curve. In this situation, the test is called one-tailed test. If H_1 is of the type $\mu > \mu_0$, $\mu_1 < \mu_2$; $\sigma^2 > \sigma_0^2$; $\sigma_2^2 > \sigma_1^2$; etc., the critical region is towards the right tail as shown in Figure 15.3.

On the contrary, if H_1 is of the type $\mu < \mu_0$; $\sigma^2 < \sigma_0^2$, $\mu_1 > \mu_2$; $\sigma_1^2 > \sigma_2^2$, etc., the critical region lies on the left tail as depicted in Figure 15.4.

However, if H_1 is of the type $\mu = 0$; $\mu_1 = \mu_2$; $\sigma^2 = \sigma_0^2$, or $\sigma_1^2 \neq \sigma_0^2$ etc., the critical region lies on both the tails. In this situation, a test is called a two-tailed test. In a two-tailed test, an area equal to $\alpha/2$

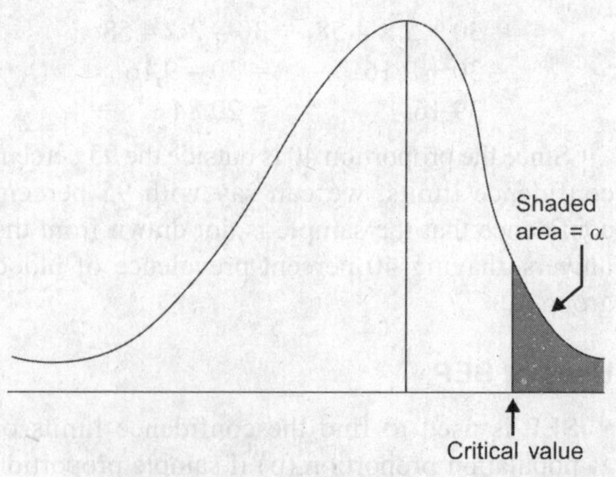

Fig. 15.3: One-sided right tailed critical region

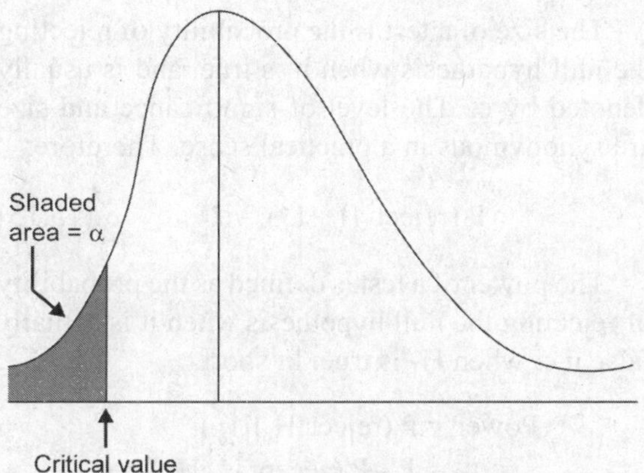

Fig. 15.4: One-sided left tailed critical region

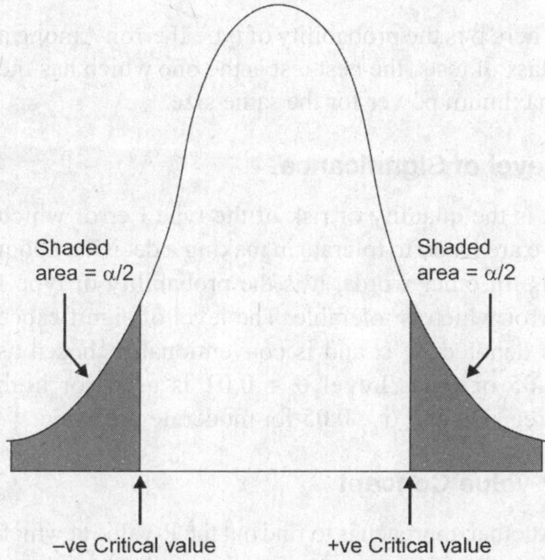

Fig. 15.5: Two-tailed critical regions

lies on both the tails, for a test of significance level α. The critical regions are shown in Figure 15.5.

Zqt Two-Tailed and One-Tailed Tests of Significance

The null hypothesis denotes that the difference between the obtained means may be either plus or minus and as often in one direction as in the other from the true (population) difference of zero. Hence for determining probabilities, both the tails of the sampling distribution are used. (See Figure 15.6). When the primary concern is with the direction of the difference rather than with its existence in absolute terms, the situation calls for a one-tailed test and only one-tail of sampling distribution is used. The procedure for picking up the values of the critical ratio, *t*, for a particular significance level under one-tailed, test are as follows:

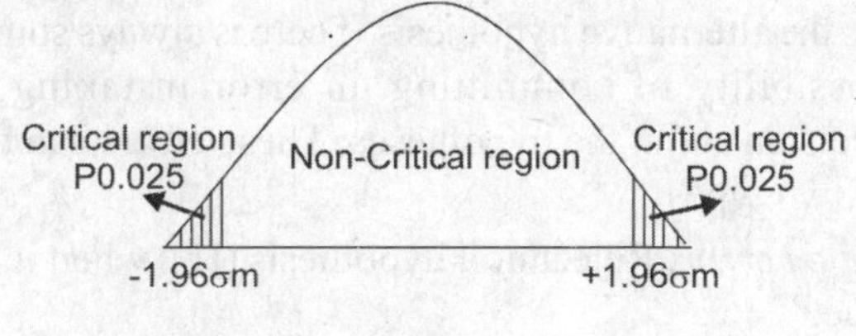

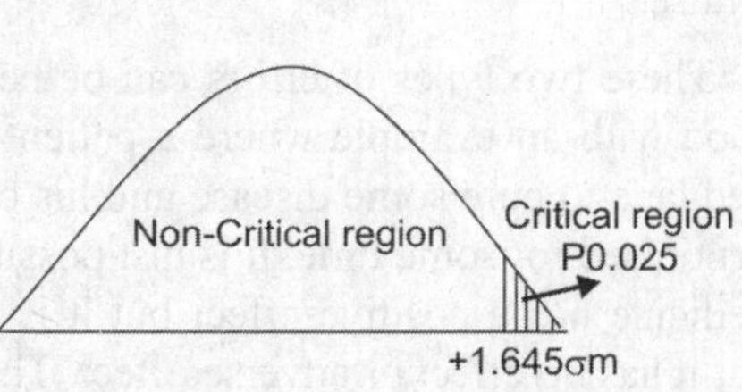

Fig. 15.6: Two sampling distribution of means showing the critical regions and non-critical regions in (A) Two-tailed or non-directional test and (B) One-tiled or directional test

Level of significance	*Column of the table to be consulted*	*Reason*
0.05	0.10	$p/2 = 0.05$
0.01	0.02	$p/2 = 0.01$

The *t* tables given in book on statistics are generally meant for a two-tailed situation and the probability is distributed equally in the two tails (For 0.05, $p = 0.025$ is in each of the two tails; and For 0.01; $p = 0.005$ in each of the two tails). Hence, the probability must be doubled to obtain the correct value of the critical ratio in a two-tailed test.

Two Types of Errors

After applying a test, a decision is taken about the acceptance or rejection of null hypothesis vis-a-vis the alternative hypothesis. There is always some possibility of committing an error in taking a decision about the hypotheses. These errors can be of two types:

Type I error: Reject null hypothesis (H_0) when it is true.

Type II error: Accept null hypothesis (H_0) when it is false.

These two types of errors can be better understood with an example where a patient is given a medicine to cure some disease and his condition is scrutinised for some time. It is just possible that the medicine has a positive effect but it is considered that it has no effect or adverse effect. Thus, it is the first kind of error or type I error. On the contrary, if the medicine has an adverse effect but is considered to have a positive effect, it is called the second kind of error or type II error. Now, let us consider the implications of these two types of error. If type I error is committed, the patient will be given another medicine, which may or may not be effective. But if type II error is committed, i.e. the medicine is continued in spite of an adverse effect, the patient is likely to develop some other complications or may even die. This means that the type II error is much more severe than the type I error. Hence, in drawing inference about the null hypothesis, practice is followed that type II error be minimized even at certain risk of type I error.

Research requires testing of hypothesis. In this process, two types of wrong inferences can be drawn. These are called Type I and Type II errors.

Type I error is committed when we reject a null hypothesis by marking a difference significant, although no true difference exists.

Type II error is committed when we accept a null hypothesis by marking a difference not significant when a true difference actually exists. These can be diagrammatically shown as below:

	Decision	
	Reject H_0	*Accept H_0*
Ho True:	Type I Error	No Error
Ho false:	No Error	Type II Error

The size of a test is the probability of rejecting the null hypothesis when it is true, and is usually denoted by α. The level of significance and size are synonymous in a practical sense. Therefore,

$$P\text{ (reject } H_0|H_0) = \alpha \qquad ...(15.15)$$

The power of a test is defined as the probability of rejecting the null hypothesis when it is actually false, i.e. when H_1 is true. In short,

$$\begin{aligned} \text{Power} &= P\text{ (reject } H_0|H_0) \\ &= 1 - P\text{ (accept } H_0|H_0) \\ &= 1 - \text{(Probability of type II error)} \\ &= 1 - \beta \qquad ...(15.16) \end{aligned}$$

where β is the probability of type II error. Among a class of tests, the best test is the one which has the maximum power for the same size.

Level of Significance

It is the quantity of risk of the type I error which we are ready to tolerate in making a decision about H_0. In other words, it is the probability of type I error which is tolerable. The level of significance is denoted by α and is conventionally chosen as 0.05 or 0.01. Level $\alpha = 0.01$ is used for high precision and $\alpha = 0.05$ for moderate precision.

P-value Concept

Another approach is to find out the P-value at which H_0 is significant, i.e., to find the smallest level α at which H_0 is rejected. In this situation, it is not inferred whether H_0 is accepted or rejected at level 0.05 or 0.01 or any other level. But the statistician only gives the smallest level α at which H_0 is rejected. This facilitates an individual to decide for himself as to how much significant the data are. This approach avoids the imposition of a fixed level of significance. About the acceptance or rejection of H_0, the experimenter can himself decide the level α by comparing it with the P-value. The criterion for this is that if the P-value is less than or equal to α, reject H_0 otherwise accept H_0.

Randomized Test

A randomized test (T°) is one in which no test statistic is used. The decision about the rejection of H_0 is taken, if it satisfies some predecided criterion. For instance, if it is decided that H_0 will be rejected if on tossing a coin it falls with the head on the upper side and will be accepted if it falls with the tail on the upper side. Since randomized test is rarely used it is not explained further.

Non-Randomized Test

A test T of a hypothesis H is said to be non-randomized if the hypothesis H is rejected on the basis that a test statistic belongs to the critical region c_T, i.e. ψ_T $(X_1, X_2, \ldots X_n) \in c_T$. Some of the commonly used non-randomized tests are given in this chapter as well as in the next chapter.

Degrees of Freedom

Degrees of freedom (*df*) is the number of independent observations in a set.

It is apparent from the discussion made so far that in a test of hypothesis, a sample is drawn from the population of which the paramter is under test. The size of the sample varies since it depends either on the experimenter or on the resources available. Moreover, the test statistic involves the estimated value of the parameter which depends on the number of observations. Hence, the sample size plays an important role in testing of hypothesis and is taken care of by degrees of freedom.

Degrees of freedom are calculated as follows:

1. In unpaired '*t*-test' of difference between the means, $df = n_1 + n_2 - 2$, where n_1 and n_2 are the number of observations in each series. In paired "*t*-test" $df = n - 1$.
2. In Chi-square (x^2) test, for independence of two classifications, $df = (r - 1)(c - 1)$ where "*r*" and "*c*" are the number of rows and number of columns in the table.
3. In testing the significance of correlation, $df = n - 2$, where *n* is the number of paired measurements. However, there are exceptions to each of the above rules. In paired or unpaired series, if the estimated or calculated '*t*'-value is higher than the tabulated '*t*'-value, the difference is statistically significant, if it is less, the difference is insignificant.

Formula:

i. The unpaired sample,

$$t = \frac{\bar{x}_1 - \bar{x}_2}{\text{SE of difference between means}}$$

$$= \frac{\bar{x}_1 - \bar{x}_2}{\text{SE}\,(\bar{x}_1 - \bar{x}_2)}$$

ii. For paired samples,

$$t = \frac{\bar{d}}{\text{SE of } d}$$

Where d = difference in the two values for each pairs (total number of pairs being *n*)

$\bar{d}$ = mean of the *n*-values for *d*.

It may be remembered here that $\text{SE of } d = \dfrac{\text{SE of } d}{\sqrt{n}}$

Note: The table values for the distribution of test statistics are provided in the Appendix B for various levels of significance and degrees of freedom. These table values make us decide about the rejection of H_0.

Student's *t*-Test

Student-*t* is the deviation of estimated mean from its population mean expressed in terms of standard deviation.

t-distribution has already been discussed in Chapter 8 where sampling distribution of $\bar{x}/s\,\bar{x}$ was discussed. Here, we shall make use of *t*-distribution in testing of hypothesis about the population mean or two population means.

Suppose, a small random sample ($X_1, X_2, \ldots, X_n$) of size *n* has been drawn from a normal population having mean μ and variance σ^2 which are unknown. We want to test the hypothesis.

$$H_0 : \mu = \mu_0 \text{ against } H_1 : \mu \neq \mu_0$$

where μ_0 is some assumed value considered fit for μ. Let the observed values on random sample (X_1, X_2, ..., X_n) be (x_1, x_2, ..., x_n). Statistic t is given as,

$$t_{n-1} = \frac{\bar{x} - \mu_0}{s_{\bar{x}}} \quad ...(15.17)$$

For the sample values, expression for t is,

$$t_{n-1} = \frac{\sqrt{n}(\bar{x} - \mu_0)}{s} \quad ...(15.17.1)$$

where $\bar{x}$ is the sample mean, s is the standard deviation of the sample, $(n - 1)$ in suffix indicates the *df* of t.

On substituting formula (15.17.1) for s, (15.17.1) can be written as,

$$t_{n-1} = (\bar{x} - \mu_0)\sqrt{\frac{n(n-1)}{\Sigma_i (x_i - \bar{x})^2}} \quad ...(15.17.3)$$

where $i = 1, 2, ..., n$.

To decide about the acceptance or rejection of H_0 vis-a-vis H_1, the calculated value of t is compared with the table value of t for $(n - 1)$ *df* and level of significance α. t-distribution table is provided in Appendix B (Table V) for different *df* and various levels of significance. The tabulated t-value gives the critical value of t. More clearly, if $t_{cal} \geq t_{\alpha/2}$ for $(n - 1)$ *df*, reject H_0, otherwise accept it.

Note:

1. In the above situation, a two-tailed test has to be applied since H_1 is $\mu \neq \mu_0$.
2. In case of a one tailed test, i.e., for the alternative hypothesis, $H_1: \mu > \mu_0$ reject H_0, if $t_{cal} \geq t_\alpha$ for $(n-1)$ *df* CR lies on the right tail. If the alternative hypothesis is, $H_1: \mu < \mu_0$ reject H_0 if $t_{cal} < -t_\alpha$ for $(n-1)$ *df*. The CR lies on left tail.
3. If t-table is provided for a two-tailed critical region, it should be consulted as such. If a one tailed t-table has been provided, we should consult the table for level $\alpha/2$, where α is a prefixed level of significance.
4. If H_0 is rejected at $\alpha = 0.01$, calculated t-value is called a highly significant value.

Assumptions about *t*-Test

t-test is based on the following five assumptions:

1. The random variable X follows normal distribution. In other words, the random sample has been drawn from a normal population.
2. All observations in the sample are independent.
3. The sample size is not large. There is no hard-and-fast rule which can be given to call a sample large. But, as a practice, a sample of size 30 or more is considered, a large sample. At the same time one should note that at least five observations are desirable for applying a t-test.
4. The assumed value μ_0 of the population mean is the correct value.
5. The sample values are correctly taken and recorded.

In case the above assumptions do not hold good, the reliability of the test decreases. Further, some tests are very sensitive and some are not. The test which gives quite a satisfactory result in spite of some departure from the basic assumptions is called a *robust test*. It is interesting to point out that the Student's t-test is a robust test.

Example: The life expectancy of people in the year 1970 in Brazil is expected to be 50 years. A survey was conducted in eleven regions of Brazil and the data obtained are given below. Do the data confirm the expected view?

Life expectancy: (years)	
54.2	58.2
50.4	56.6
44.2	61.9
49.7	57.5
55.4	53.4
57.0	

Here we have to test

$$H_0 = \mu = 50 \text{ against } H_1: \mu \neq 50$$

To test H_0, the statistic t is

$$t_{n-1} = \frac{\sqrt{n}(\bar{x} - \mu_0)}{s}$$

Now, we first compute $\overline{x}$ and s.

$$\overline{x} = \frac{598.5}{11} = 54.41$$

$$s^2 = \frac{1}{10}(32799.91 - (598.5)^2 / 11)$$

$$= \frac{1}{10}(236.07) = 23.607$$

$$s = 4.859$$

$$t = \frac{\sqrt{11}(54.41 - 50)}{4.859}, \quad t = \frac{14.626}{4.859} = 3.01$$

The table value of t at $\alpha = 0.05$ and 10 *df* is 2.228. Since $t_{cal} > 2.228$, reject H_0. It means that the life expectancy is more than 50 years. The chance of this result holding good for the whole population is 95 percent.

Indications for Statistical Tests

This question is considered by way of numerical calculations. If the frequency distribution is normal or Gaussian, the *standard deviation*, which is more descriptive than range, can be used to study a set of measurements. The *standard error* of the mean allows one to compare two or more sets of measurements. Unfortunately, there is no simple test for skew or non-parametric distributions, sometimes drawing a graph may be helpful.

Are Two Sets of Results "Significantly" Different?

1. Nominal (Classified) Measurements

Most nominal data takes the form of graded categories of response as in Table 15.5. Your eyes will tell you that this analgesic is working but the result could have been due to chance. The 15 "pain worse" patients could have been distributed in this way had we picked them out of a hat, as also could the other categories. A chi-square calculation using the formula:

$$\sum \frac{(O - E)^2}{E}$$

will tell you through the use of appropriate tables (see the references) how likely a chance result (0 stands for the observations actually observed and E for the expected observations had the assignments been random). If the number of observations is small it may be necessary to amalgamate adjacent columns or in a 2 × 2 contingency table apply Yates' Correction or Fisher's Exact Test. Yates' correction is applied in a four-fold contingency table if the numbers are greater than 40 or between 20 and 40 with no expected frequency less than 5. Fisher's Exact test is used if the numbers are less than 20 or 20–40 with one or more expected frequencies less than 5.

The McNemar test for paired data: The previous example showed the results of a group comparative study where 50 patients received an analgesic and 50 a placebo. Quite often, however, the patients can receive both and make a comparison—a "cross-over comparison". This then provides a pair of responses one for the analgesic and one for the placebo. This could take the form shown in Table 15.6, of the 50 patients, 10 obtained relief with both analgesic and placebo and 10 had no relief from either. Clearly these 20 do not help us to decide between the two treatments. Of the other 30, 5 were relieved by placebo but not by the analgesic and 25 by the analgesic but not by the placebo. This difference can be examined by the McNemar test:

$$\frac{(|A - D| - 1)^2}{A + D}$$

where A and D are the two usable results

$$\frac{(25 - 5 - 1)^2}{25 + 5}$$

$$\frac{19^2}{30} = \frac{361}{30} = 12$$

This result is a χ^2 and can be looked up in the tables under "one degree of freedom", which will tell you that the probability of such a result occuring by chance is less than 1 percent ($P < 0.01$). For small numbers of comparisons (less than 20) the

Table 15.5

A contingency table for nominal data obtained from response in a drug trial

	No pain	Partly relieved	No relief	Pain worse	Total
Analgesic	20	20	5	5	50
Placebo	5	10	25	10	50

Table 15.6

A "cross-over" comparison providing a pair of responses, one for the analgesic and one for the placebo

	Analgesic pain relief	No pain relief	
Placebo			
Pain relief	10	5	
No pain relief	25	10	Total 50

"sign test" should be used together with the table of binomial frequencies ("*c*" table).

2. Ordinal (Ranked) Measurements

Wilcoxon's tests for ranked measurements: This is used for ordinal data. The data have both direction and magnitude and are amenable to statistical tests which use the additional data. The magnitude is indicated by the rank order of the results, small differences in treatment response having low ranks and big differences high ranks. If the data are from comparative group trials these may be analyzed by the Wilcoxon's sum of ranks test or the Mann-Whitney U test. With paired data from perhaps a cross-over trial the Wilcoxon matched pairs signed rank test can be used.

3. Interval (Numerical) Data

Interval data are analyzed by plotting a frequency distribution and using the standard deviation and standard-error of the mean. Other tests are as follows:

Student's t-test: The *t*-test was developed by WS. Gosset, who wrote many papers under the pseudonym "Student". He was not a professional mathematician (his work was, in fact, in the Guinness's brewery in Dublin where he went after studying chemistry and mathematics) but his hobby was statistics and he published his paper in 1908. The *t*-test depends on a comparison of means from a group comparisons study, and associates these means with a scatter of the results (SE) using the formula

$$t = \frac{m_1 - m_2}{\sqrt{\frac{s^2}{n_1} + \frac{s^2}{n_2}}}$$

where m_1 and m_2 are the two sample means and the denominator is the combined estimate of the variance of the means (S^2) divided respectively by the number in each sample, the square root being taken out of the whole. The significance of t can then be looked up in appropriate tables.

Paired t-tests: If the data are paired as in a cross-over study, the mean of the difference between the results in each half of the cross-over can be divided by its own standard error, as in the following formula:

$$t = \frac{\text{mean difference}}{\text{SE of the mean}}$$

There are many statistical tests which depend on the normal distribution, of which the most familiar is analysis of variance or the F-test.

EXERCISES

1. Two groups of students selected randomly from two different colleges, were administered an attitude scale, and the following data was collected:

	N	M	SD	
College: I	40	30.5	6.0	Do the two groups differ significantly in their attitudes?
College: II	50	25.4	5.0	

2. A group of 10 students was given four trials on a test of physical efficiency. Their scores on the I and IV trials are given below. Test whether there was a significant gain from the first to the fourth trials.

Students	*Trial-I*	*Trial-IV*
1	15	20
2	16	22
3	17	22
4	20	25
5	25	35
6	30	30
7	17	21
8	18	23
9	10	17
10	12	20

3. A group of nursing students was administered a test of intelligence twice. The data so collected is given below: Test whether there was a significant difference in the means on the two testings.

	M	SD
Testing I	25	8
		$r = 0.65$
Testing II	35	5

4. Define the following as precisely as possible:
   i. Level of significance
   ii. Correlated samples
   iii. Standard error of the mean
   iv. Sampling distribution
5. a. Given two random samples of size 450 and 550 respectively each with sample values $p_1 = 0.66$ and $p_2 = 0.50$. Test the significance of the difference between p_1 and p_2.
   b. Test the difference between $p_1 = 500/600$ and $p_2 = 150/200$ (independent samples)
6. Given are two independent samples of size 200 each with $\sigma_1^2 = 121$ and $\sigma_1^2 = 400$, test the hypothesis that the variances are significantly different from each other.
7. If the groups are correlated and the $\sigma_1 = 15$ and $\sigma_2 = 10$ and $r = 0.6$, with $N = 100$, test the hypothesis that the standard deviations are significantly different.

8. a. Calculate the values of r's for $r = 0.60$; $r = 0.55$; $r = 0.25$; and $r = -0.85$
   b. Why is the conversion of r's into Z's required in calculating SE of r?
   c. Who devised this method of conversion?
9. Compare the following pairs of r's for significance of differences. Use 0.05 level of significance
   a. $r_1 = 0.60$; $r_2 = 0.40$: N = 84
   b. $r_1 = 0.80$; $r_2 = 0.00$: N = 83
   c. $r_1 = 0.20$; $r_2 = 0.70$: N = 124
   d. $r_1 = 0.60$; $r_2 = 0.40$: N = 84
   e. $r_1 = 0.60$; $r_2 = 0.40$: N = 84
10. Three psychological tests are administered to a sample of 100 students. The correlations obtained are $r_{12} = 0.80$; $r_{13} = 0.50$; and $r_{23} = 0.40$. Is r_{12} significantly different from r_{13}?

CHAPTER 16 The Chi-square Test and Other Nonparametric Methods

Introduction

The term **nonparametric statistics** is used to describe inferential statistics that do not require the same rigorous assumptions as parametric statistics. Nonparametric statistics are most often used when samples are small and/or when the data are measured on the nominal or ordinal scales.

Because there are literally dozens of nonparametric statistical tests available, only a few of the more commonly used will be discussed: chi-squared. Mann-Whitney U, Kruskal-Wallis one-way ANOVA, and Friedman two-way ANOVA.

Chi-square

'χ' is a Greek letter, not equivalent of English letter "X", written as "chi", pronounced as "Kye" and typed as "χ".

This test involves the calculation of a quantity, called "χ^2" in a qualitative data. χ^2-test was developed by Karl Pearson.

Perhaps the most commonly used nonparametric statistics is the chi-square (χ^2, also called chi-square) measure. This statistics can be applied to nominal or higher levels of measurement and can be used in one or more samples. Essentially, the chi-squared test is used to determine whether the observed frequencies of events in certain categories fall within the range of frequencies expected to fall in these categories.

Chi-squared tables contain information similar to parametric statistics tables. Table 16.1 is a fictitious table meant to demonstrate the information commonly found in a chi-squared table (this table is for illustrate purposes only; there has been no attempt to calculate χ^2 scores). This table shows the color preferences of a fictitious group of 84 nursing students. The numbers listed in the rows and columns show the selection and the totals by groups. By comparing the actual numbers of color selection with the expected numbers of color selection (this is done mathematically), the chi-squared statistic is computed. Degrees of freedom (*df*) are also computed, and a chi-squared table is read to determine the level of significance. In this instance,

Table 16.1

Preference of colors between male and female nursing students

	Yellow	*Blue*	*Green*	*Total*
Male	10	20	15	35
Female	12	24	13	49
Total	22	44	28	84

$\chi_2 = 1.98$, $df = 4$: $p > 0.05$

$p > 0.05$ means that the differences between male and female nursing students' preference in colors is not statistically significant at the 0.05 level.

Brown (1997) used the chi-squared statistic to analyze differences between individuals complaining of chest pain and preserving in an emergency facility over a period of 6 months. The researcher found that there were statistically significant differences in the use of different kinds of licit and illicit drugs, including cocaine, and in complaints concerning cardiac and noncardiac chest pain.

The chi-square test is applicable to test the hypotheses of the variance of a normal population, goodness of fit of the theoretical distribution to observed frequency distribution, in a one way classification having *k*-categories. It is also applied for the test of independence of attributes, when the frequencies are presented in a two-way classification called the contingency table. The chi-square test dates back to 1900, when Karl Pearson used it for frequency data classified into *k*-mutually exclusive categories. It is also a frequently used test in genetics, where one tests whether the observed frequencies in different crosses agree with the expected frequencies or not. Now chi-square tests of various hypotheses in sufficient details are given one by one.

The chi-square test is a useful measure of comparing experimentally obtained results with those expected theoretically and based on the hypothesis. It is used as a test statistic in testing a hypothesis that provides a set of theoretical frequencies with which observed frequencies are compared. The measure of chi-square enables us to find out the degree of discrepancy between observed frequencies and theoretical frequencies and thus, to determine whether the discrepancy so obtained between observed frequencies and theoretical frequencies is due to error of sampling or due to chance.

Problems in Nursing research frequently involve the counting of a number of persons, objects or responses as they occur under various categories of classifications. For example, Nursing students may be classified and counted according to their ability in theory, ability in practicals or their modes of behavior. Adult citizens may be classified according to whether they are "in favor of", "indifferent to", or "opposed to" a particular social reform. The Chi-square test is suitable for analyzing data and problems like those mentioned above. When data are in the form of discrete categories and frequencies. Chi-square is, perhaps, the most suitable test to compare the obtained set of *observed* frequencies in given categories with a set of *theoretical* or *expected* frequencies occurring within them. The number of categories may be two or more and the theoretical frequencies may be determined in a number of different ways depending upon the nature of the problem under consideration. *Chi-square is the statistic which measures the "divergence" of fact from hypothesis in the sample at hand.* The Chi-square, needed to test this and a wide variety of similar hypothesis, may be defined as

$$\chi^2 = \frac{\Sigma(f_o - f_e)}{fe} \quad ...(16.1)$$

in which,

f_o = Observed frequency in a single category

f_e = Expected, theoretical or hypothetical frequency

Σ = Sum of

From the formula, it is evident that chi-square is an index of the divergence of fact from hypothesis. If each of the observed frequency agreed exactly with the corresponding theoretical frequency, the value of χ^2 would be zero. The larger the divergence between the observed and theoretical frequency, the larger the value of chi-square. Chi-square is based on the squares of the deviations, $(f_o - f_e)^2$ and hence does not take the direction of the deviations into account. This is a limitation of the chi-square.

Steps

1. First, a table is prepared out of the qualitative data. Actual observed frequencies of 2 sets of events are entered in a two-way table, which is also known as "Contingency table". (Latin, con = together; tangere = to touch). Since this table also helps to know the association between two sets of events, the table is also called as

"Association table". Because there are only two events and two groups or classes, it is called 2×2 or four-fold or four-cell contingency table.

2. Null Hypothesis is set up stating there is no association between the events.

   x^2-text can also be applied when there are more than two classes or groups, such as social classes I, II, III and IV among smokers and non-smokers.

3. Then expected frequency for each cell is calculated on the assumption of no association, using the formula

$$fe = \frac{\text{Row total} \times \text{Column total}}{\text{Grand total}}$$

4. Then the difference between the observed and the expected frequencies for each cell is found (i.e. $fo - fe$).

5. x^2-value for each cell is calculated by using the formula

$$x^2 = \frac{(fo - fe)^2}{fe}$$

6. Then the total of x^2 for all the four cells is calculated by the formula (Summation of all 4 cell x^2-values)

$$\text{Total } x^2 = \sum \frac{(fo - fe)^2}{fe}$$

   Alternate formula for

$$x^2 = \frac{(ad - bc)^2 \times G}{(a+b)(c+d)(b+d)(a+c)}$$

   where, a, b, c and d are observed frequencies of 4 cells and G is the sample total (or grand total).

7. Next the degree of freedom (df) is calculated by using the formula, $df = (C - 1)(r - 1)$, where C = number of columns, r = number of rows.

8. Lastly to know whether the calculated x^2-value is significant or not, (i.e., whether the relation between the events smoking and cancer, for example, is by chance or a real one) we have to refer to "Fisher's x^2-table" (Annexure IV) for a particular degree of freedom, for a probability of 0.05, 0.01 etc. If the calculated value is higher than the table-value, it is concluded that it is significant and the Null hypothesis is to be rejected and accept the hypothesis (for example no association between smoking and lung cancer is ruled out and accept the hypothesis that there is significant association between smoking and cancer). If the calculated x^2-value is lower than the table value Null hypothesis is accepted.

The form of sampling distribution of chi-square depends only upon the degrees of freedom in the table from which chi-square has been calculated. In other words, chi-square shows the same distribution for all random samples in which the number of degrees of freedom is the same, regardless of the size of the sample (so long it is fairly large, say 50 or more and no theoretical frequency is very small, say 10 or less). Karl Pearson gave the concept of Chi-square and worked out its sampling distribution on the basis of the following:

$$y = yac^{-1/2 \times 2}(\chi^2)^{(df-1)2} \quad \text{...(16.2)}$$

Chi-square tables (Table F) have been prepared on the basis of this equation. Figures 16.1A to D show the distribution of chi-square for different degrees of freedom.

The value of chi-square is always positive, a circumstance which results from squaring the difference between observed and theoretical frequencies. Values of χ^2 range from 0 to infinity. The right hand tail of the curve is asymptotic to the ordinate as well as to the abscissa. This statistics is used in tests of significance in much the same way as the normal distribution, t distribution or F distribution.

Applications of χ^2-test

A. It is an alternate method of testing the significance of the difference between two proportions.

B. As a test of goodness of fit:
   By χ^2-test we can find whether the observed frequency distribution fits in a hypothetical or theoretical distribution of a qualitative data. The χ^2-test determines whether the observed fre-

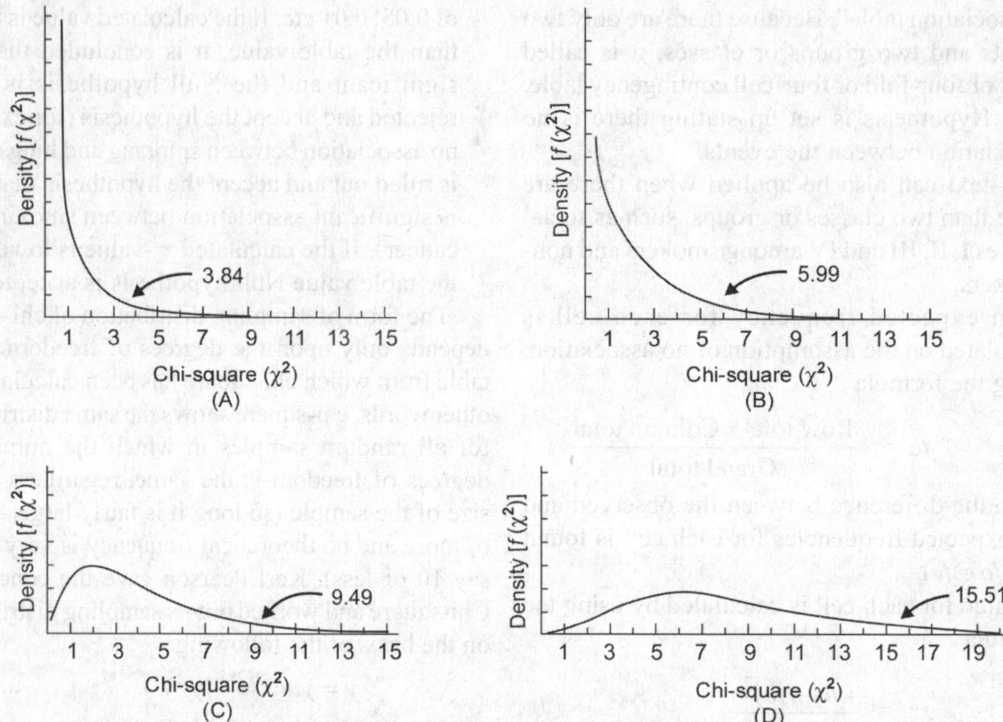

Figs 16.1A to D: χ^2 distributions for *df* = 1, 2, 4 and 8 (arrow indicates critical value at $\alpha = 0.05$): (A) *df* = 1; (B) *df* = 2; (C) *df* = 4; (d) *df* = 8

quency distribution differs from the theoretical distribution by chance or the sample is drawn from a different population.

(Theoretical distribution such as normal, binomial or poisson).

If the calculated value of χ^2-test of the sample is higher than the table-value, it is significant. (Null hypothesis is rejected) and vice-versa.

Example: The ratio of male to female births in nature is 1:1. If 52 male and 58 female children are born in a small town, could this difference be due to chance?

	Male	*Female*
Observed frequencies	52	48
Expected frequencies	50	50

$$x^2(a) = \frac{(\text{O} - \text{E})^2}{\text{E}} = \frac{(52-50)^2}{50} = \frac{4}{50}$$

$$x^2(b) = \frac{(48-50)^2}{50} = \frac{4}{50}$$

$$a + b = \frac{4+4}{50} = \frac{8}{50} = 0.06$$

Degree of freedom = 1

x^2 table value, with a *df* at 5 percent level of significance = 3.841.

Since the calculated value is much less than the table value, it is insignificant. That means the observed sex difference is by chance.

C. To find any association between two attributes (e.g. smoking and lung cancer), is real or by chance.

Similar examples are association between blood group and incidence of leprosy, age and blood pressure, nutritional status of the mother and weight of the newborn, obesity and diabetes etc. There are only two possibilities, either the attributes are associated or not associated. The χ^2-test measures the probability of association by chance.

According to Null hypothesis, the assumption of no association between two characters is made. (No relation between smoking and cancer). If the x^2-value is higher than the table value of x^2 (Annexure-IV) against a probability of 0.05, for the particular degrees of freedom, the Null-hypothesis is rejected and the association is not apparent but real, at 5 percent level of significance.

The x^2-test can also be applied to find the association in two classes or groups, as in multinomial samples (or a sample with multiple characters, e.g. a group with < 10 smokes/day, 11 to 20, 21 to 30 > 30 smokes per day and the incidence of lung cancer).

Degrees of Freedom, *df*

The number of degrees of freedom in a table of frequencies is the number of those frequencies to which we may assign arbitrary values and still satisfy the external requirements in terms of row and column totals. If we consider each frequency as occupying a cell in the contingency table, the degrees of freedom is the number of cells that may be filled at will. For example, we may have a 2 × 2 contingency table, like the following:

(a) 10	(b) 20	30
(c) 15	(d) 25	40
25	45	

The restriction imposed is that the cell frequencies in each row and column must add up to a fixed total for that row or column. We may note here, that the frequencies of only one cell can be varied at will. Others get fixed immediately to make up the row and column totals. Suppose we change *f* of 10 to 12. The frequencies of cell (b) and cell (c) will be fixed to 18 and 13 respectively to conform to the marginal totals of 30 and 25. The frequencies in cell (d) will also be fixed to make up the marginal totals. Hence, in this table, we have only one degree of freedom. In 2 × 2 or larger contingency tables, the *df* may be calculated as below:

$$df = (r - 1)(c - 1).$$

(Degree of freedom in contingency tables)

Where,

r = number of rows;

c = number of columns.

In a 3 × 3 contingency table, $df = (3 - 1)(3 - 1) = 4$.

There are other types of restrictions that might be imposed on a table besides those concerned only with totals. An illustration of these will be given in a test of goodness of fit for normality. The steps involved in the use of the Chi-square are as follows:

1. State the null hypothesis. H_0, and the alternative hypothesis, H_1
2. State the level of significance (a) and the sample size (n).
3. Determine the critical region based on df and state the decision rule. Critical value of Chi-square will be found from the Chi-square table (Table F)
4. Compute the value of Chi-square by using formula
5. Take a decision to reject or not to reject the null hypothesis.

We shall take a few illustrations to clarify the purpose.

Example 1: Apply x^2-test to find efficacy of a drug from the data given below.

Outcome (Result) of treatment with drug and placebo:

Group	***(Efficacy of the drug) Result Died***	***Survived***	***Total***	
A. Control (no placebo	(*fo*)10 (a) (*fe*)(5.25)	(O) 25 (b) (E)(29.75)	35	(a+b)
B. Experimental (on drug)	(*fo*)05 (c) (*fe*)(9.75)	(O) 60 (d) (E)(55.25)	65	(c+d)
Total	15(a+c)	85 (b+d)	(G)100	

The above values are all observed values.

The null hypothesis that the drug has no effect (drug and placebo are same). (i.e., there is no difference between the sample proportions and the population/universe proportion of 100).

The Expected (E) value and x^2-value is calculated for each cell as follows.

a. Expected number and x^2-value of "died" in the control group

$$fe_a = \frac{\text{Row total} \times \text{Column total}}{\text{Grand total}}$$

$$= \frac{35 \times 15}{100} = 5.25$$

$$x^2 = \left(\frac{fo - fe}{fe}\right)^2$$

$$= \frac{(10 - 5.25)^2}{5.25}$$

$$= \frac{(4.75)^2}{5.25} = \frac{22.5226}{5.25} = 4.29$$

b. Expected number and x^2-value of "survived" in the control group

$$fe_b = \frac{85 \times 35}{100} = 29.75$$

$$x^2 = \frac{(\text{O} - \text{E})^2}{\text{E}}$$

$$= \frac{(25 - 29.75)^2}{29.75} = \frac{(-4.75)^2}{29.75}$$

$$= \frac{22.56}{29.75} = 0.76$$

c. *fe* number and x^2-value of "died" in the experimental group

$$\text{E}_c = \frac{15 \times 65}{100} = \frac{39}{4} = 9.75$$

$$x^2 = \frac{fo - fe}{fe}$$

$$= \frac{(05 - 09.75)^2}{29.75} = \frac{(-4.75)^2}{29.75}$$

$$= \frac{22.56}{9.75} = 2.31$$

d. E number and x^2-value of survived in the experimental group

$$\text{E}_c = \frac{85 \times 65}{100} = 85 \times 0.65 = 55.25$$

$$x^2 = \frac{(\text{O} - \text{E})^2}{\text{E}} = \frac{(60 - 55.25)^2}{55.25} = \frac{(5.25)^2}{55.25}$$

$$= \frac{22.56}{55.25} = 0.408$$

$$\Sigma x^2 = \text{Total } x^2 \text{ value of all 4 cells}$$

$$= 4.29 + 0.76 + 2.31 + 0.41$$

$$= 7.77$$

$$df = (c - 1)(r - 1)$$

$$= (2 - 1)(2 - 1) = (1 \times 1) = 1$$

where

df = Degree of freedom

C = number of (vertical) columns

r = number of (horizontal) rows

On referring to Fisher's x^2-table, with 1 *df*, the tabulated x^2-value, corresponding to probability of 0.05 (at 95% significance level) is 3.84.

Since the calculated value (7.77) is more than the table-value (3.84), the null hypothesis is rejected, accepting the alternate hypothesis, i.e. the assumption that the drug is not efficacious (no difference between drug and placebo) is ruled out and accepted that the drug is efficacious (i.e., the difference between the two death rates is significant).

(Note: If the calculated value becomes lesser than x^2-table values, null-hypothesis has to be accepted).

Test of Hypothesis for Population Variance

Suppose, on the basis of previous knowledge, we have a preconceived value, σ_0^2, of variance of a normal population. Draw a random sample of size n ($n < 30$) from this population. On the basis of n sample observations ($x_1, x_2, ..., x_n$), the postulated value σ_0^2 of the population variance σ^2 is to be either substantiated or refuted with the help of a statistical test. For this the hypothesis

$$H_0 = \sigma^2 = \sigma_0^2 \text{ vs } H_1 : s^2 \neq \sigma_0^2$$

is tested by the statistic

$$\chi = \frac{\Sigma_i (x_i - \overline{x})^2}{\sigma_0^2} \quad ...(16.3)$$

$i = 1, 2, ..., n$

$$= \frac{(n-1)s^2}{\sigma_0^2} \quad ...(16.3.1)$$

where s^2 is the variance of the sample, χ^2-statistic has $(n - 1)$ *df*. Reject H_0 at pre-decided level of significance α if $\chi^2_{cal} \geq \chi^2_{\alpha/2, n-1}$ or if $\chi^2_{(1-\alpha/2), n-1}$.

In case of one-tailed test, i.e. testing H_0 against $H_1 : \sigma^2 > \sigma_0^2$, the test criterion is that reject H_0 if $\chi^2_{cal} \leq \chi^2_{\alpha/2, n-1}$

Again for testing H_0 against $H_1 : \sigma^2 < \sigma_0^2$, the test criterion is that reject

H_0 if $\chi^2_{cal} \leq \chi^2_{(1-\alpha), n-1}$

Example: An owner of a big firm agrees to purchase the product of a factory, if the produced items do not have variance of more than 0.5 mm^2 in their length. To make sure of the specifications, the buyer selects a sample of 18 items from his lot. The length of each item was measured to be as follows:

Length (mm)					
18.57	18.10	18.61	18.32	18.33	18.46
18.12	18.34	18.57	18.22	18.63	18.43
18.37	18.64	18.58	18.34	18.43	18.63

On the basis of the sample data, the hypothesis

$$H_0 : \sigma^2 = 0.5 \text{ vs } H_1 : \sigma^2 > 0.5$$

can be tested by the statistic

$$\chi^2 = \frac{\Sigma_i (x_i - \overline{x})^2}{\sigma_0^2}$$

$i = 1, 2, ..., 18$

We calculate,

$$\Sigma_i (x_i - \overline{x})^2 = \Sigma_i x_i^2 - \frac{(\Sigma_i x_i)^2}{n}$$

For the given data,

$$\Sigma_i x_i^2 = 6112.64; \Sigma_i x_i = 331.69$$

$$\therefore \Sigma_i (x_i - \overline{x})^2 = 6112.64 - \frac{(331.69)^2}{18}$$

$$= 6112.64 - 6112.125$$

$$= 0.515.$$

$$\text{Thus, } \chi^2 = \frac{0.515}{0.5} = 1.03$$

For $\alpha = 0.05$, $\chi^2_{0.05,17} = 27.587$. Since the calculated value of χ^2 is 1.03 which is not greater than 27.587, we accept the null hypothesis, $\sigma^2 = 0.5$ at $\alpha = 0.05$. It means that the buyer should purchase the lot.

Test of the Hypothesis of Equal Probability

Example: Sixty post-graduate students were asked to express an opinion on the issue "Should India make an atomic bomb?" by marking on a three point scale – "Yes?", "No". Thirty of the group marked "Yes"; 12 "?"; 18 "No". Do these results indicate a trend significantly different from equal probability of opinion in each of the three categories?

The solution is given in Table 16.2.

Test of Hypothesis of Independence (Difference)

Chi-square can be used to test whether two variables or attributes were *independent* or unrelated. Suppose we wish to know whether the variable of internal-external control was independent of sex of the subjects. We have three categories of subjects on internal-external control and two categories of subjects on sex. The obtained frequencies are shown below. Independence values or expected frequencies have also been given in parentheses. Each cell has been marked by a letter for identification purposes only.

	Externality			
	High (H)	*Middle (M)*	*Low (L)*	
Boys	(a) 20 (12)	(b) 10 (12)	(c) 10 (16)	40
Girls	(d) 10 (18)	(e) 20 (18)	(f) 30 (24)	60
	30	30	40	

Steps of procedure are given below:

Steps

1. *State the Hypothesis:* The null hypothesis H_0 is:

The proportion of males in three alternative categories of externality is the same as the proportion of females in these three categories or externality is independent of sex. The statistical alternative hypothesis (H_1) is: The proportion of males in the three alternative classifications of externality is not the same as that of the females in these categories or the externality is related to sex.

In symbolic form

$$H_0 = : P_{BH} = P_{BM} = P_{BL}$$
$$P_{GH} = P_{GM} = P_{GL}$$
$$H_0 = : P_{BH} \neq P_{BM} \neq P_{BL}$$
$$P_{GH} \neq P_{GM} \neq P_{GL}$$

2. *Decision Rule:* Given: $a = 0.05$ and $df = (3 - 1)(2 - 1) = 2$
   If $\chi^2_{obs} < 5.99$, accept H_0.
   If $\chi^2_{obs} \geq 5.99$, accept H_0.
3. *Computation:* Computation of independence values or expected frequencies for each cell may be found by multiplying the marginal totals common to a particular cell and then dividing this product by the grand total of frequencies in the table. The calculation of the same is shown below; The f_e are then shown in parentheses in each cell.

Table 16.2

Computation of chi-square test of hypothesis of equality (example about need of national Nursing University)

Hypothesis

$H_0 = f_{yes} = f_? = f_{No}$

$H_0 = f_{yes} = f_? = f_{No}$

Decision rules

Given: $a = 0.05$; and a 3 × 2 contingency table with $df = (r - 1)(c - 1) = (2 - 1)(3 - 1) = 2$

If $\chi^2_{obs} < 5.99$, accept H_0

If $\chi^2_{obs} \geq 5.99$, accept H_0

Computation:

The data is arranged in a contingency table

	Responses			
	Yes	*?*	*No*	
Observed (f_o)	30	12	18	60
Expected (f_e)	20	20	20	60
($f_o - f_e$)	10	8	2	
$(f_o - f_e)^2$	100	64	4	
$\frac{(f_o - f_e)^2}{f_e}$	5	3.2	0.2	

$$X = \frac{\Sigma(f_o - f_e)^2}{f_e} = 8.4$$

Interpretation

Reject H_0. The responses indicate a trend significantly different from equal probability.

Calculation of expected frequencies or independence values for various cells:

$$\text{(a) } \frac{40 \times 30}{100} = 12; \quad \text{(b) } \frac{40 \times 30}{100} = 12;$$

$$\text{(c) } \frac{40 \times 40}{100} = 16; \quad \text{(d) } \frac{60 \times 30}{100} = 18;$$

$$\text{(e) } \frac{60 \times 30}{100} = 18; \quad \text{(f) } \frac{60 \times 40}{100} = 24;$$

4. *Chi-square:*

$$\frac{(20-12)^2}{12} + \frac{(10-12)^2}{12} + \frac{(10-16)^2}{16} + \frac{(10-18)^2}{18}$$

$$+\frac{(20-18)^2}{18}+\frac{(30-24)^2}{18}+\frac{(30-24)^2}{24}$$

$= 5.33 + 0.33 + 2.25 + 3.56 + 0.22 + 1.50$
$= 13.19$

6. *Interpretation:* Reject H_0 and accept H_1. It shows that the distribution of externality is not independent of sex. It may further be concluded that the distribution of externality differs significantly between the two sexes.

Test of the Hypothesis of Normality

Chi-square can be used to test significance of divergence of the observed results from those expected on the hypothesis of a normal distribution. The hypothesis may be set up in such a way that it asserts, that the observed frequencies of an event follow a normal distribution instead of being equally probable.

Example: Fifty children were rated on "malnutrition" by a group of nurses in the community. The ratings were done by consensus on a threefold classification: generally aggressive (10 children); moderate malnutrition (28 children), and severe malnutrition (12 children). If aggressiveness is presumed to be normally distributed in this population of students, does this distribution of ratings differ significantly from normality?

Steps of Procedure

1. Hypothesis

H_0: The observed frequencies are normally distributed.
H_1: The observed frequencies are not normally distributed.

2. Decision Rule

Given $a = 0.05$; and a 2 × 3 contingency table with $df = (2 - 1)(3 - 1) = 2$

If $\chi^2_{obs} < 5.99$, accept H_0
If $\chi^2_{obs} \geq 5.99$, accept H_0

3. Computation

	Mild malnutrition	*Moderate malnutrition*	*Severe malnutrition*	
Observed (f_o)	10	28	12	50
Expected (f_e)	8	34	8	50
$(f_o - f_e)$	2	6	4	
$(f_o - f_e)^2$	4	36	16	
$(f_o - f_e)^2$	0.50	0.94	2	($\chi^2 = 3.44$)

In the contingency tble above, entries in row 1 give the number of children classified in each of the three categories. Entries in row 2 have been calculated with the help of a table of area under the normal curve (Table A) given in the Appendix. The baseline of the normal curve (taken to extend over 6's has been divided into segments of 2's each and the proportions enclosed by these limits found.

Segment	*Proportion*	*Frequencies out of 50*
Between +3σ and +1σ	0.16	0.16 x 50 = 8
Between +1σ and –1σ	0.68	0.68 x 50 = 34
Between –1σ and –3σ	0.16	0.16 x 50 = 8

These frequencies have been entered in the contingency table in the second row against f_e. *Other steps of computation are self-evident.*

4. *Interpretation:* The value of observed Chi-square is less than the critical value of Chi-square required for significance at 0.05 level and with $df = 2$. Hence, accept H_0. It may be concluded that the distribution of observed frequencies is not significantly different from normality.

Problems on normal distribution requiring larger classifications can also be tackled in the same manner.

Contingency Table

The data are often based on counting of objects of units. These numbers fall in various categories of attributes in a two-way classification and are very well displayed systematically in a table known as contingency table. We can express a contingency table as a rectangular array of order ($m \times p$), having *mp* cells. Where *m* denotes the number of rows which are equal to the number of categories of an attribute or criterion A, and *p* denotes the number of columns equal to the number of categories of attributes or criterion B. The matrix notation for contingency Table 16.3 is as follows:

Table 16.3

Contingency table

Attribute	Attribute B B_1	B_2...	B_j...	B_p	Total
A_1	O_{11}	O_{12}	O_{1j}	O_{1p}	R_1
A_2	O_{21}	O_{22}	O_{2j}	O_{2p}	R_2
⋮	⋮	⋮	⋮		⋮
A_i	O_{i1}	O_{i2}	O_{ij}	O_{ip}	R_i
⋮	⋮				⋮
A_m	O_{m1}	O_{m2}	O_{mj}	O_{mp}	R_m
Total	C_1	C_2...	C_j...	C_p	n

In Table 16.3 cell frequency O_{ij} in (i, j)th cell represents the number of objects, units or individuals possessing the characteristics of A_i and B_j. Any of the row total R_i and column total C_j is called the marginal total, where $i = 1, 2, ..., m$; $j = 1, 2, ..., p$ and n is the grand total. Such a table eases out the process of calculations of corresponding expected frequencies and subsequently the value of Chi-square statistics.

Example: In a large manufacturing concern, an opinion survey was conducted regarding three types of bonus schemes. Total employees were divided into four categories, namely-laborers, clerical, technical and executives. The results obtained by way of opinion survey are presented in the form of contingency table as given below:

Employees category	Bonus schemes Type I	Type II	Type III	Total
Laborer	190	243	197	*630*
Clerical	82	44	44	170
Technical	23	78	34	135
Executive	5	12	8	25
Total	300	377	283	960

The table indicates that out of 960 employees, 190 belonging to labor class, preferred type I scheme, and 243 preferred type II scheme. Similarly, any other cell frequency may be interpreted. 630, 170, 135 and 25 are the row marginal totals and 300, 377 and 283 are the column marginal totals.

Test of Independence of Factors

It is apparent now, that a contingency table is a rectangular array having rows and columns associated with different factors. The hypothesis, that one factor is independent of the other or not, i.e.

H_0: Two factors are independent of each other against H_1: Two factors are dependent, can be tested by chi-square test, where statistics,

$$\chi^2 = \sum_{i=1}^{m}\sum_{j=1}^{p} \frac{(O_{ij} - E_{ij})^2}{E_{ij}} \quad ...(16.4)$$

Statistic χ^2 has $(m - 1)(p - 1)$ *df*, whereas the data are presented in the form of the contingency Table 16.3. In formula (16.4). E_{ij} is the expected frequency corresponding to (i, j)th cell observed frequency O_{ij}. Under the null hypothesis H_0, the expected frequency,

$$E_{ij} = \frac{i\text{th row total} \times j\text{th column total}}{\text{Sample size}} \quad ...(16.5)$$

$$E_{ij} = \frac{R_i \times C_j}{n}$$

Once the expected frequencies are calculated, the value of chi-square is obtained with the help of formula (16.4). To make a decision about H_0, calculated value of chi-square is compared with the table value of chi-square for $(m - 1)(p - 1)$ *df* and α level of significance. If $\chi^2_{cal} \geq \chi^2_{\alpha, (m-1)(p-1)}$, reject H_0, which means that two factors are not independent.

Example: For the data presented in above example. We test the hypothesis H_0: Opinion about bonus schemes in independent of the types of employees against H_1 : H_0 is not true, as follows:

The expected values are calculated with the help of (16.5) and presented in parentheses, adjacent to the observed frequency and the value of chi-square is calculated by (16.6).

Expected frequencies are calculated as,

$$E_{11} = \frac{630 \times 300}{960} = 196.88 = 197$$

$$E_{12} = \frac{630 \times 377}{960} = 247.41 = 247$$

$$\vdots$$

$$E_{43} = \frac{25 \times 283}{960} = 7.37 = 7$$

Employees category	*Bonus schemes*			*Total*
	Type I	*Type II*	*Type III*	
Laborer	190 (197)	243 (247)	197 (186)	630
Clerical	82 (53)	44 (67)	44 (50)	170
Technical	23 (42)	78 (53)	34 (40)	135
Executive	5 (8)	12 (10)	8 (7)	25
Total	300	377	283	960

$$\chi^2 = \frac{(190-197)^2}{197} + \frac{(243-247)^2}{247} + \frac{(197-186)^2}{186}$$

$$+ \frac{(82-53)^2}{53} + \frac{(44-67)^2}{67} + \frac{(44-50)^2}{50}$$

$$+ \frac{(23-42)^2}{42} + \frac{(78-53)^2}{53} + \frac{(34-40)^2}{40}$$

$$+ \frac{(5-8)^2}{8} + \frac{(12-10)^2}{10} + \frac{(8-7)^2}{7}$$

$$= 0.2487 + 0.0648 + 0.6505 + 15.8679$$

$$+ 7.8955 + 0.7200 + 8.5952 + 11.7924$$

$$+ 0.9000 + 1.1250 + 0.4000 + 0.1428$$

$$= 48.4028$$

The table value of chi-square for, 6 *df* and $\alpha = 0.05$ is 12.59. Since χ^2_{cal} is greater than 12.59, we reject H_0. It means that the opinion about bonus scheme is influenced by the category of employees.

Calculation of Chi-square for 2 × 2 Tables

A frequently occurring type of contingency table is in 2 × 2 or four-fold contingency table. The value of the Chi-square for the test of independence can be readily obtained for such a table without calculating the expected values. The cell and marginal frequencies in the Table be designated as below:

A	B	A + B
C	D	C + D
A + C	B + D	

Chi-square can be calculated by using the formula

$$\chi^2 = \frac{N(AD-BC)^2}{(A+B)(C+D)(A+C)(B+D)} \quad ...(16.6)$$

in which,

N = Total number in the table

A,B,C,D = Frequencies in each of the four cells

AD, BC = Cross products of the cell frequencies A × D and B × C respectively

Thus, the formula may read, "Chi-square is equal to N times the square of the difference of the cross products divided by the product of the four marginal totals".

2 × 2 Contingency Table

When a contingency table is of order (2 × 2), test of independence of factors can be performed in the same manner as for ($m \times p$) contingency table. But in this situation, the value of chi-square can also be calculated directly from the observed frequencies. It is nothing but a short-cut method of obtaining the calculated value of chi-square. Suppose the contingency Table 16.4 of order (2 × 2) for two factors A and B is as presented below:

Table 16.4

2 × 2 contingency table

Factor B	Factor A		Total
	A_1	A_2	
B_1	*a*	*b*	(*a* + *b*)
B_2	*c*	*d*	(*c* + *d*)
Total	(*a* + *c*)	(*b* + *d*)	*a* + *b* + *c* + *d* = *n*

The formula for calculating chi-square from observed frequencies *a*, *b*, *c* and *d* is,

$$c_1^2 = \frac{n(ad - bc)^2}{(a+c)(b+d)(a+b)(c+d)} \quad ...(16.7)$$

Obviously, χ^2 in this case has (2 – 1)(2 – 1) = 1 *df*. The decision about independence of factors A and B can be taken by comparing calculated value of the chi-square with table value of χ^2 for 1 *df* and $\alpha = 0.05$, i.e. 3.841.

Example: Opinion about promotions, to be dependent on published work by persons interested in teaching or research was taken and displayed as below:

Interest	Promotion dependent on published work		Total
	Agree	Disagree	
Teaching	90	10	100
Research	70	30	100
Total	160	40	200

Here, H_0: Interest and promotion dependent on published work are independent. The value of statistic χ^2 by formula (16.7) is

$$\chi^2 = \frac{200(90\times30 - 70\times10)^2}{160\times40\times100\times100}$$

$$= \frac{200\times2000\times2000}{160\times40\times100\times100} = 12.50$$

Calculated value of χ^2 is greater than 3.841, the table value of χ^2 at 5 percent level of significance and 1 *df*. Hence, H_0 is rejected. Here, it is concluded that the opinion about promotion scheme, too dependent on published work, is influenced by the field of interest of persons.

Example: In the following table, 55 BSc Nursing Students have been placed in four cells according to their teachers' ratings as good performers and poor performers and success/failure on an intelligence test item. Is the performance independent of the intelligence?

	Test item: Fail	Test item: Pass	
Good performers	(A) 10	(B) 15	25 (A+B)
Poor performers	(C) 16	(D) 14	30 (C+D)
	26	29	55
	A + C	B + D	N

$$\chi^2 = \frac{55\left[(10\times14) - (15\times16)^2\right]}{(25\times30\times26\times29)} = 0.97$$

The critical value of chi-square with *df* = 1, on $\alpha = 0.05$, is 3.84. The observed value of Chi-square is not significant. Hence, the data do not provide enough evidence that the test item differentiates between individuals on the basis of their performance (as rated by their teachers).

When entries in a four-fold table are quite small (for example, 5 or less), Yates correction for continuity should be applied. Formula (16.6) then becomes:

$$\chi^2 = \frac{N(|AD - BC| - N/2)^2}{(A+B)(C+D)(A+C)(B+D)} \quad ...(16.8)$$

in which, |AD – BC| means the absolute difference of the two cross products. Other symbols, are as explained above. Applying the formula to the data given above, we have

$$\chi^2 = \frac{55(|140 - 240| - 55/2)^2}{(25\times30\times26\times29)} = 0.51$$

This value is smaller than that of the uncorrected Chi-square. Yates correction will always reduce the size of the Chi-square. Its effect is more crucial when entries are small. When χ^2 is marginally significant, the χ^2 may well fall below the level set for significance.

Yates' Correction

We know that the chi-square distribution is a continuous distribution. It has been proved that if any of the cell frequency in contingency table of order (2 × 2) is less than 5, the continuity of χ^2-distribution curve is not maintained. So to remove this discrepancy, Yates suggested a correction which is extensively used. The correction is named after him. He suggested that add 0.5 in the frequency which is less than 5 and subtract and add 0.5 to the remaining cell frequencies in such a way that the marginal totals remain the same. Then calculate the value of χ^2 by formula (16.7) using the adjusted contingency table.

Instead of adjusting the contingency table of order (2 × 2), the formula (16.7) has been amended and this takes care of the correction. The value of chi-square under correction can directly be calculated by the formula,

$$\chi_1^2 = \frac{n\left(|ad - bc| - \frac{n}{2}\right)^2}{(a+c)(b+d)(a+b)(c+d)} \qquad \text{...(16.9)}$$

Here, $|ad - bc|$ means that we consider only the absolute value of the difference. For instance $|23 - 75|$ will be taken as 52 instead of (–52).

Moreover, if one does not use the formula given specifically for the (2 × 2) contingency table, but follows the general procedure, under Yates' correction, the formula for the chi-square is,

$$\chi_1^2 = \sum_{i=1}^{2}\sum_{j=1}^{2} \frac{\left(|O_{ij} - E_{ij}| - \frac{n}{2}\right)^2}{E_{ij}} \qquad \text{...(16.10)}$$

It is worthwhile to point out that all the three approaches yield the same value of the chi-square because they are fundamentally the same.

Example: The number of licensor companies classified by the proportion of foreign profits derived from licence agreements were as follows:

Proportion of profit	*Licensor type*		*Total*
	Dominant product	*Diversified*	
Less than 5 percent	1	6	7
5 percent or more	7	6	13
Total	8	12	20

The hypothesis,

H_0: Proportion of profit and licensor types are independent

vs. H_1: H_0 is not true

can be tested by chi-square test

Since one cell frequency is 1, the formula is to be used.

$$\chi^2 = \frac{20\times\left(|6\times1 - 7\times6| - \frac{20}{2}\right)^2}{8\times12\times7\times13}$$

$$= \frac{20\times(36-10)^2}{8\times12\times7\times13} = \frac{13520}{8736} = 1.55$$

Since the calculated value of χ^2 is less than 3.841, the table value of $\chi^2_{0.05,1}$, H_0 is not rejected. It means that the proportion of profit and licensor types are independent.

Yates' Correction for Continuity

When the expected frequency in any cell of the four-fold (2 × 2) table is less than 5, a correction suggested by Yates, known as "correction for continuity" or Yate's correction, should be applied, for the calculation of x^2, to obtain a more accurate value of Chi-square, by using the formula.

$$x^2 = \frac{[(fo - fe) - 1/2]^2}{fe}$$

Alternate formula

$$x^2 = \frac{[(ab - bc) - G/2]^2 \times G}{(a+b)(c+d)(a+c)(b+d)}$$

Chi-square is subject to considerable error in the following two situations and requires the use of Yates correction for continuity.

1. *When working with 2 × 2 tables.* Chi-square is based on the assumption that adjacent frequencies are connected by a continuous and smooth curve (like the normal curve) and are not discrete numbers. In 2 × 2 tables this continuity of the curve is broken and needs a correction.
2. *When entries are very small.* Chi-square is not stable like any other statistic based on probability. When computed from a table in which experimental frequency (f_o) is less than 5. Hence a correction of continuity is required.

Failure to use the correction causes the probability greatly under estimated and the chances of it being called *significant* considerably increased.

Yates correction for continuity requires subtracting of 0.5 from each ($f_o - f_e$) difference are shown in the following

	Right	Wrong	
f_o	8	2	
f_e	5	5	
$(f_o - f_e)$	3	3	
Correction (–0.5)	2.5	2.5	
$(f_o - f_e)^2$	6.25	6.25	
$\frac{(f_o - f_e)^2}{f_e}$	1.25	1.25	$2.50 = \chi^2$

Falls far below the 0.05 significance level which requires a critical value of 3.841. However, the uncorrected value of χ^2, if calculated comes to 3.6, which approaches nearer to the critical value.

Example: In a case-control study of oral contraceptive use and risk of myocardial infarction, it was found that out of 156 women with myocardial infarction, 23 were oral contraceptive users at the time of their hospital admission. Of the 3120 control women without myocardial infarction, 304 were current oral pill users.

A. Construct an appropriate 2 × 2 table

B. Calculate the measure of association between the oral contraceptive use and myocardial infarction.

C. Interpret the results.

A. Construction of the appropriate 2 × 2 contingency table

		Disease Case (Disease present)	*(MI) Control (Disease absent)*	*Table*
Oral pill	Yes	23 (a)	304 (b)	327 (a+b)
users	No	133 (c)	2816 (d)	2949 (c+d)
Total		156 (a+c)	3120 (b+d)	(G) 3276 (a+b+c+d) = G

B. *Null hypothesis:* There is no association between oral pills and myocardial infarction.

$$\text{Expected } (fe) \text{ value} = \frac{\text{Column total} \times \text{Row total}}{\text{Grand total}}$$

$$fe_a = \frac{156 \times 327}{3276} = 15.50$$

$$x^2 = \frac{(O-E)^2}{E} = \frac{(23.0-15.5)^2}{15.5} = 3.62$$

$$fe_b = \frac{3120 \times 327}{3276} = 311.40$$

$$x^2 = \frac{(304-311.4)^2}{311.4} = 0.17$$

$$fe_c = \frac{156 + 2949}{3276} = 140.40$$

$$x^2 = \frac{(133-140.4)^2}{140.44} = 0.39$$

$$fe_d = \frac{3120 + 2949}{3276} = 2808.50$$

$$x^2 = \frac{(2816-2808.5)^2}{2808.5} = 7.50$$

$df = (C-1)(r-1)$ $\quad \Sigma x^2 = 11.68$
$= (2-1)(2-1)$
$= 1$

x^2-value (table value with 1 *df* at *p* value 0.05 is 3.841).

C. *Results:*

i. Since the observed or calculated value 11.68 is more than the table value 3.841, null hypothesis (H_0) is rejected and the alternate hypothesis is accepted that there is significant association between ($p < 0.05$) oral pills and myocardial infarction

ii. Odd's ratio $= \dfrac{ad}{bc} = \dfrac{23 \times 2816}{304 \times 133} = 1.6$

Oral contraceptive users are 1.6 times at a greater risk of getting myocardial infarction than non users.

iii. Exposure rate among cases and controls are compared.

Exposure rate among cases

$$= \frac{a}{a+c} = \frac{23}{156} = 0.15$$

Exposure rate among controls

$$= \frac{b}{b+d} = \frac{304}{3120} = 0.09$$

Since the exposure rate among the cases is greater then that of controls, there exists a relation between the oral pills and the myocardial infarction.

Chi-square from Percentage

Chi-square test can be used when table entries are in terms of percentages or proportions. However, in such cases, a correction for size of the sample becomes essential. It is because of the fact that percentage does not indicate whether the actual frequency from which percentage has been calculated was large enough. A frequency of 6 out of 10 gives the same percentage as a frequency of 60 out of 100. However, the latter is more significant. The calculation of Chi-square from percentage is shown with the help of an example below. N in this case is equal to 10.

	Right	Wrong	
f_o	80%	20%	100%
f_e	50%	50%	100%
$(f_o - f_e)$	30%	30%	
Correction (–5%)	25%	25%	
$(f_o - f_e)^2$	625	625	
$\dfrac{(f_o - f_e)^2}{f_e}$	12.5	12.5	

$\chi^2\%$ 25

$\chi^2 = \chi^2\% \times N/100 = 25 \times 10/100 = 2.5$

The $\chi^2\%$ based on percentage must be brought back to its proper value in terms of original numbers by multiplying it by N/100 as shown above.

General Observations on Chi-square

- **Assumption of the chi-square test:** Chi-square test is based on the following assumptions:
  i. The two samples are independent from one another. This implies that different and unrelated sets of subjects are selected.
  ii. The subjects within each group must be randomly and independently sampled.
  iii. Each observation must qualify for one and only one category. It implies that f's in each cell must be distributed in mutually exclusive categories.
  iv. The sample size must be relatively large.

  The two important assumptions of normality of distribution and homogeneity of variance which underly all important parametric tests do not apply to Chi-square.
- **One-tailed and two-tailed situations:** Tables of chi-square used for significance are based on one tailed-tests only, using the tail to the right of the sampling distribution of χ^2. Although one tail only for the sampling distribution of χ^2 is used, the table values are those required for testing the significance of a difference regardless of direction, i.e., for two-tailed tests. This is because of the fact that, in effect, χ^2 is the square of the normal deviate for 1 degree of freedom, thus incorporating both tails of the normal curve in the right tail of the χ^2 curve. In many

situations, where chi-square is applied, the idea of a directional or one tailed test has little meaning. In tests of independence and goodness of fit, we are usually not concerned with the direction of the difference observed. However, if a one tailed test is required, the proportionate areas in the chi-square table should be halved.

- **Reduction of an R × C table to a 2 × 2 table:** Sometimes a table with more than two rows and more than two columns may be reduced to a 2 × 2 table by combining the tail frequencies. The procedure is statistically legitimate provided the points of division (dichotomy) of the two variables are picked up independently of the cell frequencies and not for maximizing the association in the data to obtain a significant chi-square.
- **Additivity of chi-square:** In many experimental studies, chi-square from different samples may be added to provide an overall test of hypothesis. In such cases, the df for the new chi-square will be the sum of the separate *df*'s. Each repetition of the experiment should be done on samples of almost equal size and drawn independently and at random. Suppose a sex difference with respect to an attitude to a certain question is expected. A test is run separately in grades 10, 11 and 12 for the purpose and the separate chi-squares are found to be not significant. The chi-squares for the three classes may be combined to test an overall hypothesis covering all the three classes with greater likelihood of obtaining a significant result.

The application of chi-square table described in this chapter are fundamental and elementary ones generally applicable to simple research problems. Several tests which are required in more complex situations make use of chi-square to test significance. Some such tests are comparable to those of analysis of variance, repeated measures, trend analysis, matched pairs, etc. These tests make up a whole separate area of study known as non-parametric or distribution-free statistics.

Non-Parametric Statistical Tests

When the variables are distributed normally, tests like *t*-test and x^2-tests are applied to test the hypothesis. But at times, there are variabls like ran kings, which do not conform to any probability distribution. In such situation the above tests may not be applicable but the so called "Non-parametric tests" may be applicable. These are the Sign test, the Wilcoxon's signed rank test and Mann-Whitney test.

So far we cover a number of tests of hypotheses. All these tests are based on the assumption that the variable follows normal distribution or that the sample has been drawn from a normal population. The importance of the normal distribution theory is justified under the umbrella of the central limit theorem. However it is often doubtful whether the basic distribution is such that the central limit theorem is applicable and hence the estimates and tests based on the assumption of normal distribution are not accurate to the desired degree, the hypotheses about the parameter(s) of the distribution(s) were tested and the decision about the hypothesis taken with the help of the critical region which is determined by the distribution that is not known, one needs statistical methods which do not require the form of the parent distribution. Such methods are called *nonparametric or distribution-free methods*.

The two terms, nonparametric and distribution-free are not synonymous though they are used in the same sense and cover the same statistical techniques. The term 'nonparametric' is used in the sense that no hypothesis is established about the indexing parameters of the density function, whereas the term 'distribution-free' is used in the sense that no assumption is made about the form of the population density and thereby the decision about a hypothesis is not based on the density of the parent population.

Some problems are categorized as parametric and others as nonparametric. The distinction, however, is not very clear. Interestingly, the chi-square test is taken as a parametric as well as a nonparametric test.

Whichever technique be adopted for testing a hypothesis, the definitions and implications of terms like hypothesis, two types of error, critical region, level of significance and degrees of freedom remain the same, as on Tests of Significance. The desired significance level α in nonparametric tests is called the nominal α. It cannot, usually, be determined exactly because of the discreteness of the sampling distribution. It should be noted that nonparametric statistics are applicable to the set of observations which are either ranked or ordered. Let a random sample of n observations $X_1, X_2, ..., X_n$ be drawn from a population. These observations can always be arranged in ascending or descending order. However, the observations in this chapter will usually be arranged in ascending order, i.e. from the lowest to the highest value in increasing order of magnitude. Suppose the observations arranged in increasing order of magnitude are $x_{(1)}, x_{(2)}, ..., x_{(n)}$, where $x_{(1)}$ is the lowest value of x and $x_{(n)}$ the largest value of x. Numerically $x_{(1)} \leq x_{(2)} \leq ... \leq X_{(n)}$.

In performing any nonparametric test, it is required to know whether the random variable follows continuous or discrete distribution. It is well known that the area of the density curve between any two ordered observations is free from the form of the density function. Also, it is always possible to divide the total area under the density curve into $(n + 1)$ equal parts such that the area of each part is equal to $1/(n + 1)$. Therefore, techniques like quartiles, deciles, percentiles, rank correlation, etc. come under the category of nonparametric techniques although they are concerned with estimation. This chapter contains only some popular nonparametric tests.

Most of the tests of significance so far described in previous chapters are referred to as parametric tests because these involve the estimation of at least one population value or parameter. For example, in F test a population variance estimate is needed as the error term. The tests to be described in this chapter are sometimes called non-parametric because they do not involve the estimation of any parameter on population value. Moreover, the assumption of normality of distribution which is a pre-requisite in such tests as F, t and Z, is also not made. Therefore, the techniques presented in this chapter are sometimes called *distribution-free* meaning thereby, that in the application of these techniques the population distribution need not necessarily be normal.

Assumptions

1. For nonparametric tests, the only assumption is about the continuity of the distribution function. This is postulated to determine the sampling distributions.
2. Median is as good an index of central tendency as mean. We know, for symmetrical distributions, mean and median coincide. Hence, in nonparametric statistics median is taken as a measure of location parameter instead of mean.

One-Sample Nonparametric Tests

A random sample of size n is drawn from a population and the sample values are arranged in order of magnitude and ranked accordingly, if need be. Different tests evolved in one sample case for the test of hypothesis are discussed here. These tests lead us to decide whether the sample has come from a particular population. Also, we test whether the median of the population is equal to a known value or not. Such tests are classified as tests for goodness of fit like chi-square test.

Non-parametric tests are generally preferred to parametric tests in the following situations:

1. Whenever there are doubts that the distribution is not normal or the non-normality has been established through some statistical procedure. When samples are not from a normal distribution, the use of a normal theory test with level of significance, α, does not assure that the probability of an error of the first kind is controlled at level α. Such probability is indeterminate because generally there is no way of

knowing the direction and degree of departure from α. On the other hand, if a non-parametric test is used with level of significance α then for any parent population the probability of an error of the first kind is actually equal to α or less than α because of discreteness.

2. When measurements are in terms of nominal and ordinal scales, the use of non-parametric tests will be more appropriate. A nominal scale does not involve any measurement as such and classifies individuals into categories that are qualitatively different with no ordering implied. The categories may be assigned numerical designations and number of persons in each category expressed as proportion or percentage. Ordinal measurements are in terms of rank order based on qualitative or quantitative considerations. The level of measurements and type of data available do restrict the type of statistical techniques that can be used. Chi-square test can be used for handling nominal data and data in terms of ranks can be handled through Spearman's rho or Kendall's tau or the tests to be described in this book.

Ordinary Sign Test

Let a random sample $X_{(1)}, X_{(2)}, ..., X_{(n)}$ of size n be drawn from a population $F(x)$ where $F(x)$ is assumed to be continuous in the close vicinity of the median. Suppose the median of $F(x)$ is M. In this situation, $P(X = M) = 0$.

The hypothesis which has to be tested by sign test is,

$$H_0 : M = M_0 \text{ vs. } H_1 : M \neq M_0$$

where M_0 is a given value of the population median. We know,

$$P(X > M_0) = P(X < M_0) = 0.5$$

Hence, the null hypothesis H_0 under test is equivalent to

H_0: $P(X > M_0) = P(X < M_0)$ vs. H_1: $P(X > M_0) \neq P(X < M_0)$.

If the randomly selected sample comes from a population having the median value equal to M_0 on the average, half of the observations will be below M_0 and half above M_0. To perform the sign test, we take the differences $(X_{(i)} - M_0)$ for $i = 1, 2, ..., n$ and consider their signs. Let the number of positive signs be r and negative signs $(n - r)$. For the test statistic, we consider only the positive signs. In this way the data have been dichotomized which consist of the number of positive and negative signs. The distribution of r given n is a binomial distribution with $p = P(X > M_0)$. Thus, the null hypothesis H_0 changes to $p = 0.5$. So now we test,

$$H_0: p = 0.5 \text{ vs. } H_1 : p \neq 0.5$$

It is not necessary to use the two-sided alternative. In case there is pre-information that the sample will have an excess number of positive signs, we may use the one-sided alternative, i.e. $H_1 : p > 0.5$. The only difference between one-sided and two-sided tests is that of critical values for a prefixed α. Similarly, the alternative hypothesis H_1: $p < 0.5$ will be chosen when it is expected that the sample will have few positive signs.

The decision criterion for a two-sided test is, reject H_0 if $r > r'_{\alpha/2}$ where $r'_{\alpha/2}$ is the critical value at significance level α.$r_{\alpha/2}$ is the smallest integer which satisfies the condition,

$$\sum_{r=r_{\alpha/2}}^{n} \binom{n}{r} \left(\frac{1}{2}\right)^r \left(\frac{1}{2}\right)^{n-r} \leq \alpha/2 \quad ... (16.11)$$

or $r \leq r'_{\alpha/2}$ where $r'_{\alpha/2}$ is the largest integer such that,

$$\sum_{r=0}^{r'_{\alpha/2}} \binom{n}{r} \left(\frac{1}{2}\right)^r \left(\frac{1}{2}\right)^{n-r} \leq \alpha/2 \quad ... (16.12)$$

For the one-sided alternative H_1: $p > 1/2$, reject H_0 if $r \geq r_\alpha$ where r_α is the smallest integer such that,

$$\sum_{r=r_\alpha}^{n} \binom{n}{r} \left(\frac{1}{2}\right)^r \left(\frac{1}{2}\right)^{n-r} \leq \alpha \quad ... (16.13)$$

and for $H_1 : p < 1/2$, reject H_0 if $r \leq r'_\alpha$ where r'_α is the largest integer such that,

$$\sum_{r=r_\alpha}^{r'_\alpha} \binom{n}{r} \left(\frac{1}{2}\right)^r \left(\frac{1}{2}\right)^{n-r} \leq \alpha \quad ...(16.14)$$

In any problem, the probability of the event $X \leq r$ is computed by the binomial probability provided $n < 25$. For ease, the probabilities are tabulated and given in Appendix B. Table X for different values of n and r. If the calculated value of $P(X \leq r)$ is less than the predecided significance level α, H_0 is rejected.

For a two-sided test, the calculated probability is doubled and then compared with level α. The decision about H_0 is taken as per the criterion given above.

If $n \geq 25$, the value of Z is computed and the normal test is applied to decide about H_0. Z is given by the statistic,

$$Z = \frac{(r + 0.5) - np_0}{\sqrt{np_0(1 - p_0)}} \text{ when } r < np_0 \qquad ...(16.15)$$

or $$Z = \frac{(r - 0.5) - np_0}{\sqrt{np_0(1 - p_0)}} \text{ when } r > np_0 \qquad ...(16.16)$$

Remember that $p_0 = 0.5$.

If $Z \leq Z_{\alpha/2}$ or $Z \geq Z_{1-\alpha/2}$, H_0 is rejected. For the one-sided test, adjustment is made, as discussed, with parametric tests.

Theoretically, none of the differences $(X_{(i)} - M_0)$ should be zero since $F(x)$ has been assumed continuous. But, in practice, there are zero differences in some problems. In such a situation, the zero differences are omitted and the sample size is reduced by the number of zero differences. For instance, there are 18 observations in the ordered sample. On taking the deviation from M_0, two zero deviations occur. Then the sample size is taken as 16 ignoring two zeros.

Example: Following are the data arranged in order of magnitude of a random sample drawn from a continuous population with median M = 13.

9.62 10.19, 10.27 11.13, 12.26, 13.55, 14.16
14.46, 15.02, 15.92, 16.26

The test of the null hypothesis,

$H_0 : M = 13$

against $H_1: M > 13$

at significance level $\alpha = 0.10$ can be performed by the ordinary sign test in the following manner. The signs of difference $(X_{(i)} - 13)$ are,

-----------++++++

In the case, $n = 11$ and number of positive signs, $r = 6$.

With the help of Table X in Appendix B, the probability $P(X \leq r)$ is 0.7256. The given alternative hypothesis leads to one sided test. Since the calculated value of $P(X \leq r)$ is greater than the prefixed level $\alpha = 0.10$, the null hypothesis, M = 13 is not rejected.

Sign Test

This is applied under the following circumstances, for example, there are two diagnostic procedures of a disease, which are to be tested for their difference or significance. The two procedures are applied on a random sample of patients of the disease. The observations are categorized as follows.

It is categorized as 'one' when a person is considered as a patient of that particular disease or as "Zero" when not considered as a patient, based on the diagnostic procedure. Thus there are 2 sets of ranks, is terms of "one" and "zero".

The difference between one and zero correspond to the two test procedures, applied on a single individual.

The significance of difference between the two procedures can be tested using the usual x^2-test.

The sign test is the simplest of all distributions-free statistics and carries a very high level of general applicability. It is applicable in situations in which the critical ratio, t, tests for correlated samples cannot be used because the assumptions of normality and homosedasticity are not fulfilled. The students are aware of the fact that certain conditions in the setting of the experiment introduce the element of relationship between the two sets of data. These conditions generally are a pretest, post-tests situation; a test re-test situation; testing of one group of subjects on two tests; formation of

Table 16.5

Ratings of two groups on leadership qualities

Matched pair	*Experimental*	*Control*	*Sign of difference*
1	20	18	+
2	15	10	+
3	25	21	+
4	28	17	+
5	10	12	–
6	18	10	+
7	11	6	+
8	9	8	+
9	7	7	0
10	14	16	–

Number of zero differences = 1
Number of negative differences = 2
Number of positive differences = 7

'matched groups' by pairing on some extraneous variables which are not the subject of investigation, but which may affect the observations.

Suppose an experimenter selects a group of 20 persons and divides them into two groups, control and experimental, by matching pairs of subjects on intelligence. One of the groups is then randomly assigned to a leadership training camp. The control group receives no such training. On completion of the camp, independent observes rate the leadership qualities of each of the 20 subjects on a 30-point scale. The rating scale is an extremely crude one and the assumption of equality of intervals and the shape of the distribution of scores cannot be safely made. The only assumption we can safely make is that any difference between two paired scores is valid indicator of the direction and not the magnitude of the difference.

The data have been arranged in Table 16.5. The null hypothesis to be tested is that the probability that any difference will be positive is equal to the probability that it will be negative. Since it is a two category population of differences (Positive differences and Negative differences) H_0 can be expressed in precisely the same manner as in the binomial test with P = Q = 0.5.

Hypotheses:

$$H_0: P_{negative} = P_{positive} = \frac{1}{2}$$

$$H_1: P_{negative} = P_{positive} = \frac{1}{2}$$

If χ^2 $P_{obs} < 0.05$, accept H_0

There are 10 differences in all, 7 are plus, 2 are minus and one is zero. Since the zero differences are neither plus nor minus, they are excluded from N as well as either of the two categories of + and – signs. In our example, we now have 9 pairs out of which 7 are positive (or 2 are negative). To test the hypothesis we shall first expand the binomial $(p + q)^9$, in which the probability of *a*+ is denoted by *p* and the probability of *a*– by *q*.

$$(p + q)^9 = p^9 + 9p^8q + 36p^7q^2 + 84p^6q^3 + 120p^5q^4 + 126p^4q^5 + 84p^3q^6 + 36p^2q^7 + 9pq^8 + q^9$$

The total number of combinations is $2^N = 2^9 = 512$. Now by adding the numerical coefficients of the first three terms (namely, $p^9 + 9p^8q + 36p^7q^2$) the number of combinations which contain 7 or more plus signs out of 9 is obtained which is 46. The probability, under the binomial, of the occurrence of 7 or more + signs out of 9, can now be determined by dividing the number of combinations having 7 or more + signs by the total number of combinations. In our example, it is 46/512 = 0.089 or 0.09 (rounded to two decimal places). For convenience this value can also be obtained by referring to Table G in Appendix in which cumulative probabilities under the binomial are given. Entering Table G with N = 9 and *x*, the number of signs having smaller value, i.e. – signs, $x = 2$, the probability given is 0.09 which checks with the one calculated above.

It is a one tailed probability. The two tailed probability then, 2 × 0.09, i.e., 0.18. Using $\alpha = 0.05$ for two tailed test, we accept H_0 because $p > 0.05$. For one tailed test also, the H_0 cannot be rejected because $p > 0.10$.

Sign Test with Large Samples

When the number of pairs is 20 or more an approximation to the exact probabilities can be obtained by calculating χ^2 corrected for continuity by using a 2 × 2 contingency table. The theoretical frequencies in each cell will be N/2 (N here does not exclude the pairs having zero differences). The example solved in the previous section though has N < 20, yet is repeated here for demonstrating the technique and the computational steps involved in it.

	+	–
$f_{obtained}$ (f_o)	7	2
$F_{theoretical}$ (f_e)	5	5
$f_o - f_e$	2	3
– 0.05	1.5	2.5
$(f_o - f_e)^2$	2.25	6.25
$\frac{(f_o - f_e)^2}{f_e}$	0.45	1.25 (χ^2 =1.70)

For a two tailed tests and $df = 1$, this value is significant at $\alpha = 0.18$ approx. Which is a good approximation to the value found in the previous section. In cases involving $df = 1$,

$$z = \sqrt{\chi^2} \qquad \text{...(16.17)}$$

Applying this formula to the problem above, we have

$z = \sqrt{1.70}$ or $z = 1.304$.

Referring to a normal probability table, we find that for a two tailed test this is significant at $a = 0.19$ approximately. The difference in this value and the values obtained earlier can be attributed to the smallness of N.

Walker and Lev (1965) reported another procedure for calculating χ^2 corrected for continuity by using the following formula and regarding it as a normal deviate:

$$\text{z} = \frac{2m \pm 1}{\sqrt{\text{N}}} - \sqrt{\text{N}} \qquad \text{...(16.18)}$$

(m stands for the number of signs smaller in number).

The 1 in the numerator is added or subtracted in such a way as to change 2 m to a value nearer N. Thus, in our example, $m = 2$, N = 9, we should have

$$z = \frac{2(2) \pm 1}{\sqrt{9}} - \sqrt{9} = 1.33$$

This provides a very close approximation to the value of z computed previously.

Assumptions of Sign Test

The assumptions underlying the sign test are:

i. The differences are continuously distributed, and
ii. The differences are independent of each other

As stated earlier, no assumption regarding the form of the distribution or homogeneity of variance is required.

Some Other Uses of the Sign Test

The Sign Test can be applied to test certain more general hypotheses. It involves an additional assumption that the measurements are on a scale of equal units. By subtracting a constant C, from each difference (Difference = $X_{Ai} - X_{Bi} - C$) the null hypothesis is that the median difference $X_A - X_B$ in the population is at least C. The hypothesis is rejected if too many differences are positive.

If the data fulfill another assumption, i.e. of a zero point on the measurement scale, the difference can be calculated as follows;

$$\text{Difference}_i = X_{Ai} - X_{Bi} - KX_{Bi} \qquad \text{...(16.19)}$$

and the hypothesis

$H_0 = P(X_A > KX_B) \leq 0.5$ can be tested

As it is clear from the above two assumptions—equal units and a zero point–these extensions of the sign tests can be used only with continuous variables.

Wilcoxon Signed-Rank Test

This test is useful for testing the significance of difference in paired observations (e.g. serum fibrinogen degradation product in mg/mL among 12 patients were noted before and after prostate operation). The difference in the paired values of each unit/patient is ranked according to the size of the difference and the signs of the original differences are also assigned to the ranks. Under the null hypothesis, it is equally likely that any difference can have + or –. The sums of all ranks with + sign and –ve sign are obtained separately.

The smaller sum out of the above two is referred to Wilcoxon's table, without considering the sign, against the number of pairs observed.

When the calculated smaller rank sum is less than the tabulated value, at 5 percent level, conclusion is made that the difference between the two groups of observations, is significant at 5 percent level.

Suppose there are more than one pair of common values for the differences, they are "tied values". Then each of the tied difference is assigned the average of the ranks that would be assigned if there is no tie. When the number of pairs exceeds 16, which is the limit of number of pairs in the tables given by Wilcoxon, the normal approximation for getting the probability of rejection of null hypothesis is obtained by the formula.

$$Z = \frac{[(1\mu - T) - 1/2]}{\sigma}$$

Where, T = Smaller rank sum

n = Numebr of pairs of observations

$\mu = n(n + 1)/4$

$$\sigma = \frac{\sqrt{(2n + 1)\mu}}{4}$$

P is obtained from the normal distribution table corresponding to the value of calculated Z. As a rule of thumb $Z > 1.96$ signifies rejection of the null hypothesis at $P < 0.05$.

The ordinary sign test was based on only the sign of the deviations of the ordered sample values from the hypothesised median M_0. No heed was paid to the magnitude of the differences. The Wilcoxon signed rank test utilizes the signs as well as the magnitudes of the differences. This test is more sensitive and powerful than the ordinary sign test.

If we are prepared to assume that the population is continuous and symmetric, the Wilcoxon signed-rank test is a much improved test in comparison to the ordinary sign test for testing the same null hypothesis against an alternative hypothesis discussed with the sign test. In this case also we have a random sample $X_1, X_2, ..., X_n$ from a continuous and symmetric population with median M. The null hypothesis is,

$$H_0 : M = M_0$$

where M_0 is the hypothesised value of M. Let the difference $X_i - M_0$ be denoted by d_i, i.e. $d_i = X_i - M_0$ for $i = 1, 2, ..., n$. The difference d_i will be distributed symmetrically about the median zero so that positive and negative differences of equal absolute magnitude have equal probabilities of occurrences. First arrange the differences in ascending order ignoring their signs and rank them from 1 to n. Now assign the same sign to the ranks which their original differences possessed. In this way, the data consist of a set of n integers and a corresponding set of plus and minus signs. Let the sum of the ranks of positive d_i's be denoted by T^+ and that of ranks of negative d_i's by T^-. For a symmetrical distribution it is expected that T^+ will be approximately equal to T^-. Obviously $T^+ + T^-$ is equal to the sum of n integers, i.e.,

$$T^+ + T = \sum_{i=1}^{n} i = n(n+1)/2$$

Since the sum of all the ranks is a constant, the tests based on T^+, T^- and $T^+ - T^-$ will be equivalent. In practice, the smaller of T^+ and T^- is used for conducting the test. However, the test is discussed further taking T^+.

Let the rank of the absolute differences $|d_i|$ be denoted by r ($|d_i|$ and a variable Z_i be defined as,

$$Z_i = \begin{cases} 1 & \text{if} \quad d_i > 0 \\ 0 & \text{if} \quad d_i < 0 \end{cases}$$

T^+ may be written as,

$$T^+ = \sum_{i=1}^{n} Z_i r(|di|) \qquad ...(16.20)$$

If we take the subscripts on the original sample such that all $|d_i|$, $i = 1, 2, ..., n$ are ordered statistics, replace $r(|d_i|)$ by i and Z_i by $Z_{(i)}$ where

$$Z_{(i)} = \begin{cases} 1 & \text{if } d_i \text{ with rank } i \text{ is positive} \\ 0 & \text{if } d_i \text{ with rank } i \text{ is negative} \end{cases}$$

Now T^+ may be given as,

$$T^+ = \sum_{i=1}^{n} iZ_{(i)} \quad ...(16.21)$$

$Z_{(i)}$'s are independent Bernoulli random variables but are not identically distributed, $Z_{(i)}$ has mean p_i and variance $p_i q_i$ for $q_i = 1 - p_i$ and cov $(Z_{(i)}, Z_{(j)}) = 0$ for $i \neq j$.

Thus, the variable T^+ is distributed with mean $\sum_{i=1}^{n} ip_i$ and variance $\sum_{i=1}^{n} i^2 p_i(1-p_i)$.

Under H_0, $p_i = 1/2$ and hence,

$$E(T^+) = \sum_{i=1}^{n} ip_i = \frac{1}{2}\sum_{i=1}^{n} i = \frac{1}{2} \cdot \frac{n(n+1)}{2}$$

$$= \frac{n(n+1)}{4} \quad ...(16.22)$$

$$V(T^+) = \frac{1}{4}\sum_{i=1}^{n} i^2 = \frac{n(n+1)(2n+1)}{24} \quad ...(16.23)$$

Similar expressions may be developed for T^-. It has already been stated that it is convenient to perform the test with smaller values of T^+ and T^-. Let T be min (T^+, T^-). If t_α is a number such that $P(T \leq t_\alpha) = \alpha$, the nominal, the regions of rejection of size α for the test of H_0: $M = M_0$ are given as,

$$T^+ \leq t_\alpha \text{ for } H_1 : M < M_0$$

$$T^- \leq t_\alpha \text{ for } H_1 : M < M_0$$

$$T^+ \leq t_{\alpha/2} \text{ or } T^- \leq t_{\alpha/2} \text{ for } H_1 : M \neq M_0$$

The sample space contains 2^n points which are equally likely under H_0.

Thus,

$$P[T]^+ = t|H_0| = k_t/2^n \quad ...(16.24)$$

where k_t is the number of ways of assigning the plus and minus signs to the ranks 1, 2, ..., n such that $T^+ = t$. The critical values of T may either be calculated or obtained directly from Table XIII prepared by Wilcoxon. For large n, say $n \geq 25$, the sum T^+ follows normal distribution. Under H_0, the statistics

$$Z = \frac{T^+ - n(n+1)/4}{\sqrt{n(n+1)(2n+1)/24}} \quad ...(16.25)$$

where $Z \sim N(0, 1)$ as $n \to \infty$

The decision about H_0 is taken in the same manner as discussed with the large sample test previously.

The Median Tests

It compares the median of two independent samples and is a non-parametric replacement of its parametric t tests for comparing the means of two independent samples. It provides a procedure for testing whether two independent samples differ in central tendencies. In other words, the use of the median test allows for testing whether two independent groups have been drawn from populations with the same median. The test can be used for unequal groups also. The hypothesis to be tested can be stated either in non-directional (two tailed test) or directional terms (one tailed test). The pre-requisite of the test is measurement at least on an ordinal scale. The computation requires the following steps of procedure:

1. Determine a common median for both the groups combined
2. Dichotomize both sets of scores separately at the common median and put the data in a 2×2 contingency table as given below:

	Group I	Group II	Total
Number of scores above combined median	A	B	A + B
Number of scores below combined median	C	D	C + D
	A + C	B + D	

The rationale of the test is that if both Group I and Group II are samples from populations whose median is the same, we would expect about half of each group scores to be above the combined median and about half to be below the combined median.

3. Use the chi-square test
4. If the P yielded by the test is equal to or smaller than α, reject H_0.
5. If some scores fall at the combined median then (i) drop them from analysis if they are only a few and $n_1 + n_2$ is large, or (ii) dichotomize the groups as those scores which exceed the median

and those which do not. The troublesome scores may be included in the second category. The steps are illustrated in Table 16.6.

Kolmogorov-Smirnov (K-S) One-Sample Test

A random sample $X_1, X_2, ..., X_n$ of size n is drawn from an unknown population having the cumulative distribution function (cdf) F(x). Let the ordered values be $x_{(1)}, x_{(2)}, ..., x_{(n)}$. The K-S test is based on the Glivenko-Cantelli theorem which states that the step function $S_n(x)$, with jumps occurring at the values of the ordered statistics $x_{(1)}, x_{(2)}, ..., x_{(n)}$ for the sample, approaches the true distribution for all x. Making use of this theorem, the comparison of the empirical distribution function $S_n(x)$ of the sample for any value x is made with the population *cdf* under H_0, $F_0(x)$. This comparison is made by defining the distance between the two comulative distribution functions which is taken as the supremum[2] of the absolute deviations, i.e. Sup $|S_n(x) - F_0(x)|$ over all x. The hypothesis for the test of goodness of fit is,

$$H_0 : F(x) = F_0(x) \text{ vs. } H_1: F(x) \neq F_0(x)$$

where F_0 is a completely specified continuous distribution.

Table 16.6

Computation of a median test for two samples

Hypotheses: H_0: No. of scores below combined median in sample I = No. of scores below combined median in Sample II

H_1: No. of scores below combined median in sample I ≠ No. of scores below combined median in Sample II

Decision Rule:

Given $\alpha = 0.05$, $n_1 + n_2 > 20$ and no $f_e < 5$; $df = 1$

If $\chi^2_{obs} < 3.84$, accept H_0

If $\chi^2_{obs} \geq 3.84$, accept H_0

Computation Scores:

Sample I: 3, 6, 6, 7, 8, 8, 8, 10, 12, 13, 13, 16, 16, 18, 20.

Sample II: 6, 8, 9, 13, 13, 14, 15, 16, 18, 18, 19, 19, 24, 26.

Combined median = (14+15)/2 = 14.5

	Group I	Group II	
No. above combined Median	(A) 6	(B) 9	15 A + B
No. below combined Median	(C) 11	(D) 4	15 C + D
	17 A + C	13 B + D	N = 30

Formula: Chi-square $= \dfrac{N(|AD - BC|N/2)^2}{(A+B)(C+D)(A+C)(B+D)}$

$$= \frac{30(|6 \times 4 - 9 \times 11| - 30/2)^2}{(15)(15)(17)(13)}$$

$= 2.3$

Interpretation: Since the observed Chi-square of 2.3 is less than 3.84, accept H_0. The two samples do not differ significantly with respect to their medians.

To test H_0, the actual numerical difference $|S_n(x) - F_0(x)|$ is used in K-S test. Since this difference depends on x, the K-S statistics is taken to be the supremum of such differences, i.e.

$$D_n = \text{Sup. } |S_n(x) - F_0(x)|$$

1. The empirical (sample) distribution function of an ordered random sample $x_{(1)}, x_{(2)}, \ldots, x_{(n)}$ of size n, denoted by $S_n(x)$ for all real x, is the proportion of sample values which do not exceed x. $S_n(x)$ is a set function which increases by $1/n$ at the jump points which are the values of the ordered sample. $S_n(x)$ is also known as the statistical image of the population distribution function.

   Symbolically, $S_n(x)$ is defined as,

$$S_n(x) = \begin{bmatrix} 0 & \text{if} & x \le x_{(1)} \\ k/n & \text{if} & x_{(k)} \le x \le x_{k+1} \text{ for } k = 1, 2, \ldots n-1 \\ 1 & \text{if} & x \ge x_{(n)} \end{bmatrix}$$

2. Supremum (sup) means least upper bound. Similarly, infimum (inf) means greatest lower bound.

   where D_n is known as the K-S statistic. Under H_0, the statistic D_n has a distribution which is independent of the *cdf*. $F(x)$ that defines H_0. The statistic D_n is distribution-free. To decide about H_0, the test criterion is, reject H_0 if D_n (max $|S_n(x) - F_0(x)|$, exceeds the tabulated value for given n and prefixed significance level α. Otherwise, H_0 is not rejected. The critical values of D_n for prefixed α are given in Appendix B, Table IX.

Example: On tossing five coins 192 times, the frequencies of 0 to 5 heads are:

Number of heads:	0	1	2	3	4	5
Frequency:	6	26	73	66	14	7

The fairness of the coin by the K-S test can be ascertained. The null hypothesis under test is,

$$H_0 : F(x) = F_0(x) \text{ vs. } H_1 : F(x) = F_0(x)$$

The hypothetical frequencies are calculated with the help of the binomial function, $\binom{n}{r} p^r q^{n-r}$. Here, $n = 5, p = 0.5$.

Thus, the frequencies for $r = 0, 1, 2, 3, 4, 5$ are

$$f_0 = \binom{5}{0}\left(\frac{1}{2}\right)^0\left(\frac{1}{2}\right)^5 \times 192 = 6,$$

$$f_1 = \binom{5}{1}\left(\frac{1}{2}\right)^1\left(\frac{1}{2}\right)^5 \times 192 = 30, \text{ and similarly,}$$

$f_2 = 60, f_3 = 60, f_4 = 30, f_5 = 6$. Actual and theoretical frequencies, the sample or empirical cdf, theoretical cdf and the difference are tabulated below.

Number of heads	0	1	2	3	4	5
Actual frequencies	6	26	73	66	14	7
Empirical cdf	$\frac{6}{192}$	$\frac{32}{192}$	$\frac{105}{192}$	$\frac{171}{192}$	$\frac{185}{192}$	$\frac{192}{192}$
Theoretical frequencies	6	30	60	60	30	6
Theoretical cdf	$\frac{6}{192}$	$\frac{36}{192}$	$\frac{96}{192}$	$\frac{156}{192}$	$\frac{186}{192}$	$\frac{192}{192}$
Difference: D_n	0	$\frac{4}{192}$	$\frac{9}{192}$	$\frac{15}{192}$	$\frac{1}{192}$	0

$$\text{Max. } D_n = \frac{15}{192} = 0.078$$

Suppose the prefixed significance level $\alpha = 0.1$. The critical value of D_n from Table IX is $\frac{1.22}{\sqrt{192}}$ $= 0.088$. Since the value of statistic D_n does not exceed the critical value 0.088, H_0 is not rejected. This means that the sample cdf is similar to the hypothetical distribution function.

Run Test

In statistical theory, it has normally been assumed that a sample drawn from a population is random.

Whether the assumption of randomness is true or not needs verification. The run test is one device to test randomness. Before discussing the test, it is essential to discuss the runs.

A run is a sequence of like symbols which are followed and preceded by other kinds of symbols or no symbol at either side. For clarity, a vertical line is drawn in between two consecutive sequences of symbols to mark the runs. A sequence of symbols exhibiting a pattern of symbols is usually indicative of lack of randomness. For instance, looking at a queue of persons waiting for the bus at a bus-stop, we observe the following sequence of males (M) and females (F).

M|F|M|F|M|F|M|F|M|F|M|F|M|F|

This sequence shows a definite pattern, i.e., the males and females are standing alternately. This sequence clearly shows a lack of randomness. Again a sequence of type,

MMMMMMM|FFFFFFF

shows clustering of males and females which is again indicative of lack of randomness. From this, it may be deduced that an excessive number of runs or too few runs for a given set of symbols provide the basis for nonrandomness.

It is not always that we have sequences of symbols. Any data at hand can be converted into runs. Take the deviation of each observation of the set from the median (any other constant) and denote the positive and zero difference by *a* and negative difference by *b*. In this way we get a sequence of symbols *a* and *b*. For example, the marks of 15 students are 55, 52, 43, 49, 36, 61, 44, 47, 67, 78, 63, 57, 41, 28, 50. On taking the deviations from 50, the following sequence is obtained.

aa|bbb|a|bb|aaaa|bb|a

The above sequence has seven runs. Positive and negative signs may also be taken in place of *a* and b taking zero as positive quantity, to mark the runs.

Test for Randomness

The null hypothesis, H_0: the symbols *a* and *b* occur in random order in the sequence against the alternative, H_1: symbols *a* and *b* do not occur in random order, can be tested by the run test. Let the sample of size *n* contain n_1 symbols of one type, say *a*, and n_2 symbols of the other type, say *b*. Thus, $n = n_1 + n_2$. Also suppose the number of runs of symbol *a* is r_1 and that of symbol *b* is r_2. Suppose $r_1 + r_2 = r$. In order to perform a test of hypothesis based on the random variable R, we need to know the probability distribution of R under H_0. The probability distribution function of R is given as,

$$f_R(r) = 2\binom{n_1-1}{r/2-1}\binom{n_2-1}{r/2-1}\Big/\binom{n_1+n_2}{n_1}$$

when *r* is even.

For *r* even, the number of runs of both types must be the same, i.e., $r_1 = r_2 = r/2$. Again,

$f_R(r) =$

$$\left\{\binom{n_1-1}{\frac{r-1}{2}}\binom{n_2-1}{\frac{r-3}{2}}+\binom{n_1-1}{\frac{r-3}{2}}\binom{n_2-1}{\frac{r-1}{2}}\right\}\Big/\binom{n_1+n_2}{n_1} \quad \text{...(16.26)}$$

when *r* is odd.

For *r* odd, $r_1 = r_2 \pm 1$. In this situation, the sum is taken over two pairs of values, $r_1 = (r-1)/2$ and $r_2 = (r+1)/2$ and vice versa.

To decide about H_0 the critical number of runs are obtained from Tables XI-F_i and XI-F_{ii} given in Appendix B. Table XI-F_i and XI-F_{ii} provide the lower and upper critical values of the number of runs at level 0.05 respectively. If the number of runs in the sample lies between these critical values, the hypothesis H_0 is not rejected, otherwise rejected. Rejecting H_0 means that the data are not in random order.

Example: Given the following sequence as given in the above text.

aa|bbb|a|bb|aaaa|bb|a

The null hypothesis H_0: the observations occur in random order, against H_1: the observations do not occur in random order, can be tested by runs test as follows:

$$n_1 = 8, n_2 = 7, n = 15$$

$r_1 = 4, r_2 = 3, r = 7$

For $\alpha = 0.05$, $n_1 = 8$, $n_2 = 7$, the lower critical value = 4 (see Table XI-F_i)

For $\alpha = 0.05$, $n_1 = 8$, $n_2 = 7$, the upper critical value = 13 (see Table XI-F_{ii}). The number of runs in the sample is 7 which lies between 4 and 13. It means that the observations occur in random order with five percent significance level.

A General New Parametric Test for Two Independent Samples – Run Test

The Sign Test and the Median Test were introduced as non-parametric tests for location in which two samples were compared in terms of central tendency to test whether they were drawn from the same population.

The Run Test to be described below is a general two sample test for testing the null hypothesis that two independent samples come from identical populations against the alternative hypothesis that the two populations differ in any manner whatsoever, i.e., in central tendency, in dispersion, in skewness, in kurtosis or in any other way. The Run Test is less powerful in disclosing differences of a particular kind, for it is a test of any sort of differences and not for a particular type of difference. Hence, if we are interested in testing whether the two populations differ only in one particular respect, say either in central tendency or in dispersion, then we should use a test of location or dispersion from amongst the tests described earlier.

In 50 tosses of a coin, the following distributions of Heads (H's) and Tails (T's) was obtained. Use a run test to see whether the coin was a biased one which produced a non-random distribution of H's and T's.

HHHTTHTTTTHHHTHTTTTHHHTTTTH

TTHHTTTTHHHTTTTHTTHTHHT

Steps

1. The observations as obtained have been listed above as H's and T's. *A run is an observation in the sequence of letters of the same kind which cannot be extended by incorporating an adjacent observation.* In the example above, the H runs have been underlined and T runs over scored. If the two samples are from a common population, the H's and T's will generally be well mixed and the number of runs will be large. Now count the number of runs and call them as v.
   Number of runs for H's = 11; and for T's = 10.
   Total No. of runs = v = 11 + 10 = 21
   $N_1 = 21$; $N_2 = 29$ (N_1 and N_2 are number of H's and T's respectively).
2. *Hypothesis:* H_0: The coin is not a biased one
   H_1: The coin is a biased one.
3. *Computation:* If $N_1 > 10$ and $N_2 > 10$, the test of significance is obtained by taking v to be normally distributed with mean

$$\mu_v = \frac{2N_1N_2}{N_1+N_2}+1 \quad ...(16.27)$$

And variance,

$$\sigma^2_v = \frac{2N_1N_2(2N_1N_2-N_1-N_2)}{(N_1+N_2)^2(N_1+N_2-1)} \quad ...(16.28)$$

in the example given:

$$\mu_v = \frac{2(21\times 29)}{21+29}+1 = 25.36$$

$$\sigma^2_v = \frac{2\times 21\times 29(2\times 21\times 29-21-29)}{(21+29)^2(21+29-1)} = 11.61$$

$$\sigma_v = \sqrt{\sigma_v^2} = \sqrt{11.61} = 3.41$$

$$z = \frac{v-\mu_v}{\sigma_v} = \frac{21-25.36}{3.41} = \frac{4.36}{3.41} = 1.28$$

4. *Interpretation:* The calculated value of z, (1.28), is less than the critical value of z required for significance at 0.05 level (critical $z = 1.96$) hence the null hypothesis cannot be rejected. Therefore the coin is not biased and has produced a random distribution of H's and T's.

A correction for continuity as given below may be used when $N_1 + N_2$ is not very large.

$$z = \frac{|v - \mu_v| - 5}{\sigma_v} \quad ...(16.29)$$

If scores of two samples are given, the scores can be arranged in an ascending order in a common arrangement keeping the identity of the score as to which group it belonged. Then the runs for group I and group II can be counted and the procedure given above repeated. For example:

Group A: 5, 6, 7, 8, 12, 12, 12, 13, 18, 19

Group B: 2, 3, 4, 10, 10, 10, 11, 11, 14, 15

The arrangement for counting of runs will be as follows:

Group BBB AAAA B B B B B A A A A

Score 2,3,4 5,6,7,8 10,10,10,11,11 12,12,12,13

Group B B A A

Score 14,15 18,19

Number of runs for Group A = 3, and for B = 4

Total No. of runs or $v = 3 + 4 = 7$

Repeat the other steps.

Two-Sample Nonparametric Tests

Kolmogorov-Smirnov Two-Sample Test

It is an extension of the one sample K-S test as applied to a two-sample problem. In the one-sample test, the empirical distribution was compared with the population *c, d, f,* but in the two-sample K-S test, the two empirical distributions of two samples are compared and a decision is taken on the basis of the distance between these empirical distributions.

Let two random samples of sizes n_1 and n_2 be drawn from two continuous populations F_1 and F_2, respectively. Also, it is assumed that the two samples are independent. The observations are taken at least on ordinal scale. If these assumptions hold good, K-S two-sample test can be performed in the following manner. Let the empirical distribution functions be given by $S_{n_1}(x)$ and $S_{n_2}(x)$.

The hypothesis,

H_0: $F_1(x) = F_2(x)$ for all x

vs. H_1: $F_1(x) \neq F_2(x)$ for some x

can be tested by the K-S statistics

$$D_{n_1,n_2} = \max_x |S_{n_1}(x) - S_{n_2}(x)| \quad ...(16.30)$$

In a real problem, obtain the cumulative step functions of two samples and find the maximum difference. Compare this value with the critical value of D_{n_1,n_2} given in Table XII of Appendix B. Table XII gives the acceptance limits of D_{n_1,n_2} for $n_1, n_2 \leq 15$ at two significance levels $\alpha = 0.05$ and $\alpha = 0.01$. Reject H_0, if calculated D_{n_1,n_2} exceeds the tabulated value, otherwise not.

For large values of $n_1, n_2 > 15$, acceptance limits of D_{n_1,n_2} are calculated by the approximate formulae given below the table for various levels of significance α. The decision about H_0 is taken in the same way as for small samples.

If there is any prior information whether $F_1(x) > F_2(x)$ or $F_1(x) < F_2(x)$, the one-tailed K-S test will be applied. Now we calculate either $D^+_{n_1,n_2} = \max |S_{n_1}(x) - S_{n_2}(x)|$ or $D_{n_1,n_2} = \max_x |S_{n_2}(x) - S_{n_1}(x)|$ as the case may be and perform the test in the usual way. Table XII can be used by doubling the level of significance.

Example: A sample of 26 male patients and another of 25 female patients suffering from respiratory tuberculosis (TB) are randomly selected. The frequency distributions according to age of males and females are given below. The cdf and the differences $|S_{n_1}(x) - S_{n_2}(x)|$ are shown simultaneously.

The hypothesis, that the age distribution of males and females in respect of susceptibility to respiratory tuberculosis is same, can be tested by the K-S statistic given by (16.30).

From the above table,

$$D_{n_1,n_2} = \max_x |S_{n_1}(x) - S_{n_2}(x)| = \frac{195}{25 \times 26} = 0.300$$

The acceptance limit for $n_1 = 26$, $n_2 = 25$ at the level $\alpha = 0.05$ with the help of the formula given in Table XII is

$$= 1.36\sqrt{\frac{n_1 + n_2}{n_1 n_2}} = 1.36\sqrt{\frac{26 + 25}{26 \times 25}} = 0.381$$

	Age group							
	0-5	*5-15*	*15-25*	*25-35*	*35-45*	*45-55*	*55-65*	*above 65*
Males suffering from TB	1	1	3	2	2	4	6	7
cdf $\{S_{n_1}(x)\}$	$\frac{1}{26}$	$\frac{2}{26}$	$\frac{5}{26}$	$\frac{7}{26}$	$\frac{9}{26}$	$\frac{13}{26}$	$\frac{19}{26}$	$\frac{26}{26}$
Females suffering from TB	1	2	4	3	6	4	2	3
cdf $\{S_{n_2}(x)\}$	$\frac{1}{25}$	$\frac{3}{25}$	$\frac{7}{25}$	$\frac{10}{25}$	$\frac{16}{25}$	$\frac{20}{25}$	$\frac{22}{25}$	$\frac{25}{25}$
Difference $\lvert S_{n_1}(x) - S_{n_2}(x)\rvert$	$\frac{1}{25\times 26}$	$\frac{28}{25\times 26}$	$\frac{57}{25\times 26}$	$\frac{85}{25\times 26}$	$\frac{191}{25\times 26}$	$\frac{195}{25\times 26}$	$\frac{97}{25\times 26}$	0

Since the calculated difference D_{n_1, n_2} does not exceed the acceptance limit, H_0 is not rejected. It means that the male and female populations have the same proportion of respiratory TB in different age groups.

The Kolmogorov-Smirnov (K-S) Test is quite useful in applications in which two distributions compared are both samples. The feature primarily compared is the numerical level on some scale. Differences in variance and kurtosis have little effect on the test. Ordered categories are sufficient refinement and no assumption about equal intervals is required. The null hypothesis is that the two distributions arose by random sampling from the same population. The test differs from small to large size samples and for one-tailed to two-tailed situations.

The K-S Test with Small Samples

When N is 40 or less in each of the two distributions, the K-S test is applied as a small sample test. It is more convenient when $N_1 = N_2$ because tables of critical K statistic exist to facilitate its use.

Example: Two groups of boys and girls with $n = 12$ in each case had a cricket match and scored the runs presented in two frequency distribution in Table 16.7. Have the two distributions arisen by random sampling from the same population?

Table 16.7

The Kolmogorov-Smirnov test of similarity of distributions (two independent small samples with equal *n's*)

Score	*Frequencies (f)*		*Cum.f.*		*Kc*
Number of runs made	*Boys*	*Girls*	*Boys*	*Girls*	
55-59	2	0	12	12	0
50-54	1	0	10	12	2
45-49	3	0	9	12	3
40-44	2	1	6	12	6
35-39	1	3	4	11	7
30-34	2	2	3	8	5
25-29	1	4	1	6	5
20-24	0	2	0	2	2
					K = 7

Hypotheses: H_o: There is no significant difference in the two distribution of runs scored by boys and girls.

H_1: There is a significant difference in the two distribution of runs scored by boys and girls.

Computation: The calculations are quite easy. The essential step is to find out cumulative frequency distributions for the two samples, as shown in Table 16.8. The last operation is to find the category difference or Kc. The largest Kc is statistic K. In this case K = 7.

Interpretation

Consulting Table J with $N_1 = N_2 = 12$, we find that a K = 7 is required for significance at 0.05 level in a two-tailed situation. A K = 8 is required at 0.01 level.

Since the calculated value of K = 7, the Null hypothesis is rejected at 0.05 level. However, the calculated K is not significant at 0.01 level as it is less than 8.

One-tailed Situation

Suppose our hypothesis was that the differences were in favor of boys, we would have used a one-tailed test which would require K = 6 at 0.05 level and K = 7 at 0.01 level to be significant. Since the calculated K = 7, we would have rejected H_0 at 0.01 level, which is higher than the level of rejection in a two-tailed situation.

The K-S Test with Large Samples

When both the groups have *n*'s larger than 40, a large sample K-S test is warranted. An example with unequal *n*'s has been chosen to illustrate the generality of the procedure. Both a one-tail and two-tail tests have been applied. The test uses Chi-square distribution.

Example: A test of extroversion was administered to a set of 40 students identified by their teachers as front benchers in the class and to 50 identified as back-benchers. The scores so obtained have been shown in Table 16.8 in the form of two frequency distributions. Do the two groups belong to the same population?

Hypotheses: H_0: The two groups of front benchers and back benchers belong to a common population.

H_1: The two groups of front benchers and back benchers do not belong to a common population. These are non-directional two-tail situation.

Computation: The major step is to obtain cumulative frequencies and convert them into cumulative proportions for each of the two groups. Cumulative proportions can be obtained by dividing each category cumulative *f* by the *n* of its groups. Then the d_c values or the category differences are obtained by subtracting category cumulative proportions. The largest d_c is taken as D statistic. In our case, D = 0.620.

Calculations of critical values of D in two-tailed test are obtained by using the following formulas:

Sig. level	*Critical D value*	
0.10	$1.22\sqrt{\frac{N_1+N_2}{N_1\times N_2}}$	...(16.31)
0.05	$1.36\sqrt{\frac{N_1+N_2}{N_1\times N_2}}$	...(16.32)
0.01	$1.63\sqrt{\frac{N_1+N_2}{N_1\times N_2}}$	...(16.33)
0.001	$1.95\sqrt{\frac{N_1+N_2}{N_1\times N_2}}$	...(16.34)

The radical term may be solved to facilitate the calculation of critical values for various levels. In our case, $N_1 = 40$, and $N_2 = 50$, the radical value.

$$\sqrt{\frac{N_1+N_2}{N_1\times N_2}} = \sqrt{\frac{40+50}{40\times 50}} = 0.212$$

Hence, critical values of D can be obtained by multiplying the radical with the numerical values given in the formula. If we choose 0.05 level for interpretation, we obtain

$$D = 1.36 \times 0.212 = 0.288$$

Interpretation: The obtained value of D (0.620) is larger than the critical value of D (0.288); hence the H_0 cannot be retained. The two groups differ significantly on extroversion and therefore do not come from the common population.

Table 16.8

Kolmogorov-Smirnov two-sample test with large and unequal N's

Score	*Frequency of Gr. A**	*Gr. B**	Cf_A	Cf_B	Cf_A	Cf_B	*dc*
19	3	0	40	50	1.000	1.000	0.000
18	5	0	37	50	0.925	1.000	0.075
17	6	0	32	50	0.800	1.000	0.200
16	10	5	26	50	0.650	1.000	0.350
15	8	4	16	45	0.400	0.900	0.500
14	3	8	8	41	0.200	0.820	0.620
13	2	10	5	33	0.125	0.660	0.535
12	1	13	3	23	0.075	0.460	0.385
11	2	10	2	10	0.050	0.200	0.150
10	0	0	0	0	0.000	0.000	0.000
	40	50					D = 0.620

*A = Front benchers; B = Back benchers; Scores: Extroversion scores.

Sign Test for Paired Samples

The procedure for the ordinary sign test is extended to paired-samples problems. In paired-samples problems we have random samples of n pairs say, $(X_1, Y_1), (X_2, Y_2), ..., (X_n, Y_n)$. Just like the t-test in a parametric case, take the differences of the paired observations. Here establish the hypothesis about the median of the differences. The n differences are given as,

$$D_i = X_i - Y_i \quad \text{for } i = 1, 2, ..., n,$$

If the population of D_i is assumed continuous at its median say, M_D, the $P(D = M_D) = 0$. The hypothesis which is to be tested in this case is, H_0: $P(D > M_D^0) = P(D < M_D^0)$ vs. H_1: H_0 is not true. where M_D^0 is a hypothesized value of the median of differences.

In a nutshell, it can be said that the ordinary sign test procedure is applicable for paired samples, taking D_i as X_i. Therefore, further details are omitted. One should bear in mind that the test applied for the median difference is not the same as for the difference of two medians, $(M_x - M_y)$.

Wilcoxon Paired-Sample Signed-Rank Test

Wilcoxon's test for one sample can be applied in a way to paired-samples problems as well. Consider a paired sample of size n as, $(X_1, Y_1), (X_2, Y_2), ..., (X_n, Y_n)$. As in the case of the sign test for paired samples, the differences $(X_1 - Y_1), (X_2 - Y_2), ..., (X_n - Y_n)$, which are denoted by D_i and $i = 1, 2, ..., n$, are assumed to have come from a continuous and symmetric population of differences.

In this case, the hypothesis,

$$H_0 : M_D = M_D^0 \text{ vs. } H_1 : M_D \neq M_D^0$$

where M_D is the median of the population of differences D and M^0_D is a hypothesized value of M_D.

In case there is any prior information about the differences that an excess number of difference will be less than M_D or few differences will be less than M_D, then one-sided test should be used. To apply the test, find the differences

$$D_i = X_i - Y_i \text{ for } i = 1, 2, ..., n.$$

Now, from a practical point of view, the differences D_i are as good as X_i in one-sample case. Apply Wilcoxon's signed-rank test on D's similar to one-sample case, i.e., find T^+ or T^- and test the hypothesis in a like manner as in one-sample problems. Table XIII given in Appendix B provides the critical values of T which can directly be used to take a decision about H_0.

One-tail Case

If the hypothesis was that the front benchers are likely to be more extroverted than the back benchers, a one-tail test would have been warranted. For this purpose a chi-square can be derived from D by means of the formula.

$$\chi^2 = 4D^2 \left(\frac{N_1 N_2}{N_1 + N_2}\right) \quad ...(16.35)$$

Where N_1 and N_2 are number of cases in the two groups and D is the largest difference of category proportions. In our example,

$$\chi^2 = 4(0.620)^2 \left(\frac{40 \times 50}{40 + 50}\right)$$

With df =2, the calculated chi-square is much greater than the critical value of chi-square required for significance at 0.01 level. Hence it is significant. The front benchers are significantly higher than the back benchers on extroversion and the two groups do not come from a common population.

Median Test

This test is attributed to Westenberg (1948) and Mood (1950). The sign test for two-sample problems has been applicable only when the observations are paired. But such a situation is not always possible. Often we have samples of different sizes from two populations. In such a situation, the median test is quite-efficient. Suppose two random samples $X_1, X_2, ..., X_{n_1}$ and $Y_1, Y_2, ..., Y_{n_2}$ of sizes n_1 and n_2 are drawn from two populations F_x and F_y, respectively. Suppose, $n_1 + n_2 = n$. The median test is a test of equality of location parameters of the two populations under consideration. Here, we test the hypothesis

$$F_X(x) = F_Y(x) \text{ for all } x$$

against the shift alternative.

$$F_X(x) = F_Y(x - \delta) \text{ for all } x \text{ and } \delta \neq 0.$$

where δ is the shift in the location parameter which is the median in this text.

Without indulging into the theoretical aspects of the test, the methodology of using the test has been given directly.

Combine the samples and arrange them in order. Find the median of the combined order statistics. The median may be one of the X's or Y's. Let it be denoted by θ. Again, count the number of X's and Y's to the left of the median. Let the number of X's to the left of θ be u and that of Y's be v. Obviously, the number of X's on the right side of θ is $(n_1 - u)$ and that of Y's is $(n_2 - v)$. These results are summarized in the table below:

	On the left of the median θ	*Not to be left of the median θ*	*Total*
Sample X	u	$n_1 - u$	n_1
Sample Y	v	$n_2 - v$	n_2
	$(u + v)$	$(n_1 + n_2) - (u + v)$	n

If p is the probability that any observation is less than 0, the probability of $u + v = t$ (say) is

$$f(t) = \binom{n_1 + n_2}{t} p^t (1 - p)^{n_1 + n_2 - t} \quad ...(16.36)$$

for $t = 0, 1, 2, ..., n_1 + n_2$.

The conditional distribution of u, given t, is

$$f(u/t) = \frac{\binom{n_1}{u}\binom{n_2}{t-u}}{\binom{n_1 + n_2}{t}} \quad ...(16.37)$$

for $u = 0, 2, ..., n_1$.

The distribution given by (16.37) is the hypergeometric probability distribution. It is worth pointing out that $n = n_1 + n_2$ may be odd or even. To eliminate inconsistencies in the application of this procedure, θ can be defined as the $\left(\frac{n+1}{2}\right)$ th ordered statistics if n is odd and any number between the $\left(\frac{n}{2}\right)$ th and $\left(\frac{n+2}{2}\right)$ th ordered statistics if n is even. In this way, a unique value of u is obtained for any set of n observations. That is why θ is taken to be the median of the combined sample. Expression (16.37) gives the conditional probability of u where $t = n/2$ for n even and $t = \frac{n-1}{2}$ for n odd. The test based on u, the number of observations belonging to the X-sample which are less than the median of the combined sample is called the *median test*.

If two samples are drawn from identical populations with respect to the location parameter, i.e. median in this case, the probability distribution $U = u$ for given t is

$$f_U(u) = \frac{\binom{n_1}{u}\binom{n_2}{t-u}}{\binom{n_1+n_2}{t}} \quad ...(16.38)$$

for $u = 0, 1, 2, ..., n_1$
and $t = n/2$.

The rejection regions for significance level α are obtained by the following inequalities.

Reject H_0, if $u \le C$ or $u \ge C'$ for $H_1 : \delta \ne 0$

Reject H_0, if $u \ge C'_\alpha$ for $H_1 : \delta > 0$

Reject H_0, if $u < C_\alpha$ for $H_1 : \delta < 0$

where C and C' are any two integers such that

$$P(U \le C) + P(U \ge C') \le \alpha$$

Also C_α and C'_α are, respectively, the largest and smallest integers such that $P(U \le C_\alpha) \le \alpha$ and $P(U \ge C'_\alpha) \le \alpha$.

The critical values C, C', C_α, C'_α can be obtained from (16.38) or from the tables of the hypergeometric distribution given by Lieberman and Owen in 1961. As an alternative, calculate the probability by (16.38) and compare it with a prefixed level of significance α. For a one-tailed test, if calculated probability is less than or equal to α, H_0 is rejected, otherwise not. Also, for a two-tailed test, if calculated probability is less than or equal to $\alpha/2$, reject H_0; otherwise H_0 is not rejected.

For large $n \ge 40$, the normal deviate test can be used. The distribution of U tends to normal. The mean and variance of U given t, are

$$\text{mean} = \frac{n_1 t}{n} \text{ and variance} = \frac{n_1 n_2 t(n-t)}{n^2(n-1)}$$

Thus, the distribution of

$$Z = \frac{U - n_1 t/n}{\sqrt{\dfrac{n_1 n_2 t(n-t)}{n^2(n-1)}}} \quad ...(16.39)$$

is approximately standard normal, i.e., $Z \sim N(0, 1)$. Putting $t = u + v$ in (16.39) and doing certain algebraic manipulations, the above test statistic can be rewritten as,

$$Z = \frac{\dfrac{u}{n_1} - \dfrac{v}{n_2}}{\sqrt{pq\left(\dfrac{1}{n_1} + \dfrac{1}{n_2}\right)}} \quad ...(16.39.1)$$

where $p = \dfrac{u+v}{n_1+n_2}$ and $q = 1 - \hat{p}$. 0.5 is added to u or v, whichever is less, and 0.5 is subtracted from u or v, whichever is greater. This correction leads the more reliable results. The decision about H_0 is taken in the usual way.

Example: The data of 10 plots each, under two treatment are as given below.

(Treat. 1) X: 46, 45, 32, 42, 39, 48, 49, 30, 51, 34
(Treat. 2) Y: 44, 40, 59, 47, 55, 50, 47, 71, 43, 55

The hypothesis of equality of median response under two treatments can be tested by the median test. Here we test,

H_0: $F_1(x) = F_2(x)$ vs. H_1: $F_1(x) = F_2(x - \delta)$ for $\delta \ne 0$

Arranging the data in ascending order, we have

30	32	34	39	<u>40</u>	42	<u>43</u>	<u>44</u>	45	46
<u>47</u>	<u>47</u>	48	49	<u>50</u>	51	<u>55</u>	<u>55</u>	<u>59</u>	<u>71</u>

In the above ordered statistics, the observations belonging to treatment 2 are underlined just to differentiate them from observations under treatment 1. The median of the combined data is 46.5. Here we have 10 observations on the left of the median, and 10 observations on the right of the median, i.e., $t = 10$. Also

$$n = 20,\ u = 7,\ v = 3$$

By formula (16.38),

$$P(u/t) = \frac{\binom{10}{7}\binom{10}{3}}{\binom{20}{10}} = \frac{120 \times 120}{19 \times 17 \times 4 \times 13 \times 11} = 0.078$$

Take the prefixed significance level $\alpha = 0.05$. Since $P(u/t)$ is greater than 0.05, H_0 is not rejected. This means that the treatments are equally effective with regard to their median effects.

Wald-Wolfowitz Runs Test

This test is used for testing the identity of two populations. To avoid any confusion between one-sample runs test and this test procedure, we will consider two random samples $X_1, X_2, ..., X_m$ and $Y_1, Y_2, ..., Y_n$ combine into a single sequence of ordered statistics. Assuming that the samples have come from continuous probability distributions, a unique sequence of ordered statistics is always possible as, theoretically, no ties should occur. In the combined sequence some identification mark must be put with observations of one type so as to identify whether an observation belongs to X-sample or Y-sample. The definition of runs remains the same as in the one-sample case. Let the combined sequence of order statistics with $m = 5$ and $n = 4$ be

XX|Y|X|YY|XX|Y

In this case, there are three runs of X's and 3 runs of Y's. In all we have six runs. From this it may be concluded that the two populations are identical as the total number of runs r is quite large. If the populations are different, we expect that r will be small as the two samples are not well mixed. Here we test,

$$H_0: F_X(x) = F_Y(x) \text{ for all } x.$$

$$\text{vs.} \quad H_1: F_X(x) \neq F_Y(x) \text{ for some } x.$$

We define a random variable R, the total number of runs in pooled ordered arrangement of m X's and n Y's. An already mentioned, too few runs tend to reject H_0 in favor of H_1 as this indicates that either most of the X's are greater than or less than the Y's. The Wald-Wolfowitz runs test of nominal α has a critical region given by

$$R \leq r_\alpha$$

where r_α is chosen to be the largest integer such that $P(R \leq r_\alpha) \leq \alpha$ under H_0.

Since X and Y constitute a completely random sequence under H_0 as the letters a and b do in case of single random sample, the probability distribution of R is exactly the same. In this case, $m = n_1$ and $n = n_2$. The only difference in the Wald-Wolfowitz runs test from the one-sample runs test is that only the one-sided test is being used here. Tables of critical values of r at significance level α are prepared by Swed and Eisenhart. Table XI-$F_{(i)}$ can be used for this test also at the 0.05 level.

For large $m, n > 10$, a normal approximation may be made assuming that $m/(m + n)$ and $n/(m + n)$ remain constant as $m + n \to \infty$.

The mean and variance of R are given as,

$$\text{mean (R)} = \frac{2\ mm}{m+n} + 1 \qquad ...(16.40)$$

$$\text{and var (R)} = \frac{2\ mn\ (2mn - n - m)}{(m+n)^2 (m+n-1)} + 1$$

Thus, the normal deviate is,

$$Z = \frac{R - mean\ (R)}{\sqrt{\text{var (R)}}} \qquad ...(16.41)$$

where $Z \sim N(0, 1)$.

The decision about H_0 is taken in the usual way.

In working, ties sometimes occur though theoretically it should not. This happens due to the rounding of figures. If the ties occur within same sample, there is no problem, but if they occur across samples, we face a problem as the number of runs would not be uniquely obtained. In that situation, we break the ties in all possible ways and compute for each way of breaking ties. Then, the largest r value will be used, since that is the one value least likely to lead to the rejection of H_0.

Example: The following are the rates of flow of a certain gas through two soil samples collected from two different places.

Sample X:	23,	27,	19,	24,	22,	30		
Sample Y:	21,	29,	34,	32,	26,	28,	36,	26

The hypothesis that the populations of soil types are the same with respect to the rates of flow through the soils, i.e., symbolically,

H_0: $F_X(x) = F_Y(x)$ for all x

vs. H_1: $F_X(x) \neq F_Y(x)$ for same x

can be tested by the Wald-Wolfowitz test.

The sequence of combined samples with the clearly marked runs is,

$$19|\underline{21}|22,23,24|\underline{26,26}|27|\underline{28,29}|30|\underline{32,34,36}|$$

In this case $m = 6$, $n = 8$ and the number of runs $r = 8$. The probability for $r = 8$ (even) is,

$$fr = \frac{2\binom{5}{3}\binom{7}{3}}{\binom{14}{6}} = 0.233$$

Supposing the predecided level of significance $\alpha = 0.1$. Since the probability $f(r)$ is greater than 0.1, we accept H_0 which means that the two soils have identical distributions in respect of rates of flow of a certain gas.

Mann-Whitney U-test

A very powerful nonparametric alternative to the *t*-test is the Mann-Whitney U-test. By using this statistics, a researcher can determine whether or not two groups are significantly different when the scores from two sets of data are ranked.

Lamond and Farnell (1998) compared the scores of seven novice nurses to the scores of seven expert nurses who sorted 16 cards, 8 with pictures of a variety of pressure sores and 8 others showing various dressings that might be used in dressing pressure sores. The subjects were asked to sort the cards into categories so that each category had something in common that was different from the other categories they developed. They were then asked to explain their reasons for placing the cards into the categories they had developed. The explanations were audiotaped and subjected to content analysis to determine the common categories used by the subjects. The subjects were also given a brief, fictitious case history using a photograph of a pressure sore and other data related to the factors thought to affect the healing of pressure sores for three imaginary patients. Subjects were then asked to recommend treatment on the basis of this information and were asked to explain their decisions. Their responses were also audiotaped for analysis. The investigators used a judge panel of experts in wound care to establish a "gold standard" for treatment against which the subjects' responses were measured.

The test is useful for testing the difference between unpaired observations. (For example, control and experimental group). The observations of both the groups is arranged in the order of magnitude. Tag is made for the common observations in both the groups separately. Ranks are assigned to the observations when there are common observations, average of the ranks is given to them, as in case of Wilcoxon's test. Then the sum of ranks of each of the samples (groups) is calculated separately.

The smaller rank sum out of the above two is referred to Mann-Whitney table, which gives the maximum sum of ranks required for rejection of null hypothesis, under different probability levels.

Whenever the calculated smaller rank sum is less than the tabulated value, the null-hypothesis is rejected.

The expert nurses made more accurate decisions than the novice nurses; when these data were analyzed using the Mann-Whitney U-test, this was statistically significant at the level of $p < 0.05$. The researchers concluded that experts organize data in different ways than novices, and additional instruction on wound care and treatment decisions might result in benefits to patients.

Just like the Wald-Wolfowitz runs test, the Mann-Whitney U-test is based on the idea that the pattern of C's and Y's exhibited by combined ordered statistics provides information about the relationship between their parent populations. Unlike previous runs test, the Mann-Whitney test is based on the criterion of magnitudes of Y's in relation to X's, or vice-versa. If most Y's are greater or less than X's, the null hypothesis of equality of two populations is most likely to be refuted.

Let the two independent random samples of sizes n_1 and n_2 be $X_1, X_2, ..., X_{n_1}$ and $Y_1, Y_2, ..., Y_{n_2}$ and be drawn from two populations having the distribution functions F_X and F_Y respectively. It has been assumed that F_X and F_Y are continuous. This assumption avoids, theoretically, the chances of tied observations.

The hypothesis

$H_0: F_X(x) = F_Y(x)$ for all x

vs. $H_1: F_X(x) \neq F_Y(x)$ for some x

or $H_1: F_X(x) \leq F_Y(x)$

or $H_1: F_X(x) \geq F_Y(x)$

can be tested in the following manner. Write the combined sequence of n_1X's and n_2Y's in order of increasing magnitude. Let the combined sequence for $n_1 = 5$ and $n_2 = 3$ be

$$Y_1\ X_5\ X_1\ Y_3\ X_2\ X_3\ X_4\ Y_2$$

The Mann-Whitney U-statistic is defined as the number of times the Y's precede the X's in the combined sequence of $(n_1 + n_2)$ variables. The Mann-Whitney U-statistic can be defined with the help of an indicator variable D_{ij} where,

$$D_{ij} = \begin{cases} 1 \text{ if } Y_j < X_i & \text{for } i = 1, 2, ..., n_1 \\ 0 \text{ if } Y_j > X_i & j = 1, 2..., n_2 \end{cases}$$

and
$$U = \sum_{i=1}^{n_1} \sum_{j=1}^{n_2} D_{ij} \quad ...(16.42)$$

The random variables D_{ij} are Bernoulli variables with

$$P(D_{ij} = 1) = P(Y < X) = \pi \text{ (say)}.$$

If H_0 is true for all x, $P(Y < X) = P(X < Y) = \frac{1}{2}$ $= \pi$ and H_1 can be given any one of the alternatives $\pi = \frac{1}{2}$ or $\pi < \frac{1}{2}$ or $\pi > \frac{1}{2}$ for some x as the situation demands. Also, mean $(D_{ij}) = \pi$ and var $(D_{ij}) = \pi(1 - \pi)$.

The critical values of U for nominal α are obtained by making use of the null probability distribution of U. Instead of deriving the null probability distribution of U, we would advise readers to make use of the tables given in Appendix-B for small values of n_1 and n_2. An alternative approach to determine the value of U is also given here. Readers may find it simpler than the procedure of D_{ij}.

In the ordered sequences of combined samples, the ranks of either X's and Y's are found out. In case, the ranks of Y's are taken into consideration (the case when Y precedes X) and their sum is S_2, the Mann-Whitney U-statistic is given as,

$$U = n_1 n_2 + \frac{n_2(n_2+1)}{2} - S_2 \quad ...(16.43)$$

Similarly, if the ranks of X's are counted, i.e., the case when X precedes Y and their sum is S_1, the statistic U is given as,

$$U' = n_1 n_2 + \frac{n_1(n_1+1)}{2} - S_1 \quad ...(16.44)$$

It is interesting to point out that both the approaches yield the same value of U. For instance, consider the ordered sequence given earlier for $n_1 = 5$ and $n_2 = 3$.

Sequence:	Y_1	X_5	X_1	Y_3	X_2	X_3	X_4	Y_2
Ranks:	1	2	3	4	5	6	7	8

First we consider $D_{ij} = 1$ when $Y_j < X_i$, otherwise zero. In the given sequence,

Y_1 is less than X_5, X_1, X_2, X_3, X_4, hence, $D_{i_1} = 5$

Y_3 is less than X_2, X_3, X_4 and hence, $D_{i_3} = 3$

Y_2 is less than none and hence, $D_{i_2} = 0$

$$U = \sum_{j=1}^{3} \sum_{i=1}^{5} D_{ij} = 5 + 3 + 0 = 8$$

Now, from (16.43), statistic U can be calculated as follows:

$$n_1 = 5, n_2 = 3, S_2 = 1 + 4 + 8 = 13.$$

$$U = 5 \times 3 + \frac{3 \times 4}{2} - 13 = 8$$

Similarly, if we consider $D_{ij} = 1$ for $X_i < Y_j$, otherwise zero, we get,
$D_{5j} = 1 + 1 = 2$, $D_{ij} = 1 + 1 = 2$, $D_{2j} = 1$, $D_{3j} = 1$, $D_{4j} = 1$

and $U = \sum_{i=1}^{5}\sum_{j=1}^{3} D_{ij} = 2+2+1+1+1 = 7.$

From (16.44),

$$U' = 5 \times 3 + \frac{5 \times 6}{2} - 23$$

$$= 7$$

Since, $S_1 = 2 + 3 + 5 + 6 + 7 = 23$

From the above discussion, it is evident that the value of the statistic U remains the same, no matter which of the two approaches is adopted.

For small values of n_2, say, 8 or less, Table XIV-a given in Appendix B provides the probability associated with the calculated value of U and n_1. One should make it a point to note that n_2 in the table is the size of the Y sample for which the sum of ranks have been used. If the probability obtained from the table is less than or equal to the significance level α, we reject H_0, otherwise H_0 is not rejected.

If the probability for the given value of U is not provided in the table, the value of U' for the other group can be calculated by the relation,

$$U' = n_1 n_2 - U \qquad ...(16.45)$$

Also, $P(U' \geq U) = P(U \leq n_1 n_2 - U')$

Now the test is applied to U'.

For n_2 lying between 9 and 20 and $n_1 \leq 20$, the critical value of U can be seen in Table XIV-b for the desired nominal α. The table is provided for $\alpha = 0.05$ only for a two-tailed test. If the calculated U is less than or equal to the tabulated value of U, H_0 is rejected at level α, otherwise not.

When n_1 and n_2 are so large that the critical values cannot be determined by Table XIV-a and XIV-b, a normal approximation may be made under H_0. Under the null hypothesis,

$$\text{mean (U)} = \frac{n_1 n_2}{2} \text{ and var (U)} = \frac{n_1 n_2 (n_1 + n_2 + 1)}{12}$$

The large sample test statistic is,

$$Z = \frac{U - n_1 n_2/2}{\sqrt{n_1 n_2 (n_1 + n_2 + 1)/12}} \qquad ...(16.46)$$

where $Z \sim N(0, 1)$.

The approximation has been found accurate enough for equal sample sizes as small as 6. The decision about H_0 can be taken in the same way as we have been doing previously, in case of normal deviate test.

Example: The following are the scores of certain randomly selected students at mid-term (MT) and final examinations.

MT scores X:	55, 57, 72, 90, 57, 74
Final scores Y:	80, 76, 63, 58, 56, 37, 75

The hypothesis H_0 that the distribution of scores at two occasions is same against H_1, i.e.,

$$H_0: F_Y(x) = F_X(x) \text{ vs. } H_1: F_Y(x) \neq F_X(x)$$

can be tested by the Mann-Whitney U-test.

The combined scores in a sequence in increasing order of magnitude are,

	37	55	56	57	57	58	63	72	74	75	76	80	90
	Y	X	Y	X	X	Y	Y	X	X	Y	Y	Y	X
Ranks of Y:	1		3			6	7			10	11	12	

Considering the ranks of Y's, the Mann-Whitney statistic for $n_1 = 6$, $n_2 = 7$ is,

$$U = 7 \times 6 + \frac{7 \times 8}{2} - 50 = 20$$

From Table XIV-a, for $n_2 = 7$, $n_1 = 6$ and U = 20, the probability is 0.473. Suppose that the test has been performed at significance level $\alpha = 0.05$. The tabulated probability is greater than 0.05, hence we infer that the distribution of scores at two occasions is same.

K-Sample Problem (K ≥ 3)

The tests given so far are confined to one or two sample cases. But in real life one comes across many problems involving more than two independent samples. The analysis of variance is most commonly used.

But analysis of variance is based on the assumptions that the samples are drawn from normal populations and their variances are same. When these assumptions are not likely to hold good, the F-test cannot be applied. In such a situation nonparametric tests come to our rescue. The nonparametric tests for K-sample porblems require no assumption except that the populations are continuous. Three nonparametric tests for three or more sample problems are given here.

Median Test for Three or More Samples

This is an extension of the median test for two sample problems. The test is applied in the same way with little modification. Let k samples of sizes $n_1, n_2, ..., n_k$ be selected independently from k populations $F_1(x), F_2(x), ..., F_k(x)$, respectively. The hypothesis that the k samples have come from identical populations, i.e.,

$H_0: F_1(x) = F_2(x) = ... = F_k(x)$

vs. H_1: at least two of them are not identical.

can be tested by the median test.

All the samples are pooled and the overall median of the combined ordered statistics is found out. Track should be kept as to which observation belongs to which sample in the pooled sequence of observations. Let the median be designated by θ. Suppose $\sum_{i=1}^{k} n_i = N$. Obviously, θ will be the $\left(\frac{N+1}{2}\right)$ th observation if N is odd, and an average of the $\frac{N}{2}$ th and $\left(\frac{N+2}{2}\right)$ th observations when n is even. Again, the observations are dichotomized according as they are less than θ or more than θ. Consider a random variable U_i defined as the number of observations which are less than θ in the i-th sample for $i = 1, 2, ..., k$. Supposing

$$r = \sum_{i=1}^{k} U_i = \begin{cases} N/2 & \text{if N is even} \\ \frac{N-1}{2} & \text{if N is odd} \end{cases}$$

Under null hypothesis, all the $\binom{N}{r}$ possible sets of observations are equally likely which are in the less than θ category. Therefore, the null probability function of U's is a multivariate hypergeometric distribution given as,

$$f(U_1, U_2, ..., U_k \mid r) = \frac{\binom{n_1}{U_1}\binom{n_2}{U_2}\cdots\binom{n_k}{U_k}}{\binom{N}{r}} \quad ...(16.47)$$

If one or more U'_i they differ largely from their expected value, H_0 should be rejected. For an exact test, the best way is to calculate the probabilities for observed and extreme values of $U_1, U_2, ..., U_k$ and cumulate these probabilities. In practice, if the sum of probabilities so obtained is less than the desired significance level a, reject H_0; otherwise H_0 is not rejected.

The calculation of probabilities is a tedious process. Hence an alternative test criterion is used which is sufficiently accurate for N as small as 25 and no individual sample is of size less than 5. Each element in the combined sequence is classified according to two criteria, the sample number to which it belongs and whether it is less than θ. Hence, the test statistic is approximately chi-square. Thus, we find out the observed and expected frequencies as in the k-classification case. Let an observed frequency be denoted by f_{ij} and the expected frequency be e_{ij} for $i = 1, 2, ... k$ and $j = 1,2$.

$f_{i1} = U_i$, the no. of observations in sample i which are less than θ.

$f_{i2} = n_i - U_i$, the number of observations in sample i which are not less than θ. Similarly, the expected frequencies,

$$e_{i1} = \frac{r}{N} n_i \text{ and } e_{i2} = \frac{N-r}{N} n_i$$

The test statistic for $2k$ categories is,

$$q = \sum_{i=1}^{k} \sum_{j=1}^{2} \frac{(f_{ij} - e_{ij})^2}{e_{ij}} \quad ...(16.48)$$

Substituting the values of f_{ij} and e_{ij} in terms of U_i, N and r, we obtain

$$q = \frac{N^2}{r(N-r)} \sum_{i=1}^{k} \frac{\left(U_i - \frac{r}{N} n_i\right)^2}{n_i} \quad ...(16.48.1)$$

q has an approximately chi-square distribution with $(k-1)$ *df*.

The approximation is improved if q is multiplied by the fraction $(N-1)/N$.

The test criterion is, reject H_0 if the value of $(N-1)\,q/N$ is greater than or equal to the tabulated value of χ^2 for $(k-1)$ *df* and desired level α. Otherwise, H_0 is not rejected.

In actual problems, if two middle values in the combined sequence are equal to θ, a conservative approach is adopted, i.e. the ties are broken in a way which leads to the maximum value of q.

Kruskal-Wallis Test

The Kruskal-Wallis statistical test allows for a one-way ANOVA with ordinal data by establishing a rank order by examining the data. The Kruskal-Wallis statistic is reported as H.

Elnitsky and associates (1997) used the Kruskal-Wallis one-way ANOVA test to determine whether there were differences of opinions among nurses in their reporting of incidents in a hospital setting. They found there was a significant difference in incident reporting behaviors based on educational background: "nurses with the lower educational levels were less likely to agree with appropriate incident reporting behaviors than were nurses with higher education levels".

This is a nonparametric test for one-way classification just like one-way analysis of variance. The Kruskal-Wallis test is an improvement on the median test. In the median test, the magnitude of the observations was compared with one value only, i.e., the median. But in this method the magnitude of observations is compared with every other observation by considering the ranks.

Again the pooled sequence of k samples of size n_i, $i = 1, 2, ..., k$, in order of increasing magnitudes, will have ranks from 1 to N. The sum of the ranks is equal to $N(N+1)/2$. Under H_0, the sum of the ranks would be divided in proportion to sample size among k samples. For the ith sample of size n_i, the expected sum of ranks is,

$$\frac{n_i}{N} \cdot \frac{N(N+1)}{2} = \frac{n_i(N+1)}{2}$$

Suppose R_i is the actual sum of ranks of the elements in sample i. A reasonable test based on a function of the deviations between the observed and expected rank sums has been given by Kruskal and Wallis. The Kruskal-Wallis test statistic is

$$H = \frac{12}{N(N+1)} \sum_{i=1}^{k} \frac{R_i^2}{n_i} - 3(N+1) \quad ...(16.49)$$

The statistic H is distributed as chi-square with $(k-1)$ *df*. Reject H_0 at significance level α if,

$$H = \chi^2_{\alpha,\, k-1}$$

Otherwise H_0 is not rejected.

Example: The green yield (kg) under four treatments is as tabulated below:

Number of plots	*Treatments*			
	1	*2*	*3*	*4*
1	3.17	3.44	3.15	2.48
2	3.40	2.88	2.69	2.37
3	3.50	2.97	3.10	2.58
4	2.87	3.27	2.80	2.84
5	3.88	3.94	3.45	3.00
6	4.00	3.87		2.48
7	3.60	3.25		

The hypothesis that there is no difference among four treatments can be tested by the median test.

Here $k = 4$, $n_1 = 7$, $n_2 = 7$, $n_3 = 5$, $n_4 = 6$ and $N = 25$. The ordered statistics of the pooled samples is, (2.37), (2.48), (2.48), (2.58), 2.69, 2.80, (2.84), 2.87, 2.88, 2.97 (3.00), 3.10, 3.15, 3.17, 3.25,

3.27, 3.40, 3.44, <u>3.45</u>, 3.50, 3.60, 3.87, 3.88, 3.94, 4.00

$$M_d = 3.15$$

For treatment 1; $U_1 = 1$
For treatment 2; $U_2 = 2$
For treatment 3; $U_3 = 3$
For treatment 4; $U_4 = 6$

$$r = \sum_{i-1}^{4} U_i = 1 + 2 + 3 + 6 = 12$$

To show the method of calculations, the test will be performed at 5 percent significance level by using (i) hypergeometric distribution and (ii) chi-square statistic.

(i) The probability,

$$f(U_1, U_2, U_3, U_4/r) = \frac{\binom{7}{1}\binom{7}{2}\binom{5}{3}\binom{6}{6}}{\binom{25}{12}} = \frac{21}{74290}$$

$$= 0.00028$$

The calculated probability is less than 0.05. Hence, we reject H_0 which means that the treatment differ significantly.

(i) Observed frequencies in the two categories are,

Treatments		Category 1 (Less than q)	Category II (More than q)	
	Observed frequency	Expected frequency	Observed frequency	Expected frequency
1	1	$\frac{12}{25} \times 7 = 3.4$	6	$\frac{13}{25} \times 7 = 3.6$
2	2	$\frac{12}{25} \times 7 = 3.4$	5	$\frac{13}{25} \times 7 = 3.6$
3	3	$\frac{12}{25} \times 5 = 2.4$	1	$\frac{13}{25} \times 5 = 2.6$
4	6	$\frac{12}{25} \times 6 = 2.8$	0	$\frac{13}{25} \times 6 = 3.2$

By formula (16.48)

$$\chi^2 = 11.86$$

By formula (16.48.1)

$$\chi^2 = \frac{25 \times 25}{12 \times 13}(0.796 + 0.264 + 0.072 + 1.622)$$

$$= 11.03$$

Tabulated value of $\chi^2_{0.05,3} = 7.815$

Again, the conclusion is the same as in procedure (i)

Example: For the experimental data given in previous example we test H_0 by the Kruskal-Wallis test.

The sequence of the combined sample in increasing order of magnitude is,

(2.37)	(2.48)	(2.48)	(2.58)	2.69	2.80	(2.84)
1	2.5	2.5	4	<u>5</u>	<u>6</u>	7
2.87	2.88	2.97	(3.00)	3.10	3.15	3.17
8	9	10	11	<u>12</u>	13	14
3.25	3.27	3.40	3.44	3.45	3.50	3.60
15	16	17	18	19	20	21
3.87	3.88	3.94	4.00			
22	23	24	25			

The sum of ranks for each individual treatment is–

Treat.—1; $R_1 = 8 + 14 + 17 + 20 + 21 + 23 + 25 = 128$

Treat.—2; $R_2 = 9 + 10 + 15 + 16 + 18 + 22 + 24 = 114$

Treat.—3; $R_3 = 5 + 6 + 12 + 13 + 19 = 55$

Treat.—4; $R_4 = 1 + 2.5 + 2.5 + 4 + 7 + 11 = 28$

The Kruskal-Wallis test statistic by formula (16.49) is,

$$H = \frac{12}{25 \times 26}\left(\frac{128^2}{7} + \frac{114^2}{7} + \frac{55^2}{5} + \frac{28^2}{6}\right) - 3 \times 26$$

$$= \frac{12}{25 \times 26} \times 4932.81 - 3 \times 26$$

$$= 91.067 - 78 = 13.067$$

The table value of $\chi^2_{0.05,3} = 7.815$

The hypothesis of quality of treatments effect is rejected.

Friedman's Test

Occasionally there is a need to use a nonparametric ANOVA, such as the Friedman two-way ANOVA by ranks. The researcher ranks the scores on repeated measures of subjects and then compares the ranks of these repeated measures. Scores on the Friedman test are reported as χ^2_r, and tables that report this statistics are similar to the chi-squared statistic table.

This is a nonparametric test for *k*-related samples of equal size, say *n,* parallel to two-way analysis of variance. Here we have *k*-related samples of size *n* arranged in *n* blocks and *k* columns in a two-way table as given below:

Blocks	Samples (treatments) 1 2		Block totals k
1	R_{11}	R_{12} .... R_{1k}	$k(k+1)/2$
2	R_{21}	R_{22} .... R_{2k}	$k(k+1)/2$
3	R_{32}	R_{32} .... R_{3k}	$k(k+1)/2$
.	.		.
.	.		.
.	.		.
n	R_{n1}	R_{n2} .... R_{nk}	$k(k+1)/2$
Col. Total	R_1	R_2 .... R_k	$\frac{nk(k+1)}{2}$

where R_{ij} is the rank of the observation belonging to sample *j* in block *i* for $j = 1, 2..., k$ and $i = 1, 2...., n$. This is the same situation in which there are *k* treatments and each treatment is replicated *n* times. Here it should be carefully noted that the observations in a block receive ranks from 1 and *k.* The smallest observation receives rank 1 at its place and the largest observation receives rank *k* at its place. Intermediary observations receive ranks accordingly. Hence, the block totals are constant and equal to $\frac{k(k+1)}{2}$, the sume of *k* integers.

The null hypothesis H_0 to be tested is that all the *k* samples have come from identical populations. In case of experimental design, the null hypothesis H_0 is that there is no difference between *k* treatments. The alternative hypothesis H_1 is that at least two samples (treatment) differ from each other.

Under H_0, the test statistic is,

$$F = \frac{12}{nk(k+1)} \sum_{j=1}^{k} R_j^2 - 3n(k+1) \qquad ...(16.50)$$

The statistic F is distributed as chi-square with $(k - 1)$ *df.* At level α, reject H_0 if $F \geq \chi^2_{\alpha, k-1}$, otherwise H_0 is not rejected.

Example: The iron determinations (ppm) in five pea-leaf samples, each under three treatments, were as tabulated below.

Samples (Blocks)	Treatments number 1	2	3	Block total
1	591 (1)	682 (2)	727 (3)	6
2	818 (2)	591 (1)	863 (3)	6
3	682 (2)	636 (1)	773 (3)	6
4	499 (1)	625 (2)	909 (3)	6
5	648 (1)	863 (3)	818 (2)	6
Col. total	7	9	14	30

The null hypothesis H_0, that the iron content in leaves under three treatments is the same against H_1, that at least two of them have different effect, can be tested by Friedman's test. The ranks of observations in each block are shown below them in parentheses. Friedman's test statistic by formula (16.50) is,

$$\begin{aligned} F &= \frac{12}{5 \times 3 \times 4}\left(7^2 + 9^2 + 14^2\right) - 3 \times 5 \times 4 \\ &= -65.2 - 60 \\ &= -5.2 \end{aligned}$$

For $\alpha = 0.05$, the table value of $\chi^2_{0.05,2} = 5.99$. Since the calculated F-value is less than 5.99, H_0 is not rejected. This means that there is no difference in the iron content of pea leaves due to the treatments.

Many other tests have appeared in the literature. But they are not commonly used and are beyond the scope of the prescribed curriculum. Hence, they are not included in this chapter.

McNemar Test

The McNemar test uses an adaptation of the chi-square formula to test the direction of change. Only the two cells that include changes are included in the analysis, therefore, *df* = 1.

The McNemar test can be used with two dichotomous measures on the same subjects. It is used to measure change. Figure 16.2 contains an example of a computer printout produced by SPSS for Windows, using data collected by Wood (1997). In this example, we are interested in subjects' ability to identify lumps in models of breasts before and after training. There were 8 lumps in the model. Those who detected 0–3 lumps were scored 0, and those who detected 4–8 lumps, were scored 1. Looking at the cells, we see that 311 people did not change in their ability to detect the lumps, 199 scored low both times (0), and 112 scored high (1) both times. Among those who changed, 100 who scored low on the pretest, scored high on the post-test, whereas only 15 people who scored high on the pretest scored low on the posttest. Thus, for those who changed their scores, more moved from low to high (100) than from high to low (15). This change is statistically significant at the 0.000 level. This indicates that the training provided to these women improved their ability to detect lumps in a model of a breast.

McNemar Test
Lumps pretest and lumps post-test

Lumps pretest	*Lumps post-test* 0	1
0	199	100
1	15	112

Test Statistics (b)

	Lumps pretest and lumps post-test
N	426
Chi-square (a)	61.357
Asymp. sig.	0.000

a Continuity corrected
b McNemar Test

Comments

Row Totals—lumps found on pretest
299 women (199 + 100) found 0 to 3 lumps (0)
127 women (15 + 112) found 4 to 8 lumps (1)
Columns Totals—lumps found on post-test
214 women (199 + 15) found 0 to 3 lumps (0)
212 women (100 + 112) found 4 to 8 lumps (1)
Cells
Reflecting no change
199 women found 0 to 3 lumps both times (0)
112 women found 4 to 8 lumps both times (1)
Reflecting change
199 women who found 0 to 3 lumps at pretest, found 4 to 8 at post-test
15 women who found 4 to 8 lumps at pretest, found 0 to 3 at post-test

Fig. 16.2: Computer output of McNemar test

Precautions to Use of Nonparametric Test

In the use of the nonparametric tests, the student is cautioned against the following lapses:

1. When measurements are in terms of interval and ratio scales, the transformation of the measurements on nominal or ordinal scales will lead to the loss of much of information. Hence, as far as possible parametric tests should be applied in such situations. In using a nonparametric method as a shortcut, we are throwing away dollars in order to save pennies.
2. In situations where the assumptions underlying a parametric test are satisfied and both parametric and nonparametric tests can be applied, the choice should fall on the parametric test because most parămetric tests have greater power in such situations.
3. Nonparametric tests, no doubt, provide means for avoiding the assumption of normality of distribution. But these methods do nothing to avoid the assumption of independence on homoscedasticity wherever applicable.
4. The behavioral scientist should specify the null hypothesis, alternative hypothesis, statistical test, sampling distribution and level of significance in advance of the collection of data. Hunting around for a statistical test after the data have been collected tends to maximize the effects of any chance difference which favor one test over another. As a result, the possibility of

Table 16.9

A general guide for the selection of non-parametric tests

Level of measurements	*Non-parametric Statistical Test*					*Non-parametric measure of Correlation*
	One-sample case	*Two-sample case*		*K-sample case*		
		Related samples	*Independent samples*	*Related samples*	*Independent samples*	
Nominal	Binomial test, χ^2 one-sample test	McNemar test for the signficance of changes	Fisher exact probability test; χ^2 two independent samples	Cochran Q test	χ^2 test for k independent samples	Contingency coefficient: C
Ordinal	Kolmogorov-Smirnov one-sample test, one-sample runs test	Sign test, Wilcoxon matched pairs signed ranks test	Median test, Mann-Whitney U test, Kolmogorov Smirnov two-sample tests, Wald-Wolfowitz runs test, Moses test of extreme reactions	Friedman two-way analysis of variance	Extension of the median ests, Kruskal Wallis one-way analysis of variance	Spearman rank correlation coefficient: r Kendall rank correlation coefficient: r Kendall partial rank correlation coefficient: $r_{xy.zs}$ Kendall coefficient of concord-ance: W
Interval	Walsh test, Randomization test for matched pairs	Randomizati-on test for two independent samples				

rejecting the null hypothesis when it is true (Type I error) is greatly increased. However, this caution is applicable equally to parametric as well as non-parametric tests.

5. We do not have the problem of choosing statistical tests for categorical variables. Non-parametric tests alone are suitable for enumerative data.
6. The F and t tests are generally considered to be robust tests because the violation of the underlying assumptions does not invalidate the inferences. It is customary to justify the use of a normal theory test in a situation where normality cannot be guaranteed, by arguing that it is robust under non-normality.

A Guide for the Selection of Non-parametric Tests

In this chapter, only a few more popular non-parametric tests have been used. However, a general guide for a selection of nonparametric tests is presented in Table 16.9. It is based on the level of measurement, single or multiple samples, and correlated or independent samples. Several volumes are available in which these tests have been described.

EXERCISES

1. Seventy-nine urban and 83 rural college students were asked to respond on a three-point scale—Approve, Neutral and Disapprove—to a question "Should sex education be included in the college courses". Their number in each category is shown below:

	Urban	*Rural*
Approve	58	35
Neutral	11	25
Disapprove	10	23

2. Eighty-two teachers were classified into three categories—very good, average, and poor by a consensus of team of inspectors. If the teaching proficiency is distributed normally, does, this distribution differ significantly from the normal distribution? The observed frequencies are:
   Good = 32; Average = 40; Poor = 12
3. Two hundred students were asked whether open book examinations be instituted at the Post-graduate stage. Their responses are given below:

Strongly Disapprove	46
Approve	36
Indifferent	48
Disapprove	34
Strongly Disapprove	36

   Do these results differ significantly from equal preferences in the group?
4. The following are observations for two independent samples:
   Sample I: 5, 6, 8, 10, 14, 15, 19, 22, 25, 25
   Sample II: 8, 10, 12, 16, 18, 18, 27
   Use Median test to find out if the two samples came from the same population with respect to their medians.
5. The number of attempts taken by members of two groups of boys and girls with 20 persons in each group, in hitting a shooting target is given below. Find out if the two groups differed significantly in their shooting ability (or the boys are more efficient than the girls)

Number of attempts

Persons	*Boys*	*Girls*
1	1	8
2	2	8
3	3	8
4	3	9
5	4	10
6	5	11
7	7	12
8	7	12
9	7	12
10	7	14
11	8	14
12	8	14

Contd...

Contd...

Persons	*Boys*	*Girls*
13	8	16
14	8	16
15	9	16
16	14	18
17	14	18
18	14	20
19	15	20
20	15	22

6. On the last day of depositing the college fee for the month of January 1985, a large queue of boys and girls was seen at the fee counter. Their sex was recorded according to their position in the queue. Use of Run Test to see whether the arrangement of their position differed significantly from randomness.
   Position; 1 2 3 4 5 6 7 8 9 10 11 12 13
   Sex B B G B G B B G G G G B B
   Position 14 15 16 17 18 19 20 21 22 23 24 25
   Sex B G B G G B B B B G G G
7. Two groups of boys and girls were administered a test of attitude towards sex in the movies. The higher score means greater preference for sex. Distributions of their scores are given below. Do the two groups belong to a common population with regard to their attitude towards sex in movies?
   Attitude score 10 11 12 13 14 15 16 17 18 19 20
   Boys 1 5 6 8 7 10 2 1 0 0 0
   Girls 0 0 0 2 3 5 8 10 1 1 0
   Use One-tail and Two-tail tests.
8. What is ordered statistics? Describe the role of ordered statistics in nonparametric tests.
9. Write a short essay on the uses of nonparametric tests.
10. Throw some light on the implication of ties in the samples. Also describe the ways in which ties can be tackled.
11. Describe three nonparametric tests for two-sample problems. Also discuss their salient features.
12. How is the Wilcoxon-signed rank test superior to ordinary sign-test?
13. Justify the statement that Runs test is good for testing the randomness of a sample.
14. Differentiate between critical region and critical value.
15. Which nonparametric tests are substitutes for the analysis of variance? Describe their methodology.
16. A die was rolled 132 times and the following results were obtained.

Number of spots	1	2	3	4	5	6
Frequency	12	24	38	32	16	10

Use Kolmogorov-Smirnov statistic to test the hypothesis that the die is perfect.

17. Two quality control laboratories independently collected samples of 25 articles from a number of sales depots and tested them. The number of defectives per sales depot were as follows:

Lab A:	9	3	1	3	0	7	2	11
Lab B:	12	6	6	4	8	5	4	

18. The following 30 numbers are taken from a two-digited numbers table:

51	68	30	81	90	46	99	98	11	06
19	43	95	82	65	85	65	81	00	50
53	69	51	97	79	69	60	15	05	35

Test the randomness of the numbers by the Runs test on the basis of runs up and runs down.

19. Given the following ten-paired sample observations.

X-sample:	42.7	50.4	44.2	49.7	49.4	55.3	46.1	49.8	48.7	45.9
Y-sample:	54.2	43.7	34.0	46.1	55.4	58.2	53.4	43.6	57.0	61.9

Test the hypotheses that the two samples have come from identical populations by (a) ordinary sign test that (b) Wilcoxon signed rank test

20. On tossing a coin 15 times, the following sequence of heads (H) and tails (T) was obtained.

T T H H H T H T H H H T T H H

Test whether the coin is unbiased by the Run test.

21. School children taking coaching in three private schools secured the followng scores out of 100.

Number of chidren	*Schools*		
	1	*2*	*3*
1	33	32	55
2	38	15	68
3	39	87	27
4	48	32	88
5	58	22	46
6	70	63	52
7	61	56	76
8	41	57	
9	45	44	
10	49		

Test the hypothesis that the students studying in the three private schools have identical distribution of marks by applying the (i) Median test and (ii) Krushal-Wallis test, at significance level $\alpha = 0.1$.

22. The quantity of serum albumin (gms) per 100 mL in lepers under three different drugs and the control group was as follows:

Group No.	*Control*	*Drug I*	*Drug II*	*Drug III*
1	4.30	3.65	3.05	3.90
2	4.00	3.60	4.10	3.10
3	4.10	2.70	4.20	3.20
4	3.80	3.15	3.70	4.20
5	3.30	3.75	3.60	3.00
6	4.50	2.95	4.80	3.40

Apply Friedman's test to confirm whether the content of serum albumin in different groups of persons is same.

CHAPTER 17 The Analysis of Variance

Introduction

The term parametric statistics is used to describe inferential statistics that assumes a normal distribution of the variables and the use of interval or ratio measures. The most frequently used parametric tests include *t* tests, analysis of variance, and analysis of covariance.

The *t* test of significance is adequate for any experiment that involves only two groups and only a single factor. It provides only a test of a single mean difference. But suppose we have an experimental design involving three groups, A, B, and C, with each group tested after a different experimental treatment or under a different set of experimental conditions. The use of *t* as a relatively simple statistical technique would still be possible and would involve taking two group means at a time and testing the significance of the difference. The number of mean comparisons in this case would be three viz, A and B; A and C; and B and C. However, the problem arises when the number of groups is larger say five or more. If we have ten groups, the number of comparisons which would be required under the *t* test would be given by the formula.

$$\frac{N(N-1)}{2} = \frac{10 \times 9}{2} = 45$$

Obviously, some methods of testing differences among all of the means at the same time would prove very valuable. The analysis of variance and the corresponding test of significance based upon F distribution permits us to do this. Another important consideration which rules out the use of *t* test and warrants the use of the more sophisticated F test of significance, is the case of situations in which two or more experimental variables or one experimental and one or more control variables are simultaneously operating and not only comparison of means within each variable is required, but also the joint operation or interaction of two or more variables is of interest.

t Tests

To determine whether the differences between the means of two different sets of scores are statistically

Table 17.1

Paired *t* test results on Fictitious Test

Variables	*N*	*Test 1*	*Test 2*	*Mean difference*	*p value*
Part A	31	25	30	+ 5	0.04*
Part B	31	41	27	– 14	0.001*
Part C	31	56	57	+ 1	0.37

$^*p < 0.05$ level

significant, the researcher can use the *t* test, a parametric statistical measure to determine the differences between the means of two groups. The researcher first determines whether the two samples are independent (such as in the case of an experimental and a control group) or dependent (using the same group of individuals and their responses before and after a treatment). This must be done because there are several ways to compute the *t* statistic. If an inappropriate method is used, the researcher might obtain incorrect results in either accepting or rejecting the hypothesis.

For example, consider Table 17.1 (this is for illustrative purposes only; there has been no attempt to calculate *t* scores). This table shows that on part A of a factitious test, the probability of achieving this difference is less than 0.05, or $p < 0.05$. If the investigator sets a level of confidence at $p < 0.05$, then the differences in the scores between test 1 and test 2 are considered significant. The differences between the mean scores on part B of test 1 and part B of test 2 is –14. There are many reasons for negative numbers to occur in research design, and confidence levels can be assigned directionally—that is the hypothesis indicates that there will be an increase or decrease in what is being tested, or the investigator may simply state that the difference is significant regardless of whether the results show a positive or negative probability. An asterisk (*) shows that the result is significant. Part C shows that there is no significant difference between the two tests at the 0.05 level of confidence.

An example of the use of the *t* test statistic can be found in the study done by Sliwa (1997), in which the researcher used the paired *t* test to determine whether there was a significant difference between the mean hematocrit values of blood drawn through a saline lock device and blood drawn by traditional venipuncture. The investigator found that there was no significant difference in the hematocrit values of blood drawn by either method. This led to the conclusion that patients would be exposed to less pain and staff would have less difficulty in locating venipuncture sites if blood were drawn routinely through a saline lock. This study is also an example of establishing a probability level (in this case, $p < 0.05$) that the researcher hopes will not be met.

The technique of analysis of variance was first devised by Sir Ronald Fisher, an English statistician who is also considered to be the Father of Modern Statistics as applied to social and behavioral sciences. It was first reported in 1923 and its early applications were in the field of agriculture. Since then it has found wide applications in many areas of experimentation. The analysis of variance, as the name indicates, deals with variances rather than with standard deviations and standard errors. It is a method of dividing the variation observed in experimental data into different parts, each part assignable to a known source, cause or factor. We may assess the relative magnitude of variation resulting from different sources and ascertain whether a particular part of the variation was greater than expectation under the null hypothesis. However, it must be remembered that analysis of variance divides the total sum of squares, $\Sigma(X - X)^2$, into additive parts which are then converted into *mean square* simply by dividing the sum of squares by the relevant degrees of freedom. The main difference between variance and mean square is that the former is obtained by dividing the sum of squares by *n* while the latter is obtained by dividing the sum of squares by degrees of freedom. Hence, it is advisable to keep this fact in view while understanding the rationale of the analysis of variance.

In its simplest form, the analysis of variance is used to test the significance of the differences among means of a number of different groups supposed to have come from different populations. The total sum of squares is analyzed into two parts: a sum of squares based upon variation *within the several groups:* and a sum of squares based upon variation *between the group* estimates of the population variance are computed. The value of F is, then, the ratio between the two estimate, of the population variance.

$$F = \frac{\sigma^2 \text{ Between groups}}{\sigma^2 \text{ Within groups}} \text{ or } \frac{\sigma^2 \text{ B}}{\sigma^2 \text{ W}} \quad ...(17.1)$$

in which σ^2 is the standard symbol of population variance.

Analysis of Variance (Anova)

It is observed that '*t*' test is applied to know whether the differences in the mean values of two groups of observations are arising out of sampling variation or the two groups are coming out of a homogenous population.

But when there are more than two groups to be tested, we have to test in terms of two means at a time. However, a comparison of three or more series of observations can be made by "Analysis of Variance". This analysis is based on the assumption that the total variation present in a set of observations may be partitioned into a number of components associated with the classification of the data.

For example, when the Hb levels of antenatal mothers in three villages are to be compared, it can be seen that the total variability in the hemoglobin values of the antenatal mothers is measured as "sum of squares of deviation of the Hb values of all the observations."

However, there may be two types of variabilities, responsible for this total variability, one type is due to differences between mothers within each village (intra village difference) while the second type is due to differences in the mothers between the three villages (inter-village difference). When these types of variabilities are combined together to get the total variability of the observations, this estimate will be bigger than the sum of two components. By an analysis of variance, the total variability can be partitioned into two components one between the villages and the other within the villages. Using this partitioned components, one can test the hypothesis whether the mean hemoglobin levels of antenatal mothers in three villages are different from the overall mean or not.

The above example is a two way classification and the analysis of variance is applicable to more than two way classification also.

When a number of populations are under study and from each population a random sample or a group of units is selected, analysis of variance is a powerful tool to analyze the data. The purpose of analysis of variance is two-fold:

1. The total variance with respect to a variable (factor) is spitted into number of independent component variances, which are responsible for the total variance. Still, the sum of variances due to component factors never equals the total variance. Such a difference is attributed to error variance. This is the variance that occurs due to certain extraneous factors which cannot be held responsible for any known component.
2. The next step is to test the null hypothesis about each of the component factors individually. This hypothesis is tested by finding out the ratio of variance of a component factor to the error variance. In ANOVA table, estimated variances are termed as *mean sum of square* (MS). The skeleton of analysis of variance table is given in Table 17.2.

Table 17.2

ANOVA

Source of variation	*Degrees of freedom*	*Sum of squares*	*Mean sum of square*	*F-value*
Due to	*df*	*SS*	*MS*	*F-value*
A				
B				
Error				
Total				

Table 17.2 in practice is given with abbreviated notations. Degrees of freedom for various components are written in the usual way. Error degrees of freedom are obtained by subtracting the components df from total *df* similarly, the error SS is obtained by subtracting the components SS from total SS, whereas the total sum of squares is calculated by taking the total of the squares of each individual value and subtracting from it a factor which is known as *correction for mean or correction factor* (CF). Hence, the sum of squares for testing equality of k = population means, using the same notations as given in the preceding section are,

$$\text{(Correction for mean) CF} = \left(\sum_{i=1}^{k}\sum_{j=1}^{n_i} x_{ij}\right)^2 / n = G^2/n$$

$$\text{Total SS} = \sum_{i=1}^{k}\sum_{j=1}^{n_i} x_{ij}^2 - \frac{G^2}{n} = T_{xx}$$

$$\text{Between samples SS} = \sum_{i=1}^{k}\frac{x_i^2}{n_i} - \frac{G^2}{n} = S_{xx}$$

$$\text{Error SS} = \sum_{i=1}^{k}\sum_{j=1}^{n_i} x_{ij}^2 - \sum_{i=1}^{k}\frac{x_i^2}{n_i} = T_{xx} - S_{xx} = E_{xx}$$

Mean sum of squares is obtained by dividing the sum of squares by its corresponding *df* F-value for a component is obtained by taking the ratio of component MS to error MS. Analysis of variance table with full details is as presented in Table 17.3.

The calculated value of F is compared with the table value of F for α level of significance and $(k-1, n-k)$ *df* Traditionally α is chosen to be 0.05, and for more precision, α is chosen to be 0.01, through there is no hard and fast rule about it. We may choose any other value of α if it sounds more logical.

The above ANOVA is meant for one way classification. The ANOVA table may be extended for two or more way classification. In that situation, the component factors will increase in the ANOVA table accordingly. The methodology of analysis of variance is further explicated through a numerical example.

Example: The Table 17.4 gives the gain in body weight (kg) per heifer during four grazing treatments.

The hypothesis that the mean gain in weight of heifers under four treatments is equal or not, can be tested by F-test, i.e. the hypothesis,

$$H_0 : \mu_1 = \mu_2 = \mu_3 = \mu_4$$

against H_1 : at least two means are different, can be tested through analysis of variance technique.

For the given data, $n_1 = 7$, $n_2 = 6$, $n_3 = 6$, $n_4 = 5$, and $n = 24$,

$G = 1286.5$, $x_1 = 394.6$, $x_2 = 348.0$, $x_3 = 297.2$, $x_4 = 246.7$

Table 17.3

ANOVA

Due to	*df*	*SS*	*MS*	*F-value*
Bet. samples	$(k-1)$	$\sum_{i=1}^{k}\frac{x_i^2}{n_i}\ \ \frac{G^2}{N} = S_{xx}$	$\frac{S_{xx}}{k\ \ 1} = S_x$	$S_x/E_x = F$
Within sample (Error)	$(n-k)$	$\sum_{i=1}^{k}\sum_{j=1}^{n_i} x_{ij}^2\ \ \sum_{i=1}^{k}\frac{x_i^2}{n_i} = E_{xx}$	$\frac{E_{xx}}{n\ \ k} = E_x$	
Total	$n-1$	$\sum_{i=1}^{k}\sum_{j=1}^{n_i} x_{ij}^2\ \ \frac{G^2}{n} = T_{xx}$		

$$\sum_{i=1}^{4}\sum_{j=1}^{n_i} x_{ij}^2 = (67.3^2 + 36.9^2 + \ldots + 38.8^2 + 48.2^2)$$

$$= 74357.57$$

$$\frac{G^2}{n} = \frac{(1286.5)^2}{24} = 68961.76$$

Total SS = 74357.57 – 68961.76

$$= 5395.81$$

$$\sum_{i=1}^{4}\frac{x_i^2}{n_i} = \frac{(394.6)^2}{7} + \frac{(348.0)^2}{6} + \frac{(297.2)^2}{6} + \frac{(246.7)^2}{5}$$

$$= 22244.16 + 20184.00 + 14721.31 + 12172.18$$

$$= 69321.65$$

Between treatment SS,

$$\sum_{i=1}^{4}\frac{x_i^2}{n_i} - \frac{G^2}{n} = 69321.65 - 68961.76$$

$$= 359.89$$

Error SS = 5395.81 – 359.89

= 5035.92

From Table VII (ii), value of $F_{0.05, (3, 20)} = 3.10$.

Since the calculated value of F is less than the table value, H_0 is not rejected. It leads to the result that the mean increase in weight of heifers, under four grazing treatments, is not significantly different at 5 percent level of significance.

One Way or Single Classification ANOVA

In its simplest form ANOVA can be used when a number of treatments based on a single factor are involved. For example, in a field experiment, three randomly selected groups have been assigned randomly to three different experimental treatments say, traditional method; programmed learning method; and multi-media method. At the end, the criterion scores are obtained. The mean scores of three groups can then be compared by using ANOVA. Since only one factor, i.e. method of teaching (of course with three variations of the method) is involved, the situation warrants a single classification or one way ANOVA and can be diagrammed as below:

Table 17.4

Heifer No.	Gain in body weight (kg) during Treatments				Total
	T_1	T_2 (x_{ij})	T_3	T_4	
1.0	67.3	74.2	63.1	48.7	
2.0	36.9	42.2	32.9	49.0	
3.0	63.2	58.6	59.2	62.0	
4.0	36.8	36.6	42.4	38.8	
5.0	54.8	54.6	34.0	48.2	
6.0	64.2	81.8	65.6		
7.0	81.4				
Total	394.6	348.0	297.2	246.7	1286.5

Table 17.5

Due to	df	SS	MS	F-value
Treatments	3	359.89	119.96	$\frac{119.96}{251.79} = 0.48$
Error	20	5035.92	251.79	
Total	23	5395.81		

Programmed learning method	*Multi-media method*	*Traditional method*
X_{11}	X_{12}	X_{13}
X_{21}	X_{22}	X_{23}
X_{31}	X_{32}	X_{33}
$Xn_1{}^1$	$Xn_2{}^2$	$Xn_3{}^3$

In which X stands for scores; subscripts, for individuals and columns; and n_1, n_2, n_3, for number of persons in each groups.

As stated earlier, in the simplest case, the total variance is partitioned into two components: *The between variance* which is the variance of the means of the experimental groups about the grand mean of the total sample; this component includes the contribution of the various experimental treatments plus variance due to the sampling fluctuations or error variance. The other component, *the within variance* is an average of the variance within the experimental groups. It is often termed as *error variance* also because it results from sampling fluctuations, i.e., due only to individual differences. It may be expressed as $S_e{}^2$ or variance due to random fluctuations in sampling. However, in the formula for F-ratio, $\sigma_w{}^2$ instead of $\sigma_e{}^2$ is generally used.

The between variance can be expressed as:

$$\sigma_B{}^2 = \sigma_e{}^2 + \sigma_{Tr}{}^2 \qquad ...(17.2)$$

In which $S_{Tr}{}^2$ stands for variance due to experimental treatment; $\sigma_e{}^2$ for error variance:

The value of F is simply the ratio between the two variances – between and within. This ratio generates a new sampling distribution of F. The test whether the experimental treatment caused significantly different results is made by comparing $S_B{}^2/S_W{}^2 = (S_e{}^2 + S_{Tr}{}^2) / S_e{}^2$ to the F distribution with appropriate degrees of freedom for numerator and denominator. If the scores are truly scores from the same population, the two variance estimates, the $S_B{}^2$ and $S_W{}^2$, will be the same. However, from actual experimental data, it is difficult to find samples, though randomly and independently chosen, having exactly the same means and variances. Therefore, random differences between the numerator and denominator of the F ratio are to be expected and are given in the tables of F-distribution. If the treatments of the experiment produce decided differences in variance among criterion measures, then the between variance will be increased leading to the increase in the value of F-ratio which would then be greater than one. A comparison of this F-ratio with the appropriate value in the F-distribution table can establish whether the former arose due to chance or due to real differences among the various treatments. With an initial arbitrary decision concerning the acceptable level of the probability, one can decide to reject or not to reject the null hypothesis.

In a one-way ANOVA situation, the total variance is equal to the variance within groups and variance between groups. This concept will be demonstrated through a numerical example given in Table 17.6. There are two procedures of calculating total, between, and within variances – one through a raw score approach and the other through a deviation score approach. Both these approaches will be demonstrated below:

Deviation Score Method

Table 17.6

Work-sheet for One-Way Analysis of Variance on Hypothetical Scores using Deviation Score Method

Step I: The Measurements

	Set I	*Set II*	*Set III*
	10	3	10
	7	3	11
	6	3	10
	10	3	5
	4	3	6
	3	3	8
	2	3	9
	1	3	12
	8	3	9
	9	3	10
ΣX_s	60	30	90, $\Sigma X = 180$
M_s	6	3	9 $M_s = 6$

Step II: Deviations within sets (x_s)

+4	0	+1
+1	0	+2
0	0	+1
+4	0	–4
–2	0	–3
–3	0	–1
–4	0	0
–5	0	+3
+2	0	0
+3	0	+1

It checks with the value obtained by adding sum of squares within sets, and sum of squares between sets. The student should thus understand the following relationships:

i. Total sum of squares = Within sum of squares + Between sum of squares
or $SS_T = SS_W + SS_B$ ...(17.3)

ii. Between sets sum of squares = Total sum of squares – Within sum of squares
or $SS_B = SS_T - SS_W$ ...(17.4)

iii. Within sets sum = Total sum of squares – Between sum of squares
or $SS_W = SS_T - SS_B$ ...(17.5)

Step III: Squares of deviations within sets (x_s^2)

16	0	1	
1	0	4	
0	0	1	
16	0	16	
4	0	9	
9	0	1	
16	0	0	
25	0	9	
4	0	0	
9	0	1	
100	0	42	$\Sigma x_s^2 = 142$

Step IV: Deviations of set means from grand mean (d)

d	0	3	–3	
d^2	0	9	9	$\Sigma d^2 = 18$
nd_2	0	90	90	$n\Sigma d^2 = 180$

In Table 17.6, fictitious data have been given. In set II, all values have been kept equal. The purpose is to explain an important point later in the discussion. The three sets of scores were hypothetically obtained under three different conditions or treatments. The hypothesis to be tested is whether all the observations came by random sampling from the same general population or were there systematic overall differences among the three set means. In symbolic terms:

$$H_0: \mu_1 = \mu_2 = \mu_3 = \mu$$
$$H_0: \mu_1 \neq \mu_2 \neq \mu_3 \neq \mu$$

In verbal terms, the null hypothesis states that the means of the three populations do not differ among themselves and are equal to the mean of the general population. The alternative hypothesis expresses that these means are not equal.

Steps of Computation (Deviation Score Method)

A. *Calculation of Sum of Squares within Sets:*

I. Compute the sums and means of all the three sets, the grand total ΣX_s, and the grand mean M_t.

II. For every set, compute deviations from the set mean M_x by using the formula $x = (X - Mt)$. Designate them as X_s or deviations within sets.

III. Square the deviation within sets to find each X_s^2. Add them to obtain ΣX_s^2. These are sum of squares of deviations within sets.

B. *Calculation of Sum of Squares between Sets:*

IV. For each set, take the deviation between each set mean and grand mean, $(M_s - M_t)$, and call

Table 17.7

Summary of analysis of variance

Component of (sources of variation)	Sum of squares (SS)	Degrees of freedom (df)	Mean square (MS)	F
Between sets	180.00	2	90.00	17.11
Within sets	142.00	27	5.26	
Total	322.00	29		

them *d*. Square each *d* and sum them up to obtain Σd^2. Multiply each d^2 by *n*, the number of scores in each set and sum them up to obtain $n\Sigma d^2$. This value is sum of squares between sets.

C. *For the Calculation of Total Sum of Squares:* The total sum of squares can be obtained by adding the sum of squares within sets and the sum of squares between sets. However, for the purpose for verification of the relationship among these three types of sums of squares, the total sum of squares can be calculated directly by subtracting each score from the grand mean, squaring the deviation and summing all the deviations up. In our example,

The total sum of squares $= (10 - 6)^2 + (7–6)^2 + ... + (10 - 6)^2 = 322.00$

D. *Calculation of Degrees of Freedom and Mean Square:*

Degree of freedom can be calculated as follows:

df_{total} = (Total number of scores – 1); or (N – 1): or (30 – 1)

$df_{between}$ = (No. of sets – 1): or (*s*–1); or (3 – 1) = 2

df_{within} = (number of scores in each set minus 1, multiplied by number of sets); $s(n - 1)$; $3(10 - 1) = 27$

The sum of degrees of freedom for between and within sets should add up to the total degrees of freedom. The mean squares for each source of variation can be obtained by dividing the sum of squares by their respective *df*.

With all the above computational results at our command, we can set up a table of summary ANOVA results as given in Table 17.7:

$$F = \frac{MS_{between}}{MS_{within}} = \frac{90.00}{5.26} = 17.11;$$

$df = 2, 27$

Interpretation: The calculated F value of 17.11 is to be compared with the value of F required for significance at 0.05 and 0.01 level. For this purpose, Table K in Appendix is to be consulted. Reading of any F value from the table depends upon the *df* for greater mean square i.e., the within mean square. The former are given vertically in the columns, and the latter horizontally in the rows. The value at the intersection of the two is the value of F at a particular level of significance with *df* as mentioned above. In Table K, the upper values are at 0.05 level, while the lower ones are at 0.01 level. In our case, the values of F from the table are ${}_{0.05}F_{(2, 27)} = 3.35$: ${}_{0.01}F_{(2, 27)} = 5.49$.

The calculated value of F is higher than both the values of F at 0.05 and 0.01 levels. Since 0.01 level is higher, we can interpret that the calculated value of F is significant at 0.01 level. *Hence the H_0 cannot be accepted. It can be said that the overall differences among the three set means are significant and not due to chance.* The three sets do not belong to the same population with regard to their means.

As pointed earlier, all sources in set II were purposely kept equal. The main objective was to explain an important point. This set has a zero within variance because all scores are equal to the set mean and hence it does not contribute anything to the variance within sets. In the same manner, the mean of set I is equal to the grand mean, and

Table 17.8

Worksheet for one-way ANOVA on hypothetical scores (Raw Score Method)

	Set I		*Set II*		*Set III*	
	X_1	X_1^2	X_2	X_2^2	X_3	X_3^2
	10	100	3	9	10	100
	7	49	3	9	11	121
	6	36	3	9	10	100
	10	100	3	9	5	25
	4	16	3	9	6	36
	3	9	3	9	8	64
	2	4	3	9	9	81
	1	1	3	9	12	144
	8	64	3	9	9	81
	9	81	3	9	10	100
Σ's	60 (ΣX_1)	460 (ΣX_1^2)	30 (ΣX_2)	90 (ΣX_2^2)	90 (ΣX_3)	852 (ΣX_3^2)
M's						

$N = 30$; $n_1 = n_2 = n_3 = 10$; ΣX or $T = 60 + 30 + 90 = 180$

hence does not contribute anything to the variance between sets.

Raw Score Method

A. Sum of Squares

1. Correction term,

$$C = \frac{(\Sigma X)^2}{N} = \frac{T^2}{N} \quad ...(17.6)$$

$$= \frac{(180)^2}{30} = 1080$$

2. Total sum of squares, $SS_T = \Sigma X^2 - C$ ...(17.7)

$$\therefore\ SS_T = 10^2 + 7^2 + 6^2 + \ldots + 12^2 + 9^2 + 10^2 - 1080 = 322$$

3. Sum of squares among set means,

$$SS_B = \frac{(\Sigma X_1)^2}{n_1} + \frac{(\Sigma X_2)^2}{n_2} + \frac{(\Sigma X_3)^2}{n_3} - 1080 \quad ...(17.8)$$

$$= \frac{(60)^2}{10} + \frac{(30)^2}{10} + \frac{(90)^2}{10} - 1080$$

$$= 1260 - 1080 = 180.00$$

4. Sum of squares within sets,

$$SS_W = SS_T - SS_B$$

$$= 322 - 180$$

$$= 142$$

B. Summary of Analysis of Variance

Source of variation	*df*	*Sum of squares SS*	*Mean square (Variance)*
Between sets	2	180	90
Within sets	27	142	5.26
Total	29	322	

$$F = \frac{90}{5.26} = 17.11$$

Steps for Computation (Raw Score Method)

I. Set up the scores under X_1, X_2, and X_3 as shown in Table 17.8.

II. Square the scores of all the sets and write under X_1^2, X_2^2 and X_3^2.

III. Obtain all sums by adding up the individual columns of the table. Obtain grand sum of scores, Σx, T also.

IV. After these intermediate calculations, we are now ready for the calculation of various sums of squares.

V. Calculate correction term, C as it is required for the adjustment of origin when raw scores are used for the calculation of variance. In fact, the assumed mean here is zero and all scores form deviations from zero.

VI. Calculate SS_T which is sum of squared scores minus correction.

VII. Square each set sum and divide by respective n, and over all the three sets. Deduct C, to obtain SS_B. In case of equal n's a common denominator, n, can be used as below:

$$SS_B = \frac{(\Sigma X_1)^2 + (\Sigma X_2)^2 \ldots + (\Sigma X_k)^2}{n} - C \qquad \ldots(17.9)$$

VIII. Subtract SS_B from SS_T to obtain SS_w. SS_W can also be calculated directly without computing SS_T.

$$SS_W = \frac{\Sigma X^2 - [(\Sigma X_1)^2 + (\Sigma X_2)^2 \cdots + (\Sigma X_k)^2]}{n} \qquad \ldots(17.10)$$

IX. Table of summary of ANOVA can be set up as explained earlier in the case of deviation score method. Degrees of freedom, MS and F can also be calculated similarly.

All sums of squares, mean square and the value of F are the same as obtained by using the deviation score method. The raw score method is to be preferred when score values are small, the means are not whole numbers, and a calculating machine is to be used. However, with small data and means as whole numbers the deviation score method can be used with profit.

Post-Anova Test of Differences by Use of '*t*'

After a significant F has been obtained, one can look for significant pairs of means. For this purpose, *t* test can be used. Since MS_W, the best estimate of the population variance, is available from the ANOVA summary table, the standard deviation can be readily computed as below:

$$\sigma_W = \sqrt{MS_W} \qquad \ldots(17.11)$$

Standard error of difference of means is given by,

$$SS_D = \sigma_W \sqrt{\frac{1}{n_1} + \frac{1}{n_2}} \qquad \ldots(17.12)$$

$$SS_D = 2.29 \sqrt{\frac{1}{10} + \frac{1}{10}} = 1.024$$

Value of t with $df = 27$ (Related with MS_W)
At 0.05 level = 2.05; at 0.01 level = 2.77

Now *critical mean difference* can be calculated for comparison with all mean difference to find out the significant pairs of means.

$$d_{0.05} = t_{0.05} \times SS_D \qquad \ldots(17.13)$$
$$= 2.05 \times 1.024 = 2.099$$

$$d_{0.01} = t_{0.01} \times SS_D \qquad \ldots(17.14)$$
$$= 2.77 \times 1.024 = 2.836$$

Now set up a table of mean differences as below:

Sets	*Mean difference* *I*	*II*	*III*
Means	6.0	3.0	9.0
6.0	–	3.0*	3.0*
3.0	–	–	6.0*
9.0			_

* Significant at 0.01 level

All the mean differences are larger than the critical mean difference, 2.836 (at 0.01 level). Hence, all the mean differences are significant at 0.01 level. When number of sets is large, the above procedure saves time and shows, at a glance, the pairs of means which are significant.

Two-way or Double Classification ANOVA

In experiments more than one experimental factor or one experimental and one or more control factors may be used. For example, in a field experiment, three different methods of teaching – programmed learning, multi-media, and traditional – may be tried out as an experimental factor. At the same time, two different teachers (teacher factor), may be used as a control factor. Thus, we have three levels of method-factor and two levels of teacher-factor and there are in all 3 × 2 = 6 combinations of these two factors. This situation is termed as a 3 × 2 factorial design. Depending upon the number of factors and the number of levels of each factor, several variations of the factorial designs are possible. In this section, only two-way or double classification analysis will be presented. The hypothetical data used in one-way classification ANOVA in Table 17.9 has been once again used by introducing a second factor of teacher. The three sets of scores have been designated as programmed learning (M_1), multi-media (M_2) and traditional (M_3) and the two levels of the teacher-factor as Teacher I (T_1) and Teacher II (T_2).

The factorial design will thus be as follows:

		Method		
		M_1	*M_2*	*M_3*
Teacher	T_1	M_1T_1	M_2T_1	M_3T_1
	T_2	M_1T_2	M_2T_2	M_3T_2

The mathematical model for this example will be:

$$X = m + d_m + d_t + d_{mt} + e_r \quad ...(17.15)$$

In which symbols are:

X = Any raw score; m = Population mean or grand mean; d_m = deviation due to method factor; d_t = deviation due to teacher factor; d_{mt} = deviation due to combined effect of m and t or interaction of m and t; and e_r = random error.

In verbal expression, any raw score is a combination of the population mean (here grand mean), plus variation due to method factor plus variation due to teacher factor, plus variation due to the combined effect of method and teacher factors plus random error due to sampling fluctuations. This model can be further extended to three factors or larger factorial designs. The model makes it obvious that the various effects are additive and through a process of analysis, variance due to various effects can be separately determined and tested for significance. The population mean, m is the grand mean of the scores empirically obtained, and is a constant value and thus does not contribute to any variation in the data.

The procedure of calculation of various effects in the two way ANOVA is illustrated in Table 17.8. The notation for the purpose is also given therein.

Total Number of observations, N = 30

Number of observations in each cell, $n = 5$

Number of columns (teaching methods), $m = 3$

Number of rows (teachers), $t = 2$.

Table 17.9

Worksheet for two-way analysis of variance on hypothetical data (Raw Score Method)

	Teaching Methods						*Total*
	Programmed Learning (M_1)		*Multimedia (M_2)*		*Traditional (M_3)*		
	X_1	*X_1^2*	*X_2*	*X_2^2*	*X_3*	*X_3^2*	
Teacher I (T_1)	10	100	3	9	10	100	
	7	49	3	9	11	121	
	6	36	3	9	10	100	
	10	100	3	9	5	25	
	4	16	3	9	6	36	
Σs	37	301	15	45	42	382	94
Teacher II (T_2)	3	9	3	9	8	64	
	2	4	3	9	9	81	
	1	1	3	9	12	144	
	8	64	3	9	9	81	
	9	81	3	9	10	100	
Σs	23	159	15	45	48	170	
Σ	60	460	30	90	90	852	180

The student should be able to calculate and identify various sums of scores and sums of squared which are required in the further calculations of sums of squares:

Sums of Method Factor

$\Sigma X_{M1} = 60$; $\Sigma X_{M2} = 30$; $\Sigma X_{M3} = 90$; Total 180

Sums for Teacher Factor

$\Sigma X_{T1} = 94$; $\Sigma X_{T2} = 86$; Total 180

Sums for Cells (Method X Teacher)

$\Sigma X_{M1T1} = 37$; $\Sigma X_{M1T2} = 23$; $\Sigma X_{M2T1} = 15$;
$\Sigma X_{M2T2} = 15$; $\Sigma X_{M3T1} = 42$; $\Sigma X_{M3T2} = 48$;
Total 180

Sums of Squared Scores

$$\Sigma^2_1 + \Sigma^2_2 + \ldots + \Sigma X^2_N = 10^2 + 7^2 + \ldots + 10^2 = 1402$$

A. *Sum of Squares*

1. Correction term,

$$C = \frac{(\Sigma X)^2}{N} = \frac{T^2}{N} = \frac{(180)^2}{30} = 1080.00$$

2. Total sum of squares = $\Sigma X^2 - C$

$$SS_{total} = (10^2 + 7^2 + 6^2 + 10^2 + \ldots + 9^2 + 12^2 + 9^2 + 10^2) = 1080$$

Now 1402 – 1080 = 322.00

3. Sum of the squares between cells,

$$SS_{teacher\text{-}method} = \frac{\Sigma(\Sigma X_m)^2}{nt} - C \quad \ldots(17.16)$$

$$= \frac{(37)^2 + (15)^2 + (42)^2 + (23)^2 + (15)^2 + (48)^2}{5} - 1080$$

$$= \frac{1369 + 225 + 1764 + 529 + 225 + 2304}{5} - 1080$$

$$= \frac{6416}{5} - 1080$$

$$= 1283.2 - 1080 = 203.2$$

4. Sum of squares between rows (teacher)

$$SS_{teacher} = \frac{\Sigma(\Sigma X_t)^2}{nm} - C \quad \ldots(17.17)$$

$$= \frac{(94)^2 + (96)^2}{5 \times 3} - 1080$$

$$= 1082.13 - 1080 = 2.133$$

Source of variation	*df*	*SS*	*MS*	*F*	*Sig*
Teacher	$(t - 1) = 1$	2.133	2.133	0.431	n.s.
Method	$(m - 1) = 2$	180	90.00	18.182	0.01
Interaction	$(t - 1)(m - 1) = 2$	21.067	10.5335	2.128	n.s.
Within	$tm(n - 1) = 24$	118.8	4.95		
Total	29	322.00			

One-way ANOVA			*Two-way ANOVA*		
Source of variation	*df*	*SS*	*Source of variation*	*df*	*SS*
Between sets (methods)	2	180.00	Methods	2	180.00
Within	27	142.00	Teacher	1	2.133
			Interaction	2	21.067
			Within	24	118.80
Total	29	322.00	Total	29	322.00

5. Sum of squares between columns (Method)

$$SS_{method} = \frac{\Sigma(\Sigma X_m)^2}{nt} - C$$

$$= \frac{(60)^2 + (30)^2 + (90)^2}{5 \times 2} - 1080$$

$$= 1260 - 1080 = 180$$

6. Sum of squares for interaction

$$SS_{teacher \cdot method} = SS_{teacher \cdot method} - SS_{teacher} - SS_{method}$$

$$= 203.2 - 2.133 - 180$$

$$= 203.2 - 182.133$$

$$= 21.067$$

7. Sum of squares within cells

$$SS_W = SS_{total} - SS_{teacher \cdot method}$$

$$= 322 - 203.2$$

$$= 118.8$$

B. *Summary of analysis of variance*

Calculation of F values:

For Teacher:

$$\frac{MS_{Teacher}}{MS_{Within}} = \frac{2.133}{4.95} = 0.431$$

For Method:

$$\frac{MS_{method}}{MS_{Within}} = \frac{90.00}{4.95} = 18.182$$

For Interaction:

$$\frac{MS_{Interaction}}{MS_{Within}} = \frac{10.5335}{4.95} = 2.128$$

Interpretation: To determine the significance of these F values, we have to consult Table K with appropriate *df*. The following values are obtained from Table K:

For $df = (1, 24)$, value of F to be significant
at $0.05 = 4.26$
at $0.01 = 7.82$

For $df = (2, 24)$, value of F to be significant
at $0.05 = 3.40$
at $0.01 = 5.61$

In the last column of the table of summary of ANOVA above, the interpretation of the F values has been given. The Teacher factor and the interaction are not significant (n.s.) while only the method factor is significant at 0.01 level. Hence the three methods have been found to be significantly different in their effects on the criterion scores. This result is consistent with one obtained in one-way ANOVA problem presented in a previous section in Table 17.8. Similar one shown in the bottom.

For Teacher:

$$\frac{MS_{Teacher}}{MS_{Within}} = \frac{2.133}{4.95} = 0.431$$

Effect of Introduction of a Second Factor

Since the data used in the one-way ANOVA problem was repeated here by introducing a second factor of 'teacher' and thus increasing the number of cells from three to six, a comparison of the sums of squares obtained in the two situations will be revealing.

The following observations can be easily made:

1. The SS for method factor (between sets) remains the same in both situations.
2. The SS for within in the one-way situation has been further broken down into three components – SS for teacher, SS for interaction and SS within. If we add up these three sums of squares from the two-way situation, we obtain a value equal to the SS within of the one-way situation.

	Method₁		*Method₂*		*Method₃*	
	Teacher₁	*Teacher₂*	*Teacher₁*	*Teacher₂*	*Teacher₁*	*Teacher₂*
$School_1$						
$School_2$						
$School_3$						

3. Addition of a second or further factor leads to the reduction of the value of SS_{within} and consequently of error variance. Since the error variance is the denominator of the F-ratio, the values of F will go up and thus increase the likelihood of the rejection of the null hypothesis.
4. The SS_{total} remains the same in both the situations.
5. Reduction in error variance increases the precision of the experimental results.
6. The degrees of freedom for within variance in the one way problem have also been shared by the additional factor of teacher, interaction and within, in the two-way problem. The total *df* remains the same in both the situations.
7. However, selection of the additional factors for introduction in the experiment should be done carefully. Otherwise, a lot of labor and expense will go waste. Only those factors which have a known relationship with the criterion may be used for the purpose.

Notation for Three-way ANOVA

The notation and procedure of calculation used in the two-way analysis of variance problem can be extended for application to three-way or larger designs of ANOVA. However, the notation for a three-way analysis problem is presented below.

The factorial design may also be diagrammed as under:

The various sources of variation are:

Main effects

Source	*df*
Method (M)	$m-1$
Teacher (T)	$t-1$
School (S)	$s-1$
Interactions	
Method × Teacher	$(m-1)(t-10)$
Method × School	$(m-1)(t-1)$
Teacher × School	$(t-1)(s-1)$
Method × teacher × School	$(m-1)(t-1)(s-1)$
Within cells	$mts\,(n-1)$
Total	$n-1$

Notation

The notation for the three-way analysis of variance design is given below. The meaning of small letters *m*, *t*, *s*, and *n* have already been given above.

Correction Factor,

$$C = \frac{\Sigma(\Sigma X_{mts})^2}{N}$$

$$SS_{method} = \frac{\Sigma(\Sigma X_m)^2}{nts} - C$$

$$SS_{teacher} = \frac{\Sigma(\Sigma X_t)^2}{nms} - C$$

$$SS_{school} = \frac{\Sigma(\Sigma X_t)^2}{nmt} - C$$

$$SS_{M\times T} = \frac{\Sigma(\Sigma X_{mt})^2}{ns} - \frac{\Sigma(\Sigma X_m)^2}{nts} - \frac{\Sigma(\Sigma X_t)^2}{nms} + C$$

$$SS_{M\times S} = \frac{\Sigma(\Sigma X_{ms})^2}{nt} - \frac{\Sigma(\Sigma X_m)^2}{nts} - \frac{\Sigma(\Sigma X_s)^2}{nmt} + C$$

$$SS^*_{MTS} = \frac{\Sigma(\Sigma X_{mts})^2}{n} - C$$

$$SS_{within} = \Sigma X^2_{mts} - \frac{\Sigma(\Sigma X_{mts})^2}{n} - C$$

$$SS_{total} = \Sigma X^2_{mts} - C$$

*SS between cells of M, T and S. Direct calculation of $SS_{M\times S\times T}$ interaction was not possible except by subtracting SS for all main effects and interaction from total SS.

The student should understand the simple rules on which the above notation has been based.

Σ = Sum of

X = Any raw score or observation

ΣX^2_{mts} = Sum of all X scores taken over all combination of factors M, T and S. In fact, the correct term should be $\sum^{m}\sum^{t}\sum^{s} X_{mts}$ – However, to avoid $m = 1, t = 1, s = 1$ complications, multiple signs of summation with their limits have been left out.

ΣX_m = Sum of all X scores within various levels of M. Hence, there will be as many sums as there are levels of M factor.

ΣX_{mt} = Sum of all X scores within various cells composed of Method and Teacher factors. If M = 3; T = 2; there will be 3 × 2 such cells and hence six sums.

Denominators of the terms can be mechanically determined. This will be the product of small letter not used in the numerator. For example, in SS_{Method} $= \frac{\Sigma(\Sigma X_{mts})^2}{n}$, the small letter m has been used in the numerator leaving n, t and s for insertion into the denominator. Further more in $SS_{M \times S}$ = $\frac{\Sigma(\Sigma X_m)^2}{nts}$, m and s have been used in the Numerator, leaving n and t for the denominator. These small letters as explained already stand for:

m = number of levels of factor M or Method factor
t = number of levels of factor T or Teacher factor
s = number of levels of factor S or School factor
n = number of observations in each cell.

Interaction

In any discussion of analysis of variance, a consideration of the meaning and interpretation of the interaction of variables or factors becomes important. These interactions may be between two or more independent variables and could be the main effects and make the interpretation of their significance difficult. The interaction of Method and Teacher on the criterion variable of achievement may be encountered if one teacher is more efficient on one method while the other teacher is more efficient on the other method. To illustrate,

Table 17.10

Interaction of Method and Teacher (Hypothetical Mean Achievement Scores)

(A)	M_1	M_2	Av	(B)	M_1	M_2	Av	(C)	M_1	M_2	Av
T_1	16	4	10	**T_1**	16	6	11	**T_1**	16	8	12
T_2	4	12	8	**T_2**	6	4	5	**T_2**	12	4	8
Av	10	8	9	**Av**	11	5	8	**Av**	14	6	10

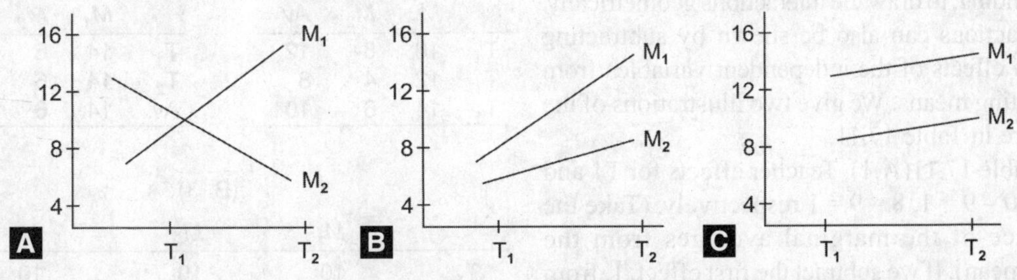

Figs 17.1A to C: Geometrical representation of the interactions based on the data of Table 17.9

let M_1 and M_2 represent two methods of teaching a foreign language. Let T_1 and T_2 represent the two teachers participating in the experiment. Hypothetical mean achievement scores of three experiments are given in Table 17.10:

In Table 17.10 (A), it is obvious that M_1 (with an average of 10) is better than M_2 (with an average of 8). But on closer inspection, one may see that M_1 gives better results than M_2 when used by T_1.

In Table 17.10 (B), M_1 results are better than those of M_2, but M_1 is not nearly as effective with Teacher$_1$ as it is with Teacher$_2$.

In Table 17.10 (C), M_1 is equally more effective than M_2 with Teacher$_1$ and Teacher$_2$.

These situations are diagrammed below in Figures 17.1A to C.

Figures 17.1A and 17.1B indicate presence of interaction in the two factors of method and teacher. In Figure 17.1A, the two graphs intersect each other. It is called as *disordinal* interaction and is very difficult to interpret. The interaction represented by non-parallel and non-intersecting lines as in Figure 17.1B is called *ordinal* interaction. Figure 17.1C shows parallel lines or lines with equal slopes, and represent absence of any interaction. Interaction occurs when the vertical differences between the lines in the geometrical representation are not equal. In the case of disordinal interaction, the direction of these differences is reversed from one level to the other. In the latter case, one cannot say that either method is superior to the other without qualifying the statement as to where the superiority lies in relation to the other variable. It is, therefore, advisable, for a clearer understanding, to draw the interactions geometrically.

Interactions can also be shown by subtracting the main effects of the independent variables from the resulting means. We give two illustrations of the procedure in Table 17.11.

In Table 17.11(A.1), Teacher effects for T1 and T2 are 10 – 9 = 1, 8 – 9 = 1 respectively. (Take the difference of the marginal averages from the general mean). If we subtract the first effect, 1, from all averages in the first row and add 1 to all averages in the second row, we have Table 17.11(A.2). Similarly, we can take out the main effects due to method by subtracting 10 – 9 = 1 from the first column and adding 1 to the second column. Table 17.11(A.3) gives the resultant averages which show the direction of the interaction. Moreover, statistical tests can also be used to test their significance.

In Table 17.11(B), the process of subtracting the main effects from the data of Table 17.10(C) has been demonstrated with the result that in Table (B3) all averages have become equal to the grand mean. This shows absence of any interaction.

Table 17.11

Subtraction of the Main Effects

A. *Interaction Exists*

(A.1) Original Data

	M_1	M_2	Av
T_1	16	4	10
T_2	4	12	8
Av.	10	8	9

(A.2) Teacher effects subtracted

	M_1	M_2	Av
T_1	15	3	9
T_2	5	13	9
Av.	10	8	9

(A.3) Teacher effects subtracted

	M_1	M_2	Av
T_1	14	4	9
T_2	4	14	9
Av.	9	9	9

B. *No Interaction Exists*

(B.1)

	M_1	M_2	Av
T_1	16	8	12
T_1	12	4	8
T_1	14	6	10

(B.2)

	M_1	M_2	Av
T_1	14	6	10
T_2	14	6	10
Av.	14	6	10

(B. 3)

	M_1	M_2	Av
T_1	10	10	10
T_2	10	10	10
Av	10	10	10

It may, however, be remembered that the graph or adjusted averages can give us an idea only of the presence or absence of an interaction. But, whether the interaction was significant or not would require an appropriate test of significance.

Assumptions Underlying the Analysis of Variance

As is the case of all parametric statistical tests, in the mathematical development of the analysis of variance, a number of assumptions have been made. It is important to take a look at the procedures of collecting data and the nature of the distribution of the data obtained before taking a decision to use this technique. Normally, the data should satisfy the following assumptions:

1. *Normality of Distribution:* The dependent variable in the population from which the samples have been drawn should be normally distributed. Generally, a test of goodness of fit is used to ascertain the fulfillment of this pre-requisite. Violation of this assumption will make the results appear somewhat more significant than they actually are. However, this deficiency can be made up by using a somewhat more rigorous level of confidence that usual. In case of very large N, near normality may be obtained without much difficulty.
2. *Homogeneity of Variance:* Homogeneity of variance means that the variance in the different sets of scores does not differ beyond chance. The H_0: $S_1^2 = S_2^2 = S_k^2$ is generally tested by using either Hartley's procedure or Bartlett's Test. Gross departures from homogeneity may lead to results which are seriously in error. However, mild departures from homogeneity of variance may not affect the results much. Transformation of scores to generate homogeneity or the use of a non-parametric test instead of ANOVA are generally recommended to avoid the violation of this assumption.
3. *Additivity of Effects:* As stated in an earlier section, the basic model of ANOVA states that a given observation or score is a sum of certain components each due to the effect of a particular identifiable source of variation. In most cases, this assumption is generally met.
4. *Random Sampling:* The sampling within the various sets should be random. It usually means that observations are mutually independent and with equal chance of selection.

General Uses and Limitations of ANOVA

Since the very inception of this wonder technique, the researchers have found it useful for the interpretation of experimental and observational data. It has been widely used in social and biological sciences. Since problems in these areas are generally multi-dimensional, ANOVA provides an appropriate and a powerful technique of analysis in which several factors can be simultaneously used and their effects tested. The research has now advanced from the single-variable classical experiments to the factorial designs in Fisher's tradition.

ANOVA, not only provides us an overall tests of significance among several means, but also allows us to test their interactions, which is not possible with *t* test. Sometimes only interactions are of interest to the researcher.

The rationale of ANOVA allows for the extension of the single classification model to a multiple classification model using three, four or more factors at a time. Thus, ANOVA has opened up the possibilities of research and statistical analysis in situations which require the use of multiple treatments.

Several new experimental designs randomized blocks designs, repeated measure designs. Latin squares designs, Greco-Latin squares designs and a host of other designs have been devised.

Based on very sound mathematical assumptions and model, ANOVA provides a very powerful parametric test of significance. However, this technique suffers from the following *limitations:*

i. It is based on four rigorous assumptions. If these assumptions are not fully met by the data, the results may be in error.

ii. It may become difficult to interpret the results of triple or quadruple interactions. They may turn out to be significant.
iii. Set of data may not always be independent and thus involve correlated means.
iv. It imposes a very strict set of requirements in designing experiments, which may not be always possible to achieve.
v. The minimum number of cases in each cell should be 10 to have confidence in the results.
vi. ANOVA provides an overall test of significance among various means. We may need post ANOVA *t* test to locate the significant pairs of means.
vii. In case of comparison of two means, F test provides no additional information as compared with the *t* test. The relationship between the two in such situation is:

$$t = \sqrt{F} \text{ or } F = t^2.$$

Relation between *t*, χ^2, F and *z*

It is worth pointing out that for some hypothesis, more than one test can be used. For instance, the equality of two population means can be tested by *t*-test as well as F-test. The reason is that some relationship exists between *t*, χ^2 and and F-distribution in particular situations and hence these tests become equivalent, permitting the use of either of these.

Thus, the relationship for $k_1 = 1, k_2 = n$ is,

$$t_n^2 = F_{1,n} \quad \ldots(17.18)$$

$$t_n = e^z = \sqrt{F_{1,n}} \quad \ldots(17.18.1)$$

If $k_1 = n, k_2 = \infty$, z is related to chi-square and the relation is

$$z = \frac{1}{2}\log_e\left(\frac{\chi^2}{n}\right) \quad \ldots(17.19)$$

$$e^{2z} = \chi^2/n \quad \ldots(17.19.1)$$

or

$$F = \chi^2/n \quad \ldots(17.19.2)$$

Since we know, $F = e^{2z}$

If $k_1 = n, k_2 = \infty$, then

$$F_{1,\infty} = \chi_1^2 \quad \ldots(17.20)$$

where suffix 1 donetes the *df* for χ^2.

Also from (17.18),

$$t_\infty^2 = \chi_1^2 \quad \ldots(17.21)$$

If F-table is available only for the upper percentage points, the following identity enables us to obtain the F-values on the left-tail distribution. Let α be the level of the test and F be distributed with (k_1, k_2) *df*, the identity is,

$$F_{\alpha,(k_1,k_2)} = F_{\alpha-1,(k_1,k_2)} \quad \ldots(17.22)$$

The identity (17.22) is very useful and easy to prove.

If the degrees of freedom for a chi-square are large, i.e. more than 100, then the chi-square can be approximated to a standard normal variate using the relation,

$$z = \sqrt{2\chi^2} - \sqrt{2k-1} \quad \ldots(17.23)$$

where *k* is the *df* for a chi-square and $z \sim N(0, 1)$. In this situation, the significance of null hpothesis can be tested by using the normal table for one tail.

These tests will be used in subsequent chapters also as and when the need arises to test various hypotheses.

Table 17.12

Type I and Type II Errors

Decision	*If statement of the H_0 is really true*	*If statement of the H_0 is really false*
Accept H_0	Correct decision	Type II (Beta)
Reject H_0	Type I (Alpha)	Correct decision

Table 17.13

Dependent variable by HIV status interaction

Variable	*F*	*p*
Stress	0.197	0.658
Coping	3.276	0.075
Social support	10.391	0.002*

Note: Univariate F test with (1,66) *df.*
$*p < 0.05$

Sometimes the researcher has more than two means to test to determine whether there are significant differences between them. In this instance, using the *t* test statistic could be exceedingly tedious because of the number of possible permutations of the *t* test. Also, the more individual *t* tests conducted, the greater the possibility of what is called a **type I error** or a **type II error** (Table 17.12).

A type I error, also called the alpha error, means that the investigator has rejected the null hypothesis when it should be accepted. A type II error, also called the beta error, occurs when the investigator accepts the null hypothesis when it should be rejected.

Consequently, the statistical analysis of variance (ANOVA) is often used. With this technique, it is possible to determine whether there is a significant difference between several means simultaneously. The literature will report these differences as the F test, the F ratio, or the F statistic.

Also, when many means have been tested, the researcher will want to know exactly which means were significantly different from the other means. There are other methods, such as Sheffe's test or the Tukey HSD test, that can be applied to determine which means were significantly different from the other means.

Table 17.13 has been modified from the original table in the research report in Appendix C. When examining tables such as this, the critical reviewer needs to concentrate on the asterisks. These indicate footnotes that tell which findings are significant, and the level of significance (in this case, $p < 0.05$). The term *df* stands for degrees of freedom. Degrees of freedom are used when calculating many statistics and refer to the number of values in a set that are free to vary.

Sometimes additional information concerning sums of squares and mean squares is presented in an ANOVA table (Table 17.14) (this is fictitious table; no effort was made to calculate F ratios). Sometimes such tables also include other footnotes that contain additional explanations of the findings and the meanings of various abbreviations used in the table. The researcher should discuss the important parts of the findings in the text but probably would not include all of the details shown in the table.

The use of ANOVA can be found in a study conducted by Gaffney and Associates (1997) of

Table 17.14

Fictitious table of nursing students' test scores comparing three different methods of instruction

Source of Variation	*Degrees of Freedom*	*Sum of Squares*	*Mean Square*	*F Ratio*
Between groups	2	24.38	12.19	11.5*
Within groups	42	987.44		

$*p < 0.05$

pregnant Salvadoran women in the United States. The researchers compared stressful events occurring in the lives of women from three cultural groups, Salvadoran-Hispanic, non-Salvadoran-Hispanic, and non Hispanic. By using ANOVA and the Tukey B test to identify specific group differences, the investigators found that Salvadoran women had significantly different kinds of life stress when compared to non-Salvadoran and non-hispanic women.

ANOVA may be applied when there is more than one dependent variable to be examined. Statisticians call this multiple analysis of variance or multi-variate analysis of variance (MANOVA). MANOVA was used by the researchers whose report is found in Appendix C. This type of statistical analysis can become quite complex. The researcher reports the results of MANOVA using the F statistic, just like the researcher using ANOVA. The tables used by researchers reporting MANOVA are similar to those using ANOVA.

Gwele (1996) used MANOVA to examine how the imposition of curriculum reform on schools of nursing by legislative edict affected nurse educators in four institutions in south Africa. Using the Concerns-Based Adoption Model, the investigator examined the nurse educators' concerns about the new curriculum by testing six hypotheses that compared inexperienced users and "old hands" in determining differences in their levels of concern in reacting to the government's mandate for change. Gwele found that coercing staff to adopt change impedes the development of staff concerns, which may affect student learning. Gwele concluded that "legislated change is not the best means for facilitating adoption and implementation".

EXERCISES

1. What do you mean by analysis of variance? Justify this nomenclature and give the theoretical rationale of ANOVA.
2. Compare F-ratio test and *t* test in terms of their relative merits and limitation. What is the mathematical relationship between the two?
3. State the assumptions of ANOVA. Discuss what happens when these assumptions are violated?
4. Apply ANOVA on the following sets of scores. State the H_0 and H_1. Set the summary table and interpret the results.

a. *Set I*	*Set II*	*Set III*	*Set IV*
3	5	8	2
4	5	7	3
6	5	8	1
8	5	7	
4		4	

(There are unequal n's in this case)

b. *Set I*	*Set II*	*Set III*	*Set IV*	*Set V*
10	5	3	6	7
6	2	8	9	7
4	1	4	8	7
5	1	0	6	7
10	1	0	1	7

(Use deviation score method and also the raw score method. Do they give similar results?)

c. An experiment wanted to see the relative effects of three drugs on the physical growth of rats. Three groups of rats were randomly selected from the same species. In each group, the number of male and female rats was kept equal. The gain in ounces in the weights of the rats is given below. By using an appropriate statistical technique, find out if the effects due to drugs, sex and the interaction of the two-were significant.

	Drug 1	*Drug 2*	*Drug 3*
Male	2	5	4
	3	3	4
	1	3	4
	0	3	3
	2	4	5
Female	4	2	5
	3	2	5
	0	2	5
	0	1	3
	1	0	2

d. An experiment on the relative effectiveness of three different methods of teaching and map-reading was conducted. Three teachers participated in the experiment. Groups of three students each selected randomly were assigned to various treatments. At the end of the experiment, criterion scores were obtained which are given below. Test the two main effects and interaction for significance.

	Method 1	*Method 2*	*Method 3*
Teacher 1	0	3	5
	1	5	1
	2	6	2
Teacher 2	1	0	0
	3	4	5
	5	0	7
Teacher 3	5	3	0
	3	3	4
	2	3	2

e. Four groups of 8 students each having an equal number of boys and girls were randomly selected and assigned to four different conditions of an experiment. Use ANOVA to test the main effects due to conditions and sex, and the interaction of the two:

	Condition 1	*Condition 2*	*Condition 3*	*Condition 4*
Boys	7	9	12	12
	0	4	6	14
	5	5	10	9
	8	6	6	5
Girls	3	4	3	6
	3	7	7	7
	2	5	4	6
	0	2	6	5

5. On the data of 4 (b) above, use post-ANOVA t test to locate the significant pairs of means.
6. How many degrees of freedom are associated with the variation in the data for:
   a. A comparison of four means for independent samples, each containing 15 cases?
   b. A comparison of three means for independent samples, each containing 10 cases?
   c. In a $3 \times 2 \times 4$ factorial experiment, with three factors A, B and C, and $n = 5$; all independent samples?
7. State five situations from education and psychology in which the use of ANOVA can be recommended.
8. What are the limitations of ANOVA?
9. What is an Interaction? Define ordinal and dis-ordinal interactions. Draw the graphs of the following data:

(A)			*(B)*		
	M_1	M_2		M_1	M_2
S_1	18	10	Boys	10	6
S_2	16	8	Girls	2	10

Subtract main effects from each table and show the presence or absence of interaction in the adjusted means.

CHAPTER 18 The Analysis of Covariance

Introduction

Experimental designs, very often, require control of the intervening variables so that the results observed can be attributed, within certain limits of sampling error, to the treatment variable and to no other casual factor. Random assignment of subjects to various experimental treatments and matching of subjects for making up equivalent groups are two important procedures for this purpose. However, the experimenter may fail to control one or two conditions experimentally due to administrative difficulties or through ignorance of their relationship with the criterion measures. In such cases, where experimental control of a covarying variable or covariate has not been done, analysis of covariance (ANCOVA) provides a method of statistical control of the differential in the criterion scores attributable to the covariate.

Frequently, because of the nature of the research setting, it is impossible for a researcher to place subjects into truly randomly assigned groups. In this case, there may be variables that confound the variable under consideration. This means that the researcher's data may or may not show significant differences unless the confounding variable(s) is accounted for.

To account for the confounding variable(s), the researcher may use analysis of convariance (ANCOVA), which is also reported as an F statistic or F ratio. This procedure may also be used in place of the *t* statistic when two groups are involved and there is no way to achieve the requirements of randomness necessary for appropriate use of the *t* statistic. ANCOVA may also be used on more than two sets of subjects or when there is more than one dependent variable. The tables used by the researcher reporting ANCOVA are similar to those used to report ANOVA.

An example of the use of ANCOVA can be found in the 1997 study by Kerr and associates about the effect of short-duration hyperventilation during endotracheal suction on intracranial pressure in adults with severe head injury. The researchers compared the level of intracranial pressure resulting from severe head injuries in adults during endotracheal suctioning after providing short-term hyperventilation before the suctioning process. They found that there was a significant difference in the level of intracranial pressure and that short-duration hyperventilation helped to reduce intracranial pressure.

Examples of multiple analysis of covariance (MANCOVA) may also be found in the literature. For more information on this subject, discuss it with your instructor or find information in a statistics text.

Analysis of Covariance

An extremely useful tool for analyzing experimental data is the **analysis of covariance**. As normally presented within for context of the analysis of variance, the analysis of covariance appears to be unpleasantly cumbersome, especially so when there is more than one covariate. Within the framework of multiple regression, however, it is remarkably simple, requiring little, if any, more work than does the analysis of variance.

Covariate

Suppose we wish to compare driving proficiency on three different sizes of cars to test the experimental hypothesis that small cars are easier to handle. We have available three different groups of drivers, but we are not able to match individual subjects on driving experience, which varies considerably within each group. Let us make the simplifying assumption, which will be discussed in more detail later, that the mean level of driving experience is equal across groups. Suppose further that using the number of steering errors as our dependent variable, we obtain the somewhat exaggerated data plotted in Figure 18.1. In this figure the data have been plotted separately for each group (size of car), as a function of driving experience (the **covariate**), and the separate regression lines have been superimposed.

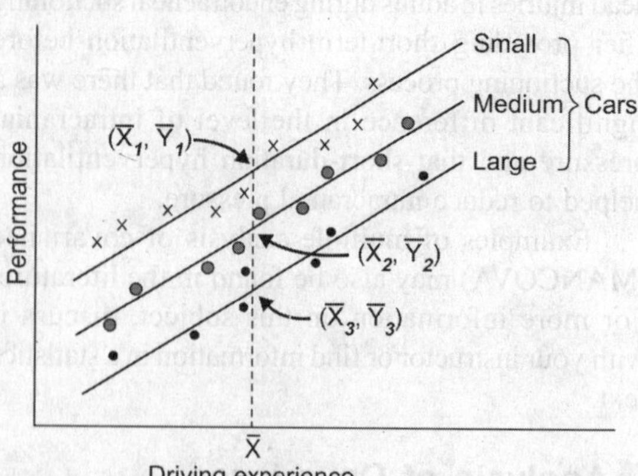

Fig. 18.1: Hypothetical data illustrating error-reduction in analysis of covariance

One of the most striking things about Figure 18.1 is the large variability in both performance and experience within each treatment. This variability is so great that an analysis of variance on performance scores would almost certainly fail to produce a significant effect. Most of the variability in performance, however, is directly attributable to differences in driving experience, which has nothing to do with what we wish to study. If we could somehow remove (partial out) the variance that can be attributed to experience (the covariate), we would have a clearer test of our original hypothesis. This is exactly what the analysis of covariance is designed to do, and this is precisely the sitation in which it does its job best—its job in this case being to reduce the error term.

Adjusted Y Means

A more controversial use of the analysis of covariance situations in which the treatment groups have different covariate (driving experience) means. Such a situation (using the same hypothetical experiment) is depicted in Figure 18.2, in which two of the treatments have been displaced along the *X*-axis. At the point at which the three regres-

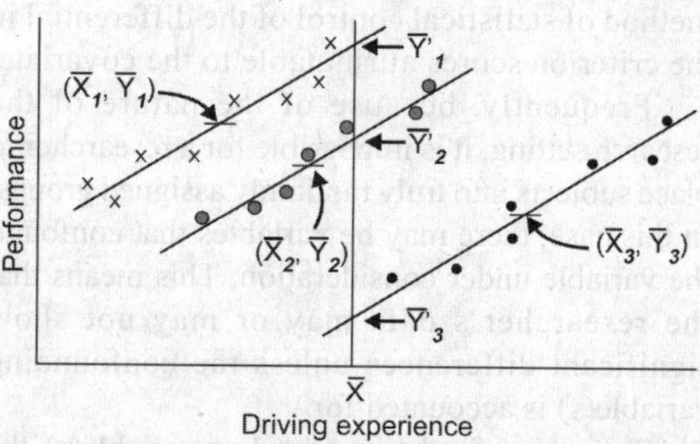

Fig. 18.2: Hypothetical data illustrating mean adjustment in analysis of covariance

sion lines intersect the vertical line X = $\overline{X}$, you can see the values $\overline{Y}_1'$, $\overline{Y}_2'$ and $\overline{Y}_3'$. These are the **adjusted Y means** and represent our best guess as to what the Y means would have been *if the treatments had not differed on the covariate*. The analysis of covariance then tests whether these *adjusted* means differ significantly, again using an error term from which the variance attributable to the covariate has been partialled out.

Although the structure and procedures of the analysis of covariance are the same regardless of whether the treatment groups differ on the covariate means, the different ways of visualizing the problem as represented in Figures 18.1 and 18.2 are instructive. In the first case, we are simply reducing the error term. In the second case, we are both reducing the error term *and* adjusting the means on the dependent variable. We will have more to say about this distinction later in the chapter.

Homogeneity of Regression

Aside from the usual analysis of variance assumptions of normality and homogeneity of variance, we must add two more assumptions. First we will assume that whatever the relationship between Y and the covariate (C), this relationship is linear. Second, we will assume **homogeneity of regression**—that the regression coefficients are equal across treatments—$b^*_1 = b^*_2 = b^*_3 = \cdots = b^*$. This is merely the assumption that the three lines in Figures 18.1 or 18.2 are parallel, and it is necessary to justify our substitution of one regression line (the pooled within-groups regression line) for the separate regression lines. As we shall see shortly, this assumption is testable. Note that no assumption has been made about the nature of the covariate; it may be either a fixed or a random variable (It can even be a categorical variable if we create dummy variables to represent the different levels of the variable, as we did in the earlier parts of this chapter).

Calculating the Analysis of Covariance

When viewed within the framework of multiple regression, the analysis of covariance is basically no different from the analysis of variance, except that we wish to partial out the effects of the covariate. As Cohen (1968) puts it, "A covariate is, after all, nothing but an independent variable which, because of the logic dictated by the substantive issues of the research, assumes priority among the set of independent variables as a basis for accounting for Y variance."

If we want to ask about the variation in *Y* after the covariate (C) has been partialled out, and if the variation in Y can be associated with only C, the treatment effect (α), and error, then $SS_{regression_{C,\alpha}}$ represents the total amount of accountable variation. If we now compare $SS_{regression_{C,\alpha}}$ with $SS_{regression_C}$ the difference will be the variation attributable to treatment effects over and above that attributable to the covariate.

We will take as an example a variation on the study by Conti and Musty (1984). As you may recall, in that study the authors were interested in examining.

For illustration, suppose an experiment is conducted to compare the relative effectiveness of traditional method, programmed learning method, and multi-media method in teaching geography. Random formation of three groups of students for instructional purposes was not possible. Hence, intact classes were used. These classes may differ in intelligence which is an important and known covariate or correlate of academic achievement (The Criterion). Intelligence, thus remained an uncontrolled variable. If intelligence scores of the groups were available from the records or could be obtained otherwise, analysis of covariance provides a method of statistical control of the variation or differential due to intelligence; the adjusted means could then be compared meaningfully.

Analysis of covariance which is an extension devised by RA Fisher, of his methods of analysis of variance, enables us even to dispense with the inconvenient procedure of matching of groups and secure the same increase in precision by the use of statistical controls. The hypothesis to be tested is that there are no differences in the various treatments, and that any differences in final criterion mean scores of the treatment groups, after allowances have been made for chance differences in the covariate mean scores, are due entirely to chance fluctuations in random sampling. The allowance for criterion measure on covariate measures. Under ANCOVA, it is assumed that there is homogeneity of regression which means that there is one true regression of criterion scores on covariate scores which is the same for all the groups.

To sum up, the method of analysis of covariance enables us:

1. To estimate the true regression of criterion scores on covariate scores with the assumption that there is no real difference in regression from group to group.
2. To use this regression coefficient to correct or 'adjust' the criterion means so as to allow for differences in the covariate measures, and
3. To test the differences remaining in the adjusted means.

In a one-way analysis of variance for comparing means, each criterion score, Y, can be expressed as

$$Y = \mu + \text{treatment effect} + \text{error} \quad ...(18.1)$$

If the purpose is to separate difference due to covariate from the criterion differences and do an analysis of covariance, the model changes. The covariate score (in our example intelligence) is denoted by X. It is related to the criterion measure, Y, by the regression equation.

$$Y - M_y = \beta (X - M_x) \quad ...(18.2)$$

β here denotes, regression coefficient.

Model for ANCOVA, then would be

$$Y = \mu + \text{treatment effect} + \beta (X - M_x) + \text{error} \quad ...(18.3)$$

In one-way classification with two covariates, the model extends to

$$Y = \mu + \text{treatment effect} + \beta_1 (X_1 - M_{x1}) + \beta_2 (X_2 - M_{x2}) + \text{error}$$

Increase in precision of results ANCOVA depends on the degree of correlation between criterion (Y) and covariate (X). Some statisticians say that ANCOVA will result in no appreciable

Table 18.1

Worksheet for covariance analysis

Group I					*Group II*					*Group III*				
X_1	Y_1	X_1Y_1	X_1^2	Y_1^2	X_2	Y_2	X_2Y_2	X_2^2	Y_2^2	X_3	Y_3	X_3Y_3	X_3^2	Y_3^2
6	8	48	36	64	8	10	80	64	100	3	2	6	9	4
3	7	21	9	49	6	15	90	36	225	6	2	12	36	4
8	5	40	64	25	3	14	42	9	196	2	3	6	4	9
2	3	6	4	9	8	8	64	64	64	2	1	2	4	1
1	2	2	1	4	5	3	15	25	2	2	2	4	4	4
Sums														
20	25	117	114	151	30	50	291	198	594	15	10	30	57	22
M's														
4	5													

For all groups:

$\Sigma X = 65$; $\Sigma Y = 85$; $\Sigma X^2 = 369$; $\Sigma Y^2 = 767$; $\Sigma XY = 438$;

change in the adjusted means if this correlation is below.

Computation of ANCOVA

In order to illustrate the computational procedure of analysis of covariance, let us assume that three methods of teaching 'NURSING' are applied to three randomly chosen groups of five subjects each and the criterion measures, Y, are obtained. From the COLLEGE records, their intelligence score or covariate measures, X, are also taken. The scores and the procedural steps in the analysis of covariance are given in Table 18.1.

Step 1: Correction terms

$$C_x = (65)^2/15 = 281.67$$
$$C_y = (85)^2/15 = 481.67$$
$$C_{xy} = (65 \times 85)/15 = 281.67$$

Step 2: Total SS

$$X = 369.00 - 281.67 = 87.33$$
$$Y = 767.00 - 481.67 = 285.33$$
$$XY = 438.00 - 368.33 = 69.67$$

Step 3: Between Group Mean SS

$$\text{For } X = 20^2 + 30^2 + 15^2$$
$$= 281.67 = 23.33$$
$$Y = 25^2 + 50^2 + 10^2$$
$$= 481.67 = 163.33$$
$$XY = (20 \times 25) + (30 \times 50) + (15 \times 10)$$
$$= 368.33 = 61.67$$

Step 4: Within Groups SS

$$X = 87.33 - 23.33 = 64.00$$
$$Y = 285.33 - 163.33 = 122.00$$
$$XY = 69.67 - 61.70 = 8.00$$

Step 5: Analysis of Variance of X and Y scores taken separately.

Summary of ANOVA as given below:

Source of variation	df	SS_x	SS_y	MS_x	MS_y
Between Means	2	23.33	163.33	11.67	81.67
Within Groups	12	64.00	122.00	5.33	10.17
Total	14	87.33	285.33		

$F_x = 11.67/5.33 = 2.18$; $F_y = 81.67/10.17 = 8.03$.

From Table K, F values with *df* (2, 12); at 0.05 = 3.88 at 0.01 = 6.93.

F for Y is significant at 0.01 level. F for X is not significant which shows that there are no significant differences among the covariate, X, means. Hence the experimenter was successful in getting random samples in Groups I, II and III.

Step 6: Computation of Adjusted SS for Y, i.e. SS_{y-x}

$$\text{Total } SS_{y-x} = 285.33 - \frac{(69.67)^2}{87.33} = 229.75$$

$$\text{Within } SS_{y-x} = 122.00 - \frac{(8)^2}{64.00} = 121.00$$

$$\text{Between } SS_{y-x} = 229.75 - 121 = 108.75$$

$$MS_{y-x} = 54.38/11.00 = 4.94$$

(significant at 0.05 level but not at 0.01)

$$SD_{y-x} = \sqrt{V_{Y-X}} = \sqrt{11} = 3.32$$

Step 7: Correlation and Regression

$$T_{total} = \frac{69.67}{\sqrt{87 \times 285.33}} = 0.44$$

The summary of ANCOVA as shown below:

Summary of ANCOVA

Source of variation	df	SS_x	SS_y	SS_{xy}	SS_{y-x}	MS_{y-x} (V_{y-x})
Between Means	2	23.33	163.33	61.67	108.75	54.38
Within Groups	11	64.00	122.00	8.00	121.00	11.00
Total	13	87.00	285.33	69.67	229.75	

$$T_{\text{between means}} = \frac{61.67}{\sqrt{23.33 \times 163.33}} = 0.98$$

$$T_{\text{within groups}} = \frac{8.00}{\sqrt{64.00 \times 122.00}} = 0.09$$

$$b_{\text{within groups}} = \frac{8.00}{64.00} = 0.125$$

Step 8: Calculation of Adjusted Y Means

Adjusted Y Means are shown below:

Group	N	M_X	M_Y	M_{y-x} (Adjusted)
I	5	4	5	5.04
II	5	6	10	9.79
III	5	3	2	2.17
General Mean		4.33	5.67	

$$M_{y-x} = M(y-b)(M_x - GM_x) = M_y - b_x \quad ...(18.4)$$

(Y means adjusted for X variations)

b: denotes regression coefficient,

x: denotes deviation of M_x from GM_x other symbols are as before.

For Group I: $M_y - b_x = 5 - 0.125\ (4 - 4.33) = 5.04$

For Group II: $M_y - b_x = 10 - 0.125\ (6 - 4.33) = 9.79$

For Group III: $M_y - b_x = 2 - 0.125\ (3 - 4.33) = 2.17$

Step 9: Comparison of Adjusted Means

Post ANCOVA *t* test can be used for the purpose Adjusted MS_W for *y-x* is the estimate of the population variance available. Hence

$$SD_{Y-X} = \sqrt{11} = 3.23$$

$$SE_{MD} = \sigma_W \sqrt{\frac{1}{n_1} + \frac{1}{n_2}} \quad ...(18.5)$$

$$= \sigma_W \sqrt{\frac{1}{5} + \frac{1}{5}}$$

$$= 2.04$$

t values:

$$M_1 - M_2 = \frac{5.04 - 9.79}{2.04} = 2.33 \text{ Significant}$$

at 0.05.

$$M_1 - M_3 = \frac{5.04 - 2.17}{2.04} = 1.41 \text{ Significant}$$

$$M_2 - M_3 = \frac{9.04 - 2.17}{2.04} = 3.73 \text{ Significant}$$

at 0.01.

Notation and Description of Computational Steps

The actual computational steps with results have been presented above. However, for a better understanding, the same are described below and the relevant notation and formulas are presented to outline the procedure.

Step 1: Corrective Term (C)

There are now three sets of data in each group – Covariate X; Criterion Y; and Cross products XY. Keeping this fact in view, we need three correction terms:

$$\text{Correction for X, } C_X = \frac{(\Sigma X)^2}{N} \quad ...(18.6)$$

$$\text{Correction for Y, } C_Y = \frac{(\Sigma Y)^2}{N} \quad ...(18.7)$$

$$\text{Correction for products, } C_{XY} = \frac{\Sigma X \times \Sigma Y}{N} \quad ...(18.8)$$

Step 2: SS for Totals

We have three SS's for total: Sums of squared scores over all the groups are used:

For $X = \Sigma X^2 - C_X$ ...(18.9)

For $Y = \Sigma Y^2 - C_Y$ ...(18.10)

For $XY = \Sigma XY - C_{XY}$ ...(18.11)

SS_{XY} were obtained by multiplying pairs of X and Y scores, summing over the entire range and subtracting C_{XY}: thus $(6 + 8 + 3 \times 7 + \ldots + 2 \times 2)$. In the worksheet col. 3 of each group shows the cross products which were summed up over all the three groups.

Step 3: SS between Means

SS between means for X and for Y follow the method of ANOVA while SS between means for XY is the sum of the corresponding X and Y column totals divided by *n*, i.e., 5, and minus C_{XY}.

Thus SS between means for

$$XY = \frac{\sum^{k}(\Sigma X \times \Sigma Y)}{n} \quad \ldots(18.12)$$

in which *k* stands for number of groups, which is three in this case.

Step 4: SS within Groups

These SS's for X, Y and XY were found by subtracting between mean SS's from total SS's.

For X = Total SS for X – between means SS for X

For Y = Total SS for Y – between means SS for Y

For XY = Total SS for XY – between means SS for XY.

Step 5: Preliminary Analysis of Variance

A preliminary analysis of variance on X and Y scores separately was done and results presented in a summary table. The groups did not differ significantly on the covariate, X. However, there were significant differences among the Y means. This analysis is done to have a pre-adjustment view of the differences in the criterion means and also to see the differences in the covariate over the various groups.

Step 6: Adjusted SS for Y

This step is taken to remove from Y scores, any variability contributed by X scores. The adjusted SS_Y are symbolized as SS_{Y-X}. The generalized formula is

$$SS_{Y-X} = SS_Y - \frac{(SS_{XY})^2}{SS_X} \quad \ldots(18.13)$$

(Sum of squares of Y adjusted for X differences)

Thus, SS_{Y-X} total would be given by

$$\text{Total } SS_{Y-X} = \text{Total } SS_Y - \frac{\text{Total } SS^2{}_{XY}}{\text{Total } SS_X} \quad \ldots(18.14)$$

And

$$\text{Total } SS_{Y-X} = \text{Within } SS_Y - \frac{\text{Total } SS^2{}_{XY}}{\text{Total } SS_X} \quad \ldots(18.15)$$

Between means SS_{YX} cannot be readily calculated directly. Hence these are to be obtained by subtracting between mean SS_{YX} from total SS_{YX}. Thus,

Between Mean SS_{YX} = Total SS_{YX} – Within SS_{Y-X} ...(18.16)

The variance (MS_{YX}) was computed from the various adjusted sums of squares by dividing the latter by appropriate *df*. Owing to the adjustment of Y scores, and the additional restriction imposed by formula, 1 *df* was lost, thus giving a total *df* equal to 13 instead of 14; and *df* for 'within groups' equal to 11 instead of 12.

A comparison of the F_Y (pre-adjustment) and F_{Y-X} (Adjusted) would show that the former of F which was 8.03 and significant at 0.01 level has come down to 4.94 which is not significant at 0.01 level but only at 0.05 level. Hence, one can see the utility of using ANCOVA. The pre-adjustment Y mean differences have become less sharp after adjustment of the variability due to the covariate, X. This is evident from an inspection of the values of adjusted means. The smallness of changes is due to the fact that the correlation between criterion and covariate scores for total is 0.44 only and r for within groups is very small i.e., 0.09 (See step 8) .

Step 7: Correlation and Regression

This step is taken to obtain various correlations and regression coefficients for total, between means and within groups. This helps in a better understanding of the results of step 6 above. The general formula used is:

$$r = \frac{\Sigma xy}{\sqrt{\Sigma x^2} \cdot \sqrt{y^2}} \quad ...(18.17)$$

The regression coefficient, b, is given by

$$b = \frac{\Sigma xy}{\sqrt{\Sigma x^2}} \quad ...(18.18)$$

Σxy, Σx^2, Σy^2, denote sums of squares, respectively for cross products, x and y.

This may be applied to the appropriate SS's for total, between means and within groups.

The Within-groups correlation is a better measure of the relationship between the intelligence scores, X, and the achievement scores, Y, than the total correlation as the systematic differences have been removed from the within r. This correlation is very small, rather negligible and hence did not lead to much reduction between the Y means when variability due to X is kept constant. High correlation "between means" has reduced the numerator of the F_{X-Y} ratio, from SS_Y = 163.33 to SS_{Y-X} = 108.75 while the very low correlation within groups has almost not reduced the denominator of the variance ratio, F_{X-Y} as within groups sum of squares has come down only by one unit, i.e., from SS_Y = 122 to SS_{Y-X} = 121. When correlation among scores is high and correlation among means is low, non-significance of results of preliminary ANOVA is likely to change into significance on adjustment of SS. However, if the case is in reverse as in our example, the value of F in ANOVA is likely to come down in ANCOVA.

Regression coefficient, b_{within} was calculated as a nearly unbiased estimate of the regression of Y on X, since any systematic influence due to differences among means has been removed. Therefore, this coefficient was used in the calculation of adjusted Y means.

Step 8: Adjusted Means

After ANCOVA has been completed, criterion mean scores (Y means) can be adjusted directly for difference in the X means. The formula for the same is $M_{Y-X} = M(y - b)(M_X - GM_X)$, using regression coefficient b within which in our example is 0.125. For each group, the same formula is to be used. M_X stands for the mean of X scores of the corresponding group whose Y mean is being adjusted. GM_X is the general mean of X scores which remains the same for all groups. The adjusted mean as obtained in our example has not changed much because of the reasons explained in step 7 above.

Step 9: Comparison of Adjusted Y Means

As a post-ANCOVA step, significant pairs of adjusted Y means can be determined by using formula (18.11). For this purpose, within MS_{y-x} from the ANCOVA table is used as an estimate of the population variance and SD_{y-x} can be readily calculated by taking its square-root. The procedure has been explained in the computational step No. 9. The estimate of the population variance is readily available in the form of MS_{within} for adjusted Y scores from the ANCOVA table. Two pairs of means $M_1 - M_2$; and $M_2 - M_3$ turn out to be significant.

Assumptions Underlying ANCOVA

Analysis of covariance is based on some assumptions, warranted by the mathematical logic on which it is based. These assumptions include the usual four assumptions made for analysis of variance and two additional ones. These are:

1. Normality of distribution,
2. Homogeneity of variance,
3. Additivity of effects,
4. Mutual exclusiveness an independence of observations which may in other words be termed as random selection,
5. A linear relationship between X and Y,
6. Homogeneity of regression or similarity of the slope of the regression lines for each experimental group. For this purpose H_0: $\beta_1 = \beta_2 =$ - - - - - $= \beta_k$ is tested by using an F test. This F-ratio is based on the difference between sum of squares for pooled and separate regression lines and sum of squares for separate regression lines.

General Uses of ANCOVA

The basic model of analysis of covariance can be further extended to include a double classification in which an experiment is duplicated in randomly selected situations. For example, the experiment can be repeated in a number of randomly selected schools. The procedure in this case will be much the same as before. The principal difference, however, will be that the error estimate will be based on the interaction (Method × School) variance, rather than on the "within groups" variance of the adjusted scores. The 'adjustment' of the criterion scores will accordingly be based on a regression coefficient derived from the sum of squares of Method × School interaction rather than for "Within groups".

If it is desired to eliminate the effect of more than one uncontrolled variables in the experiments of the type described in this chapter, it may be done by an extension of the methods described in the preceding pages. The use of multiple regression equation will be required for adjustment of criterion means by eliminating the influence of the uncontrolled variables. As the number of covariates increases, the computational labor will be tremendous. However, the advantage gained depends upon the magnitude of the multiple correlation coefficient. Hence, it is advisable to select the best combination of variables. Some of the uses of ANCOVA were pointed out in the section on introduction. Some other uses of ANCOVA are given below:

1. It leads to increase in the precision of randomized designs or experiments. It is very useful in situations where a chance assignment of a particular treatment to group already better than other groups has taken place.
2. It allows for the adjustment of sources of bias in observational studies. For example, the differential effects of covariates of age and weight can be eliminated from the dependent variable of time taken in covering a distance.
3. It allows for probing into the nature of treatment effects after significant main effects have been obtained.
4. It permits, as a by-product, the study of regression in multiple classification.

To conclude, analysis of covariance is a powerful technique for removing bias, effects of disturbing variables and environment sources of variations. However, this holds good when the assumptions of ANCOVA are met and a good combination of variables achieved and the interaction between the treatment and covariate is absent. ANCOVA, in no way, be taken as an answer or a substitute for ability to randomize and provide an experimental control. Stratified random sampling is preferable to ensure pre-experimental equivalence of groups and thus to eliminate the need of using ANCOVA.

EXERCISES

1. Three intact groups were taken and randomly assigned to three treatments. Pretest and posttest measures were obtained as follows:

Treatment A		*Treatment B*		*Treatment C*	
Pre-test X	*Post-test* Y	*Pre-test* X	*Post-test* Y	*Pre-test* X	*Post-test* Y
10	15	16	15	15	22
12	19	18	18	15	21
16	20	17	16	14	20
11	18	15	14	13	18
11	18	14	17	13	19
60	90	80	80	70	100
12	18	16	16	14	20

   a. Do analysis of variance and then analysis of covariance. Compare the results.
   b. Explain the possible reasons for the differences in results.
2. On what single factor does the gain, in precision, in ANCOVA depends?
3. If the covariate mean is greater than the X grand mean in one group, what would be the effect on the adjusted Y means for that group?
4. Why would a randomized-block-analysis be more robust than an ANCOVA?
5. State and explain the assumptions underlying ANCOVA.
6. Give some uses of ANCOVA in educational and psychological research.

CHAPTER

19 Reliability and Validity of Test Scores

Reliability

The term "reliability" as used in everyday language conveys a meaning which is somewhat parallel to the meaning ascribed to it by the measurement expert. Suppose we say that a worker was reliable. What does this convey? It might be supposed that the worker reports at the same time everyday, appears in the same condition and performs consistently. This similarity of behavior from time to time would be comparable to one of the tester's approaches to reliability. "Trustworthiness" is another word used by the common man to signify the term reliability of human beings. Reliability pertains to a class of test characteristics. These are stability, equivalence and internal consistency. These are time-associated and form-associated bases of reliability. Reliability is not concerned with the appropriateness of measurements, an issue that falls within the scope of the meanings of another test characteristic called validity. The main concern of reliability is an accurate repeatability of scores overtime and parallel forms of a test. Reliability of physical measurements using steel tape, etc. is high as the instruments give consistent results with high accuracy. However, psychological tests and instruments are less reliable as many measurement errors are bound to creep in. The *coefficient of reliability* of a test forms the basic index of reliability reported in the literature. It is based on self-correlation of a test.

Reliable people are people whose behavior can be relied onto be consistent and predictable. Reliability of a research instrument likewise is defined as the extent to which the instrument yields the same results on repeated measures. Reliability is then concerned with consistency, accuracy, precision, stability, equivalence and homogeneity. Concurrent with the questions of validity or after they are answered, the researcher and the critiquer of research ask the question of how reliable is the instrument. A reliable measure is one that can produce the same results if the behavior is measured again by the same scale. Reliability then refers to the proportion of accuracy to inaccuracy in measurement. In other words, if we use the same or comparable instruments on more than one occasion to measure a set of behaviors that ordinarily remain relatively constant, we would expect similar results if the tools are reliable. The three main attributes of a reliable scale are *stability*, *homogeneity*, and *equivalence*. The stability of an instrument refers to the instrument's ability to produce the same results with repeated testing. The homogeneity of an instrument means that all the items in a tool measure the same concept or characteristic. An instrument is said to exhibit equivalence if the tool produces the same results when equivalent or parallel instrument or procedures are used. Each of these attributes and the means to estimate them will be discussed. Before these are discussed, an understanding of how to interpret reliability is essential.

Methods of Estimating Reliability

There are basically four different procedures generally used for computing reliability:

1. Test-retest method (Repetition of the same test or measure overtime)
2. Alternate or parallel forms method (Administration of a second 'equivalent' form of the test)
3. Split-half technique (Subdivision of the test into two or more equivalent fractions)
4. Rational equivalence method
5. Measures used to test reliability include:
   - Stability: Test-retest reliability
     Parallel or alternate form
   - Homogeneity: Item-total correlation
     Split-half reliability
     Kuder-Richardson coefficient
     Cronbach's alpha
   - Equivalence: Parallel or alternate form
     Inter-rater reliability

All these methods furnish estimates of the reproductivity of test scores and one method may be preferred to another according to the demands of the structure. These methods are described below:

Test-Retest Method

This method involves (i) repetition of a test on the same group immediately or after a lapse of time, and (ii) computation of correlations between the first and second set of scores. The correlation coefficient thus obtained indicates the extent or magnitude of the agreement between the two sets of scores is often called the *coefficient of stability.* Although test retest is sometimes the only available method, this procedure is open to several serious objections. Immediate repetition of a test may involve (i) immediate memory effects, (ii) practice effects and (iii) confidence effects induced by familiarity of contents. Intervals of six months or longer in young children may show "growth effects". The factors of intervening learning and under learning may lead to lowering of self correlations. It may not be possible to control conditions on the second testing.

Memory, practice and other carry overeffects may be offset by increasing the time interval between the two testings.

Test-retest reliability is the administration of the same instrument to the same subjects under similar conditions on two or more occasions. Scores on the repeated testing are compared. This comparison is expressed by a correlation coefficient, usually a Pearson r. The interval between repeated administrations varies and depends on the phenomenon being measured. For example, if the variable that the test measures is related to the developmental stages in children, the interval between tests should be short. The amount of time over which the variable was measured should also be recorded in the report. An example of an instrument that was tested for test-retest reliability is the Work Impediment Scale (WAS) (Gulick, 1991), which was designed to rare situations that impede or enhance work capabilities of persons with multiple sclerosis (MS). Test-retest correlation coefficients for WAS subscales (mobility, hand function, congnitive, general body state, pain, environmental barrier, heavy labor) obtained at 1 and 3 weeks for 51 MS subjects were 0.91, 0.88, 0.83, 0.76, 0.88, 0.77, and 0.81 respectively. The magnitude of these correlations supports the idea that the WAS has the attribute of stability.

Alternate or Parallel Form Method

This method involves the administration of two equivalent or parallel forms of the test instead of repetition of a single test. This avoids, to a great extent, the disadvantages of the test-retest method involving short or long intervals of time. The two equivalent forms are so constructed as to make them similar (but not identical) in content, mental processes involved, number of items and the difficulty levels of the items. The subjects take one form of the test and then, as soon as possible, the other form. The correlation coefficient between the two sets of scores determines the agreement and is generally called as *coefficient of equivalence.* Alternate forms should be drawn very carefully by matching test material for content, difficulty and form. An interval of at least two to four weeks should be allowed between the two administrators of the test, to offset the carryover due to familiarity of content. The method has some other limitations also. The second form of a test may not be available. A second testing may place heavier demands on the time and resources of the researcher and the subjects. The psychometricians have devised another technique called the split-half method which takes care of some of these defects.

Parallel or alternate form reliability is applicable and can be tested only if two comparable forms of the same instrument exist. It is like test-retest reliability in that the same individuals are tested within a specific interval, but it differs because a different form of the same test is given to the subjects on the second testing. Parallel forms or tests contain the same types of items that are based on the same domain or concept, but the wording of the items is different. The development of parallel forms is desired if the instrument is intended to measure a variable for which a researcher believes that "test-wiseness" will be a problem. For example, there are two alternate forms of the Partner Relationship Inventory (Hoskins, 1988) that may be used in a repeated-measures design. An item on one scale ("I am able to tell my partner how I feel") is consistent with the paired item on the second form ("My partner tries to understand my feelings").

Another example of a parallel test is the Multidimensional Health Locus of Control Scale (Wallston, Wallston and DeVellis, 1978), which was designed to measure three dimensions or sources of reinforcement for health-related behaviors. This scale has parallel forms for studies that incorporate a repeated-measures design. Examples of parallel items are "If I get sick, it is my own behavior that determines how soon I get well". This term compares with "If I get sick, I have the power to make myself well again". As can be seen, the two items, although worded differently, reflect the same idea. Practically speaking, it is difficult to develop alternate forms of an instrument when one considers the many issues of reliability and validity of an instrument. If alternate forms of a test exist, they should be highly correlated if the measures are to be considered reliable.

The Split-half Method

The most widely used procedure for estimating reliability from a single testing divides a particular test into two presumably equivalent halves. The test is divided into two halves only for the purpose of scoring and not for administration. It means that a single test is given at a single sitting and with a single time limit. However, two separate scores are derived – one by scoring one-half and the other, by scoring the other half. The correlation between these two sets of scores provides the accuracy with which the test is measuring the individual. A sensible procedure generally used for splitting the test into two halves is the odd-even split technique. The odd numbered items, 1, 3, 5, 7, etc; and the even numbered items, 2, 4, 6, 8, etc. form two different sets of items for scoring. This procedure is better than others like first half and the second-half and splits into blocks of 5 or 10 items, etc. and ensures balancing out of factors of item form, content covered, and difficulty level in tests having 60 or more items.

Split-half reliability involves dividing a scale into two halves and making a comparison. The halves may be odd-numbered and even-numbered items or a simple division of the first from the second half, or items may be randomly selected as to the halves that will be analyzed opposite one another. The split-half provides a measure of consistency in terms of sampling the content. The two halves of the test or the contents in both halves are assumed to be comparable, and a reliability coefficient is calculated. If the scores for the two halves are approximately equal, the test may be considered reliable. A formula called the Spearman-Brown formula is one method used to calculate the reliability coefficient. In a study investigating the appraisal of pain and coping in cancer patients, Arathuzik (1991) obtained a split-half reliability rating of 0.85 from a pilot test of the Pain Experience Inventory with 30 patients with metastatic breast cancer who were experiencing pain.

The computed correlation, in this technique, is between two half-length test. This value is not directly applicable to the full length test which is the actual instrument prepared for use. Hence, Spearman Brown Prophecy formula is used to estimate the reliability of the full length test from the self-correlation of the half-tests.

$$r_{11} = \frac{2r_{1/2-1/2}}{1 + r_{1/2-1/2}} \quad ...(19.1)$$

(Spearman Brown Prophecy formula for estimating reliability from two comparable halves of a test.

Where, r_{11} = reliability coefficients for the full length test

$r_{1/2-1/2}$ = reliability coefficients for the half-test found experimentally.

For example, if correlation between the two halves of a test is 0.60, the reliability of the full test will be

$$r_{11} = \frac{2(0.60)}{1+0.60} = \frac{1.20}{1.60} = 0.75$$

This split-half method is regarded to be the best by many psychometricians. The main argument in favor of this method is the single shot approach, leading to no place for errors due to repetition and lapse of time. Convenience and saving of time and expense are some other important considerations. However, this method suffers from some *limitations.*

- It is not useful for speeded tests
- Splitting of the test can be done in several ways, thus leading to the noncomparability of reliability indices from these
- It is not so useful for tests having a small number of items, i.e. less than twenty
- Chance errors may affect scores on two halves equally and thus lead to higher correlations.

Kuder-Richardson (KR-20) Coefficient

The Kuder-Richardson (KR-20) coefficient is the estimate of homogeneity used for instruments that have a dichotomous response format. A dichotomous response format is one in which the question asks for a yes/no or a true/false response. The technique yields a correlation that is based on the consistency of responses to all the items of a single form of a test that is administered one time. Strauss and Sawin (1990) developed the Krantz Health Opinion Survey (KHOS), which is designed to measure one's preferences for information and control over one's health care. Because the response format for the KHOS and the Information and Behavior Control subscales in binary (yes/no), the KR-20 was used to determine the internal consistency of the items. Kuder-Richardson 20 reliability coefficient for KHOS subscales ranged from 0.68 to 0.70, indicating a moderate level of internal consistency reliability.

Cronbach's Alpha

The fourth and most commonly used test of internal consistency is Cronbach's alpha. Many tools used to measure psychosocial variables and attitudes have a Likert scale response format. A Likert scale format asks the subject to respond to a question on a scale of varying degrees of intensity between two extremes. The two extremes are anchored by responses such as "strongly agree" to "strongly disagree" or "more like me" to "least like me". The points between the two extremes may range from 1 to 5 or 1 to 7. Subjects are asked to circle the response closest to how they feel. Following items provide examples of items from a tool that uses a Likert scale format. Cronbach's alpha compares each item in the scale simultaneously with each other.

	Definitely yes	*Yes*	*Uncertain*	*No*	*Definitely no*
I am uncertain about being pregnant	5	4	3	2	1
The baby seems to know when I feel tense or anxious	5	4	3	2	1

"Rational Equivalence" Method

The three methods described above suffer from some limitations. The method of rational equivalence is an approach to avoid some of these objections. This method is based upon intercorrelations of the items in the test and the correlations of the items with the test as a whole. Several formulas for calculating reliability by this method have been suggested. However, the formula, given below, is the most popular.

$$r_{11} = \frac{n}{(n-1)} \times \frac{\sigma_1^2 - \Sigma pq}{\sigma_1^2} \quad ...(19.2)$$

(Kuder-Richardson formula based on difficulty and intercorrelations of test items).

In which,

r_{11} = reliability coefficient of the whole test

n = number of items in the test

σ_t = SD of the test scores

p = the proportion of the group answering a test item correctly

$q = (1 - p)$ = the proportion of the group answering a test item incorrectly

Another formula which is a simple approximation to the above formula is as follows:

$$r_{11} = \frac{n\sigma_t^2 - \mathrm{M}(n - \mathrm{M})}{\sigma_t^2(n-1)} \quad ...(19.3)$$

(Approximation to formula 19.2)

where, r_{11} = reliability of the whole test

n = number of items in the test

σ_t = SD of the test scores

m = Mean of the test scores

Formula (19.3) saves labor as it is based on the mean, SD and number of items. Correlation coefficient between two halves is not required.

These formulas are based on the assumption of equal difficulty of items which may not be generally met in power tests. The formulas provide a minimum estimate of reliability thus giving an underestimation.

Equivalence is either the consistency or agreement among observers using the same measurement tool or the consistency or agreement among alternate forms of a tool. An instrument is thought to demonstrate equivalence when two or more observers have a high percentage of agreement of an observed behavior or when alternate forms of a test yield a high correlation. There are two methods to test equivalence: *inter-rater reliability* and *alternate or parallel form*.

Inter-rater Reliability

Some measurement instruments are not self-administered questionnaires but are direct measurements of observed behavior. Instruments that depend on direct observation of behavior that is to be systematically recorded need to be tested for inter-rater reliability. To accomplish inter-rater reliability, two or more individuals should make an observation or one observer observes the behavior on several occasions. The observers should be trained or oriented to the definition of the behavior to be observed. In the method of direct observation of behavior, the consistency or reliability of the observations between observers is extremely important. In the instance of inter-rater reliability, the reliability of consistency of the observer is tested rather than the reliability of the instrument. Inter-rater reliability is expressed as a percentage of agreement between scores or as a correlation coefficient between the scores assigned to the observed behaviors.

An example of inter-rater reliability is given in the study conducted by Stewart Fahs and Kinney (1991), who studied the differential effect of three injection sites for low-dose heparin therapy in relation to thromboplastin time and bruising. The bruises measured in this study were soft tissue injuries resulting from the trauma of subcutaneous injections of heparin. Over a 4-month period, 105 injection sites were used to calculate inter-rater reliability with respect to occurence and size of bruises. Ratings were done by the principal investigator and three research assistants. The Pearson correlation coefficient ranged from $r = 0.94$ to 0.99, indicating a high degree of inter-rater reliability.

Parallel or alternate form was described under the heading *Stability*. Use of parallel forms is then a measure of stability and equivalence. The procedure for assessing equivalence using parallel forms are the same.

Factors Affecting Reliability

Length of Test

Other things being equal, the reliability of a test is a function of its length. Longer tests tend to be more reliable than shorter tests. Logically, the more samples we take of a given area of knowledge, skill, behavior and the like, the more reliable will be our appraisal of that area. Lengthening the test means adding more items or having several applications of the test or use of parallel forms. The Spearman Brown Prophecy Formula for calculating the reliability of a test with increased length is

$$r_{nn} = \frac{nr_{11}}{1+(n-1)r_{11}} \quad ...(19.4)$$

in which, r_{nn} = the correlation between n forms of a test and n alternate forms

r_{11} = the reliability coefficient of Test 1.

Example: Suppose for a test of 50 items, the reliability coefficient is 0.80. What would be the reliability of a test if its length is doubled to 100 items; tripled to 150 items; and quadrupled to 200 items?

The calculations are as below:

First Situation (Doubling the Length)

$$r_{22} = \frac{2\times 0.80}{1+(2-1)\times 0.80} = 0.889$$

Second Situation (Triplicating the Length)

$$r_{33} = \frac{3\times 0.80}{1+(3-1)\times 0.80} = 0.923$$

Third Situation (Quadruplicating the Length)

$$r_{44} = \frac{4\times 0.80}{1+(4-1)\times 0.80} = 0.941$$

Spearman-Brown formula shows that after we have reached a high degree of reliability, additional items do not improve the reliability enough to justify the extra time and effort required for building items for testing pupils. The increase in the values calculated above are not appreciable above the doubling of the test.

Range of Talent

The range of talent, achievement or ability of the pupils on whom the reliability is based has a direct effect on the reliability coefficients. The greater the variability in the group, the higher the reliability coefficient.

Testing Conditions

The conditions in which the test is administered and scored may affect reliability in either side. Other such factors are: mental set of pupils, level of their motivation, speed of work, emotional stability, distractions and accidents, and cheating by pupils.

Stability

An instrument is thought to be stable or to exhibit stability when the same results are obtained on repeated administration of the instrument. Researchers are concerned with the stability of an instrument when they want the instrument to be able to measure the concept consistently over a period of time. Measurement over time is important when an instrument is used in a longitudinal study and therefore will be used on several occasions. Stability is also a consideration when the researcher is conducting an intervention study that is designed to effect an alteration in a specific variable. In this case the instrument is administered once and again later after the alteration or change intervention has been completed. The tests that are used to estimate stability are *test-retest* and *parallel or alternate form*.

Homogeneity

Another attribute of an instrument related to reliability is the internal consistency or homogeneity with which the items within the scale reflect or measure the same concept. This means that the items within the scale correlate or are complementary to each other. This also means that a scale is unidimensional. A unidimensional scale is one that measures one concept. For example, a scale that is designed to measure anxiety should not be designed to measure depression as well. There are scales, such as the Interpersonal Relationship Inventory (Tilden et al, 1990), that do contain two or more concepts or dimensions within them. If that is the case, the researcher should identify this for the reader and should also have tested separately each concept within the scale. The internal consistency of items allows the investigator to tally the items and obtain a total score for the concept. The total score is then used in the analysis of data. Homogeneity can be assessed by using one of four methods: *item-total correlations, split-half reliability, Kuder-Richardson (KR-20) coefficient, or Cronbach's alpha.*

Item to Total Correlations

Item to total correlations measure the relationship between each of the items and the total scale. When item to total correlations are calculated, a correlation for each item on the scale is generated (Table 19.1). Items that do not achieve a high correlation may be deleted from the instrument. Usually in a research study, not all the items to total correlations are reported unless the study is a report of a methodological study. Typically the lowest and highest correlations are reported. An example of an item to total correlation report is "item-total correlations ... were computed for the 15 item HRHS. A minimum total criterion item-total correlation level of 0.25 was set for inclusion in the scale. Ten items failed to meet the criterion level and were dropped. Of the remaining 41, all but 5 items had item-total correlations above 0.30. An examination of the correlation matrix showed no redundant items. Correlations ranged from ± 0.01 to 0.51" (Pollack and Duffy, 1990).

Table 19.1

Examples of item to total correlations from computer-generated data

Item	*Item to total correlation*
1	0.5096
2	0.4455
3	0.4479
4	0.4369
5	0.4139
6	0.4016

The investigators eliminate items that have too low a correlation, whereas they examine others to ensure that they are high enough to be measuring the same concept without being redundant. If item to total correlations are found to be too high, they are considered to be redundant and therefore not complementary to each other (Anastasi, 1988). This is unlike the other errors of reliability in which a higher correlation is generally a better correlation.

Reliability Coefficient Interpretation

Because all the attributes of reliability are concerned with the degree of consistency between scores that are obtained at two or more independent times of testing, they often are expressed in terms of a correlation coefficient. The reliability coefficient ranges from 0 to 1. The reliability coefficient expresses the relationship between the error variance, true variance, and the observed score. A zero correlation indicates that there is no relationship. When the error variance in a measurement instrument is low, the reliability coefficient will be closer to 1. The closer to 1 the coefficient is, the more reliable the tool. For example, a reliability coefficient of a tool is reported to be 0.89. This tells the reader that the error variance is small and the tool has little measurement error. On the other hand, if the reliability coefficient of a measure is reported to be 0.49, the error variance is high and the tool has a problem with measurement error. For a tool to be considered reliable, a level of 0.70 or higher is considered to be an acceptable level of reliability. The interpretation of the reliability coefficient depends on the proposed purpose of the measure.

There are five major tests of reliability that can be used to calculate a reliability coefficient. The test(s) used depends on the nature of the tool. They are known as test-retest, parallel or alternate form, item-total correlation, split-half, Kuder-Richardson (KR-20), Cronbach's alpha, and inter-rater reliability. These tests are discussed as they relate to the attributes of stability, equivalence, and homogeneity. There is no best means to assess reliability in relationship to stability, homogeneity, and equivalence. The critiquer of research should be aware that the method of reliability that the researcher uses should be consistent with the investigator's aim.

Validity in Experimentation

An experiment is conducted with two aims: (i) to draw valid inferences about the effects of treatments (independent variable) on the subjects under investigation, and (ii) to generalize our results to a larger population of interest. The first aim concerns **internal validity** whereas the second to ***external validity***. Now both the validities will be discussed in brief.

Internal Validity

It is mainly concerned with drawing the correct conclusion that whatever variation is observed in the dependent variable is really due to the effect of the treatment(s). Thus, internal validity checks whether the observed effect on the subjects or test group could have occurred due to some extraneous factors. If the observed effects are confounded with the extraneous variable(s), then it would not be reasonable. Hence, internal validity is a must for correct and valid inferences. To ensure internal validity, extraneous factors should be controlled.

There are many threats to internal validity. We discuss here some of them.

1. **History:** In many experimental designs, measurement (O_1) about the criterion variable is taken on the test units prior to the manipulation *x*. When the manipulation is over, an after measurement (O_2) on the same criterion variable is taken. The difference ($O_2 - O_1$) measures the effect of X. But there is a possibility that in the mean time between O_1 and O_2, many events might have occurred which could have influenced O_2 besides X. Such events are known as ***history***. For instance, the management of a company wants to convince his workers about a new bonus scheme. Managers give a test to all its employees to know their existing opinion (O_1) about the bonus scheme. Again at the end of a campaign, a test is conducted to known their present opinion (O_2) about the bonus scheme. Diagrammatically the experiment can be depicted as follows:

Pretest	Treatment	Post-test
O_1	X	O_2

   Such experiments are called *one-group Pretest–Post-test design experiment*. But between O_1 and O_2, many events could have occurred like some union leaders might have conveyed their views, some articles would have appeared in withdraw from the test group as they do not like the changes in their compensation. So the comparison of the test group with the control group would be distorted. As a remedy, random assignment of group may reduce the treatment to internal validity to a great extent.

2. **Limitation of treatment:** In many studies, the independent variable entails varied information as treatment levels that is passed on selectively to the subjects. In case, the subjects under various information levels communicate with each other, then the differences in responses under various treatment levels get compromised. To overcome this problem, the researcher should not allow the subjects to meet and discuss with one another about the topics under study.

3. **Resentful Demoralization:** If the subjects come to know that the treatment levels assigned to them are inferior in terms of benefits, goods or services, they may feel demoralized and hence, show their resentment. They are very likely to perform very low. This will create larger difference than the real one between desirable and undesirable treatment levels. Confidentiality of treatment levels be maintained to reduce this type of threat.

External Validity

External validity is concerned with the generalization of research findings to and across the population from which we select the subjects or settings. In other words, external validity means to ensure whether the cause and effect relationship established in the experiment can be generalized to other similar populations beyond the subjects involved in the experiment. In applying the results of an experiment to populations in general, there are many threats to external validity. Some of the important ones are enucleated below.

1. **Interaction of testing and treatment (X):** It refers to sensitizing the subjects to a topic via a pretest as it may focus attention on the topic. So this may very likely either enhance the effectiveness of X or reduce the effectivity of X. Hence, pretesting be done on the subjects of the population other than the selected subjects.
2. **Interaction of selection and X:** The process by which the test subjects are selected for an experiment may not be a representative of the population to which the researcher wishes to generalize the research findings. For instance, the opinion of a buyer about a product in the mall cannot be generalized to the public.
3. **Reactive factors:**
   i. If the subjects know, that they are being observed, they will act and respond differently than those who are not being observed. So, the results cannot be generalized.
   ii. There are situations in which the experimental settings are such that they may have biasing effect. For example, a group of workers receiving incentive pay are kept away from the control group to avoid any likely menace. The new environment will create a strong reactive condition and the results cannot be generalized "newspapers". Such intervening events are called *history* and have an influence on O_2. So the difference $(O_2 - O_1)$ cannot be taken exclusively due to campaign because the campaign effect might have been confounded with history. For valid conclusion history must be controlled lesser the gap between O_2 and O_1, better is the check on history.
4. **Maturation:** It concerns to the changes occurring within subjects or test units themselves with the passage of time. These changes are not due to the effect of the treatment at all. For instance, a subject may get bored, tired, uninterested, more experienced. Maturation is more vulnerable when the study continues for a long time, such as tracking and market studies span overmonths. Maturation effect can also happen in cases other than persons. For example, malls may also change in respect of decoration, prices, counters, etc. Possibility of maturation can be minimized by conducting interviews at the convenience of the respondents and completing the studies in short periods.
5. **Testing effects:** The effects which are caused due to taking a measure on the dependent variable before and after the application of the treatment on the test units are called testing effects. These are further classified into two types of effects, (i) main

testing effect (MT), (ii) interactive testing effect (IT).

The effect that occurs when a prior observation (O_1) affects a latter observation (O_2) is known as *main testing effect*.

An effect in which a prior measurement (O_1) has an influence on the independent variable and hence, affecting the test unit response is called *interactive testing* effects.

6. **Instrumentation (I):** Any changes made in the calibration of measuring instrument during interviews cause threats to internal validity.
7. **Selection bias (Sr):** The differential selection of subjects to experimental and control groups is a major threat to the internal validity. Selection bias is almost eliminated, if the subjects are assigned to control and experimental groups randomaly or matching the members of both the groups on key factors.
8. **Statistical regression (SR):** This refers to the threat where the measurements of the dependent variable have a tendency that the extreme scores regress towards mean scores. To elucidate further, if we select 25 percent workers (ω_1) of a factory which have minimum output (scores) and 25 percent workers (ω_2) with maximum output (scores) and then they are exposed to certain treatment. It is observed that the scores of ω_1 tend to increase and that of ω_2 tend to decline towards the average output (scores). Such a tendency is termed as *statistical regression* and is inversely related to the validity of the test.
9. **Experimental mortality:** This term does not refer to only death of the experimental unit(s) but also pertains to the changes in composition of the study group(s) during experimentation. Such changes often occur due to death of subjects or some subjects refuse to continue in the experiment. This alters the distribution of the subjects and one cannot ensure that the units lost would have responded to the treatments in the same manner as the remaining ones. Suppose various compensation schemes have been tried on workers. External validity can be secured by selecting the subjects from a population to which the research findings are to be generalized and also controlling reactive factors as far as possible.

Conclusion Validity

It refers to the threats to draw valid inferences that can be made from random error and adopting inadequate statistical procedures. Well known threats for conclusion validity are as follows:

1. **Low statistical power:** If the power of a test is low, then a research will very likely fail to reject a false null hypothesis. This may hapen due to inadequate test.
2. **Violation of assumptions:** All tests are based on certain assumptions. If such assumptions are violated, then there is every likelihood that incorrect inferences will be drawn.
3. **Reliability of measures:** If the reliability of measure on dependent variable is low, it results into increase of error variance, a false null hypothesis will not be rejected. In this way one would be drawing wrong conclusion.
4. **Random irrelevancies:** If the conditions, in which the treatment levels are administered, change during experimentation, then error variance may inflate. This may result into nonrejection of false null hypothesis. This is obviously a threat to conclusion validity.
5. **Respondents random heterogeneity:** Idiosyncratic variation of the respondents may inflate the error variance which may lead to acceptance of a false full hypothesis. So idiosyncrasy is threat to conclusion validity. Above mentioned threats to conclusion validity can be minimized by strictly observing the rules and requirements of a good design.

Types of Validity

Validity of a test or evaluation device can be defined as the degree to which the test measures what it is intended to measure. A test which is meant to measure achievement in mathematics should not measure achievement in history or any other subject. In physical sciences, validity of measuring instruments like scales, thermometers, chronoscopes and ammeters is found by comparing their measurements with standard measures. The validity of a psychological test is also found by comparison with standard (and sometimes arbitrary) measure. However, the validity of a physical instrument can be estimated accurately while it can never be done in the case of a mental test.

Validity is a relative term and has reference to a particular purpose or situation. The question "Is the test valid"? can be answered only by replying to the question "Valid, for what"? Hence, there are different types of validity meant for different purposes.

Content Validity

Content validity is evaluated by showing how well the content of the test samples the class of situations or subject matter about which conclusions are to be drawn. It is based on a comparison of the analysis of test content with the analysis of the course content and the instructional objectives. It is seen as to how well the former represents the latter. The analysis is done essentially through logical, rational, and judgmental process. That is why, sometimes the content validity may be referred to as *rational or logical validity*. Content validity is important primarily for measures of achievement. The test maker first determines the widely accepted goals of instruction in the subject and then prepare a blueprint for the test. Test content is drawn from the course content and weighted according to the weightage of the objectives of the course and the course content. An appraisal of the content validity of a test involves a careful and detailed examination of the actual test tasks.

Face Validity

Face validity has something to do with the mere appearance of a test. A test is said to have face validity when by appearance it "looks like" measuring what it is meant to measure. The appearance of reasonableness is spoken of as "appears to" correspond to that of the course. A test of Mathematics should have numerical questions; and a test of History, questions about kings, movements, wars, etc. The relevance of the test items to specific situations, age groups, language groups, etc. is also a matter of concern. However, no single numerical index of the face validity of a test can be calculated.

Concurrent Validity

Concurrent validity is evaluated by showing how well the test scores correspond to already accepted measure of performance or status made at the same time. For example, scores on a test of knowledge of basic concepts in Geography can be validated against the teachers ratings of the students on this aspect. Intelligence tests were first validated against school grades, teacher's ratings, etc. A newly constructed test of intelligence may be validated by finding its correlation with another already existing well-accepted test in this area. In these cases, a correlation coefficient between the two sets of measures is calculated as an index of validity. The main problem is to set up a criterion which is independent and reliable.

Criterion Related Validity

In a discussion of concurrent validity as given above, the test is validated against a criterion at the same point of time. However, we may be interested in using a test to predict some future outcome. A test of aptitude for teaching may be used to admit students to teachers training college and be expected to predict success at the job as teachers. A scholastic aptitude test may be used to predict how likely will the high school students be successful at a college. A clerical aptitude test may be used to predict success on the job as clerks. We are thus interested in success or performance in the future. This process is also called *Predictive Validity.* A correlation coefficient between the test scores and the criterion scores is calculated. The higher the correlation, the better the test as a predictor. However, the problem of selecting "an appropriate criterion" is very ticklish. The main problem arises when the criteria of success on the job is to be determined; the records are not available, time interval between completion of training and placement, working on the job for a period long enough to allow proper evaluation of success and the like. The success or failure of a worker may depend on conditions external to his own personality and skill. Ratings of success by superiors may be influenced by many factors other than the proficiency of the worker being rated. However, the following qualities are desired in a criterion measure:

- Relevance
- Freedom from bias (providing equal opportunity to all to perform well)
- Reliability, and
- Availability.

Construct Validity

Sometimes questions like the following are asked, "What does this test mean or signify?" "What does the score tell us about the individual?" "Does it correspond to some meaningful trait or construct that will help us in understanding him?" These questions are related with the construct validity of the test. The term "construct" is used in psychology to refer to something that is not observable, but is literally "constructed" by the investigator to summarize or account for the regularities or relationships that he observes in behavior. Thus, most names of traits refer to constructs. Intelligence, sociability, extroversion, aggressiveness, need-achievement and verbal reasoning are some examples of constructs. Tests of these functions are valid in so far as they behave. A "theory" about a trait will lead to predictions of three types.

- A theory may make predictions about correlations with other accepted measures of the function in question.
- It may make predictions about differences in the groups which are supposed to or known to possess the trait in high degrees and those in low or nonexistent degrees, just as delinquent and nondelinquents, intellectually superior and intellectually inferior groups.
- A theory may predict modifications of a human characteristic as a result of certain experimental conditions or treatments.

For any test that presumes to measure a trait or quality, we can formulate a network of theory leading to definite predictions as explained above. In so far as they are borne out, the validity of the test as a measure of the trait or construct is supported. In so far as the predictions fail to be verified, we are led to doubt the validity of our test or our theorizing, or both. Evidence of construct validity is partly rational and partly empirical judgment and evidence join together in the validation enterprise.

Factorial Validity

Factorial validity is, in a way, extension of the construct validity discussed above. The intercorrelations of a large number of tests are examined and if possible accounted for in terms of a much smaller number of more general "factors" or trait categories. Sometimes 3 to 4 factors may account for the intercorrelations among 15 to 20 tests. The factorial validity of a test is defined by its correlation with a factor, called factor loadings. A word comprehension test may correlate. Eighty two with the verbal factor extracted from a test battery. This coefficient will then be the tests for factorial validity.

Factors Affecting validity

The following are some of the factors which affect test validity. The test users should recognize factors that tend to make their test invalid.

i. *Cultural factors* such as socioeconomic status, social class structure, differential sex roles affect performance on various tests.
ii. *Response sets* or test-taking habits of the examines may differentially affect the validity estimates.
iii. *An increase in the number of test items* may boost up reliability but may bring down the validity.

iv. *Difficult and ambiguous directions* to the pupils may render the test a measure of something different than the test author intended.

Relation between Reliability and Validity

Reliability and validity are the two important aspects of the same quality of a test, called test efficiency. Reliability is concerned with the stability of the test score and does not go beyond the test. Validity, on the other hand, implies evaluations in terms of outside—and independent-criterion. A test, to be reliable, need not be practically valid while a test to be valid must be reliable. A clock which gains twenty minutes in a day is a perfectly reliable instrument as it will repeat the same gain every day. However, judged against a standard time piece, the clock is not valid.

Item Analysis

Item analysis of a test comes after the preliminary draft of a test has been constructed, administered on a group of students and scored. A tabulation is done to determine the following two important characteristics of each item.

i. Level of difficulty or item difficulty, and
ii. Discriminating power of the test items or item discrimination.

The above two indices help in item selection for the final draft of the test. Another step which precedes the calculation of item difficulty and item discrimination of a test is *item selection* based upon the judgment of component persons as to the suitability of the item for the purpose of the test. This is, in brief, a step towards establishing the 'content validity' and face validity of the test items (already described). The procedure involves a referral of the items to the experts and obtaining of their consensus on each. There are several methods of item analysis described in various texts exclusively based on construction of tests. However, for the purpose of the present book, only a few generally more popular techniques will be presented.

Item Difficulty

Item difficulty can be gauged in various ways:

i. Expert ranking of the items in order of difficulty
ii. Quickness by which the item can be solved, and
iii. Calculation of the proportion of students solving the item correctly.

While the first two are based on the judgmental process, the last one is based on empirical evidence and generates a numerical index and is hence, widely used.

Item difficulty may be defined as the proportion of the examinees that marked the item correctly. The numerical term which indicates the level of difficulty is called *difficulty index.* It may range between 0 and 100. An item answered correctly by 65 percent students has a difficulty index of 0.65. If 90 percent of a standard group pass an item, it is easy; if only 10 percent pass the item it is hard or too difficult. Generally, items of moderate difficulty (40–60% passing) are to be preferred to those which are much easier or much harder. If p is the proportion passing an item; q is $(1 - p)$ or proportion failing, the SD of the item (its variability) is square pq and its variance (σ^2) is pq. The variance of an item is at its maximum when $p = q = 0.5$. Hence, to bring out more individual differences (a greater spread), the item difficulty may be kept near 0.5.

Correction for Guessing

In multiple choice objective items guessing plays an important role and boosts up the result of those who do not understand the item nor know its correct answer and hence, indulge in guesswork. Thus, chance success must be corrected. A formula for the purpose is:

$$P_c = \frac{R - \dfrac{W}{(k-1)}}{N - HR} \qquad \text{...(19.5)}$$

In which,

P_c = the percent of examinees who correctly know the answer (corrected index of item difficulty)

R = the number of examinees who get the right answer
W = the number of examinees who get the wrong answer
N = the number of examinees in the sample
HR = the number of examinees who do not reach the item and hence could not try solving it
k = number of alternatives in the item

As an example, consider the following data: A sample of 200 students took a test of 100 items. Each item had 5 choices. Item number 28 was answered correctly by 60 and incorrectly by 96; 44 could not reach the item. Now the item difficulty can be calculated as below:

$$P_c = \frac{60 - \frac{96}{5-1}}{200 - 44} = \frac{60 - 24}{156} = 36/156 = 0.23$$

The uncorrected index of item difficulty would have been R/N or 60/200 or 0.30. The use of the formula for correction for guessing has brought it down to 0.23.

The student should be aware of the fact that as the number of options or choices increases the effect of guessing on success decreases. This effect is the largest in a true-false item. The formula given above is based on two assumptions: (i) Wrong answers are due to lack of knowledge, and (ii) to an examinee who does not know the correct answer, all the options or choices are equally attractive.

Item Discrimination

Item discrimination or the discriminating power of a test item refers to the degree to which success or failure on an item indicates possession of the ability being measured. It determines the extent to which the given item discriminates among examinees in the function or ability measured by the item. The procedure involves the following steps:

i. Administration of the draft test on a sample of about 300
ii. Identification of upper 27 percent and bottom 27 percent examinees (having highest and lowest scores in rank order respectively on the total test)
iii. Calculation, in respect of each item, of the percentage/proportion of the examinees attempting it correctly
iv. The discrimination index, DI will be given by the following formula:

$$DI = P_u - P_L \qquad ...(19.6)$$

In which,

DI = Discrimination index
P_u = Proportion in the upper group passing the item
P_L = Proportion in the lower group passing the item

v. The DI can be tested for significance by using a critical ratio test and items with positive and significant difference retained
vi. The value of the determination index can range from –1.00 through zero to +1.00
vii. An item is said to have negative discrimination power if poor students answer it correctly more often than the good students or $P_u < P_L$
viii. Items having negative discrimination are rejected. Items having discrimination index above 0.20 are ordinarily regarded satisfactory for use in most tests of academic achievement.

Several other indices of discrimination based on upper and lower 27 percent groups can be calculated. These include calculation of normalized biserial coefficients which can be readily read from a table prepared by JC Flangan.

The size of an acceptable item validity index will depend upon the length of the test, the range of difficulty indices and the purposes for which the test has been designed. The poor items are removed or improved for inclusion in the final test.

EXERCISES

1. What do you mean by reliability? How is it established?
2. Must all test be reliable?
3. What is the effect of lengthening of a test on reliability?
4. A test of 60 items has a reliability coefficient of 0.60. What will be the reliability coefficient of the test if
   i. the number of items is increased to 120?
   ii. the number of items is increased to 180?
5. Estimate the reliability of a test of 100 items if $\sigma_t = 10.00$; $\Sigma pq = 20.00$. Which method of reliability is applicable here?
6. What does the term 'validity' stand for? Explain various types of validity that a test can have.
7. Give the following data for 4 items. Calculate difficulty and discrimination indices for each.

Item No.	*% right in upper 27%*	*% right in lower 27%*	*Difficulty index*	*Discrimination index*
10	80	60		
15	45	40		
21	50	26		
38	79	21		

CHAPTER

20 Health Information and Vital Statistics

Introduction

Health information is a basic tool of management and a main input for the progress of any community or nation. Health information system is a mechanism in the collection, processing, analysis and transmission of information required for organizing and operating health services, and also for research and training. The main objective of health information system is to provide reliable relevant up-to-date adequate, timely information for health managers at all levels.

Statistics in Health

Basically, vital statistics are derived from legally registrable events without including population data or morbidity statistics. In general, the benefits of statistics in the health may be summarized as given below:

- It helps to describe the level of community health.
- It helps to diagnose community ills or factors influence on health.
- It helps to discover solutions to health problems and find clues for administrator action, i.e. planning, implementing, followings, etc.
- It helps to determine priorities for health programs.
- It helps to direct or maintain control during execution of programme.
- It helps to develop procedures, definitions, classifications and technique such as recording systems, sampling schemes, etc.
- It helps to promote health legislation.
- It helps to create administrative standards of health activities.
- It helps to determine the met and unmet health needs.
- It helps to disseminate reliable health information on this health situation and health program.
- It helps to determine success or failure of specific health programme or undertake overall evaluation of public health work; and
- It helps to demand public support for health activities in the community.

Health Statistics

Statistics covering various aspects of health, nutrition and demographic picture of population can be included under vital statistics. The term 'health statistics' should include all statistical information required for the administration of health agency, and so would comprise not only vital statistics but also good deal of other numerical information. Since health is a function of social, economic, political and environmental factors, any data pertaining to these in relation to health and disease are useful. In addition, the statistics on health services such as health and disease are useful, In addition, the statistics on health services such as health manpower and recipients of health care also constitutes health statistics; benefits of health statistics will include the following:

- It gives information that how many people suffering from particular diseases, how after, for how long and how fatal of different diseases, and to what extent people are prevented by these diseases carrying on their normal activities, financial loss due to disease.

- It gives information regarding to what extent diseases are concentrated in particular group of population according to age, sex, ethnic groups, occupation or place of residence.
- It gives information regarding seasonal variation of diseases from time to time and what is the effect of medical care and health service on the control of disease incidence. The above information is available statistics falls into three categories, relating to:
   i. Health status of persons and population in a given area providing it with indices of vitality and health.
   ii. Physical, environmental and other conditions and factors having a more or less direct bearing on health status of the population–indices of social and environmental factors.
   iii. Health services and activities directed at the improvement of health condition–indices of health activities and facilities.

The health information system is composed of several related subsystems. A comprehensive health information system requires **information** and **indicators** on the following subjects:

1. Demography and vital events
2. Environmental health statistics
3. Health status: mortality, morbidity, disability and quality of life
4. Health resources: facilities, beds, manpower
5. Utilization and non-utilization of health services: attendance, admissions waiting lists
6. Indices of outcome of medical care
7. Financial statistics (cost, expenditure) related to the particular objective

The important uses to which health information may be applied are:

1. To measure the health status of the people and to quantify their health problems, medical and health care needs
2. For local, national and international comparisons of health status. For such comparisons, the data need to be subjected to rigorous standardization and quality control.
3. For planning, administration and effective management of health services and programs
4. For assessing whether health services are accomplishing their objectives in terms of their effectiveness and efficiency
5. For assessing the attitudes and degree of satisfaction of the beneficiaries with the health system, and
6. For research into particular problems of health and disease.

The human population plays a very important role in the development of a country. Hence, its study is very important. Demography is the science which pertains to the study of population. Demography covers a large number of aspects concerning the human population like births, age, sex, caste, literacy and educational level, workers and non-workers, income patterns, marital status, natality and fecundity, immigration emigration, disease, death, etc. Such studies reveal a number of facts and figures which help in the planning so as to achieve the desired socio-economic standards. For centuries, many theories have been propounded regarding population growth. The Malthusian theory is one of the most famous theories. This theory is based on the proposition that population, when unchecked, increases in a geometrical ratio while subsistence increases only in an arithmetical ratio. If population grows in a geometrical ratio, it is inevitable that the population would ultimately outstrip the available resources. Food grains, particularly, will become scarce and population growth would not be limited by any means other than starvation. Hence, the study of population is a must.

Demography has many facets and vital statistics is one of them. Vital statistics deal exclusively with marriages, births, morbidity and deaths in the human population. These factors are mainly responsible for population growth. In other words, we limit our discussion to population growth. For a marked region, immigration and emigration affect population growth and thus these two factors also come within the purview of vital statistics. Births depend on the age at marriage, fertility and fecundity – still-births, infant mortality and birth intervals are some other factors responsible for the growth rate.

Deaths due to epidemics like plague, cholera, small pox, malaria, dengue, etc. and fatal diseases like cancer, tuberculosis and heart diseases cannot be ruled out. In the last few decades, a check has been made on the spread of epidemics like plague, cholera and small pox. But many other diseases are still prevalent among the masses. Tuberculosis and cancer are taking a great toll. Natural calamities like cyclones, earthquakes, floods and famines are no less disastrous. In the modern age, wars cause innumerable deaths within no time. However, discussion of these factors is out of the scope of this chapter. Of course, deaths due to various diseases are recorded to maintain vital statistics.

Now-a-days, family planning is one of the most important programs of the governments of various countries. In India, it has attracted special attention of the government due to population explosion. The study of vital statistics enables the government to assess the impact of family planning on population growth.

Though, a general idea of vital statistics has been given in the preceding paragraphs, a few definitions of vital statistics are quoted below:

Vital statistics is one among the many facts of demography. Demography is the scientific study, measurement of human population with respect such as death, marriage, morbidity and migration. It encompasses two different aspects of quantification, i.e. static and dynamic. Static refers to a technique concerned with characteristics of population at a fixed time, for example, census and Dynamic refers to a technique concerned with the changing nature of a population, for vital events, i.e. births, death, marriage, divorce and migration. Now demography focuses on three readily observable human phenomena:

- Changes in population size (growth decline)
- Composition of population, and
- Distribution of population in space.

Concepts of Vital Statistics

The term "Vital Statistics" means the "data and analytical methods for describing vital events occuring in communities". Vital events are those pertaining to human life such as births, deaths, sickness, marriages, divorces, migration etc. So vital statistics means it covers various aspects of health nutrition and demography.

The term 'vital statistics' has been used to denote facts systematically collected and compiled in numerical form relating to vital events. Vital events are all those events which have to do with an individual's entrance into or departure from life altogether with changes in civil status which may occur to him/her during his/her life time such as birth, death, marriage, sickness, divorce, adoption, legitimation, recognition, annulment, or legal separation. These events may be required to be permanently registered with authorized offices for legal and documentary purposes as well as to provide national statistical data. The definitions of vital statistics are given below:

- Vital statistics are conventional numerical records of marriages, births, sickness and deaths by which the health and growth of a community may be studied (Benjamin).
- Vital statistics is the branch of biometry which deals with data and laws of human mortality, morbidity and demography (Arthur Newsholme).
- Vital events are those pertaining to human life such as births, death, sickness, marriage, divorce, migration, etc.

Arthur Newsholme gave two definitions of vital statistics:

1. The branch of biometry which deals with data and the laws of human mortality, morbidity and demography.

2. Vital statistics may be interpreted in two ways—in a broader sense it refers to all types of population statistics collected by whatever mode, while in a narrower sense it refers only to the statistics derived from the registration of births, deaths, and marriages.

According to Benjamin:

"*Vital statistics are conventional numerical records of marriages, births, sickness and deaths by which the health and growth of a community may be studied.*"

From the above description, it is amply clear that vital statistics are useful to individuals, various agencies, medical sciences, business communities, planners, policy makers and researchers.

Ajudicious discussion of the factors which fall within the framework of vital statistics have been covered in this chapter.

Generally the advantages of vital statistics are given below:

- Vital statistics is very handy for authentication of some vital events such as births, deaths, marriages, etc. to individual.
- The role of vital statistics in planning and evaluation is of most important use to which this body of data may be placed to improve public administration.
- The life-table known as "biometer" of public health and longevity enables the insurance agency in fixing the life insurance premium rates at various levels and can be used by insurance agency. The data on life expectancy at various age levels is useful in actuarial calculations of risk on life policies.
- Vital statistics are indispensable in demographic research. The information regarding fertility, mortality, morbidity, urban density is indispensable for planning and evaluation schemes of health, family planning and other civic amenities by the government.

Methods of Vital Statistics

There are five methods usually adopted for collecting data for vital statistics:

1. Registration method.
2. Census enumeration method.
3. Survey method.
4. Sample registration system.
5. Analytical method.

Registration Method

This method is a perpetual process which entails the registration of vital events such as, births, marriages, deaths, etc. A large number of countries have adopted this system which is a legal binding on each individual. Registration is done with the proper authorities as appointed by the government of a country. In India, registration of births and deaths is compulsory by legislation, through an act known as 'The Registration of Births and Deaths Act, 1969'. It came into force throughout the country through a Gazette notification in 1970. In case of birth, the information with regard to the date of birth, place, name of father, sex of the newborn, nationality, religion and profession of the parents has to be reported to the appropriate authority in the area. In case of death of a person, information in respect of date of death, name of the deceased, his/her father's/husband's name, place at which the death occurred, age, sex, marital status, religion, nationality, permanent address and cause of death has to be supplied to the registering authority. In the act, various terms are defined as follows:

Birth: Means livebirth or still births.

Livebirth: Means the complete expulsion or extraction from its mother of a product of conception, irrespective of the duration of pregnancy, which, after such expulsion or extraction, breathes or shows any other evidence of life. Each product of such birth is considered live born.

Still Birth: Means fetal death where a product of conceptions has attained at least the prescribed period of gestation.

Death means the permanent disappearance of all evidence of life at any time after livebirth has taken place.

Fetal death means presence of all evidences of life prior to the complete expulsion of extraction from its mother of a product of conception, irrespective of the period of pregnancy.

The legal responsibility of giving the information in respect of births and deaths to the registering authority lies with the following persons:

a. Head of the household and in absence of any such person, the eldest male present therein during the said period.
b. In case of births and deaths in a hospital, health center, nursing home or other like institutions, the medical officer in charge or any person authorized by him or his behalf.
c. In respect of births and deaths in a jail, the jailor incharge.
d. In respect of births and deaths in a choultry, hostel, dharamsala, boarding house, lodging house, tavern, barrack or place of public resort, the person in charge thereof.
e. In respect of a newborn child or dead body found deserted in a public place, the headman or other corresponding officer of the village, in case of a village and the officer in charge of the local police station, elsewhere.
f. In any other place, such person as may be prescribed.

The registration office issues a certificate on registration of a birth or death. This certificate is of great use. The birth certificate is a legal document and helps a person at the time of entering a school, taking a job, insurance policy and ration card. Similarly, a death certificate helps in getting insurance money and in disputes of land and property.

The registration method is easy in operation and very effective. Yet it suffers from the lacuna that a large number of births and deaths are not reported to the registration office as the law has not been enforced effectively.

Sources of Health Statistics

The statistics required for health activities can be obtained from varied sources. These sources depend upon the type of the health statistics. The raw data of vital statistics are generally obtained through the sources of population census, sample surveys, and vital statistics register.

Population Census: A major source of information for population analysis is the census data. According to United Nations, Population Census is defined as "the simultaneous recording of demographic data by the government, at a particular time, pertaining to all persons who live in a particular territory".

Census is a process of complete counting of all individuals in a country on a fixed data or period. In census, in addition to counting of total number of people, certain other informations of importance are collected. The information pertaining to the individuals such as age, sex, religion, occupation, literacy, housing, income, etc. are also obtained at the time of census. Published census reports contain the information pertaining to the population according to the above categorization of each geographical area in the country in addition to the total population of each place at the time of census.

The first official census was undertaken in the world at Sweden in year 1749. In India, the first countrywide census took place in 1872 although the population census were conducted for individual areas prior to that data also. Subsequently census is taking place once in every ten years with the years ending with one. In India, the census count was taken either to as of sunrise on 1 March, every ten years beginning from March 1, 1881. The last census was taken as of sunrise of March 1, 2011. With a population of 1210 million, India is the second most populous country in the world, next only to China, whereas seventh in land area. With only 2.4 percent of the world's land area, India is supporting about 16.87 percent of the world's population. The population of India since 1901, average annual exponential growth rate (%), and the decadal growth of population (%) is as shown in Table 20.1.

Census operations are calculated in almost all countries at intervals of ten years. In a census, the enumeration of every individual of all habitational

Table 20.1

Demographic trends in India for 1901 to 2011

Year	*Total population (in million)*	*Average annual exponential growth rate (%)*	*Decadal growth rate (%)*
1901	238.4	–	–
1911	252.1	0.56	0.75
1921	251.3	(–) 0.03	(–) 0.31
1931	279.0	1.04	11.00
1941	318.7	1.33	14.22
1951	361.1	1.25	13.31
1961	439.2	1.96	21.64
1971	548.2	2.20	24.80
1981	683.3	2.22	24.66
1991	843.9	2.14	23.86
2001	1027.0	1.93	21.34
2011	1210.99	1.41	17.64

areas is carried out at a specific time. Information is collected on community, sex, age, literacy, economic conditions, etc. This information is analyzed in the form of various tables based on regions and characteristics. The scope and contents of the Indian census have been expanding over the decades to cater to the needs of various ministries of the Government of India, the State Government and other institutions.

Census Enumeration Method

A census presents a comprehensive profile of a country's population. Census operations are conducted in almost all countries at intervals of ten years. In a census, the enumeration of every individual of all habitational areas is carried out at a specific time. In India, the 1991 census record was updated by the enumeration from March 1 to March 5, 2001. So was the census 2011. Census enumeration usually covers data regarding age, sex, marital status, educational level, occupation, religion and other factors needed for vital statistics. But this information is available for the census year only. Hence, census data fail to produce vital statistics for intercensal years, whereas population growth rate is needed from time to time. Moreover, the data obtained in respect of births and deaths are not complete even for the census year. Hence, the census enumeration method fails to provide data suitable for vital statistics.

Vital Statistics Registration

The records of births and deaths are fundamental necessities of health statistics as they are most helpful in working out indices like birth and death rates which are useful in estimating the population of a community. Death records are also useful in knowing the causes of mortality. Such registrations were recognized long before 1250 BC in Egypt. Churches started maintaining the records of baptisms, marriages and deaths. However, Sweden and Finland were the first countries to make these registrations as a civilian affair and they were used for vital statistical indices. In various other countries both in Europe and America, the system of registration developed in 18th and 19th centuries. By 1933 the registration laws covered about half of world's population and by 1955 it was about 60 percent.

In India, before independence in some states the registration of births and deaths were not compulsory. After the dawn of independence in India, even though, these registrations were compulsory in every state, the laws pertaining to them varied from State to State and were not uniform. However, an act of Parliament has been enforced for the compulsory registration of births and deaths, throughout the country and this has come into force from April 1970.

The channel of compilation of births and deaths are slightly different in urban and rural areas and are as follows.

In *urban areas* such as municipalities, cantonments, there will be certain notified number of wards and ward registrars to maintain these records in each ward. Heads of the families in which a birth and death occurs are bound by obligation of law to report, any birth or death occurring in his family, to these ward registrars within seven days for births and three days for deaths from the occurrence of the event. In bigger towns there are registration offices at the burial and burning ghats and they keep the record of deaths. Heads of hospitals, *dharmasalas* and maternity homes should also report the events to the ward registrars. To avoid omissions, sweepers, midwives and dais have to report every occurrence that comes to their knowledge. These ward registrars send the returns, once in a week, to the Municipal Health Officer and in the absence of such health officer to the Executive officer of the municipality. The weekly returns are sent direct to the State Directors of Health by the municipal medical officer by health once a month.

In *rural areas*, the primary unit of registration is a *Grama Sabha*. The *pradhans* of the village get the information about births and deaths from the heads of the families in which the event occurs. The *panchayat secretary* maintains the births and death registers, who copies down these information into the registers during visits to the Pradhans. Then these reports are sent to the Block Development Officer at the Block level. From here the returns are sent to the State Director of Medical and Health Services once a month. This state level return is then sent to the Registrar General of Vital Statistics attached to the Director General of Health Services at the national level where the returns are compiled for the whole country.

The international level report is compiled by the World Health Organization at Geneva.

The Registrar General of Vital Statistics at the national level and the State Directors of Medical and Health Services at the State level publish these data once a year.

Lapses in the Registration System

In India, only in 1970 a uniform law for the registration of births and deaths have come into force. Previous to this period, the laws were not uniform from State to State. The under-registration of births and deaths ranged up to 80 percent. The situation was almost similar in rural as well as in urban areas. The main lapses in the registration system are as follows:

- Both in rural and urban areas, the primary responsibility of reporting rests with the head of the family where the event has occurred. With high illiteracy rate prevailing in the country, the public are not conscious of the importance of these statistics and as such most of the times they never report the statistics.
- Even though the laws exist for imposing punishment for non-reporting, the laws are rarely enforced.
- In rural areas, the *pradhan* and the *panchayat secretary* who are primarily responsible for maintenance of these records, are multifarious workers and they never give much importance for maintaining these records. Further they are not employees of the health department.
- The death records which are the main source of information of age at death as well as the cause of death, are never complete. The age and the cause of death are seldom recorded correctly.
- There is a time lag in the compilation and transmission of these statistics from one agency to the other in the channel of compilation, as such the statistics at the higher levels are mostly under compiled.

Thus, the coverage of vital statistics registration is defective both quantitatively and qualitatively.

Improvement of Registration System

Various schemes have been implemented in the recent years to improve the quality and quantity of vital statistics. Both long-term and short-term schemes have been in operation, to get quick and reliable estimates of vital statistics and also statistics relating to the causes of death. The two important schemes in this direction are mentioned below.

Sample Registration Scheme

This scheme is implemented to provide reliable estimates of birth and death rates at both the State level as well as at all India level, separately for rural and urban areas. In this scheme about 150 rural units in terms of villages and about 60–100 urban units in terms of census enumeration blocks are selected on random basis within each State. The sample size has been determined on the basis of estimate of the birth and death rates of 40 and 20 respectively. 1 percent and 2 percent permissible errors have been allowed for the estimates. The selection of the rural units is done by a unistage stratified random sampling procedure from the list of villages, while the urban units are selected by a two-phase stratified random sampling procedure with urban areas and enumeration blocks serving as the units of selection in the two stages respectively. Villages and towns are stratified according to population size.

Local residents like teachers, midwives, village level worker, etc., are appointed as part-time enumerators and are given intensive training. They are paid monthly honorarium. These enumerators maintain a layout map of their respective areas. The population base is collected on a household schedule. They also maintain a list of pregnant women. Every birth or death is recorded as and when they occur. This information is collected through reliable informants like barber, village dai, washerman, village priest, etc. These events are recorded by him only after satisfying himself of the occurrence of the event.

A half yearly survey cum enumeration is carried out by the supervisor and the lists prepared by the enumerator and the supervisor are matched. Unmatched events in the two lists are verified jointly by them or by a third person. The final lists are transmitted to the Registrar General of India, where the countrywide statements are prepared.

Thus SRS has the unique feature of recording the vital events both in a longitudinal manner as well as through a periodical survey. The longitudinal method of recording avoids the bias inherent in recall lapse. The events are recorded on *de jure* basis and proper accounting of these events according to permanent residents and visitors are also done.

Model Registration

The scheme mainly envisages collection of data on deaths by para-medical staff. For this purpose certain primary health centers are provided with *field agents* who contact *local informants* regularly at short intervals and correct the addresses of the dead persons. Then each of these field agents visits these households in his area and obtains necessary information and ensures that the event has occurred within the village and not outside, irrespective of the fact that the event pertains to a person resident of the village or not and then assigns a probable cause of death. He also collects information about births in the village so as to keep watch over infant deaths and deaths due to child birth and complication of pregnancy. For assigning the cause of death he consults the Manual of Instruction provided to him. At the end of each month the field agent is required to prepare a report and send it to the *Recorder* at PHC who after scrutinizing submits it to the Medical Officer for checking and onward transmission to the State headquarters. The monthly returns received at the State headquarters are compiled and a consolidated statement is sent to the Registrar General of India for further checking, processing and analysis.

At the end of half year, i.e. 30th June and 31st December of every year, the field agent rechecks occurrence of any death or birth by house to house enquiry and matches with similar information collected during continuous recording. The events recorded wrongly are deleted. The Medical Officer of the PHC is also expected to check ten percent of the deaths reported by the field agent. Thus, the model registration aims more at quantitative rather than qualitative assessment of mortality pattern. The number of primary health centers selected for this scheme is approximately equal to the quotient obtained by dividing the population by one lakh.

There is no machinery for the collection of morbidity data as it exists for vital statistics. Still major health institutions compile the outpatient and in-patient records according to the names of the diseases. From these reports, the *Central Health Intelligence Bureau* attached to the Director General of Health Services publishes periodical reports after compiling and collating health data from various sources.

Periodical surveys are also undertaken by organizations like Central Statistical Organization, National Sample Survey wing of Central Secretariat, Indian Council of Medical Research, etc., to obtain information on various morbidities.

Further information regarding communicable diseases is compiled from the reports of infectious diseases.

Process for Collection of Vital Statistics

It is by no means an easy task to set up a system that will ensure accurate recording of information for each vital event occurring in a country, in each and every town, village, institution, and individual home. In many of the less developed countries a system of this kind does not exist; and even where considerable advances have been made, and improvements are still being effected. There are thus many countries in which statistics have yet to be 'sold' to the government and the people. It has to be clearly understood that this is the only way in which the level of health can be measured, and effective comparisons made.

In countries where the machinery for the collection of statistics for rural areas has been set up, the village is generally the smallest administrative unit for which an agent is appointed to report the events, and in some cases he may also be responsible for registering them. The responsibility for registration in rural areas generally rests with the head of the houshold in the developed countries. The primary responsibility for each village may rest with the village headman, the police officer, village watchman or revenue office. Sometimes one of the local inhabitants is appointed registrar of vital statistics whose duty is not only to keep himself informed about all vital events occurring in the area, but also to be the custodian of legal records.

Regulations for reporting and registering vital events differ from one country to another.

The Health Survey and Development Committee (Bhore Committee) in 1946 brought out that vital statistics in India had three main defects, viz.,

i. Incompleteness in the recording of the events
ii. Inaccuracy in the cause of death; and
iii. Faulty compilation.

These defects were attributed to poor collection of vital occurrences at the periphery (in villages) by illiterate Chowkidar or by the lowest grades of local body employees, registration by agencies other than health such as police, village headman, passage of the recorded vital statistics through a series of stages before they reached the Directorate of Public Health of each Province. Thus the data on vital events were poorly collected, improperly handled and scarcely used for either operating or evaluating projects in the country. The Bhore Committee gave several recommendations to improve these defects.

Since this report, a number of conferences have been held emphasizing the importance and role of health statistics. Pilot schemes with training facilities have been set up. The steps already taken by the Central Government in this direction are the establishment of the Office of the Registrar General of India, the Central Statistical Organization, National Sample Survey Unit and the Bureau of Health Intelligence in the Directorate General of Health Services, New Delhi. Each state government is also expected to have its own department of Vital and Health Statistics. Attempts are being made to improve hospital statistics by establishing Medical Record

Departments in the hospitals. The Registrar-General's Office produces a report on 'Vital Statistics' each year since 1958. A number of organizational changes were made both at the centre and in the various states. However, the various stages in the collection, compilation, preservation and utilization of data on vital and health statistics are still passing through a transition. Whereas the compilation and preservation phases have improved to some extent in States and Corporations, the collection and registration phases are still that they were at the time of the Bhore Committee's recommendations. Much more effort is required to increase the quality of the statistics to serve more efficiently.

Registration method entails registration of vital events such as deaths, births, marriages, etc. Registration of vital events is done with proper authorities appointed by the government of a country. These authorities issue the certificates of respective vital events. It serves many useful purposes of authentication of these events. For example, death certificate is necessary for life insurance claim, for succession certificate, etc. Similarly birth certificate required for school admission, job, etc.

The other **different methods** of intercensal population estimates are as follows:

i. **Natural Increase Method:** This method can be applied for an area where the registration of births and deaths is satisfactory and, further, if satisfactory statistics of migration are also available. The method consists of adding to the last balance of immigration over emigration, during the period from the last census to the time when the estimate is to be made. The method does not provide estimate of the population of any future date. In countries where vital statistics and data on migration are of a high level of accuracy, the method provides good estimates.

   In the case of number of births, deaths, immigration and emigration are taken into account for estimating population during any year.

   Thus, estimated population period
   = census population + Number of (births – deaths) during the period after census + Number of (immigrants – emigrants) during the period after census.

ii. **The Arithmetic Progression or 'AP' Method:** In this method it is assumed that the population increases or decreases by a constant figure from year to year between two census years. The difference between the population figures of the two censuses gives the total increase of the population in 10 years. Dividing the number by 10 (the period between two censuses) obtained the growth for one year. As already stated in this method, population increases in an arithmetic progression from year to year or between two census period. In other words, the rate of increase of population from one year to another is a constant amount and is same from year to year between two census periods.

   To estimate the population during any year, the rate of increase is calculated from previous two census population. The annual rate of increase is used in estimating the population at any time from the following formula:

   $P_t = P_o + rt$

   P_t is the population at a period t (ten) years after last census,

   r is the annual rate of increase of population which is obtained as 1/10 of the difference between the population of two successive census estimates, and

   P_o is the population estimates at the previous census.

   Example: Population of India enumerated as on 1 April 1991 and 1 March 2001 were 843.9 and 1027.0 respectively.

   Increase in 9 years 9 months = 1027 – 843.9

   Population of India 1991 =

   Population of India 2001 =

Increase in 10 years =
Increase in one year =
Increase in population 6 years from 2001 to 2007 =
Population of India during 2007 =

iii. **The Geometric Progression or GP Method:** In this method it is assumed that the increase in population is constant throughout the period. An alternative assumption can be made that percentage rate of growth that remains constant or according to geometrical law of growth. In other words, in this method year to year will be in a geometric progression of the population increase from year to year in a constant ratio.

To estimate the population by this method, the constant ratio of increase is obtained from the previous two census population estimates and the population estimate for any year is obtained from the following formula:

$P_t = P_o + (1 + r)^t$

Where

P_t is the estimate of population at a period t year after census,

P_o is the population estimates at the previous census, and

r is the annual geometric growth rate which is estimated by substituting the population estimates of the two census, taking 't' as 10.

ω estimation of population by this method is illustrated in the following example: To estimate the population of one state during 2007 for the data given below.

First annual growth rate in estimation as follows:

$P_t = 73746401$, $P_o = 63215742$, $t = 10$

Substituting these values in the equation $P_t = P_{10}\ (1+r)^{10}$ and taking logarithm of both sides

$\log P_t = \log P_o + 10 \log (1 + r)$

$\log (1 + r) = 1/10 (\log P_t - \log P_o)$

$= 1/10 (\log 73746401 - \log 63215742)$

$= 1/10 (7.86777 - 7.80086) = 1/10 (0.06691)$

$= 0.006691$

$(1 + r) = \text{Antilog } (0.006691)$

$= 1.016$

$\therefore\quad r = 1.016 - 1.000 = 0.016$

Population of state in 2007 = 73746401 $(1 + 0.106)^6$

Taking logarithm of both sides

Log (2007 population) = log (73746401) + 6 log (1.016)

= 7.86777 + 0.04014 = 7.90791

Population 2007 = Antilog (7.90791)

= 80,000000.

Survey Method

Surveys are generally conducted in areas, or regions where the system of registration or recording of births, deaths or marriages, etc. has not been functioning properly and efficiently. The survey records make vital statistics available for that area or region. Since civil registration is deficient in India, a Sample Registration System (SRS) was initiated in 1960s to provide reliable estimates of births and death rates at the National and State levels. The SRS is a dual-record system consisting of continuous enumeration of births and deaths by an enumerator and an independent survey, every 6 months by an investigator supervision. The half-yearly survey, in addition to serving as an independent check on the events recorded by the enumerator produces the denominator required for computing rates. Now SRS covers the entire country. It is a major source of health information. Since the introduction of SRS, more reliable informations on birth and death rates, age-specific fertility and mortality rates, infant and adult mortality, etc. have become available.

The term 'health survey' is used for surveys relating to any aspects of health–morbidity, mortality, nutritional status, etc. The types of surveys covered in health survey include

- Surveys for evaluating health status of population
- Surveys for investigation of factors affecting health and disease
- Surveys relating to administration of health services.

From the point of view of the method employee for data collection, health surveys can be broadly classified into:

- Health interview survey
- Health examination survey
- Health record survey
- Mail questionnaire survey.

Ad-hoc surveys are conducted in areas or regions where the system of recording births and deaths has not been functioning properly and efficiently. It becomes necessary, particularly in those areas where registration offices have not been established. The survey records make vital statistics available for that region.

Sampling Registration System

Vital rates are needed from time to time for an idea of population growth, specially for the purpose of evaluation of family planning programs in terms of their ultimate objective of reduction in fertility.

In organizing the post enumeration check of a census, the continuing sample registration of births and deaths in a reasonably large sample covering all parts of the state or country has been taken as a useful source for recording information. Sample registration system is operated under the aegis of the Registrar General and Census commissioner. In India, the sample registration system has been in operation since June 1967 in rural areas and since July 1968 in urban areas. Under this scheme, census blocks are selected by a random sampling method in rural and urban areas, separately, as sampling units. The sample covers less than one percent of the rural and urban population. Regular information about births, marriages, deaths, etc. are collected by the recorders appointed for the purpose. Half-yearly enumeration is done for each family in the selected blocks, by a team of investigators. The anomalies found in the daily records and periodic enumeration are removed after revisiting the families under conflict by a totally new team of personnel. At present, several methods are built in SRS to aid full coverage. The scheme of permanent house marking has been introduced so that no households are missed at the time of half-yearly checking. All old sampling units have been gradually replaced by new ones based on the frame of the latest census. The following studies are undertaken by the sample registration unit.

At All India Level

a. Infant mortality.
b. Age-specific mortality rates in rural areas.
c. Sampling variability of vital rates.

At State Level

a. Differences in birth rates with education, religion and parity.
b. Extent of institutional and domiciling event.
c. Sex ratio of vital statistics.
d. Seasonality in birth and death rates.

The types of events missed by the enumerator and supervisor are:

- Volume of migration in the sample area.
- Age and sex composition of the population in sample areas.
- Errors in matching.

The sample registration system is a continuous process for estimating the vital rates and is very effective besides certain lacunae. The SRS is designed to give estimates of urban and rural vital rates separately. The estimates of vital rates based on the records provided by SRS are a good barometer in the evaluation of family planning programs.

Analytical Methods

The population estimates at a given time can be obtained without ad-hoc surveys by mathematical methods. These estimates are based on the assumption that the population grows at a constant rate during intercensal years. Analytical methods are algebraic methods which make use of available data without requiring any fresh survey.

As population is liable to change every instant due to births, deaths, immigration and emigration, the population at any time can only be obtained as an estimate. Estimates of population are required for the years falling between two census dates (intercensal estimates) or following the last census (Post-censal estimates). Most annual rates are compiled by using the population estimate referring to 1 July (Mid-year population). Sometimes, as the result of a new census or some other fresh information, there is an abrupt change of considerable magnitude in the population estimate used for calculation of vital rates. When such discontinuity occurs, references to the change should be indicated, separating the years before and after the change.

It is generally not possible to conduct ad-hoc surveys to assess the population at any period in between two censal years. The population estimates at a given time can be obtained without ad-hoc surveys by mathematical methods. The estimates are based on the assumption that the population grows at a constant rate during the intercensal years. For example, given the birth and death rates, population growth may be estimated for an intercensal period. The number of births or deaths at a given time in a population sub-group can also be estimated. Analytical methods are algebraic methods which make use of available data without requiring any fresh survey. Some analytical methods are given below:

1. Estimation of population in a given intercensal year can be done by the formula,

$$\hat{P}_t = P_o + \frac{n}{N}(P_1 - P_o) \qquad ...(20.1)$$

where,

$\hat{P}_t$ – Estimated population at some-intercensal year t.

P_o – Population in the previous census.

P_1 – Population in the succeeding census.

N – Number of years between the censuses.

n – Number of years between the given year and the previous census year.

Formula (20.1) is a linear interpolation formula and yields good estimates provided population changes occur at a constant rate all over the intercensal years.

Example: The population of Jaipur city, according to censuses 1971 and 1981, are 7, 45, 876 and 12, 50, 532, respectively. The population estimate for the year 1975 is obtained by (20.1). In this problem,

$P_1 = 12{,}50{,}532$, $P_o = 7{,}45{,}876$, $N = 10$, $n = 4$.

$$\text{Thus } \hat{P}_t = 7{,}45{,}876 + \frac{4}{10}(12{,}50{,}532 - 7{,}45{,}876)$$

$$= 9{,}47{,}738.$$

2. Population for any intercensal year can be estimated provided accurate records regarding births, deaths and migration are available. The formula is,

$$\hat{P}_t = P_o + (B - D) + (I - E) \qquad ...(20.2)$$

where,

P_t and P_o are the same as in (20.1).

B – Total number of births during the period o to t.

D – Total number of deaths during the period o to t.

I – Total number of immigrants during the period o to t.

E – Total number of emigrants during the period o to t.

3. *Compound interest formula:* Population increase takes place in a geometrical progression. In case, the population growth rate r is known, the population estimate at any time t can be obtained by the formula,

$$\hat{P}_t = P_o(1 + r)^n \qquad ...(20.3)$$

where, n is the number of years between o to t. $\hat{P}_t$ and P_o have already been explained.

If r is not known, it can be estimated by using the formula given below.

Let P_n be the known population at any period subsequent to t. Then,

$$r = \sqrt[n]{\frac{P_n}{P_o}} - 1 \qquad ...(20.3.1)$$

where, n is the gap between period o and the end period.

Example: The population of a town in two census years is as follows:

Year	*Population*
1941	54,892
1971	1,08,431

a. The rate of increase in population per thousand, per annum,
b. The estimate of the population in 1965, and
c. The estimate of the population in 1977, have been calculated.

a. By formula (20.3.1),

$$r = \sqrt[30]{\frac{108431}{54892}} - 1 = \sqrt[30]{1.9754} - 1$$

$$\log(r+1) = \frac{1}{30}\log(1.9754) - 1 = \frac{0.2956}{30}$$

$= 0.009853$

Taking antilog,

$r + 1 = 1.023$

$r = 0.023$

The rate per thousand $= 0.023 \times 1000 = 23.$

b. The population estimate for 1965 from (20.3) is,

$\hat{P}_{1965} = 54,892\ (1+0.023)^{24}$

Taking log,

$$\log \hat{P} = \log 54,892 + 24 \log (1.023)$$
$$= 4.7395 + 0.2370$$
$$= 4.9765$$

Taking antilog,

$$\hat{P}_{1965} = 94,733$$

c. As in part, (b)

$$\hat{P}_{1977} = 54,392 + (1.023)^{36}$$
$$= 1,254,460$$

4. *Geometric mean formula:* The mid-year population between any two consecutive census years can be estimated by the geometric mean formula.

$$\hat{P}_{1\text{-}2} = \sqrt{P_1 \times P_2} \qquad \text{...(20.4)}$$

where P_1 – Population at the first census.
P_2 – Population at the second census.

5. *Logistic curve:* The logistic curve was originally developed by Verhulst and later studied by Pearl, R. and Read L. The curve, is also known as the *Pearl–Read curve*. The curve, in its simplest form, is given by,

$$Y_c = \frac{K}{1+10^{a+bx}} \qquad \text{...(20.5)}$$

Where, Y_c – Estimated value of population.

$$K = \frac{2y_0 y_1 y_2 - y_1^2(y_0 + y_2)}{y_0 y_2 - y_1^2}$$

$$a = \log \frac{K - y_0}{y_0}$$

$$b = \frac{1}{n} \log \frac{y_0}{y_1}\left(\frac{K - y_1}{K - y_0}\right)$$

where, x – the year for which the value has to be interpolated.
y_0 – Geometric mean of the first 3 years of the series.
y_1 – Geometric means of the middle 3 years of the series
y_2 – Geometric mean of the last 3 years of the series

The theory propounded by Pearl and Read is not universally accepted. Moreover, this theory involves high level mathematics.

Calculation of Vital Statistics

As a matter of fact, all the significant events related to life come under the category of vital statistics. Hence, the vital statistics rates are of prime importance and can be calculated by the formulae given ahead.

$$\text{Rate of vital event} = \frac{\text{Number of cases of the event under consideration}}{\text{Total population exposed to the risk of the event}} \qquad \text{...(20.6)}$$

The rate of vital events is mostly expressed on the basis of per thousand ($^0/_{00}$) persons. Formula (20.6) may be considered a fundamental formula which leads to all the subsequent formulae.

Basic Formulae of Calculation of Vital Statistics

The number of events that occur in any place is to a large extent dependent on the people living in that area. Therefore, in assessing the state of health or change, the vital events must be considered in terms of the population that have given rise to these events. Hence, vital statistics are expressed usually either as (*a*) 'rate' or as (*b*) 'ratio'. A ratio is a static quantity; it is a proportion such as a/b, describing the state of affairs at a particular instant. A rate, on the other hand, describes the rapidity with which something is happening during a stated period of time. Thus, a rate is the proportion a/b per unit of time, usually one year.

There are some most useful and widely used rates, ratios and proportions. Definitions are provided below.

Rate

The term *rate* usually is reserved to refer to those calculations that imply the probability of the occurrence of some events. A rate is expressed in the following form,

$$\frac{a}{a+b}k$$

where,

a = The frequency with which an event has occurred during some specified periods of time,

$a+b$ = The number of persons exposed to the risk of the event during the same period of time, and

k = Numbers such as 100, 1000, 10,000 or 1,00,000.

The numerator of a rate is a component part of the denominator. The purpose of the multiplier k called the base, is to avoid results involving the very small numbers that may arise in the calculation of rates and to facilitate comprehension of the rate. The value chosen for k, will depend on the magnitude of the numerator and denominator.

Rate is a proportion with a defined denominator (here it is population) and the numerator (here it is occurence of an event in the same population) and multiplier (magnification agent), i.e., 100 or 1000 or 10000 or 100000 etc., as per magnification desired.

Example:

$$\text{Crude birth rate} = \frac{\text{Numerator}}{\text{Denominator}} \times \text{Multiplier}$$

$$\frac{\text{Total number of births in a year in a defined geographical area}}{\text{Total mid year population}} \times 1000$$

So, the rate is a measure of the speed at which new events are occuring in a community.

The rates in general are of two types: Crude and Specific. Crude rates are general rates calculated without specification of sections of the population. They measure the proportion between total events and the population over a period of time for a given geographical area.

Specific rates: These are for the specific group of the population such as for a particular age, sex, marital status, occupation, etc. The definition is as,

Specific rate =

$$\frac{\text{Number of events which occurred among specific group of the Population of a given geographic area during a given time}}{\text{Mid-year population of the specific group of population in the same geographic area during a given year}} \times 1000$$

The crude rate as well as the specific rates are usually calculated for every calendar year. They can be calculated also for periods of 5 years or 10 years or less than one year.

Annual rates or yearly rates from the events recorded for the periods shorter than a calendar year or more than a calendar year are expressed on annual basis by multiplying with the adjustment factors.

Specific rates means rate for specific groups (Age-sex groups, disease specific rates).

Commonly used rates are:

A. Mortality rates
  1. Crude death rate
  2. Standardised death rates
     - Direct method
     - Indirect method
  3. Specific death rates
     a. Age specific death rates and sex specific death rates
     b. Infant mortality rate (IMR)
     c. Neonatal mortality rate

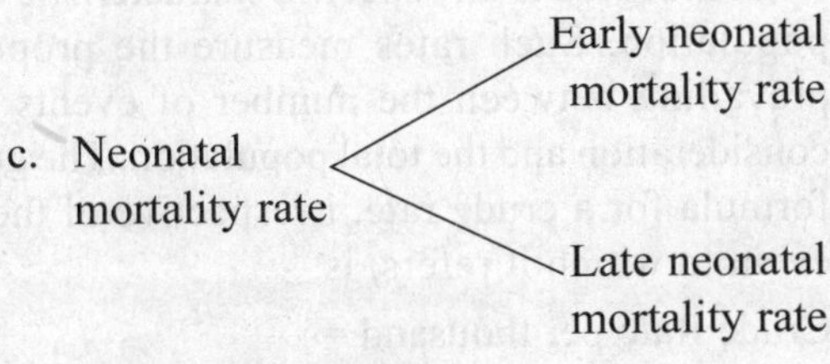

     d. Perinatal mortality rate
     e. Maternal mortality rate
     f. Proportional mortality rate
     g. Case fatality rate

B. Morbidity Rates
  1. Incidence rates
  2. Prevalence rates
     - Point prevalence rate
     - Period prevalence rate
  3. Notification rates

C. Fertility related statistics (or rates)
  1. Birth rate (crude birth rate)
  2. GFR (General fertility rate)
  3. General marital fertility rate
  4. Age specific fertility rate
  5. Age specific marital fertility rate
  6. TFR (Total fertility rate)
  7. Total marital fertility rate
  8. GRR (Gross reproduction rate)
  9. NRR (Net reproduction rate)
  10. Pregnancy rate
  11. Abortion rate
  12. Marriage rate
      - Crude marriage rate
      - General marriage rate
  13. Couple protection rate (CPR)

Ratio

In a very broad sense, a *ratio* results from dividing one quantity by another. However, it is mostly used in a more specific sense, i.e. when the numerator and the denominator are two distinct quantities. That is, the numerator is not a component part of the denominator. Two kinds of ratios are in common use:

i. A ratio is used in comparing the frequencies of two mutually exclusive classes. Examples are, (i) Sex ratio and (ii) Fetal death ratio. Definitions are as given,

$$\text{Sex ratio} = \frac{\text{Number of females}}{\text{Number of males}} \times 1000$$

Fetal death ratio =

$$\frac{\text{Number of fetal deaths in a year}}{\text{Number of live births in a year}}$$

Various populations or population groups can be compared by these ratios. In addition to these, other examples are person-doctor ratio or person-hospital bed ratio, or the person-hospital ratio or the person-hospital nurse ratio of a certain geographic area. Fraction or ratio, can be multiplied by 1000 or 100 or one lakh as per convenience.

ii. An index is a summary measure intended to reflect relationship among variables. It is often expressed as a ratio. Example are, weight/height; weight/head circumference, weight/height and weight/(height – 100). These are some of the indices utilized for the measurement of malnutrition.

Proportion

Proportion is a special type of ratio in which the numerator is a part of the denominator, i.e.

$$P = \frac{a}{a+b}$$

If the numerator and denominator are integrates and represent frequencies of certain events then '*p*' is a relative frequency. For example,

$$= \frac{\text{Number of males}}{(\text{Number of males} + \text{Number of females})}$$

given the proportion or relative frequency of males, in a given community.

In a large population, proportion may determine the probability of a certain event. For example, the quantity:

$$= \frac{\text{Number of fetal deaths}}{(\text{Number of fetal deaths} + \text{Number of live births})}$$

A given population for a given year is clearly a proportion. It is the probability that a fetus might die before it is born. This is called fetal death rate and this is different from fetal death ratio.

Generally, the numerator and denominator in ($a/a + b$) do not need to be integers. They can be measurable quantities such as weight, length, volume height, etc. In such cases, proportions are also often called fractions. For example, in chemical analysis, the mass of a given component can be expressed as a fraction of the total weight of a compound. Percentage is a proportion or a fraction per 100 units. Thus, proportion '*p*' corresponds to (100*p*) percent (100*p*%).

Ratios and proportions are useful in studies of populations by demographic factors such as age, sex, race or region or grades of nutritional status.

Most useful rates and ratios can be used (i) to measure the levels of health and nutrition; (ii) to monitor the progress made in health and nutrition; (iii) to compare fertility, mortality and morbidity of different places, times, communities and regions and (iv) to determine the expectation or longevity of life at birth or at any particular age or by sex. There are, (A) measures of fertility, (B) measures of mortality and (C) measures of morbidity. Details of these are presented in the following pages.

Ideally a rate (or ratio) should satisfy the following requirements:

i. The numerator should have arisen from the denominator
ii. Each one included in the denominator should contribute to or have an opportunity to appear in the numerator.

In reality, however, these two conditions are not strictly satisfied due to practical considerations, as will be discussed later.

Crude rates: A crude rate, sometimes known also as a general rate, total rate, or gross rate, is computed with respect to the total population, without regard to any specific characteristic of that population. Such rates measure the proportion prevailing between the number of events under consideration and the total population. The general formula for a crude rate, irrespective of the vital event to which it refers, is:

Crude Rate per thousand =

$$\frac{\text{Number of events which occurred among the population of a given geographic area during a given period}}{\text{Mid period total population of the given Geographic area during the same period}} \times 1000$$

Specific rate: Rates defined in terms of one or more characteristics of the population are known as specific rates. Any relevant characteristic of the population may be the basis for a specific rate. Those found most useful and feasible are age, sex, birth order, occupation, marital status, etc.

Specific Rate per thousand =

$$\frac{\text{Number of events which occurred among a specific period of population of a given geographic area during a given period}}{\text{Mid period population of the specific group in the given Geographic area during the same period}} \times 1000$$

The specific rate is characterized by its reference to only one special segment of the population.

Annual rate: Although a crude rate or a specific rate may be computed for any period of time, it is a general rule to express it on an annual basis. An annual crude rate is obtained when the term 'period' in the numerator and denominator of the above definition of the crude rate is replaced by the term 'year' – preferably 'calendar year'. The same substitution in the definition of the specific rate defines the annual specific rate.

Should the period be different from the one year, it is customary, in order to facilitate comparison, to adjust the rates to an annual basis. Adjustment is achieved by multiplying the rate by an appropriate factor obtained by dividing the year by the period in question.

Quinquennial rate: When long-term trends are studied, it is convenient to calculate rates for the five yearly periods. If a quinquennial rate is required, the total events that occurred in a five-year period should be divided by five, to make the rate comparable with the annual rate. The general formula is:

Quinquennial Rate =

$$\frac{\text{Number of vital events which occurred among the population of a given geographic area during the period of five years}}{\text{Population estimated at the middle of the five years}} \times \frac{1}{5} \times 1000$$

Decennial rate: This is required when a ten-year period is considered:

Decennial Rate =

$$\frac{\text{Number of vital events which occurred among the population of a given geographic area during the period of 10 years}}{\text{Population estimated at the middle of the 10 years}} \times \frac{1}{10} \times 1000$$

Weekly rate: In the study of seasonal variation of diseases, rates are calculated for periods shorter than a calender year. To express it on an annual basis, the weekly rate is multiplied by 52. The formula is:

Weekly Rate =

$$\frac{\text{Number of vital events which occurred in one week}}{\text{Total mid-year estimated population}} \times 52 \times 1000$$

This is not much affected by the use of the estimated mid-year population in the denominator, as generally variations in population size are relatively small in the course of one year. Furthermore, as a rule only one annual estimate of the total population, i.e. the mid-year population, is published.

Monthly rate: Similarly, monthly rates are calculated by using an adjustment factor equal to 12 or more exactly, using the fraction

$$\frac{365}{\text{Number of days in the month considered}}$$

Quarterly rate: For computation of a quarterly rate, the adjustment factor is 4.

Half-Yearly rate: Use is made of an adjustment factor of 2 for a half-yearly rate.

Measures of Mortality

The study of mortality can be made through the following death rates. Three types of death rates are calculated which enable us to know about the depletion of population. The rates are,

1. Crude death rate.
2. Specific death rate.
3. Standardized death rate.

Crude Death Rate

This is the simplest type of death rate and is defined as the number of deaths in a specific community or region in a given period, preferably on a yearly basis, per thousand persons. The formula is,

$$CDR = \frac{\text{No. of deaths in a specified area in the given period}}{\text{Total population of the area in that period}} \times 1000 \qquad ...(20.7)$$

or

$$CDR = \frac{\text{No.of deaths in a year}}{\text{Annual mean population}} \times 1000 \qquad ...(20.7.1)$$

$$= \frac{D_A}{T_A} \times 1000$$

The formula for CDR resembles to that for probability and thus CDR gives the probability of death of a person belonging to the population under reference in the specified year. Here, the death rate is crude in the sense that no attention has been paid to the age and sex distribution of the population. The information revealed by CDR is not complete. We know that the death rate is high in infants and old persons, but this has not been considered in CDR.

Specific Death Rate

Here the death rates are calculated for a section of the population exclusively. For instance, the death rates for males and females are calculated separately, the death rates for persons belonging to age groups, say 0 to 5 years, 5 to 15 years, 50 to 60 years, etc., are calculated.

The formula for specific death rate is,

$$SDR \times \frac{\text{No.of deaths in the specified section of the population in given period}}{\text{Mean population of the specified section in the given period.}} \times 1000 \qquad ...(20.8)$$

$$= \frac{D_s}{P_s} \times 1000 \qquad ...(20.8.1)$$

Specified death rate may be found for any section of the population. However, *Infant mortality rate* is usually calculated and may be formulated as given below.

Infant mortality rate =

$$\frac{\text{No. of deaths of children under one year of age in a population in a given year}}{\text{No. of births in the same population during the same year}} \times 1000 \qquad ...(20.9)$$

Similarly, for the neonatal mortality rate, the number of deaths of children under one month are recorded in formula (20.9). Other things remain the same.

Specific death rates can be calculated for any age group, sex, religion, caste or community. There is no end to the type of specifications. Anyway, formula (20.8) can easily be applied with a slight modification in its numerator. SDR reveals more glaring facts about various sections of a population than CDR. If the death rate is high in a situation. SDR's are very helpful in planning and research.

Example: The number of livebirths and deaths of children under one year of age, in a city, in the year 1983 are reported as given below:

Number of births = 4,721

Number of deaths = 101

The infant mortality rate by formula (20.9) is,

$$= \frac{101}{4{,}721} \times 1{,}000$$

$$= 21.39 \text{ per thousand.}$$

Standardized Death Rate

When it is required to compare the death rates of two regions or community, heterogeneity factors have to be removed. In the formulae for death rates, the overall population of the region plays a dominant role and, thus, causes heterogeneity. Hence, the population has to be standardized. For this, the population in various categories or groups of one region are taken as standard and death rates are calculated on the basis of this population classification alone.

For calculating the standardized death rate, the death rate of each group, obtained separately for each region, is multiplied by the respective population of the group of the standard region and summed up. This sum is divided by the total population of the standard region. The ratio so obtained is called the standardized death rate. The formula is,

$$S_TDR = \frac{\Sigma_x P_x^s D_x}{\Sigma_x P_x^s} \times 1000 \quad \ldots(20.10)$$

where, P_x^s – Standard population for group x

D_x – Death rate for group x in the original, i.e., SDR for a region.

Σ_x – Summation overall groups.

The comparability of S_TDR provides a logical solution of the problem and the conclusion whether the death rate of one region is lower or higher than the other is valid.

Sometimes one comes across a situation in which the SDR's of a population are not known but the distribution of population in various age groups is known. Hence, standard death rate cannot be calculated. In such a situation, an indirect approach is adopted which provides an approximate S_TDR. In this approach, known age-specific death rates, of a standard population are taken as standard values of age-specific death rates. First, a quantity known as the Index death rate (IDR) of the population is calculated. The formula for index death rate is,

$$A = \frac{\Sigma_x P_x^q D_x}{\Sigma_x P_x^q} \times 1000 \quad \ldots(20.11)$$

where, P_x^q – Population in the region under question for the group *x*.

D_x – Group specific death rate of the standard population.

Also calculate the crude death rate of the standard population. Calculate an adjustment factor A which is obtained by the formula,

$$A = \frac{\text{CDR of standard population}}{\text{IDR}} \quad \ldots(20.12)$$

The approximate standard and death rate of the population under consideration is calculated by the relation.

$$S_TDR = CDR \times A \quad \ldots(20.13)$$

Example: The rate of two districts regions for the year 2001 given in Table 20.2.

The computation of (i) The crude death rate, (ii) age specific death rates for both the districts and, (iii) the standard death rate, taking the population of district A as standard population, is shown below.

i. The crude death rate for district A by formula (20.7) is,

$$CDR = \frac{5,960}{6,16,400} \times 1000 = 9.67‰$$

The crude death rate for district B is,

$$CDR = \frac{4,283}{5,79,291} \times 1000 = 7.39‰$$

ii. Specific death rate for district A by formula (20.8) are,

Age group 0 – 5,

$$SDR = \frac{338}{45,860} \times 1000 = 7.37‰$$

Age group 0 – 15,

$$SDR = \frac{308}{99,120} \times 1000 = 3.11‰$$

Age group 15 – 35,

$$SDR = \frac{602}{1,52,050} \times 1000 = 3.96‰$$

Age group 35 – 50,

$$SDR = \frac{1,827}{1,04,600} \times 1000 = 17.47‰$$

Age group 50 and above

$$SDR = \frac{2,885}{2,14,770} \times 1000 = 13.43‰$$

Similarly, the SDR's for district B are calculated and entered in column 7 alongwith the data.

iii. Computation of standardized death rates has been explicated in Table 20.3.

The standard death rate for the district A, by formula (20.10), is,

$$S_TDR = \frac{59,90,092.5}{6,16,400} = 9.67‰$$

Similarly, for district *B*,

$$S_T DR = \frac{45,70,477.1}{6,16,400} = 7.41‰$$

The standardized dcath rate in district B is less than that in district A. Hence, it can be concluded that the health hazards in district B are less than that in district A.

Measures of Fertility

Fertility rates are the barometer for the increase in population due to births in a specified period, usually a year.

The term *fertility* refers to the actual bearing of children. The term *fecundity* indicates the capacity to bear children. Fecundity is difficulty for measurement. The knowledge of the "rate" of child-bearing in a community, region, state or a country is important to the health planners for providing health facilities and services for mothers, infants and children. The following are the useful measures of fertility:

(i) Crude birth rate, (ii) fertility rate, (iii) sex ratio and (iv) age and sex composition of populations. Details of measures of fertility are provided below.

Table 20.2

Age group (Years)	*District A*		*District B*		*Age SDR Distt. A*	*Age SDR Distt. B*
	Population	*No. of deaths*	*Population*	*No. of deaths*	D_x^a	D_x^b
(1)	*(2)*	*(3)*	*(4)*	*(5)*	*(6)*	*(7)*
0–5	45,860	338	41,169	784	7.37	19.04
5–15	99,120	308	88,163	415	3.11	4.71
15–35	1,52,050	602	1,48,440	724	3.96	4.88
35–50	1,04,600	1,827	1,02,632	977	17.47	9.52
50 and above	2,14,770	2,885	1,98,887	1383	13.43	6.95
Total	6,16,400	5,960	5,79,291	4,283		

Table 20.3

Age group	*Standard Population*	*District A SDR*		*District B SDR*	
	P_x^s	D_x^a	$P_x^s\ D_x^a$	D_x^b	$P_x^s\ D_x^b$
(1)	*(2)*	*(3)*	*(4)*	*(5)*	*(6)*
0–5	45,860	7.37	3,37,988.2	19.04	8,73,174.4
5–15	99,120	3.11	3,08,263.2	4.71	4,66,855.2
15–35	1,52,050	3.96	6,02,118.0	4.88	7,42,004.0
35–50	1,04,600	17.47	18,27,362.0	9.52	9,95,792.0
50 and above	2,14,770	13.47	28,84,361.1	6.95	14,92,651.5
Total	6,16,400		59,60,092.5		45,70,477.1

Crude Birth Rate

It is the most commonly used index of childbirth. The formula is,

Crude birth rate (CBR) =

$$\frac{\text{Number of live births which occurred in a year in a specific area}}{\text{Mid-year population of the area in the same year}} \times 1000$$

For calculation of CBR, mid-year population is considred. The mid-year population is defined as the number of living on first July which takes care of births and deaths from first January to 31st December of the year.

This measure is a crude one because the total population taken as denominator is not exposed to births but only married women are exposed. Natality is also affected by several factors like age and sex composition, socioeconomic status, marriage rates, etc. These are not considered in the definition of the crude birth rate. Also, it excludes the still births.

The crude birth rates in India and other developing countries have been higher than those observed in developed countries like USA, Japan and Sweden.

Example: In a geographical area with a population of 60 million, number of livebirths taken place were 2.4 million in one calendar year 2002. Calculate the crude birth rate:

$$\text{Crude Birth Rate} = \frac{2.4 \text{ million}}{60.0 \text{ million}} \times 1000 = 40$$

Fertility Rates

These rates are related to women in the reproductive period and are better measures of fertility in the population. They are: (a) general fertility rate, (b) general marital fertility rate, (c) age specific fertility rate, (d) total fertility rate, (e) gross reproduction rate, and (f) net reproduction rate. Definitions are as given below:

a. *General fertility rate* =

$$\frac{\text{Number of live births in a year}}{\text{Number of women aged 15-49 years}} \times 1000$$

b. *General marital fertility rate* =

$$\frac{\text{Number of live births in a year}}{\text{Number of married women aged 15-49 years}} \times 1000$$

c. *Age specific fertility rate:* Fertility rates for each specified ages of women are calculated. Age groups like 15–19, 20–24, 25–29, 30–34, 35–39, 40–44 and 45–49 years are chosen.

Age specific fertility rate =

$$\frac{\text{Number of live births in women of specified age}}{\text{Number of women of specified age}} \times 1000$$

d. *Total fertility rate:* If b_i is the number of births to women of age i and p_i is the number of women of age i in the population of a given area and in a given year, then the total fertility rate (TFR) is given by,

$$\left(\frac{b_{15}}{p_{15}} + \frac{b_{16}}{p_{16}} + \ldots + \frac{b_i}{p_i} + \ldots \frac{b_{49}}{p_{49}}\right) \times k$$

$$\sum_{i=15}^{49} \frac{b_i}{p_i} \times k$$

where k is sometimes 1000 and sometimes 1, I = 15, 16 ... 49 years. Obviously, this ratio is the sum of age specific fertility rates over the child-bearing age range of women.

If $k = 1$, this ratio can be roughly interpreted as the number of livebirths to a woman as age passed through the child-bearing age range of 15 to 49 years.

The data in Table 20.4 given the number of births only by 5-year age groups. Let us assume the births in any age group be equally distributed over the 5 ages that constitute the age groups. Thus, the age specific fertility rates are calculated as in the Table 20.4.

Table 20.4

Number of births by the age of mother in a given area and in a given year

Age of the mother (yrs)	*Number of mothers (P_j)*	*Total no. of livebirths (b_j)*	*Age specific fertility rates 5 (b_j/p_j)*
15–19	1,40,000	4,838	5 × 0.0345
20–24	1,09,000	21,656	5 × 0.1980
25–29	80,000	17,829	5 × 0.2230
30–34	81,000	12,413	5 × 0.1530
35–39	79,000	6,161	5 × 0.078
40–44	82,000	1,712	5 × 0.0210
45–49	68,000	322	5 × 0.0047
Total fertility rate	6,39,000	64,931	5 (0.345 + ... + 0.0047) = 3.561

It is easy to see that if the age specific birth rates are calculated for the 7 five-year age groups (15–19, 20–24, 25–29, 30–34, 35–39, 40–44, 45–49), then the total fertility rate would be 5 times the sum of the 7 age specific birth rates. Thus, TFR =

$$5\left(\frac{b_{15-19}}{p_{15-19}}+\frac{b_{20-24}}{p_{20-24}}+...+\frac{b_i}{p_i}+...+\frac{b_{45-49}}{p_{45-49}}\right)\times k$$

$$\text{TFR} = 5\sum_{i\text{-}1}^{7}\frac{b_i}{p_i}\times k$$

k is taken as one.

TFR for the given data is 5 (0.0345 + 0.198 + 0.223 + 0.153 + 0.078 + 0.021 + 0.0047) = 3.561

e. *Gross reproduction rate (GPR):* This is defined as,

$$\text{GRR} = \left[\frac{f_{15}}{p_{15}}+\frac{f_{16}}{p_{16}}+...+\frac{f_i}{p_i}+...+\frac{f_{49}}{p_{49}}\right]$$

Where $k = 1000$ or 1, f_i is the number of female births to women of age i in a given year and p_i is the mid-year population of women of age i in that year. If the data are given by 5-year age groups, then:

$$\text{GRR} = 5\sum_{i=1}^{7}\frac{f_j}{p_i}\times k$$

GRR is about half of the total fertility rate where $k = 1$. GRR gives an idea of the rate at which the female population in the child bearing age range is replaced. If GRR = 2.5, it means that the number of females of child-bearing age group are being replaced by 2.5 times their present number. It is assumed that the sex ratio at birth is 105 males for every 100 females, so that out of 205 births, 100 are female births.

$$\text{GRR} = \text{TFR}\times\frac{100}{205} = 3.561\times\frac{100}{205} = 1.737$$

f. *Net reproduction rate (NRR):* Since, all the females born will not survive to become women in child-bearing age group, it is desirable to apply suitable survival factors in calculating the reproduction rate. For example, out of 1000 females born to women of age group 15–19, only 965 will survive to grow up to the age 15–19, then 0.965 is the corresponding survival factor. In determining the replacement of women in child-bearing age group, the female births should, therefore, be multiplied by appropriate survival factors. If P_{oi} is the chance of survival from birth to age i according to the currently applicable life table for females, the net reproduction rate is given by:

$$\text{GRR} = \sum_{i=1}^{49}\frac{f_i}{p_i}\times p_{oi}\times k \text{ where } k \text{ is either 100}$$

or 1

If the data are by 5-year age groups, then

Table 20.5

Calculation of net reproduction rate (NRR)

S. No.	*Age group (i) (1)*	*Survial factor (P_{oi}) (2)*	*No. of births in age group (i) ÷ No. of mothers (3)*	*(2) × (3)*
1	15–19	0.9694	0.0345	0.0334
2	20–24	0.9698	0.198	0.1914
3	25–29	0.9632	0.223	0.2140
4	30–34	0.9584	0.153	0.1470
5	35–39	0.9519	0.078	0.1940
6	40–44	0.9424	0.021	0.1970
7	45–49	0.9279	0.047	0.0044

$$NRR = 5\sum_{i=1}^{49} \frac{f_i}{p_i} \times p_{oi} \times k$$

where i now denotes 5-year age group and P_{oi} is the survival probability from birth to age group i.

For the given data, we assume that the required survival factors are as given in Table 20.5. Using these, NRR is obtained easily as shown.

$$NRR = 5 \times \frac{100}{205}(0.0334 + 0.1914 + 0.2140 + 0.1470 + 0.0740 + 0.197 + 0.0444) = 1.668$$

Note: The multiplier 100/205 based on sex ratio at birth is used to get the number of female births from the total number of births.

The NRR = 1.668 shows that the female in the child-bearing age group would be replaced by 1.688 or roughly 5/3 times after number, if the existing age specific fertility rates and survival rates continue to operate.

Sex Ratio

This is also an index of fertility. It is defined as,

$$\text{Sex ratio} = \frac{\text{Number of females}}{\text{Number of males}} \times 1000$$

Sex ratio in India is 930 in the year 1991. It varies from state to state in India and country to country in the world. The sex ratio in countries like India is lower than it is observed in developed countries.

This sex ratio at birth is a better index of fertility than the overall sex ratio. It is defined as,

Sex ratio at birth =

$$\frac{\text{Number of female live births}}{\text{Number of male live births}} \times 1000$$

Composition of Population by Age

The proportion of population by age and sex is good indicator of fertility and health. In countries or regions, where there are high fertility rates, the percentage of population below the age of five years or younger ages is higher than that observed in countries or regions where fertility rates are lower. The proportion of population in older age groups of 60 years or above are higher in countries where fertility rates are low. It is also an index of health and nutritional status.

Crude Birth Rate: As an index of the relative speed at which additions are being made to the population through child birth, use is made of the crude birth rate. The formula is:

Annual Crude Birth Rate =

$$\frac{\text{Number of live births which occurred among the population of a given geographic arca during a given year}}{\text{Mid-year total population of the given geographic area during the same year}} \times 1000$$

For example: During 2010, there were a total of 4757 livebirths in a rural area and 3485 in an urban settlement. The estimated mid-year population in these 2 areas were 136303 and 113518 respectively. The *Crude Birth Rates* for the 2 areas will be:

$$\text{Rural} = \frac{4757 \times 1000}{136303} = 34.9$$

$$\text{Urban} = \frac{3485 \times 1000}{113518} = 30.7$$

This rate is a measure influenced by several factors affecting natality in the population, viz. the age and sex composition, marriage rate, economic level, the true fertility, migration, etc. In spite of this limitation, the rate is widely used because of the general availability of the data.

Fertility Rate: The number of births in a population is largely dependent upon the proportion of women of child-bearing age, especially the married women. A more appropriate measure of the fertility of a population is therefore obtained if we relate livebirths to the total women as the reproductive age period, viz. 15–44 years. The rate is known as the General Fertility Rate (GFR) or age-limited livebirth rate, calculated as follows:

General Fertility Rate (GFR) =

$$\frac{\text{Number of live births in one year}}{\text{Number of women in age group 15-44 years}} \times 1000$$

The numerator consists of all livebirths, whether legitimate or illegitimate, and the denominator comprises all women of ages 15–44 years, whether married or unmarried. Since women of child-bearing ages of 15–44 constitute approximately a quarter of the total population, the General Fertility Rate (GFR) is approximately 4 times the Crude Birth Rate.

If only the married women are considered, this rate will be known as the General Marital Fertility Rate (GMFR). Thus,

General Marital Fertility Rate (GMFR) =

$$\frac{\text{Number of live births in one year}}{\text{Number of married women in age group 15-44 years}} \times 1000$$

In some countries, the age-group extends 15–49 years or 10–49 years.

Age-Specific Fertility Rates (ASFR): These take account of the age-sex composition of population and therefore, provide better basis for comparisons of natality. They are useful in analyzing the historical trend of the livebirth rate of various ages. The formula for the age-specific birth rate is:

Annual Livebirth rate Specific for Age of Mother (or Father) =

$$\frac{\text{Number of live births which occurred to mothers (or fathers) of a specified age group of the population of a given geographic area during a given year}}{\text{Mid-year female (or male) population of the specified age group in the given geographic area during the same year}} \times 1000$$

Total Fertility Rate: This is the average number of children that would be born alive to a woman during her lifetime, who would be subjected to age-specific fertility rates of a given year. Thus,

Total Fertility Rate (TFR) = (Sum of all age-specific fertility rates) × (Width of each age-group) ÷ 1000.

Gross Reproduction Rate (GRR): The average number of female livebirths that would be born to a woman during her lifetime who would be subjected to age-specific fertility rates of a given year.

Net Reproduction Rate (NRR): The average number of female livebirths that would be born to a woman who would be subjected to age-specific fertility and mortality rates of a given year.

Illustrations of Mortality Rates

Crude Death Rate: To measure the decrease of population due to death, the rate commonly used is the crude death rate described below:

Crude Death Rate =

$$\frac{\text{Number of deaths which occurred among population of a given geographic area during a given year}}{\text{Mid-year total population of the given geographic area during the same year}} \times 1000$$

Example: During 1982, there were 426 deaths in a town 'A' and 504 deaths in town 'B'. The estimated mid-year populations for 1982 for towns A and B were 34080 and 42711 respectively. The crude death rates will be:

$$\text{Town A} = \frac{426}{34080} \times 1000 = 12.5 \text{ per } 1000.$$

$$\text{Town B} = \frac{504}{42711} \times 1000 = 11.8 \text{ per } 1000.$$

The crude death rate is perhaps the most widely used of any vital rate. This is because it is relatively easy to compute, requiring only total deaths and total population, and it has value as an index to numerous demographic and public health problems. Within broad limits, the crude death rate represents the probability of dying for persons in the population. As such, it can be interpreted in terms of public health since the rate of death is the first approximate measure of the health status of a population.

Care is needed in the use of the crude death rate for inter-area comparisons. Mortality varies with age. The crude rate which masks all age differences may therefore be misleading, if the age-sex structures of the populations being compared are not similar. Populations composed of a high proportion of persons at the older ages, where mortality is higher, will naturally show a higher crude death rate than a 'younger' population. Some deaths escape registration. The degree of under-registration of deaths also greatly influences the value of the rate.

The crude death rate is valid for comparisons for the same area from year to year, since changes in the composition of the population of an area occur rather slowly. If a long-term trend is studied, the effect of population change must be allowed for. Where it is known that the population distributions are approximately similar, or where the crude rate differences are large, as in many international comparisons, the crude rate has value as an index of mortality. It is commonly utilized one without reference to age, sex, region, cause or occupation, etc.

It is defined as,

CDR =

$$\frac{\text{Number of deaths which occurred in a specific area during a given year}}{\text{Mid-year population of the specific area during the same year}} \times 1000$$

$$= \frac{D}{p} \times 1000$$

where D is the number of deaths and p is the mid-year total population of the specific area in a given year.

Crude death rate, varies in India by region. Kerala has the lowest and Uttar Pradesh has the highest death rates.

Specific Death Rate: By themselves, crude death rates are not enough for a detailed study of the mortality conditions in a community. We often need to know more about deaths ocurring in different sections of the population. For instance, people interested in infant or child welfare work, study deaths taking place under 1 year of age or in such age groups as 1–4 years, 5–9 years, etc. Those interested in maternal health, study how many

Table 20.6

Population and deaths by age

Age (years)	*Mid-year estimated population*	*Number of deaths*	*Age-specific death rate per 1000*
Under 5	11,150,000	2,23,946	20.1
5–9	9,560,000	19,998	2.1
10–14	8,710,000	10,339	1.2
15–19	8,530,000	21,472	2.5
20–24	7,710,000	36,124	4.7
25–29	6,160,000	33,096	5.4
30–34	5,190,000	26,600	5.1
35–39	5,060,000	28,364	5.6
40–44	4,490,000	29,503	6.6
45–49	4,000,000	34,082	8.5
50–54	3,390,000	40,465	11.9
55–59	2,740,000	48,533	17.7
60–64	2,290,000		
65–69	1,760,000		
70–74	1,290,000	3,55,602	55.7
75 and above	1,040,000		

deaths occurred among women of child-bearing age. Insurance companies are interested in deaths caused separately by different diseases or injuries. All these require separate classifications of the total number of deaths.

Death rates specific for age, sex, etc., can be calculated in a manner similar to the crude death rate. Computation of age-specific death rates is shown in the following example:

Example: The mid-year estimated population in an area for different age groups and the number of deaths occurring in each of them are given below in Table 20.6:

Specific death rate per 1000 population for age-group under 5 years:

$$= \frac{2,23,946}{11,150,000} \times 1000 = 20.1 \text{ per } 1000$$

Rates computed for the entire life span invariably show high mortality operating at the two ends of life, i.e. among infants and old persons.

Specific Death Rate by Sex: When age-specific death rates are calculated separately for each sex, the mortality is generally at a lower level among females than among males. However, in the reproductive age-groups mortality among women may be higher than for men because of lack of medical care of the mother.

Cause-of-death Rate: Most death rates by cause are computed on total population; the exceptions being the infant mortality rate and some age, sex specific rates. The formula for cause-of-death rate is:

Annual Cause-of-Death Rate =

$$= \frac{\text{Number of deaths from a specified cause which occurred among the population of a given geographic area during a given year}}{\text{Mid-year total population of the given geographic area during the same year}} \times 100,000$$

The numerator of this rate is often small. For this reason the formula uses a multiplying factor of 100,000 rather than the usual 1000 so that the computed rates are not expressed as small decimal fractions.

Example: There were 52 deaths due to diarrheal diseases in Town 'A' during 1982. The estimated mid-year population for 1982 was 34080. Therefore: The death rate due to

Diarrheal diseases =

$$\frac{52 \times 100,000}{34080} = 152.6 \text{ per } 100,000$$

We can calculate cause-of-death rates specific for age and sex as in the example below:

27 of those deaths occurred among children under 10 years, of which 15 were among boys and 12 among girls. The estimated mid-year populations in 1982 for these 2 groups are 6200 and 5700 respectively. Then,

Specific death rates for diarrheal diseases among girls under 10 years = 12 × 100,00/5700 = 210.5 per 100,000.

Infant Mortality Rate: For a health worker, mortality rate among infants is of special significance because it is regarded as one of the most sensitive indexes of health conditions of the general population. It is a sensitive measure of health because a baby in its extrauterine life is suddenly exposed to a multitude of new environmental factors and their reactions are reflected in this rate. Under ideal conditions of social welfare, no baby should die, except possibly the few who are born with serious handicaps such as congenital disabilities or disorders originating in uterine life. The computation of the infant mortality rate on the basis of the population of infants presents difficulty because the infants are usually under-enumerated. Sometimes the estimates of the population by age are not available. For the calculation of this rate the population of infants in the denominator is therefore substituted by the number of livebirths. The formula for its calculations is:

Annual Infant Mortality Rate =

$$\frac{\text{Number of deaths under one year of age which occurred among the population of a given geographic area during a given year}}{\text{Number of live births which occurred among population of the given geographic area during the same year}} \times 100,000$$

Example: The number of livebirths during 1980 in a rural area was 4757. The number of infant deaths during the same year was 543. The infant mortality rate for 1980 would therefore be:

$$\frac{543 \times 1000}{4757} = 114.1 \text{ per } 1000 \text{ livebirths}$$

Comparison of infant mortality rates enables one to locate populations where the rate is high and thus provides indication of the need for special action. For example, in many parts of the world, where the infant mortality rate is computed separately for urban and rural areas, the unequal distribution of health facilities is brought out sharply. But in calculating the rate for urban populations it has to be noted that frequently, owing to better hospital facilities in cities or towns, maternity cases are attracted from the adjoining rural areas. We should therefore exclude all births occurring in urban maternity institutions if the normal place of residence of the mother is outside the area.

The infant mortality rate is studied separately for geographical sub-divisions or for specific population groups. As a matter for fact, it is a problem that needs study and attack on a wider front, and the health worker should consider the effect of such factors as overcrowding, unemployment, social habits and customs, food habits, topography, occupation of parents and illegitimacy.

It is universally true that mortality in the first year of human life is high, higher than at any age except among the very old. In many countries, it is about 20 to 50 times higher than in the age-group 10–15 years.

In all the advanced countries there has been a marked reduction in the infant motality rate during recent years.

Since the infant mortality rate is of special significance in health work, its correct computation and interpretations are important. Errors in the rate arise from wrong use of the definition or under-registration of vital events. For instance, variation in the definition of the terms 'livebirth' and 'fetal death' may produce appreciable differences. Live-born infants who die at birth or very soon after, may fail to be registered as livebirths. On the other hand, by improving the registration of livebirths, a higher figure in the denominator will automatically produce a reduced infant death rate. It has therefore been said that (satistically speaking) it is possible to lower the infant mortality rate even without a reduction in infant deaths.

Neonatal Mortality Rate: Infant mortality is studied in detail by classifying deaths first by the age of the infant. In accordance with the WHO Regulations No. 1, deaths in the first year of life are classified by single days for the first week of life, by weeks up to the fourth, and then by single months up to age 1 year. For deaths occuring under 28 days, a rate called the neonatal mortality rate is calculated:

Annual neonatal mortality rate =

$$= \frac{\text{Number of deaths under 28 days of age which occurred among the population of a given geographic area during a given year}}{\text{Number of live births which occurred among population of the given geographic area during the same year}} \times 1000$$

Post-neonatal mortality rate or late infant mortality rate:

Post neonatal mortality rate (or late infant mortality rate) =

$$= \frac{\text{Deaths of infants of age 28 days to under 1 year}}{\text{Live births minus neonatal deaths}} \times 1000$$

The infant morality rate is then approximately the sum of the neonatal and the postneonatal mortality rates.

Fetal Death Ratio: For international comparability, the WHO Expert Committee on Health Statistics has recommended that fetal death ratio be computed on the basis of livebirths. As the registration of all fetal deaths is incomplete, better figures are obtained if the calculation of this ratio is limited to late fetal deaths (still births). This ratio relates the number of the fetal deaths to the number of livebirths.

Annual late fetal mortality rate =

$$\frac{\text{Number of fetal deaths under 28 or more completed weeks of gestation which occurred among the population of a given geographic area during a given year}}{\text{Number of live births which occurred among population of the given geographic area during the same year}} \times 1000$$

Another name for this ratio is the 'still-birth ratio'.

Example: The number of still-births registered from a rural area during 1980 was 128. During the same year, there were 4757 live-births.

The *Still-Birth Ratio* for 1980 will be:

$$\frac{128 \times 1000}{4757} = 26.9$$

Occassionally another measure defined as the still birth rate is used which is defined as follows:

$$\text{Still-Birth Rate} = \frac{\text{Number of still births which occurred among the population of a given geographic area during a given year}}{\text{Total number of births (live plus still) of the given geographic area during the same year}} \times 1000$$

Thus, for the example given above we can determine the *Still-Birth Rate* as

$$\frac{128 \times 1000}{4885} = 26.2$$

Perinatal Mortality Rate: Many late fetal deaths and early neonatal deaths may be attributed to similar underlying conidtions and it has been suggested that a single rate called the perinatal mortality rate be calculated by combining the deaths in both categories. The idea is to include the period of perinatal existence after the fetus is considered viable (i.e. fetal deaths occuring after 20 or 28 completed weeks of gestation), the duration of labor and the early part of the postnatal life. Some prefer to restrict the postnatal period to under 7 days, others to the neonatal period, i.e. under 28 days. No agreement has yet been reached on these points or on the denominator to be used, i.e. whether it should be only the livebirths or the sum of livebirths and fetal deaths. In setting out the rate of perinatal mortality, the terms should therefore be clearly defined. At its Sixth National Meeting in 1956, the USA Public Health Conference on Records and Statistics proposed this definition of the perinatal mortality rate for general use in analysis of vital records:

Perinatal mortality rate =

$$= \frac{\text{Fetal deaths (20 weeks or more) plus postnatal deaths under 1 week}}{\text{Fetal deaths (20 weeks or more) plus live births}} \times 1000$$

The formula used in WHO publication is as follows:

Perinatal mortality rate =

$$= \frac{\text{Fetal deaths (28 weeks or more) plus deaths under 1 week}}{\text{Live births plus late fetal deaths}} \times 1000$$

Maternal mortality rate: The risk of dying from causes associated with childbirth is measured by the maternal mortality rate. For this purpose, the deaths used in the numerator are those arising from puerperal causes, i.e. deaths falling under the code numbers 630–676 (Deliveries and complications of pregnancy, childbirth and the puerperium) of the International Statistical Classification of Diseases, the Causes of Death, Eight Revision.

The numbers exposed to the risk of dying from puerperal causes are women who have been pregnant during the period. Their number being unknown, the number of livebirths is used as the conventional base for computing comparable maternal mortality rates. The formula is:

Annual maternal mortality rate =

$$= \frac{\text{Number of deaths from puerperal causes which occurred among the female of the population of a given geographic area during a given year}}{\text{Number of live births which occurred among the population of the given geographic area during the same year}} \times 1000$$

The classification and coding of deaths as puerperal deaths vary from one country to another or even within the same country, so we must be cautious in comparing maternal mortality rates for different places.

Age or Sex Specific Death Rate

Death rates vary by age as well as sex. Age specific or sex specific death rates are useful. Studies have shown that death rates are higher in infants, toddlers and women of child-bearing age. The definition for age specific death rate is:

Age specific death rate =

$$= \frac{\text{Number of deaths in the specific age group in a year}}{\text{Mid-year population of the same age group in the same year}} \times 1000$$

Now

a. *Infant mortality rate*: This is a good index of health and nutrition and socio-economic development of a region, country or a community. It is also an index of maternity and child health services, available and utilized.

This definition is,

Infant mortality rate (IMR) =

$$= \frac{\text{Number of deaths undergone year of age in a year}}{\text{Number of live births in year}} \times 1000$$

In India, the IMR is very high. Kerala state has the lowest and Uttar Pradesh state has the highest IMR figures. IMR is lowest in the countries like Japan and Sweden. Many developing countries have very high IMR.

b. *Neonatal mortality rate (NNMR):* It is defined as the ratio of number of deaths up to 28 days of life to the total number of livebirths.

NNMR

$$= \frac{\text{Number of deaths up to 28 days of life}}{\text{Total number of live births}} \times 1000$$

c. *Post neonatal mortality rate (PNNMR):* This is defined as,

PNNMR

$$= \frac{\text{Number of deaths upto 28 days of life up to one year}}{\text{Total number of live births in a year}} \times 1000$$

This mortality is due to environmental and nutritional factors.

d. *Fetal death ratio (FDR):* It is defined as,

FDR

$$= \frac{\text{Number of fetal deaths}}{\text{Number of live births in a year}} \times 1000$$

Statistics of deaths below 28 weeks of gestation are usually not available in many countries. As a result, still-birth rate is of use in place of fetal death ratio. Still-birth rate or late fetal death rate is,

Still-birth rate or late fetal death rate

$$= \frac{\text{Fetal deaths after 28 weeks of gestation}}{\text{Live births + Still births}} \times 1000$$

e. *Perinatal mortality rate (PNMR):* This is defined as,

PNMR =

$$= \frac{\text{(Late fetal deaths after 28 weeks or more gestation) + Deaths under one week}}{\text{Total births (Live births + Still births)}} \times 1000$$

f. *Maternal mortality rate:* This is an important measure based on deaths in mothers due to puerperal or maternal causes. It is as given here.

Maternal mortality rate =

$$= \frac{\text{Number of deaths due to puerperal causes in females}}{\text{Number of live births in a year}} \times 1000$$

Puerperal or maternal deaths include those due to complications of pregnancy, childbirth and puerperium.

g. *Age and specific death rate (ASDR):* This gives the rate for specific age. It is defined as,

FDR

$$= \frac{\text{Number of deaths occuring in a specific age}}{\text{Mid-year population of a specific age}} \times 1000$$

h. *Sex specific death rate:* Death rates can be had specifically for males as well as for females. They are as given.

Male death rate =

$$= \frac{\text{Number of male deaths}}{\text{Mid-year population of males}} \times 1000$$

Female death rate =

$$= \frac{\text{Number of female deaths}}{\text{Mid-year population of females}} \times 1000$$

i. *Age and sex specific death rates* are also available. They indicate rates of risk of mortality for given age and sex. Example is, death rate in women of reproductive age 15–49 years is,

ASDR =

$$= \frac{\text{Number of female deaths due to the age 15-49 years}}{\text{Mid-year female population of age 15-49 years}} \times 1000$$

j. *Cause specific death rates* are also of use. These are calculated for specific diseases like cancer, tetanus or coronary heart disease. These death rates are calculated for the total population. These are useful for comparison between diseases by age/sex/occupation.

k. *Proportional mortality rate (PMR):* This is the ratio of the number of deaths due to a specific cause or in specific age or in specific sex or area to the total number of deaths. This ratio is multiplied by 100. By this, relative importance of factors contributing to the total deaths can be assessed.

PMR =

$$= \frac{\text{Number of deaths in a specific age/sex/region}}{\text{Total number of deaths in a year}} \times 1000$$

Proportional mortality rate in Indian infants and preschool children is higher than in developed countries. This rate together with population composition by age will indicate the inter-relationship between the mortality and fertility. Studies indicated that higher the proportion of population in younger ages, the higher is the mortality they have. This is found true in all Indian states and developing countries.

Example: Calculate the proportional mortality rate in infants and preschool children of two investigations conducted in Kerala and Uttar Pradesh (see on the next page).

PMR = Proportional mortality in age 0-5 years

$$= \frac{\text{Number of deaths in the age 0-5 years}}{\text{Total number of deaths}} \times 100$$

PMR (Proportional mortality rate)

Kerala	Uttar Pradesh
$\frac{30}{120} \times 100 = 25.0\%$	$\frac{65}{150} \times 100 = 43.3\%$

The proportional mortality rate is higher in Uttar Pradesh than in Kerala. Proportional mortality rate and population composition (%) with children below five years are lower in Kerala than in Uttar Pradesh. These proportional mortality rates can be calculated for any age group or separately by sex or any cause or region of country or world.

Population Age Pyramid

An interesting use of bars is made for studying at glance, the age and sex distribution of the population by means of what is called a *population age pyramid.* Age intervals are located on the vertical scale and the corresponding populations or percentages are shown by bars horizontally on either side for the two sexes.

Details of age (years)	*Number of deaths in*		*Percentage of population*	
	Kerala	*Uttar Pradesh*	*Kerala*	*Uttar Pradesh*
0-5	30	65	10.5	16.9
6+	90	85	89.5	83.1
Total	120	150	100.0	100.0

Pie Diagram

In pie diagram, the area of a circle is divided into different sectors, the angles of which are proportional to the percentages of the numbers in each constituent category. Such diagrams are used for comparative purposes, i.e. to study the relative importance of various quantities producing a comparable total figure. Percentage of total hospital admissions by type of disease/sex/age/season are of interest for comparison over years or between countries by pie diagrams.

Measures of Morbidity

The health workers are interested in assessing the health status of the communities through morbidity. Morbidity relates to types and varieties of diseases one faces or experiences affecting the day-to-day activity. Data for the study of the morbidity of a community are not readily available as are the data on births and deaths because of the scarcity of the facilities for registration through hospitals. The two rates most frequently used in the study of diseases in a community are the incidence rate and the prevalence rate. These are useful for initiation of curative and preventive measures for varieties of diseases. Rates which are utilized are:

i. *Incidence rate:* =

$$= \frac{\text{Total number of new cases of a specific disease during year}}{\text{Mid-year population}} \times k$$

Where the value of k depends on the magnitude of the numerator. A base of 1000 is used when convenient, but 100 can be used for the more common diseases, and 10,000 or 100,000 can be used for those which are less common or rare.

ii. *Prevalence rate:* =

$$= \frac{\text{Total number of cases, new or old existing at a point of time}}{\text{Total population at that point of time}} \times k$$

iii. *Period prevalence rate:* This is defined as,

Period prevalence rate

$$= \frac{\text{Number of cases of diseases in the population during a period of time}}{\text{Mid-year population during that period in which cases occurred}} \times k$$

The numerator includes all cases which commenced before the period and continued during the period and new cases observed during the period and continued later.

iv. *Case fatality ratio*

Case fatality ratio rate =

$$= \frac{\text{Total number of deaths due to a specific disease}}{\text{Total number of cases due to the specific disease}} \times k$$

This is useful in determining how well the treatment program for a certain disease is succeeding. The period of time covered is arbitrary. Depending on the nature of disease, it may be taken as a period of several years. It indicates the seriousness of the disease and effectiveness of the treatment.

v. *Secondary attack rate:* This rate measures the occurrence of a contagious disease among susceptible persons who have been exposed to a primary case and is defined as,

$$\frac{\text{Number of additional cases among contacts of primary cases within the maximum incubation period}}{\text{Total number of susceptible contacts}} \times k$$

This is used to measure the spread of infection and is usually applied to closed gropus such as a household or classroom where it can be assumed reasonably that all members were, indeed, contacts.

vi. *Immaturity ratio:* This is defined as,

$$\frac{\text{Number of births under 2500 grams of weight during a year}}{\text{Total number of live births during the year}} \times k$$

Illustrations of Calculations

Example 1: In two villages near Bangalore with a population of 10,000, fifty new cases of cholera occurred in February 2011 and ninety cases occurred in 2012 in the months of July, August and September. Calculate the monthly morbidity rate in 2011 and 2012.

Monthly morbidity rate in 2011

$$= \frac{\text{Number of cases occurred}}{\text{Population}} \times 1000$$

$$= \frac{50}{10,000} \times 1000 = 5.0, \text{i.e.}$$

five cases per 1000 per month.

Monthly morbidity rate in 1992

$$= \frac{\text{Number of cases occurred in these months}}{\text{(Population) Number of months}} \times 1000$$

$$= \frac{90}{10,000} \times \frac{1}{3} \times 1000 = 3.0, \text{ i.e}$$

three per 1000 per month.

There is variation in morbidity rates as observed in 2011 and 2012. This can be due to seasonal variation.

Example 2: The number of deaths due to tuberculosis, kwashiorkor and vitamin A deficiency noted in rural preschool children of two villages in a PHC of 1990 (see on the next page). Calculate the incidence rate of tuberculosis, kwashiorkor and vitamin A.

To determine the incidence rate of any disorder/ disease for any year or month, the fresh cases that occurred in that period, have to be taken into account.

Example 3: Calculate the prevalence rate of B-complex deficiency and iron deficiency anemia observed in a study on pregnant women attending the outpatient department of the Victoria Hospital Bangalore 2012.

Details	Total	Number of cases	
		B-complex deficiency	Iron deficiency
Population	250	15	80

Prevalence rate of B-complex deficiency

$$= \frac{\text{Number with B-complex deficiency}}{\text{Number of subjects surveyed}} \times 1000$$

$$= \frac{15}{250} \times 1000 = 60 \text{ per 1000 pregnant women}$$

Prevalence rate of iron

$$= \frac{\text{Number with iron deficiency anemia}}{\text{Number of subjects surveyed}} \times 1000$$

$$= \frac{80}{250} \times 1000 = 320 \text{ per 1000 pregnant woman}$$

Details	Total	Number of cases with		
		Tuberculosis	Kwashiorkor	Vitamin A deficiency
Population	1500	3	25	54

Incidence rate of Tuberculosis $= \frac{3}{1500} \times 1000 = \frac{30}{15} = 2.0$ per 1000 children

Incidence rate of Kwashiorkor $= \frac{25}{1500} \times 1000 = \frac{50}{3} = 16.7$ per 1000 children

Incidence rate of Vitamin A deficiency $= \frac{54}{1500} \times 1000 = \frac{108}{3} = 36.0$ per 1000 children

Sl.No.	Details	Kwashiorkor	Kwashiorkor with typhoid and cholera	Cholera
1	Number of cases	90	50	150
2	Number of deaths	30	40	75

Prevalence rates are determined for diseases or illness of population who are studied at a point of time.

Example 4: In a group of villages with a population of 1,00,000 there were 4,000 births and 360 infant deaths in the year 1991. 70 infants died in the first 28 days of life and 90 of them died in the first week of life. Still births were 100 in the same year. Calculate the crude birth rate, infant mortality rate, neonatal mortality rate, perinatal mortality rate and post-neonatal mortality rate.

Crude birth rate

$$= \frac{\text{Number of live births in a year}}{\text{Mid-year population}} \times 1000$$

$$= \frac{4000}{1,00,000} \times 1000 = 40.0 \text{ per 1000 population per year}$$

Infant mortality rate

$$= \frac{\text{Number of deaths in the age of less than one year}}{\text{Number of live births}} \times 1000$$

$$= \frac{360}{4000} \times 1000 = 90.0 \text{ per 1000 live births}$$

Perinatal mortality rate

$$= \frac{\text{Number of deaths in the first week of life + Number of still births in a year}}{\text{Number of live births in a year}} \times 1000$$

$$= \frac{90+100}{4000} \times 1000 = \frac{190}{4000} \times 1000$$

$= 47.50$ per 1000 livebirths.

Neonatal mortality rate

$$= \frac{\text{Number of deaths before the age 28 days of life}}{\text{Number of live births}} \times 1000$$

$$= \frac{90}{4000} \times 1000 = 22.5 \text{ per 1000 live births}$$

Post-neonatal mortality rate

$$= \frac{\text{Number of deaths of infants after the age of 28 days and above up to one year}}{\text{Number of live births}} \times 1000$$

$$= \frac{360-90}{4000} \times 1000 = \frac{270}{4}.$$

$= 67.50$ per 1000 livebirths

Infant mortality rate = Neonatal mortality rate + Post neonatal mortality

$= 22.5 + 67.5 = 90.0$ per 1000 livebirths

The figures indicate a high mortality rate in infants of this rural area.

Example 5: Calculate the case fatality rate (CFR) observed in the treatment of diseases of kwashiorkar with and without typhoid and cholera observed in an urban hospital during a year. The details are noted as given above:

CFR = Case fatality rate for a disease

$$= \frac{\text{Number of deaths due to a particular diseases}}{\text{Number of cases of the same disease}} \times 1000$$

CFR for Kwashiorkor is

$$= \frac{30}{90} \times 100 = \frac{300}{9} = 33.3 \text{ percent}$$

CFR for Kwashiorkor with typhoid is

$$= \frac{40}{50} \times 100 = 80.0 \text{ percent}$$

CFR for cholera is

$$= \frac{75}{150} \times 100 = 50.0 \text{ percent}$$

Kwashiorkor with typhoid and cholera to have fatality higher than kwashiorkar.

The CFR is useful to compare the effects of treatments and seriousness of the disease.

Example 6: Calculate the proportional mortality observed in preschool children in two villages of India, Japan and USA as given:

Details	*Number of total deaths*	*Number of deaths in 0–4 years*
India	500	156
USA	80	4
Japan	50	1

Proportional mortality (0–4 years)

$$= \frac{\text{Number of deaths in 0-4 years}}{\text{Total number of deaths}} \times 100$$

Proportional mortality (0–4 years) in India

$$= \frac{156}{500} \times 100 = 31.2 \text{ percent}$$

Proportional mortality (0–4 years) in USA

$$= \frac{4}{80} \times 100 = 5.0 \text{ percent}$$

Proportional mortality (0–4 years) in Japan

$$= \frac{1}{50} \times 100 = 2.0 \text{ percent}$$

Japan and USA have very low proportional mortality rate in preschool children as compared to India.

Example: In a city with a population of 1,00,000 there were 3,500 births and 260 infant deaths in the year 2006, 80 infant died in the first 28 days and 80 of them died in the first week of life, still births were 100 in the same year. Calculate the CBR, IMR, NMR, perinatal mortality rate and postnatal mortality rate.

Crude birth rate (CBR)

$$= \frac{\text{Number of live births in a year}}{\text{Mid-year population}} \times 1000$$

$$= \frac{3500}{1,00,000} \times 1000 = 35$$

Infant mortality rate (IMR)

$$= \frac{\text{Number of deaths in the age of less than one year}}{\text{Number of live births}} \times 1000$$

$$= \frac{260}{3500} \times 1000 = 74.286$$

Perinatal mortality rate (PMR)

$$= \frac{\text{Number of deaths in the first week of life + Number of still births in a year}}{\text{Number of live births in a year}} \times 1000$$

$$= \frac{80+100}{3500} \times 1000 = \frac{180}{3500} \times 1000 = 51.429$$

Neonatal mortality rate (NMR)

$$= \frac{\text{Number of deaths before the age 28 days of life}}{\text{Number of live births}} \times 1000$$

$$= \frac{80}{3500} \times 1000 = 28.858$$

Post-neonatal mortality rate (PNMR)

$$= \frac{\text{Number of deaths of infants after the age of 28 days and above upto one year}}{\text{Number of live births}} \times 1000$$

$$= \frac{260-80}{3500} \times 1000 = \frac{180}{3500} \times 1000 = 51.4$$

The fertility rate may be defined as, "*The number of births to the women of child bearing or reproductive ages as against the total population*".

The rates are expressed per thousand women capable of children bearing. In India's 1981 census, four questions relating to fertility were canvassed. The questions were about the age at marriage, number of surviving children, number of children ever born during the last one year. The last question was canvassed in case of newly married women. Different types of fertility rates are discussed adequately as given below:

1. General fertility rate
2. Age specific fertility rate
3. General marital fertility rate
4. Age specific marital fertility rate
5. Total marital fertility rate
6. Total fertility rate.

General Fertility Rate

This is defined as the number of children born alive per thousand women of child bearing age (in India 15–49 years), in a year and region.
The formula is,

$$\text{GFR}=\frac{\text{No. of live births}}{\text{No. of women of childbearing age}} \quad \ldots(20.14)$$

The fecundity of women in all age groups is not the same. Hence, for the control of population growth, the study of fertility rates of women in various age groups is of special interest. The marital status of women also has an impact on fertility rates. Hence, marital fertility rates and age specific fertility rates should have been studied in detail rather than being confined to the general fertility rate.

Age Specific Fertility Rate

In this, fertility rates are calculated separately for various age groups of females of child bearing age. The number of livebirths to women of a particular age group are taken into account, e.g. 15 to 20, 20 to 25, and so on. Also, the population consists of the total number of females of that group alone. The age specific fertility rate may be defined as, "*The number of children born alive during a year, per thousand women of a particular age group.*"

The formula is,

$$\text{ASFR} = \frac{\text{No. of live births to women in the age group } x \text{ to } (x+c)}{\text{Average no. of women in the age group } x \text{ to } (x+c)} \times 1000 \quad \ldots(20.15)$$

Example: The female population and livebirths with age of mother, in 1979, of a country, are given below. General fertility rates and age specific fertility rates have been calculated.

Age group (years)	*Female population*	*Livebirths*
15 – 19	1,16,410	10,468
20 – 24	1,13,610	16,983
25 – 29	1,02,930	12,522
30 – 34	98,300	7,083
35 – 39	73,920	3,456
40 – 44	62,700	1,140
Total	5,62,870	51,652

The general fertility rate by formula (20.14) is,

$$\text{GFR}=\frac{51,652}{5,62,870}\times 1000 = 91.76‰$$

Age specific fertility rates are calculated by the formula (20.15):

Age group	*ASFR*
15–19	$\frac{10,468}{1,16,410}\times 1000 = 89.92$
20–24	$\frac{16,983}{1,13,610}\times 1000 = 149.48$
25–29	$\frac{12,522}{1,02,930}\times 1000 = 121.65$
30–34	$\frac{7.083}{93,300}\times 1000 = 75.92$
35–39	$\frac{3,456}{73,920}\times 1000 = 46.75$
39–44	$\frac{1,140}{62,700}\times 1000 = 18.18$

The above ASFRs show the maximum fertility rate in the age group 20 to 24 years.

General Marital Fertility Rate

This type of fertility rate is slightly different from the general fertility rate. In General Marital Fertility Rate (GMFR), the population of married women of child bearing age only is considered, whereas in GFR, all women of child bearing age are taken into consideration. The general marital fertility rate, can be defined as, *"The number of children born alive during a year per thousand married women of child bearing age"*.

The formula is,

GMFR

$$= \frac{\text{No. of live births to married women}}{\text{No. of married women of child bearing age}} \times 1000 \quad ...(20.16)$$

As fertility varies in various age groups of married women, it is preferable to calculate the age specific marital fertility rate.

Age Specific Marital Fertility Rate

Fertility rates are considered only for married women of a specific age group. It may be defined 'as, *"The number of children born alive during a given year, per thousand married women of a particular age group"*.

The formula is,

ASMFR

$$= \frac{\text{No. of live births to married women in the age group } x \text{ to } (x+c)}{\text{Average no. of married women in the age group } x \text{ to } (x+c)} \times 1000 \quad ...(20.17)$$

Total Marital Fertility Rate

This rate gives the total number of children that would have been born alive per thousand married women, had the current schedule of age specific marital fertility rates been applicable for the entire child bearing period. It is calculated as the sum of age specific marital fertility rates in the age groups x to $(x + c)$ multiplied by c where c is interval.

The formula for this may be given as,

$$\text{TMFR} = \text{Sum of ASMER} \times c \quad ...(20.18)$$

Total Fertility Rate

In this type of fertility rate all females of reproductive age are considered. It may be as, *"The total number of children that would have been born alive per thousand women, had the current schedule of age specific fertility rates been applicable for the entire child bearing period"*.

It is calculated as the sum of age specific fertility rates in the age group x to $(x + c)$ multiplied by c, where, c is the interval. Thus,

$$\text{TFR} = \text{sum of ASFR} \times c \quad ...(20.19)$$

Example: The following are the fertility rates in Rajasthan (India) in various age groups of women of child bearing age for the census year 1981.

Age group	*Fertility rate*
15 – 19	73
20 – 24	270
25 – 29	290
30 – 34	237
35 – 39	166
40 – 44	93
45 – 49	40

The sum of the fertility rates
$= (73 + 270 + 290 + 237 + 166 + 93 + 40)$
$= 1169$

Class interval, $c = 5$.

Total fertility rate by formula (20.19) is,

TFR = 1169 × 5 = 5,845 per thousand women of child bearing age

= 5.845 per woman of child bearing age

The total fertility rate per woman may be interpreted as the average number of children produced by a woman in her entire child-bearing span of life.

Fertility rates can be worked out for different religions and regions separately to make comparisons. Such comparisons reveal interesting facts, like TFR for Jains is much lower than for Hindus and Muslims. Particularly in India, fertility rates are not very accurate as many sensitive questions on births are not canvassed in case of single, divorced or widowed women. These women might have given birth during the last one year but such births are not recorded in census operations. Women who died in the last year but gave birth are all omitted. All these limitations lead to under-estimation of fertility rates. Anyway, fertility rates presented after any census or obtained for intercensal periods are indicative of broad trends rate than actual levels. Such information is good enough for chalking out family planning operations, population projections, estimation of demand of various commodities, etc.

Life Table

A life table exhibits the numbers living and dying at each age, on the basis of the experience of a cohort. It also gives the probability of dying and living separately. The probability of dying manifests the mortality rate. The life table is mainly based on the assumption that the cohort experiences the age specific mortality in the population under consideration. More so, the deaths are evenly distributed over the whole year. The life table also reveals the expectation of life at any state or age. A life table is essentially a more detailed expression of mortality rates.

Ulpian's life table, consisting of a series of values diminishing with increasing age, came into existence first. But the manner in which it was constructed and its purpose, was uncertain. Valid life tables were developed only at the end of the eighteenth century, for the purpose of life assurance. It was soon realized that the mortality rate is not the same in all age groups. Hence, age specific mortality rates were taken into consideration. Also, the mortality rates were found to differ widely for male and female populations. Hence, life tables are prepared separately for both sexes.

It is almost impossible to predict how long a particular individual will live. In spite of this, the policy makers must be able to assess and describe the health of a nation. For many years life tables were used to serve this purpose.

Life table identifies the death rates experienced by a particular population over a given period of time by following a fictional cohort individuals (usually a group of 100,000) from birth until the last individual in the cohort has died. So, a life table describes the mortality experienced by a group over a specific period of time.

It assumes that we observe 100,000 persons from birth until death and that as they pass through each year of life, the individuals die at the rates experienced by given population in given year. Here, the number 100,000 is chosen to simplify calculations. We will end up with same results to matter which number we choose.

This measure we can use not only for mortality but also for other vital events like natality, reproduction, chances of survival (after treatment, surgery, radiation therapy etc.).

Uses of Life Table

1. Life tables are of maximum utility to actuaries to work out the rate of premium for persons of different age groups.
2. Population projections may be construed by age and sex with the help of life tables. The life table for any specific section of the society can be prepared and used to deduce many conclusions about population growth, specific death rate, etc of that section of society.
3. A life table clearly depicts the distribution of people according to age which is useful for planning in respect of education, employment, availability of persons for labor and military forces, etc.
4. The life table helps to assess the accuracy of census figures, death and birth registrations.
5. The computation of measure of intrinsic natural increase, such as net production rate and the true rate of natural increase, makes use of life tables.

6. It helps to evaluate the impact of family planning on population growth.
7. How far the new scientific inventions, sophisticated medical treatment and better living conditions have increased the span of life can be assessed through life tables.
8. Estimates of migration can also be made from life tables.
9. Useful to analyze the mortality of given population, i.e., to find number of survivors out of 100,000 (or 1000 or 10000) births at any age.
   (a) At the age of 5, to find number of children likely to enter primary school.
   (b) At the age of 15, to find number of women entering fertile period or to find number of adolescents entering into the community.
   (c) At the age of 18, to find number of persons who become eligible for voting and at 58, who become eligible for pension.
10. To compute insurance premium and annuities.
11. Useful to make international comparisons.
12. By modified life table technique we can find the survival rate after treatment in chronic diseases like TB, cancer, after cardiac surgery etc.

So, the main use of life table we can say is like this:

"Expectation of life at birth or expectation of life at age one year (or at any other age) can be calculated by using life table".

Construction of a Life Table

As expressed earlier, life tables depict the mortality vis-à-vis survival rate of cohorts or groups of people. George Barclay has rightly defined it as, *"The life table is a life history, as it diminishes gradually by deaths. The record begins at the birth of each member and continues until all have died."*

A life table usually begins with a population of one lakh people or any other convenient figure like 10,000, 1000, etc. This figure is known as the *radix* of the table. A life table consists of eight columns as expressed below.

1. The age in years = x
2. Persons living at age $x = l_x$
3. Dying between age x and $x + 1 = d_x = l_x - T_{x+1}$
4. Prob. of dying between age x and $x + 1$ = $q_x = \dfrac{d_x}{l_x}$
5. Prob. of surviving between age x and $x + 1$ = $p_x x = 1 - q_x = \dfrac{l_{x+1}}{l_x}$
6. Living between age x and $x + 1 = L_x$ = $\dfrac{l_x + l_{x+1}}{2} = l_x - \dfrac{1}{2}dx$
7. Living above the age $x = T_x = L_x + L_{x+1} + \ldots = L_x + T_{x+1}$
8. Expectation of life at age $x = e^o_x = T_x/l_x$.

Each symbol has been further explicated so that one makes their correct usage.

x – Exact age in years till last birthday.

l_x – the number of survivors at the exact age x out of the initial cohort which is usually taken 1,00,000.

d_x – the number of deaths in the interval x to $(x + 1)$ in the initial cohort. (The interval taken may be more than one year also if desired). It gives the number of those who could celebrate their xth birthday but not the $(x + 1)$th birthday.

q_x – It is the proportion of persons dying between the ages of x and $x + 1$ to the number of persons alive at the age of x, i.e. at the beginning of the interval.

p_x – It gives the proportion of persons surviving upto the end of the interval, i.e. at age $(x + 1)$ years to the number of persons alive at the beginning of the interval, i.e. at age x.

Either a person will die or remain alive.

Therefore, $p_x + q_x = 1$ or $p_x = 1 - q_x$

L_x – The number of persons lived between the age x and $(x + 1)$ in the hypothetical life table stationary population.

T_x – The number of years lived by the cohort after x years of age. In other words, T_x denotes the total future years lived by l_x persons of the cohort who have attained age x.

e_x^o – The average remaining life time. It gives the average number of years a person of age x is likely to survive under the existing mortality rate.

Assumptions Certain assumptions are made while constructing a life table.

They are:

i. There is no effect of immigration on the cohort. It means that the reduction in number of the initial cohort is merely due to deaths.
ii. The deaths occurring in between two consecutive birthdays are evenly distributed.
iii. The deaths recorded for a cohort through any method are correct without any errors and omissions.
iv. The cohort begins with a convenient figure of 1,00,000; 10,000; 1,000; etc. Now a life table is presented to understand its working for live data (Table 20.7).

Single year age returns and number of deaths are obtained from census data. The age returns for each year are converted to the base 1,00,000 and accordingly, the data for mortality are adjusted. Third to eighth columns of the life table are prepared as per the clarifications of the symbols. Table is self-explanatory.

Example: A life table with two years age returns with certain missing values is presented below.

Age (years)	l_x	d_x	p_x	q_x	L_x	T_x	e_x^0
35	9,345	?	?	?	?	1,63819	?
36	9,243	149	?	?	?	?	?

The life table has been completed using the relationship of unknown terms with other terms.

$$d_{35} = 9{,}345 - 9{,}243 = 102 \ (d_x = I_x - I_x + 1)$$

$$q_{35} = \frac{102}{9{,}345} = 0.0109, \ p_{35} = 1 - 0.01091 = 0.9891$$

Table 20.7

Life Table

x(i)	l_x(ii)	d_x (iii)	q_x (iv)	p_x (v)	L_x (vi)	T_x (vii)	e^o_x (viii)
0	1,00,000	9,872	0.09872	0.90128	95,064	57,68,318	57.68
1	90,128	3,939	0.04370	0.95630	88,158	56,73,254	62.95
2	86,189	2,654	0.03079	0.96921	84,862	55,85,096	64.80
3	83,535	2,476	0.02964	0.97036	82,297	55,00,234	65.84
4	81,059	1,772	0.02186	0.97814	80,173	54,17,937	66.84
5	79,287	1,234	0.01556	0.98444	78,670	53,37,764	67.32
6	78,053	987	0.01264	0.98736	77,560	52,59,094	67.38
7	77,066	765	0.00993	0.99007	76,684	51,81,534	67.24
8	76,301	477	0.00625	0.99375	76,062	51,04,850	66.90
9	75,824	462	0.00609	0.99391	75,593	50,28,788	66.32
10	75,362	418	0.00555	0.99445	75,153	49,53,195	65.72
–	–	–	–	–	–	–	–
–	–	–	–	–	–	–	–
–	–	–	–	–	–	–	–
96	371	158	0.42588	0.57412	292	788	2.12
97	267	104	0.38951	0.61049	215	496	1.86
98	210	57	0.27143	0.72857	182	281	1.34
99	181	29	0.16022	0.83978	166	99	0.55

$$q_{36} = \frac{149}{9,243} = 0.0161, p_{36} = 1 - 0.0161 = 0.9832$$

$$L_{35} = 9,345 - \frac{1}{2} \times 102 = 9,294$$

$$L_{36} = 9,243 - \frac{1}{2} \times 149 = 9,168.5$$

$$T_{36} = T_{35} - L_{35} = 1,63,819 - 9,294 = 1,54,525$$

$$e_{35} = \frac{1,63,819}{9,345} = 17.53$$

$$e_{36}^0 = \frac{1,54,525}{9,243} = 16.72$$

Substituting the values of unknown terms, the completed life table is,

Age (years)	l_x	d_x	p_x	q_x	L_x	T_x	e_x^0
35	9,345	102	0.9891	0.0109	9,294	1,63,819	17.53
36	9,243	149	0.9832	0.0161	9168.5	1,54,525	16.72

Measures of Population Growth

The growth of the population of a country or region can be measured by the following methods:

1. Crude rate of natural increase
2. Vital index
3. Gross reproduction rate
4. Net reproduction rate
5. Replacement index.

Crude Rate of Natural Increase

This is the simplest kind of measure of population growth and can easily by obtained by subtracting the crude death rate (CDR) from the crude birth rate (CBR). This is also known as the *crude rate of natural survival.* Symbolically,

The crude rate of natural increase = CBR – CDR.

In case the total number of births and deaths of a country or region for a given year are known, then the annual crude rate of natural increase can be calculated by the formula,

Annual crude rate of natural increase

$$= \frac{\text{Total birth} - \text{Total death}}{\text{Mid year population}} \times 1000 \quad \ldots(20.20)$$

Example: The following are the figures for the year 1982 obtained from the sample registration system under operation in Rajasthan.

Mid-year population = 3,52,72,000

Total births = 1,87,236

Total deaths = 72,299

The annual crude rate of natural increase by formula (20.20) is,

$$= \frac{187236 - 72299}{3,52,72,000} \times 1000 = \frac{114937}{3,52,72,000} \times 1000$$

=3.26 per thousand persons.

Vital Index

This is an index which takes into account the two most vital events, namely, births and deaths. For a specific period and region, the vital index is given by the formula,

$$\text{Vital index} = \frac{\text{Total births}}{\text{Total deaths}} \quad \ldots(20.21)$$

The vital index may be equal to 1 or less than 1 or greater than 1. The value 1 indicates stagnation in population growth. A value greater than 1 throws light on the expected increase in population whereas a value less than 1 is indicative of a decline in the population.

Gross Reproduction Rate

Fertility rates include the birth of children of both the sexes. But the population growth depends mainly on the birth of female children who are the future mothers. Hence, population growth is mainly a function of the fertility rate, restricted to female children. The demographic year book published by United Nations, 1954, has defined Gross reproduction rate (GRR) as, *"The gross reproduction rate indicates the average number of daughters who would be born to a group of girls beginning life together in a population where none died before the upper limit of child bearing age and where the given set of fertility rates was in operation,"*

It S_{ix} is the fertility rate at age x, restricted to the births of the female infants, the function $\sum_{x=0}^{n}$ is called the GRR, where n is the upper child bearing age. GRR is based on the assumptions,

i. There is no mortality of newly born female children till they attain the highest reproductive age. In India this is 49 years.
ii. There are no gains or losses due to migration.
iii. The current fertility rate is maintained till their highest child-bearing age.

In other words, the GRR is the sum of age specific birth rates of women of child-bearing age restricted to female births only. The working formula for GRR may be written as,

$$\text{GRR} = \frac{\begin{array}{c}\text{No. of daughters expected to be born}\\ \text{to 1000 newly born girls under the}\\ \text{current ASFR without mortality}\\ \text{and with no migration}\end{array}}{1000} \quad \ldots(20.22)$$

All GRR may be calculated from the formula,

$$\text{GRR} = \text{TFR} \times \frac{\text{No. of female births}}{\text{Total births}} \quad \ldots(20.23)$$

$$= \text{TFR} \times \frac{B_g}{B} \quad \ldots(20.23.1)$$

GRR is usually given for female births. But male births have an equal role in the reproduction system. Hence, the GRR for males can also be calculated in a like manner.

Example: The demographic year book published by the United Nations (1978–80) gives the following figures for female births and the total number in Sweden for the year 1979.

No. of female births = 46,842
Total births = 96,255

Taking the total fertility rate = 3.6, the gross reproduction rate by the formula (20.23) is,

$$\text{GRR} = 3.6 \times \frac{46842}{96255} = 1.75$$

Net Reproduction Rate

It is clear from the description of gross reproduction rate that is has its significance in relation to the replacement of one generation by the next one. This replacement may be towards increasing the population or decreasing it. But the GRR over-estimates the next generation as the loss due to mortality was ignored and it was assumed that all the newborn female children attain their maximum reproductive age. This made the GRR quite artificial. Of course, other losses like migration, unmarried persons, etc. do affect the next generation. But these factors are not so important as mortality. Hence, by making use of the life table, it is possible to make some allowance for mortality losses and obtain the reproduction rate which is devoid of the losses due to mortality. The net reproduction rate, as defined in the Demographic year book, United Nations, 1954 is, *"The net reproduction rate may be interpreted as the average number of daughters that would be produced by women throughout their life-time if they were exposed at each age to the fertility and mortality rates on which the calculation is based."*

From the above discussion, it is evident that Net reproduction rate (NRR) measures the extent to which the female infants, who continue to survive their maximum reproductive age, can reproduce infants of the same sex. The formula for net reproduction rate is,

$$\text{NRR} = \sum_{\substack{\text{all age}\\ \text{groups}}} \left(\frac{B_g}{P_g} \times S \right) \times \text{class interval of the age group} \quad \ldots(20.24)$$

where, B_g – No. of female infants born to women of specific reproductive age groups.
P_g – No. of women in each specific reproductive age group.
S – Survival rate p_x per woman, which is obtained from the life table.

In brief, vital statistics is mainly concerned with births and deaths. The accountability of births and deaths depends on the effectiveness of the registration system. Incompleteness of registration of births and deaths, in spite of the existing laws, has made it difficult to give a correct picture of fertility and mortality rates. In the absence of such correct and up-to-date information, all other statistical estimates also produce a distorted picture of the present population and population projections. The life table, which depends entirely on the number of deaths, also leads to faulty conclusions due to the lack of accurate data regarding the number of deaths. Anyway, more and more emphasis on the registration system is improving the vital statistics. Whatever vital statistics are available, they provide enough reliable information for planning.

Vital statistics have many aspects. The salient facets are covered in this chapter. For greater details, readers are advised to go through various books and reports on vital statistics.

Terms Used in Population Registration and Health Surveys

- *Sampling:* Sampling is a procedure by which some units of a population, people or things; are selected as representative of the entire population. The objective of sampling is to make some observations or measurements on the individuals or things selected from the population and to conclude or gain knowledge on the whole population. The subgroup selected to represent the population is known as a sample. *Key words:* Sample we observe, population we seek to know.
- *Random sample:* Sample drawn by this method gives every unit in the population an equal chance to be included in the sample. Selection of any unit does not influence the selection of any other unit. Haphazard selection may not lead to a random selection. The sample drawn by a non-random process is termed as non-random sample or purposive sample.
- *Techniques of random sampling:* A number of methods of drawing samples are available to make it more representative sample.
  a. Use of tables of random digits
  b. Shuffling of cards and selecting required number of cards, each card represents a unit selected.
  c. Tossing of a coin and converting it to a random number.
  d. Systematic sampling – starting point by random choice.
- *Pilot study:* In the pilot studies a small sample of the target population is subjected to all the procedures planned in the full scale investigation in order to study the field acceptability and practicability of the methods used, to provide an opportunity for training the field staff in the procedures, to pretest the schedules to be used in the study, to obtain data on the variability existing in the sample, to obtain data on the amount of labor time and resources required to complete the main survey and to develop the final research plan.
- *Protocol:* The aims or objectives and methods of the survey or experiment are described in some detail in a document called protocol. This will contain the details such as the type and number of population or patients included or admitted to the study, the type of observations intended and the method of measuring them and other administrative details specific to the study.
- *Health survey:* A health survey is a planned study to investigate the health characteristics of a population. The health surveys used to measure the prevalence of the diseases, its distribution on various factors and the distribution of the population on particular characteristics, e.g. Breastfeeding practice, contraceptive practices, cholesterol level, nutritional status, etc. It can also examine the demand and utilization of the health care facilities and the role and relationship of one or more factors in the etiology of a disease.
- *Baseline study:* Baseline studies are conducted at the beginning of a program or action plan or activity to measure the status of the target population on the related fields for which intervention is attempted. The baseline data collected through these studies serves as an

initial status from which subsequent changes are measured or evaluated.

- *Longitudinal study:* In longitudinal studies, observations are repeated in the same population over a prolonged period of time by means of follow up examinations/observations. Longitudinal studies are useful to study the natural history of diseases, to identify the risk factors and to estimate the incidence rates.
- *Cross-sectional study:* Cross sectional studies are the simplest form of observational studies and provide the distribution pattern of the disease in the population related to certain variables and provide the information about the disease prevalence.
- *Case-control study:* Case-control studies are basically comparison studies which compare case group and control group on certain factors to highlight the possible association existing between them and the disease under study. It is also used to estimate the risk associated with exposure to certain factors on a particular disease. The study proceeds backwards from effect to cause, i.e. exposure and disease have already occurred when the study is initiated.

  The constituents of case and control groups are to be identified and defined clearly and the groups must be comparable with respect to known confounding factors such as age, sex, social status, etc.
- *Cohort study:* Cohort is a group of things or animals or human beings having the same characteristics followed up for a definite period of time. Cohort studies are another type of analytical studies to provide evidence on the association of diseases with certain factors. They are generally prospective studies, observed over a period of time. The cohort study proceeds forward from cause to effect, i.e. the exposure has occurred and not the disease or the cohorts are identified prior to the appearance of the disease.

  The cohort must be well-defined before the study and include the individuals free from the disease under study.
- *Reliability and Validity:* Reliability and validity are the two desirable characteristics of the procedures or methods to collect the data or the instruments which measure.

  Reliability deals with the performance of the procedures or methods or instruments and is considered as reliable when it gives consistent or similar results on all the occasions when applied more than once on the same unit under similar conditions. It is synonymous to dependability, stability, consistency, predictability. Examples of unreliable measurements are:
  - Patients giving different answers to questions (same or related questions) at history taking, providing different age to different investigators or occasions.
  - Measurement of blood pressure or reading of X-ray films or blood slides—repeated measurements by the same reader of an object provides different readings, measurement by one or more different readers provides different results or readings of the same object.

    Key word: Repeatability.
  - Validity deals with the condition of measurement which is supposed to measure. If the measurement or the data conformed to the true value, then the data collected is called valid.

    Key word: Comparability.
- *Sensitivity and Specificity:* Sensitivity and specificity are two important components of validity. Sensitivity is defined as the ability of a test, a procedure or a measuring instrument to identify correctly all those who have the disease, that is, the true positions. The proportion of true positives correctly identified by a test.

  Specificity is defined as the ability of a test, a procedure or a measuring instrument to identify correctly those who do not have the disease, that is true negatives. The proportion of true negatives correctly identified by a test.
- *Indicators:* Indicators are variables which indicate the given situation or measure the changes. The measures may be direct or indirect. An ideal indicator should be objective, valid, sensitive and specific.

Health indicators are infant mortality rate, child mortality rate, death rate, morbidity rates, etc.

- *House:* Every structure, tent, shelter, etc. is a house irrespective of its use. It may be used for residential or non-residential purposes or both or even may be vacant. Non-residential purposes are "cattle shed", sericulture, shops, etc.
- A household is a group of persons who live together in the same dwelling unit and have their main meals prepared in the same kitchen. They may include both related or unrelated persons. A person who lives alone in a separate housing unit or who as a lodger occupies a separate room or rooms in a part of a housing unit but does not join with any of the other occupants of the housing unit to form a part of that household is termed as one person household. Others are termed as multiperson household.
- *Institutional household:* Institutional household is a group of persons living in schools, orphanages, hospitals, military installations, hotels, boarding houses, mess, penal establishment, etc. If the number of boarders and lodgers exceed five in the above institutions, they are enumerated as institutional households. However, the households of these institutional residential staff living in separate quarters in the same campus are considered as separate households.
- *Normal residents of a household (NR):* The normal residents of a household are those persons who are normally and continuously live in that household. The persons who are on a temporary visit and are likely to go back after some time are not considered as normal residents. The following cases are to be noted as under for population registration:
    i. If the place of residence of a person is different from the place of boarding, he will be treated as a member of the household with whom he resides.
    ii. A resident domestic servant or a paying guest will be considered as a member of the household with whom he resides even though he is not a member of the same family.
    iii. A non resident domestic servant will be considered in his house.
    iv. If any member of the household stays elsewhere in hostel or otherwise for studies or employment or for any other reasons, will not be considered as a member of the parents' household.

    However, for fertility surveys and MCH surveys the husband or wife stays elsewhere or in a separate house will be considered as member of one family and registered in the household along with their children provided they are considered as currently married.

    v. In certain categories of persons who migrate frequently in connection with their occupation, like laborers who move to other villages during harvesting season, laborers hired by contractors who proceed from one work-site to another, etc. their current place of residence will be treated as their place of normal residence.
    vi. A person who may be belonging to a household but was absent from the village for more than a year or absent for less than a year and has no intention of returning to the village within one year is not registered as normal resident.
- *Homeless persons (floating population):* Persons who have slept in the village the previous night but do not belong to any household in the village are termed as homeless persons. But if they continue to reside in the village open space, shades, road-side shelter they are eligible for registration as homeless persons.
- *Temporarily absent (TA):* A normal resident of a household (NR) is classified as temporarily absent if he was absent from the village the previous night and likely to return after few days.
- *Temporarily present (TP) or visitors:* A person is classified as a temporarily present or visitor to a household if he was not considered as

normal resident of any household in the village but has slept in the village the previous night and likely to go back after few days.

- *Ever married (EM):* A person is said to be ever married if she or he has been married at anytime before by any recognized custom or society.
- *Currently married (CM):* A currently married person is one whose marriage whether for the first or any other time, subsists at the time of enumeration with the spouse living. Persons who are recognized by custom or society as married and persons who are living in stable defacto union are also classified as currently married. Persons living apart from their spouses for reasons of employment or second marriage but still regarded as forming a marital union are also classified as currently married.
- *Primary sterility (PS):* A currently married woman in the age group 15–44 years and not practising any family welfare methods is classified as primary sterility if conception has never occurred within a period of five years after marriage.
- *Secondary sterility (SS):* A currently married woman in the age group 15–44 years and not practising any family welfare methods to limit the family is classified as secondary sterility if she failed to conceive within a period of five years from the date of termination of last pregnancy.
- *Early menopause (EM):* It is a state of a woman who regularly menstruates up to the age of 40 years but ceases to menstruate for more than one year in the age group period 40–45 years is considered as early menopause.
- *Widowed person (W):* A widowed person is one whose husband or wife is dead.

Separated or Divorced (S/D): A person who has been separated from his/her wife/husband and is living apart with no intention of living together again or who has been divorced either by decree of a law court or by an accepted social and religious custom but has not remarried is classified as separated or divorced.

- *Never Married (NM):* A person who has never been married at any time before is said to be never married. Very young children also classified under this.
- *Age:* Age of a person is to be recorded in completed years, i.e. age at last birth day. Very often, there is a tendency on the part of the individuals especially in the rural area to state the "years running" rather than "years completed" as age. Before recording, it should be made sure that the "years completed" is ascertained. The age as stated by the person can be taken as correct, however if it is observed that the age stated is obviously wrong, the age has to be estimated by looking at the person or by cross-examination of the person or with reference to important happenings in the past or festivals or by assessing on the basis of the age of the other members of the family.

  For infants, the age may be recorded as "0" as they have not yet completed one year of age. However if it is required by completed months the same may be recorded as 1/12 for completed one month, 2/12 for completed two months and so on.
- *Literate, Illiterate:* A person who can both read and write with understanding in any language is considered as literate irrespective of any formal education received. A person who can neither read nor write or can merely read but cannot write in any language is considered as illiterate. Ability to sign one's name is not adequate to qualify a person as being able to write with understanding. For 1991 Census, all children below 7 years of age are considered as illiterates even though they may be going to school.
- *Educational attainment:* For all literate persons the information on attainment of the educational level may be noted. The highest educational level attained or class actually passed may be recorded. The same analogy will be followed for a person who is still studying.
- *Work, Worker:* Work may be defined as participation in any economically productive activity. One who participates in such activity and contributes to nation's income is called worker.

Such participation may be physical or mental in nature. Work involves not only actual work but also effective supervision and direction of work.

Non-workers are those who have not participated in any kind of work during or part of reference period such as housewives, students, retired and disabled workers, institutional inmates, young children, beggars, and those who do not work at income producing jobs although they may receive income in the form of rents, dividents, royalty, pensions, etc.

Main workers are those who have worked for a period of more than six months and marginal workers are those who have worked for a period of less than six months.

A person may have worked in more than one activity for varying periods during the reference period. The main activity will be dicided by the more time spent on the activity or as indicated by the individual.

The following specific instances will be dealt as given.

A person who normally works but has been absent from work during the reference period on account of illness, holiday, temporary closure, strike, training, etc., must be treated as engaged in the work normally doing. A person who is engaged primarily in household duties such as cooking for the households or performing such household duties or producing or making something only for the domestic consumption of the household and not for sale is considered as non-worker.

A person engaged in full time public or social service activity is considered as a worker and treated accordingly.

- *Economically active population:* Economically active population is defined as those individuals who participate in the production of economic goods and services which contribute to the economic concept of time, income and national income. Workers of the population are considered as economically active population.
- *Urban and rural population:* For census purposes the places are classified as urban area (Towns/Cities) and rural area. The criteria used for classifying urban area are as under:
  1. All places with Municipal Corporations, Municipalities, cantonment boards and notified town area committees.
  2. All other places with
     a. Density of population 400 persons per sq. km. or more.
     b. At least 75 percent of the male working population engaged in non-agricultural activities.
     c. A minimum population of 5000.

  The urban areas with a population of one lakh and above are classified as cities and the rest are towns.

  All other places not classified as urban area are considered as rural area.

Terms Used in Morbidity Surveys

Morbidity: The terms "Illness", "Sickness" and "Morbid Condition" used in the Health Surveys by household interview are usually based on subjective rather than objective criteria and synonymous. They are basically a departure from a state of physical or mental well-being resulting from disease or injury of which the affected individual is aware. It includes not only active or progressive diseases but also impairment, that is, chronic or permanent defects and that are static in nature, resulting from disease injury or congenital malformation. Injury covers all types of damages such as cuts, wounds, hemorrhage, fractures and burns caused by accidents including bites to any part of the body. Disease or injury may not cause any disability necessitating hospitalization, confinement to bed or restricted activity.

However the following cases are excluded:

1. Normal pregnancy, delivery, puerperium and menstruation;
2. Sterilization, insertion of IUD, getting MTP, etc. under Family Planning Program;
3. Handicapped conditions (blindness, deafness, dumbness, impairment of trunk or extremities and disturbance of central nervous system with

symptoms stabilized and fixed). But abortion, natural or accidental will be treated as sickness.

Treatment: A sick person will be considered to have received medical treatment if a doctor is consulted anywhere in OPD of a hospital, PHC, PHU, doctor's chamber, private residence, etc. and obtained medical advice on his disease or injury or hospitalized as indoor patient. The doctor consulted may follow any system of medicine. Hospital may include Government, Private or Nursing Homes.

However self-medication, medical treatment or advice provided by the non-medical person including Health Workers for the diseases not covered under Health Programs are not considered as medical treatment.

Duration of illness: Duration of illness is measured from the date of onset and the date of recovery from illness. These dates are defined on the basis of uniformly applied criteria depending on the type of morbidity statistics under consideration.

Disease: It denotes a disturbance in physical or mental health, this disturbance may not be apparent but discovered only after special investigation.

Injury: It is a condition produced by an external cause such as violence, accident, poisoning or misadventure in applying a diagnostic procedure and included in codes 800-991 of the ICD.

Qualifying Terms Used for Illness

a. *New illness:* Illness commencing during defined period.
b. *Continued illness:* Illness that commensed before the defined period and continued into the defined period.
c. *Acute and chronic illness:* The distinction between acute and chronic illness is in practice based on a variety of criteria such as medical indications, severity, duration, etc. It should be defined clearly.

Normally the term acute illness is used to specify the illness which is having a short and relatively severe condition and the term chronic illness is used to specify the illness which is persisting in nature over a long period of time.

d. *Disabling or incapacitating illness:* The illness which causes any degree of interference with the ability of the patient to continue his ordinary activities.
e. *Non-disabling or non incapacitating illness:* The illness which causes no disability throughout that portion of its duration.

Another way of classifying illness according to medical advice and/or treatment is:

f. *Ill-defined:* The illness which is asymptomatic or undiagnosed complaint included in codes 773, 780-795 of the ICD.
g. *Minor illness:* The illness which is not ill-defined and does not customarily keep the patient in bed (at ages under 65 years) for as much as one day.
h. *Major illness:* The illness which is neither classified as minor nor ill-defined.

- **Impairment:** An impairment is defined as any loss or abnormality of psychological, physiological or anatomical structure or function, e.g. loss of foot, defective vision or mental retardation. An impairment may be visible or invisible, temporary or permanent, progressive or regressive.
- **Disability:** A disability is defined as any restriction or lack or ability to perform an activity in the manner or within the range considered normal for a human being. Disability is the transition of the disease process from impairment to handicap.
- **Handicap:** Handicap is defined as a disadvantage for a given individual resulting from an impairment or a disability that limits or prevents the fulfilment of a role that is normal for that individual.

Concept

Disease-Impairment-Disability-Handicap

Eg: Accident-Disease (disorder)
Loss of foot-Impairment

Cannot walk- Disability
Unemployed- Handicap

- *Handicapped children:* A child is defined as handicapped if it deviates from normal conditions physically, mentally or psychologically. Such children need special care, treatment and education.

Usually the handicapped children are classified into three groups:

i. Physically handicapped children, e.g. Polio, cerebral palsy, heart disease, road accidents burns and injuries.
ii. Mentally handicapped children, e.g. Feeble minded idiots, mental defectives, mental retardation.
iii. Psychologically handicapped children, e.g.

Orphans, maternal deprivation, emotional deprivation, maladjusted children, etc.

- *Congenital malformation:* Congenital disorders are defined as those diseases of births that are substantially determinal before or during birth and which are in principle recognizable in early life. Some of the birth defects like club foot, cleft palate and harelip are detectable obviously at birth and some other defects like congenital dislocation of hip may escape detection until walking commences, i.e. detected at early life. Some defects are classified as major which may require surgical intervention and some are classified as minor that have no functional implications like skin tags in front of the ear.

  In includes anatomical defects and molecular and cellular abnormalities present at birth.

  The term congenital malformation is normally confined to structural defects at birth and the term congenital anomaly is used to include all biochemical, structural and functional disorders present at birth.

- *Infection:* The entry and development or multiplication of an infectious agent in the body of man or animals is called infection. An infection may or may not lead to a disease state.
- *Infectious disease:* A clinically manifested disease of man or animals resulting from an infection is called infectious disease.
- *Contagious disease:* A disease that is transmitted through contact is called contagious disease, e.g. Scabies, trachoma, STD, leprosy.
- *Communicable disease:* An illness due to a specific infectious agent or its toxic products capable of being directly or indirectly transmitted from man to man, animal to animal or from the environment to man or animal is called communicable disease.
- *Incubation period:* Interval between effective exposure to an infectious agent and onset of a related disease is called incubation period. As a general rule, infectious diseases are not communicable during the incubation period with an exception of measles, chicken pox, whooping cough and hepatitis A.
- *Noncommunicable diseases (NCDs):* Noncommunicable diseases include chronic diseases such as cardiovascular, renal, nervous and mental diseases, musculoskeletal conditions such as arthritis and allied diseases, chronic non-specific respiratory diseases such as chronic bronchitis, asthma, permanent results of accidents, senility, blindness, cancer, diabetes, obesity and various other metabolic and degenerative diseases and chronic results of communicable diseases.
- *Latent period:* The term latent period is used in non-infectious diseases as an equivalent to incubation period in infectious diseases. Latent period is defined as the period from disease initiation to disease detection.
- *Epidemic:* Epidemic or outbreak of epidemic is defined as the occurrence in a community or region of a group of illness of similar in nature, clearly in excess of normal expectancy, derived from a common or propagated source, attacking many people in the region at the same time widely diffused and rapidly spreading in other words epidemic disease is a disease of high morbidity which is only occasionally present.

  Key words: Unusual occurrence in excess of expected occurrence.

Endemic: A disease is said to be endemic when it is present in a community at all times relatively at low morbidity without importation from outside. The common endemic diseases are typhoid fever, viral hepatitis, amoebiasis, filariasis, leprosy, tuberculosis, cholera, etc. Sometimes, when conditions are favorable an endemic disease may flare up into an epidemic.

Key words: Constant presence at expected frequency.

- *Persons exposed to risk:* Persons exposed to risk for any particular disease are those who would in the event of their becoming sick be recorded as sick in the context of the particular enquiry. In other words the people who stand a chance of contracting a specified disease.
- *Risk factor:* Risk factors for a disease are attributes or exposure that are significantly associated with the development of that disease.

Carrier: Carrier is an infected person or animal that harbors and transmits pathogenic parasites without showing the usual evidence of infection or symptoms, i.e. does not show clinical evidence of disease but serves as a potential source of infection for others.

In some diseases, either due to inadequate treatment or immune response, the disease agent is not completely eliminated, leading to a carrier state, carriers are less infectious than cases and epidemiologically more dangerous than cases because they escape recognition and continue to infect the population or susceptibles under favorable conditions.

- *Suspect:* A person whose medical history and symptoms suggest that he may have or be developing some communicable disease is called a suspect or suspected case.
- *Surveillance:* Surveillance is defined as the continuous scrutiny of the factors that determine the occurrence and distribution of diseases and other conditions of ill-health. Surveillance is essential for effective control and prevention of diseases. Surveillance programs include collection, analysis, interpretation and distribution of relevant data to detect changes in trend or distribution and initiate investigative or control measures. We have surveillance programs like epidemiological surveillance, nutritional surveillance, demographic surveillance, serological surveillance, etc.
- *Monitoring:* Monitoring is defined as a continuous watchover the performance of an activity or program by analyzing routine indicators to ensure that they are proceeding according to the plan.
- *Eradication:* Termination of all transmission of infection by extermination of the infectious agents through surveillance and containment actions is called eradication.

As on this day small pox is eradicated and the following diseases are amenable to eradication: Measles, diphtheria, polio and guineaworm.

Notification and registration: The term registration is defined as the legal recording with the authorized officials of the occurrence of an event together with certain identifying or descriptive characteristics of the event. For example, we have birth and death registration and marriage registration. On the other hand notification is a mere reporting of events such as sickness to the health officer and certain occupational or industrial diseases to an inspector of factories. The law, making it obligatory on certain people to notify the notifiable diseases, is enacted under Public Health Act. The government may notify from time to time the notifiable diseases.

The notified diseases at present are:

a. Cerebrospinal Fever
b. Chicken Pox
c. Cholera
d. Diphtheria
e. Enteric Group of Fevers
f. Infective Hepatitis
g. Leprosy
h. Measles
i. Plague
j. Poliomyelitis
k. Rabies
l. Small-Pox
m. Tuberculosis

n. Tetanus
o. Whooping Cough

Notifiable diseases may also include non-communicable diseases. List of notifiable diseases may vary from country to country. The reporting can be done by anybody but normally, the community health guides, multipurpose by health workers, attending physicians, head of the family, village leaders, teachers and religious, political and administrative leaders.

- *Cause of death:* The term cause of death is defined as the morbid condition or disease process, abnormality, injury or poisoning leading directly or indirectly to death. Symptoms or modes of dying such as heart failure, respiratory failure, etc. are not considered to be the cause of death.
- *Underlying cause of death:* The underlying cause of death is defined as (a) the disease or injury which initiated the train of morbid events leading directly to death or (b) the circumstances of the accident or violence which produced the fatal injury.
- *Morbidity Rates:*

i. Incidence rate (Spells): The number of spells of sickness which start during a defined period divided by the average number of persons exposed to risk during that period.
ii. Incidence rate (Persons): The number of persons who start at least one spell of sickness during a defined period divided by the average number of persons exposed to risk during that period.
iii. Period prevalence rate (Spells): The number of spells of sickness which are current at some time during a defined period divided by the average number of persons exposed to risk during that period.
iv. Period prevalence rate (Persons): The number of persons who are sick some time during a defined period divided by the average number of persons exposed to risk during that period.
v. Point prevalence rate (Spells): The number of spells of sickness which are current at a given time divided by the number of persons exposed to risk at that time.
vi. Point prevalence rate (Persons): The number of persons who are sick at a given time divided by the number of persons exposed to risk at that time.
vii. Average duration per spell: The total of the entire durations of all spells of sickness ending during a defined period divided by the number of spells ending during that period.
viii. Average duration per sick person: The total of the entire durations of all spells of sickness ending during a defined period divided by the number of persons who experienced at least one spell ending during that period.
ix. Fatality ratio: The number of deaths from a disease recorded during a defined period divided by the number of new cases of that disease recorded during the same period (or related period).
x. Proportion of time lost: The total duration within a defined period of all spells of sickness that occurred wholly or partly within that period divided by the total duration of exposure to risk in the period.
xi. Average duration per person: The total duration within a defined period of all spells of sickness that occurred wholly or partly within that period divided by the average number of persons exposed to risk during the period.
xii. Attack rate: Attack rate is a special incidence rate used when the population is exposed to risk for a limited period of time such as during an epidemic.

Attack rate =

$$\frac{\text{Number of new cases of a specified disease during a specified time interval}}{\text{Total number of people at risk during the same interval}} \times 1000$$

xiii. Secondary attack rate (SAR):

$$SAR = \frac{\text{Number of exposed persons develping the disease within the range of the incubation period}}{\text{Total number of expose/ susceptible contacts}} \times 100$$

Here primary case is excluded from both numerator and denominator. SAR is applicable to infectious diseases only. Identification of susceptibles is a limiting factor of this rate. In such cases all the exposed family members can be considered.

When the primary case is infective over a long period of time as in the case of tuberculosis, the denominator should be number of person-years or person-months of exposure since the duration of the exposure is an important factor in determining the extent of spread.

xiv. Survival rate: Survival rate is the proportion of survivors in a group of patients studied and followed over a definite period say 5 years. It is a method of describing prognosis in certain disease conditions. Survival experience can be used as a yardstick for the assessment of standards of therapy. The survival period is usually reckoned from the date of diagnosis or start of the treatment or completion of treatment.

$$\text{Survival Rate (5 years)} = \frac{\text{Total number of patients alive after 5 years}}{\text{Total number of patients diagnosed or treated}} \times 100$$

xv. Notification rate: This is the number of notifications during a defined period divided by the average number of persons exposed to risk during the same period.

EXERCISES

1. Define vital statistics.
2. What are the areas covered by vital statistics?
3. Why is vital statistics so important in national life?
4. Write short notes on:
   a. Analytical methods of estimation of population.
   b. Sample registration system.
   c. Standardized death rate.
   d. General marital fertility rate.
   e. Life table.
5. Differentiate between the following:
   a. Crude death rate and specific death rate.
   b. Gross and net reproduction rate.
   c. General fertility rate and total fertility rate.
6. a. Define crude and specific death rates. Explain why the mortality situations of two places cannot usually be compared. Describe in this connection, the construction and usefulness of standardized death rates.
   b. Distinguish between crude and specific birth and death rates. How are the two types of rates calculated? What are their uses?

7. Explain the gross and net production rate. Discuss their suitability as measures of fertility.
8. Explain the concepts of crude death rates and standardized death rates. Why is standardization necessary for comparing mortality in different populations.
   How does one select a standard population? What would you choose as the standard population for comparing the mortality levels of Madhya Pradesh and Uttar Pradesh?
9. The population and deaths of two towns, according to age groups, are given below.

Age group	*Town X*		*Town Y*	
	Population	*No. of deaths*	*Population*	*No. of deaths*
Under 5	6,040	216	93,000	904
5–15	12,645	241	1,54,100	523
15–35	13,300	294	1,86,200	618
35–50	4,625	362	81,900	1237
over 50	6,710	463	64,800	1475

   Calculate (i) the crude death rates (ii) standardized death rates taking the population of Town X as standard population and compare their health conditions.
10. Given the following information about a city.

Mid-year population	*Total livebirths*	*Total deaths*
1,96,200	13,071	3,048

   Calculate the crude rate of natural increase.
11. Complete the following incomplete life table.

Age (years)	l_x	d_x	q_x	p_x	L_x	T_x	e^0_x
72	4,412	X	X	X	X	X	X
73	3,724	X	X	X	X	X	X
74	3,201	642	X	X	X	26,567	X

12. From the following figures, calculate the gross and net reproduction rates.

Age group (years)	*No. of female children born to 1,000 women*	*Percent survival rate*
15–19	200	85
20–24	265	80
25–29	300	70
30–34	188	65
35–39	115	60
40–44	42	50
45–49	5	45

13. The following data pertain to the female population and number of livebirths in different age groups of reproductive age. Calculate the general and specific fertility rates.

Age group:	15–19	20–24	25–29	30–34	35–39	40–44	Total
Female population:	29,240	24,565	21,138	18,319	15,661	13,035	1,21,958
No. of livebirths:	2,046	6,313	5,792	4,048	2,380	1,094	21,673

14. Estimate the standard death rate for the following two countries.

Age group (years)	*Death rate per 1,000*		*Standardized population in lakhs*
	Country I	*Country II*	
0 – 4	10.1	5.0	100
5 – 14	1.0	2.0	200
15 – 24	1.4	1.0	190
25 – 34	2.0	1.0	180
35 – 44	3.3	2.0	120
45 – 54	7.0	5.0	100
55 – 64	15.0	12.0	70
65 – 74	40.0	35.0	30
75 and over	120.0	110.0	10

15. From the data given below, calculate the gross reproduction rate, assuming that for the given population, the ratio of female babies to total birth is 48.8%.

Age group (years)	16–20	21–25	26–30	31–35	36–40	41–45	46–50
Fertility rate per 1000 women	19	173	253	201	157	67	9

16. Fill up the blanks in a portion of a life table given below:

Age	l_x	d_x	p_x	q_x	L_x	T_x	e_x^0
4	95,000	500	x	x	x	48,50,300	X
5	400	X	X	X	X	X	X

17. What do you understand by net reproduction rate? Calculate such rate from the following data—

Age group of child bearing females	*No. of female children born to 1,000 women passing through each age group*	*No. of survivors out of each 1,000 female children*
15–20	50	850
20–25	190	800
25–30	450	750
30–35	500	700
35–40	300	650
40–45	100	600
45–50	40	500
15–50	1620	

18. From the data given below, calculate the gross reproduction rate assuming that the ratio of female births to total birth is 49 percent.

Age group:						
16–20	21–25	26–30	31–35	36–40	41–45	46–50
Fertility rate per 1000 women:						
20	170	242	200	167	69	9

19. Which of the two places, for which mortality data are given below, is in your opinion more healthy?

Age group	*Locality A*		*Locality B*	
	Standard population	*Population deaths*	*Local population*	*Population deaths*
Under 5	4,500	135	4,000	144
5 – 15	10,000	40	10,500	63
15 – 65	12,500	75	12,500	81
Above 65	3,000	140	2,000	102
Total	30,000	390	30,000	390

20. Compute the crude and standardized death rates of the two populations A and B item as the following data.

Age group (years)	*A*		*B*	
	Population	*Deaths*	*Population*	*Deaths*
Below 5	15,000	360	40,000	1,000
5 – 30	20,000	400	52,000	1,040
Above 30	10,000	280	8,000	240
Total	45,000	1,040	1,00,000	2,280

Terms Used in Biostatistics

Absolute risk: It is same as Risk: but contrast it with relative risk.

Abstract: A brief descriptions of a completed or proposed study, usually located at the beginning of report or proposal.

Accidental sampling: Selection of most readily available people as study participants, also called as convenient sampling.

Addition rule (of probability): The probability of occurrence of one of two or more mutually exclusive events is the sum of probabilities of their individual occurrence.

Adult literacy rate: Percentage of literates in population of age 15 years and above.

Age standardization: A procedure of adjustment to remove the effect of differences in age composition of the groups to be compared. This increases comparability. The standardization can be done by direct method or by indirect method.

Age-specific death rate: Number of deaths in one year of persons of specified age-group per thousand population of that age-group.

Age-specific fertility rate: Number of live births to the women of particular age-group per 1000 women of that age-group.

Agreement: When two procedures, two observers, or two sites, etc. tend to give same result in same group of subjects, they are said to be in agreement with one another. The extent of agreement is statistically measured by Cohen's kappa for qualitative data and by limits of disagreement for quantitative data.

Aleatory uncertainties: Uncertainties arising from variation in the factors internal to the system such as biological, psychological and environmental: contrast it with epistemic uncertainties.

Alpha error: It is same as Type I error.

Alpha error rate: The probability of Type I error.

Alpha level: It is same as significance level.

Alternative hypothesis: A hypothesis which is accepted by default when the null hypothesis is rejected.

Analysis of variance: The statistical procedure of breaking variance into its components such as within subjects and between subjects. This method is used in regression analysis and various other situations, but more commonly for comparing three or more means.

Analytical study: A study with the objective to delineate the determinants of an outcome, such as etiological factors, and their specific contribution to the outcome.

ANOVA: Acronym for analysis of variance.

ANOVA *F*-test: The criterion used to find statistical significance of difference in means in three or more groups. This is used for several other situations as well.

Antecedent: A characteristic that precedes the outcome. It may or may not be (fully or partially) responsible for the outcome.

APACHE score: Acronym for acute physiology and chronic health evaluation—a scoring system that helps to assess the prognosis in case of critical condition of a patient. This is based on state of consciousness, reflexes, eye movements, blood pressure, etc.

Apgar score: Sum total of (0 to 2) scores assigned to each of heart rate, respiration, muscle tone, skin color and response to stimulation in a newborn. A low score such as less than 4 out of possible 10 is an indication of poor prognosis.

Arithmetic mean: It is same as mean.

Arm of a trial: The case (or test or intervention) is one arm of a trial and the control group (or placebo) is the other arm.

Association: The property of change in one qualitative factor being accompanied by the change in the other. This change can be causal, incidental, or due to a third intervening factor. The association can be full or partial of various degrees, and can be negative or positive.

Attack rate: New spells during a specified time interval (such as the period of an epidemic) as percentage of the total population at risk in the same interval.

Attributable risk: The risk that can be attributed to the presence of a factor. If risk of diabetes in those with both parents diabetic is 0.30 and in those with one parent diabetic is 0.25 (no other difference) then risk attributable to the diabetes in the second parent is 0.30 – 0.25 = 0.05.

Bar diagram: A diagram appropriate for disjoint categories to show the number of subjects or mean or rates by bars of corresponding height.

Bayes' rule: The rule that converts probability of A given B to the inverse probability of B given A. Most common use of this in medicine is in obtaining the probability of disease given signs/symptoms by first obtaining the probability of signs/symptoms given disease, and in obtaining predictivities on the basis of sensitivity and specificity. This calculation requires the prevalence rate of the disease.

Bed occupancy: Percentage of patient-days the beds were occupied in a hospital or nursing home.

Bed-population ratio: Number of beds available per 1000 population, or the average population served by one bed (calculated both ways).

Bell-shaped distribution: It is same as Gaussian distribution.

Beta error: It is same as Type II error.

Beta error rate: The probability of Type II error.

Bias: A systematic error in measurement or observation or in the result: contrast it with random error.

Binary variable: A characteristic that is assessed only as present or absent (or yes/no), such as ascites present or absent. A qualitative variable is mostly binary (in some cases could be polytomous or ordinal) but a quantitative variable can also be made binary by dividing into two categories such systolic BP <140 and >140 mm Hg.

Binomial distribution: A statistical distribution that describes the probabilities of various number of subjects with a characteristic out of total when the chance of one subject being positive is known. If it is known that 30 percent of diabetics have eye problems, the probability that all five randomly selected diabetics will have eye problems is only $(0.30)^5 = 0.0024$, and the probability that 3 will have eye problems and 2 will not is ${}^5C_3\ (0.30)^3\ (0.70)^2 = 0.132$.

Biostatistics: The science dealing with medical and nursing uncertainties—their identification, measurement and control, leading to decision with less error.

Birth interval: The time elapsed between two consecutive births—also called spacing.

Birth rate: Number of live births per year per 1000 population counted at mid-year.

Births averted: Number of births averted due to contraception. This depends on the method of contraception, age at which this was adopted, and the duration of use.

Bivariate analysis: A statistical analysis of data by considering two variables together, such as age and BP, or MI and obesity. One or both variables can be either quantitative or qualitative.

Blinding: When either the experimental subject or the observer or both are kept ignorant about which subject is in the case group and which in the control group in a trial. Another term for the same concept is masking.

Body mass index (BMI): Weight in kg divided by square of height in meters: a measure of obesity in adults. A BMI <20 kg/m^2 is interpreted as lean, 20.0–24.9 as 'normal', 25.0–29.9 as overweight, and >30.0 as obese.

Burden of disease: A composite measure of premature mortality from a disease and morbidity equated to mortality through a weighting system based on age, discounted duration and severity of disease. Premature mortality is assessed in comparison to the mortality in the population with highest life expectancy.

Case: A person or unit of interest possessing a specified characteristic, such as a person with the disease or condition of interest.

Case-fatality rate: The number of cases who die out of those who are suffering from a particular disease. This measures the virulence of the disease. Case-fatality in typhoid is low and high in tetanus. For chronic diseases such as cancers, the case-fatality may be 100 percent but measures such as 5-year survival rate may be better indicators of the virulence of disease.

Case group: The group of subjects that already has the disease or the condition under study.

Case-control study: Investigation of the antecedents in a group of cases and equivalent controls without introducing any intervention. The groups are defined on the basis of presence or absence of disease or any other outcome of interest.

Case-referent study: It is same as case-control study but comparison group here could be a group with some other disease and not necessarily without disease.

Categorical data: All qualitative data are categorical. In addition, quantitative data are also summarize into categories. For example, if you measure smoking index of 300 individuals, the table for reporting these measurements may have categories such as 0, 0.1–4.9, 5.0–9.9 and 10.0+. Some times such categories are used for analysis and inference purposes also.

Cause-effect relationship: Biologically supported dependence of an outcome on an antecedent so that any change in antecedent changes the outcome. See necessary cause and sufficient cause.

Cause-specific rate: The rate obtained when at least the numerator is restricted to a cause (e.g. morbidity or of mortality). Cause-specific death rate is number of deaths due to a cause per thousand population.

Census: A complete count of the population . This is done in India once in ten years—the first year of each decade.

Centile: It is same as percentile.

Central limit theorem: A result that says that as the number of individuals increase in a sample (sample size becomes large), the chance that sample mean follows a Gaussian distribution rapidly increases in almost all practical situations. As a result of this theorem, there is no need to worry about the nonGaussianity of the underlying distribution when the sample size is large.

Central tendency: Among variations, there is still a tendency for a set of values to gather around a central value. Mean, median and mode are measures of central tendency.

Central values: The summary values of data representing the central tendency of the observations. They are mean, median and mode.

Chance: Unknown or too complex to comprehend.

Child mortality rate: Number of deaths of children below five years in one year period per thousand births in the same year.

Child-woman ratio: Number of children less than five years per woman of reproductive phase.

Chi-square test: A versatile statistical procedure that is used to test different types of hypothesis proportions, such as equality, trend and relationship.

Classification: Placing a unit to one of the two or more known classes or categories. Units within each category share some similarity among them.

Class-interval: The categories of grouped data such as 150–169 mg/dL for cholesterol level.

Clinical thresholds (of normal range): A range of values of a quantitative medical measurement in healthy subjects that has least overlap with the values found in diseased subjects so that the chance of misclassification is minimum. But the chance of error remains. For blood pressure, this is 140 mm Hg.

Clinical trial: A medical experiment on human subjects such as to find efficacy of a new regimen.

Clinimetrics: Assigning scores to clinical entities for diagnostic or rating purposes—thus qualities converted to quantities.

Close-ended question: A question for which list of possible answers is already provided.

Cluster: A group of subjects with some commonality—generally those that are available in close proximity.

Cluster random sampling: Dividing the target population into clusters of specified size and select clusters by random method.

Coding: Assigning a numeric to a qualitative characteristic, such as code 1 for hypertension, code 2 for diabetes, code 3 for cancer, etc. Codes are not quantities, and care should be exercised that they are not used as quantities at the time of analysis. These are used only for convenience in data entry.

Coefficient of determination: The percentage of variation in a variable that is explained by one or more of the others: generally obtained in a regression setup.

Coefficient of variation: SD divided by mean. This unit-free measure is used to compare dispersion of one variable with the other, such as dispersion of cholesterol level with dispersion of body temperature.

Cohen's kappa: A measure of agreement in excess of chance between two or more observers or methods used for qualitative data.

Cohort: A clearly defined subject or a group of persons with some common features that are followed for a specific period beginning from a defined common baseline.

Cohort study: A study of cohort for a specified period, generally to observe the outcome of interest.

Collation of data: The process of rearranging the data into intelligible form so that either the conclusions can be easily drawn or analysis can be easily done.

Complete enumeration: Counting or inclusion of all individuals in the target population—opposed to fraction of cases included in a sample.

Concomitant variable: It is same as confounder.

Conditional probability: The probability of occurrence of an event such as disease when some prior information such as signs-symptoms are known: denoted by P(A/B) where after slash (/) sign is what is known a-priori.

Confidence interval: The interval within which a parameter value is expected to lie with a certain confidence levels as could be revealed by repeated samples.

Confidence level: The degree of assurance for an interval to contain the value of a parameter.

Confidence limits: The upper and lower boundaries of a confidence interval.

Confounder: A factor that could be an explanation of the outcome of interest in addition to the factor under study, such as dietary factors when examining relationship between smoking and cervical cancer. Presence of unaccounted confounders decreases the validity of the study.

Confounder bias: Bias due to presence of one or more unaccounted confounders.

Consistency: It is same as reliability.

Contingency table: A table containing the frequency of subjects with different characteristics, which should be mutually exclusive, such as number of subjects with and without disease, and each with a positive or negative test. This table is used to find if one variable is associated with the other or not.

Continuous variable: A variable that can theoretically have infinite number of possible values within a short range. Age is continuous since within 8 and 12, it can be 8.17, 10.874, 9.756 years, etc. Age can be measured in terms of days, hours and minutes, although practically there is no need to do this. BP is a continuous variable but measured in integers for convenience. Parity is not a continuous variable because there is no possibility of it being 2.75 or 1.6.

Control (subject): A person or unit of interest but not possessing the specified characteristic, such as a person not having the disease of interest.

Correlates: Factors that are related in someway to an outcome of interest. They may or may not be contributors to the outcome.

Correlation: The degree or strength of relationship between two quantitative variables. Loosely used for qualitative variables also. For linear relationships, it is measured by correlation coefficient that ranges from –1 to +1. A negative correlation implies that increase in the value of one variable is accompanied by linear decrease in the other, and vice-versa. A positive correlation implies that the two move together in the same direction. A correlation close to zero implies that increase or decrease in one does not linearly affect the other. Correlation coefficient can be close to zero when a strong relationship is present but is nonlinear.

Correlation coefficient: See Pearsonian correlation coefficient. The other types of correlation are Spearman's, multiple, partial, etc.

Couple protection rate: The percentage of eligible couples with one partner sterilized or those using a contraceptive method.

Covariance: A measure of how the product of two variables behave—used in evaluating correlation.

Covariates: It is same as correlates, but generally used in a restrictive sense for quantitative variables only.

Cross-over design: A design that stipulates that same subjects will get the test and the control regimen after a washout period, but the sequence is randomized. Half the subjects get regimen A followed by B, and the 'other half B followed by A.

Cross-product ratio: It is same as odds ratio.

Cross-sectional study: A study with a format that entails eliciting information on the antecedents and the outcomes at the same time. Such a format is poor to investigate cause-effect type of relationship but is good to generate hypotheses. Also, this format is used for descriptive studies.

Cross-tabulation: The process of dividing a group of individuals by two characteristics simultaneously such as distribution of myocardial infarction cases by their lipoprotein(a) and homocysteine levels. In most cases, these levels would be in categories such as 10.0–14.9, 15.0–19.9, etc.

Crude death rate: Total deaths in one year per thousand population: the latter is generally counted at mid-point of the year.

Cumulative frequency: Total number of subjects in a category and its preceding categories: obtained by addition of frequencies in successive categories.

Cumulative relative frequency: Cumulative frequency till a category divided by the total frequency.

Curve: Opposed to straight line, the curve depicts relationship that varies at different values of two variables. For example, one variable may increase for lower values of the other and then decrease for the higher values of the other. The relationship between glomerular filtration rate (GFR) in chronic renal failure cases and plasma creatinine level is expressed by a curve. As creatinine level rises, GFR declines steeply in the beginning and slowly later on.

Curvilinear relationship: The relationship that is depicted by a curve opposed to a line but can be converted to a line through some mathematical transformation.

DALYs: See disability-adjusted life years lost.

Data: A set of observations, generally in numerical format but can be in text format also (plural of datum).

Database: A collection of items of data arranged in a predefined format.

Data entry: The process of entering data onto an input medium for computer analysis.

Death rate: Deaths in one year per thousand population at mid-year. This can be restricted to any specific group, in which case it is called age-specific.

Decile: Nine cutpoints of values of a measurement that divide total subjects into 10 equal groups-each with $n/10$ subjects, after arranging in ascending order.

Degrees of freedom: The number of observations in a dataset that can freely vary once the parameters have been estimated. This concept is used in a chi-square and a *t*-test since their distribution depends on degrees of freedom.

Delphi method: A less scientific but a quick method to arrive at an estimate by consensus among experts. In this method, the responses from a panel of experts are iteratively obtained that are progressively refined by reducing the options in successive rounds.

Demographic cycle: Over a long duration, from high birth and death rates, the changing phases of quick decline in death rate, slow decline in birth rate, and finally both rates settling down to a low level.

Demographic gap: The difference between birth rate and death rate over a long period of time.

Demographic transition: Changes in structure of the population, particularly going from one phase of demographic cycle to the other.

Demography: The study of structure of a population.

Dependency ratio: Number of people who need care (children less than 15 years and old age persons of age 60 years and above) to the people who provide care (of age 15–59 years).

Dependent variable: A variable on the left side of an equation that is sought to be explained by one or more variables on the right side of the equation. The dependent variable is generally the outcome of interest whereas independent variables are the antecedents.

Descriptive study: A study with the objective to delineate the distribution of disease or a health condition in a defined population. It also includes estimation of parameters such as mean and proportion. This does not examine causality or etiology.

Design: The format of collection, compilation and analysis of observations.

Dichotomous variable: It is same as binary variable.

Digit preference: Preference for certain like digits 0 and 5. Then they become predominant in reporting and recording. This is a bias that can affect the conclusion.

Direct standardization: A procedure of adjustment to bring the differential structure of two or more groups to a common (standard) base to increase their comparability: most commonly done for differential age structure that can affect mortality. For this the observed age-specific death rates are used on astandard population and the death rate is thus recomputed.

Disability: Restriction on ability to perform normal activities.

Disability-adjusted life years lost: The loss of years of life due to premature mortality compared to the most healthy population, plus loss of equivalent years of life due to various disabilities of different severity and different duration from morbidities or otherwise. This measures the burden of disease in a population when future years lost are discounted to bring them to their 'value' in the current year.

Disability-free life expectancy: Life expectancy based on duration lived without disease or infirmity.

Disability-adjusted life expectancy: Life expectancy when duration spent in various degree of disability are converted to equivalent healthy years.

Discrete variable: A variable that can take only small number of possible values. Parity for a woman is a discrete variable. Deaths in an area with population 200,000 is theoretically discrete but can be considered continuous for statistical purposes because it can take a large number of possible values.

Disease registry: A special database that contains information about patients diagnosed to have a specific disease of interest such as cancer.

Disease spectrum: Among many types of disease spectra, the one of special epidemiological interest is the proportion of population that is susceptible, proportion that has infection (apparent + inapparent), proportion that has disease, the proportion that has serious form of disease, and the proportion who die. Note that the subsequent proportion is nested in the preceding proportion. Disease spectrum helps to plan the health intervention accordingly.

Disease surveillance: Continuous or sporadic scrutiny of occurrence and spread of a disease to assess trends, and to initiate control measures.

Disease thresholds (of normal range): The range of values of a quantitative medical measurement beyond which there is a considerable risk of presence of disease or occurrence of disease in future. The chance of misclassification remains in this threshold also as in any other such threshold.

Dispersion: The variability or scatteredness of the values of a variable when measured for different subjects or at different times.

Distribution (statistical): The pattern of values when obtained for a large number of subjects. For incubation period of HIV, the distribution would tell how many or what percentage of cases have incubation period between 5 and 6 years, what percentage between 6 and 7, 7 and 8, etc. Thus, the distribution tells what has been the dispersion and where has been the concentration of values.

Doctor-population ratio: Number of qualified doctors per 1000 population, or the average population served by one qualified doctor (calculated both ways).

Dose-response relationship: Any kind of relationship between quantity of dose and the degree of response but generally indicating that higher the dose, higher the response, such as in smoking and lung cancer.

Double blind trial: A trial in which neither the experimental subject nor the assessor knows that the subject has received the test regimen or the control regimen. This removes the possible bias in response and in ascertainment.

Early expanding phase: The phase of demographic cycle when birth rate is high and death rate starts to decline. The difference between birth and death rate increases, and the population starts to expand.

Early neonatal mortality: Deaths from the time of birth to under 7 days of life per 1000 live births.

Effective marriage: Consummation of marriage in the sense that both the partners are leading a conjugal life as husband and wife.

Effectiveness: The extent to which a regimen is effective in meeting its objectives in actual field conditions or routine circumstances—generally measured in percentage. Field trials or post-marketing surveillance is used to evaluate effectiveness of treatment regimens.

Efficacy: The extent to which a regimen is effective in meeting its objectives in ideal conditions—generally measured in percentage. RCTs are used to evaluate efficacy of a new drug.

Efficiency: The frequency of desired outcome per unit of resource inputs such as time, money and manpower. For example, coronary angiography using 4 French catheters may be more efficient procedure than 6 French catheters because of early ambulation without sacrificing the quality of images. Case-control studies are considered more efficient, particularly for rare outcomes, than prospective studies because of lower cost. Campaign against smoking may be more efficient for avoiding deaths or for increasing life-years than treatment of lung cancer patients.

Eligible couple: A couple who is currently married and the wife is in reproductive age.

Empirical science: Science such as medicine that depends on observations and not on theories or theorems.

Empiricism: The system based on observations and evidence, opposed to theories.

Epidemiologic consistency: Consistency among incidence, prevalence, duration of sickness, mortality, etc. These affect each other and the values of various indications should adequately reflect the underlying relationship.

Epidemiology: The study of factors that affect distribution and determinants of disease or a health condition in a human population.

Epistemic uncertainties: Uncertainties arising from limitation of knowledge: contrast it with aleatory uncertainties.

Error: See random error, bias, false positive and false negative.

Ethics: A system of moral values that is concerned with the degree to which research procedures adhere to professional, legal and social obligations to the study participants.

Etiological factor: The characteristic that contributes to the occurrence of disease or a health condition. It may or may not be a causal factor.

Evidence-based medicine: Using evidence as available in literature or in records or in newly generated data for managing patients after proper accounting of risks and benefits.

Evidence-based practice: A practice that involves making clinical decisions on the best available evidence, with an emphasis on evidence from disciplined research.

Exclusion criteria: The set of conditions presence of which will exclude an otherwise eligible subject from the study. Generally these conditions are indicative of severe form of disease or complications that render a subject unsuitable for that research. Exclusion criteria are part of the case definition that delineates the target population. The other part is inclusion criteria.

Exhaustive categories: Categories such that each eligible person will definitely belong to at least one of the categories.

Expectation of life: It is same as life expectancy.

Expectation of life at any age: The estimated years of life remaining of a person of a given age considering the current death pattern.

Expectation of life at birth: The estimated years of life of a person at the time of birth considering the current death pattern.

Experiment: A study on effect of intentionally introduced intervention or alteration of a factor, under controlled conditions.

Experimental design: The structure of an experiment in terms of inclusion and exclusion criteria for subjects, method of allocation of subjects to intervention, details of assessments, their reliability and validity, etc.

Explanatory variable: Same as independent variable.

Exploding a pie: Showing all segments of a pie diagram separated from each other as if it has been exploded.

External validity: The generalisability of results to those subjects that are not included in the study, i.e. the applicability of results to a larger population and not just to the study participants.

False negative: A person with disease classified as without disease. In place of disease any other attribute can also be used.

False positive: A person without disease classified as with disease. In place of disease, any other attribute can also be used.

Family: People who are related by blood or marriage, and live together sharing a kitchen.

Fecundity: The capacity to reproduce.

Fertility: The actual reproductive performance in terms of live births taking place.

Field trial: An experiment on human subjects in a community, such as vitamin A supplementation to children less than 3 years for examining the improvement in their nutrition status.

Fetal loss: See pregnancy wastage.

Follow-up study: Same as prospective study.

Force of mortality: Hazard of death at an instantaneous point of time. In an air accident, the force of mortality is exceedingly high. In home it is very low. The force of mortality in leukemia is high relative to breast cancer.

Frequency: Used in two senses:

1. Rate of occurrence per unit of time (per month or per year, etc.).
2. Number of subjects with a particular characteristic or with values in a particular interval, such as how many have homocysteine level between 10 and 14 µmol/L.

Frequency curve: A smooth curve showing the pattern of frequencies at different levels of a quantitative measurement: a long-term perspective of frequency polygon.

Frequency distribution: A statistical distribution of subjects that says how many cases have different levels of measurement, e.g. how many have DiasBP <70 mm Hg, how many between 70–74, 75–79, etc.

Frequency polygon: A graphic depiction of frequencies in different categories of a quantitative measurement by joining the points corresponding to the frequencies.

***F*-test:** A statistical procedure to test hypothesis on equality of three or more means, and for other setups such as regression.

Garbage-in, garbage-out syndrome: The tendency of poor output or poor outcome when the input or efforts are poor.

Gaussian distribution: Distribution of values of a quantitative variable such that they are symmetric with respect to a middle value with same mean, median and mode, and the frequencies taper-off rapidly in a particular manner on both sides—a bell-shaped distribution.

General fertility rate: Number of live births per 1000 women of reproductive age-group (15–49 years).

Genuine variations: Variations that are natural and cannot be controlled such as biological variations.

Gold standard: In medical assessment, a method, procedure or a measurement with almost 100 percent sensitivity/specificity or 100 percent predictivity: an extremely difficult proposition to achieve. As a compromise, the best available is considered "gold," against which the newer tests are compared.

Goodness of fit: How well the actual observations fit into a specified model. The goodness of fit is generally tested by chi-square method.

Gross reproduction rate: Average number of female live births per woman during her entire reproductive span according to the existing age specific fertility but not adjusted for their mortality.

Grouped data: Values of metric data presented in categories alongwith number of subjects in each category.

Health: Complete physical, social and mental well-being and not merely absence of disease or infirmity.

Health expectancy: It is same as healthy life expectancy.

Health information system: A systematic approach to the generation, compilation, and analysis of health data for effective management of health. The system may have various objectives such as health situation analysis and health program evaluation.

Health policy: Statement of priorities and goals of health improvement, alongwith the strategies regarding the mechanisms to achieve those goals.

Health program evaluation: Assessment of the extent to which the objectives of the program are achieved, and the delineation of the role of different factors in this achievement (or nonachievement).

Health situation analysis: Assessment of the quality and type of health services required to improve the health status of a community.

Health-adjusted life expectancy: It is same as disability-adjusted life expectancy.

Healthy life expectancy: The remaining portion of life at any age that would be spent without any morbidity. Life expectancy at age 40 may be 36 years but healthy life expectancy would be only 33 years if 3 years on average are spent in nonhealthy state as per the current pattern of morbidities.

Herd immunity: When a large percentage of susceptibles such as more than 90% is immunized, the infection feels strangulated as it is not able to find susceptibles in its proximity. Thus the infection fails to spread.

High stationary phase: The phase of demographic cycle when both birth rate and death rate are high. The difference between birth rate and death rate is practically zero and the population is stationary.

Histogram: A diagram showing the number of subjects with values in different intervals by means of contiguous bars: used only for quantitative variables.

Historical cohort: A cohort whose common baseline is in the past, and mostly outcomes too have already occurred. But the format of investigation still is from antecedent to outcome. The past is reconstructed mostly on the basis of records.

Household: Related or unrelated persons living together and sharing a kitchen.

Human development index: A combination of the achievement on (i) education, (ii) income, and (iii) life expectancy at birth: a widely used index to measure social development.

Hypothesis: A statement of belief that is made before the investigation regarding the status of parameters under study, including those that measure relationship.

ICD: International Classification of Diseases that assigns a group and a code to each cause of morbidity, injury, mortality, etc. The objective is to promote uniformity and comparability.

Improvident maternity: Births with parity three or more that are considered avoidable to achieve family welfare objective.

Incidence: The number of cases newly occurring or arising over a defined period of time.

Incidence density: It is same as incidence but now number of new spells are counted instead of persons newly affected. One person can have more than one spell of disease such as diarrhea and angina in a defined period.

Incidence rate: Incidence per unit of time and per unit of population. If incidence of MI in a population of 100,000 adults in six months is 16 cases, the incidence rate is 0.32 per 1000 adults per year. This can also be calculated per person-year or per 100 person-years, etc.

Incident cases: It is same as incidence.

Inclusion criteria: The set of characteristics such as age, disease and severity, which are necessary in a subject to be considered eligible for inclusion in the study. Some of these subjects may become ineligible when exclusion criteria are imposed. The inclusion and exclusion criteria together define the study subject and the target population.

Independent events: If occurrence of one event does not affect the occurrence of the other, they are called independent. Body temperature is generally independent of blood pressure levels but not of heart rate. Occurrence of typhoid is independent of color blindness-none affects the other. Although, in adults, weight does not affect height but they are not independent since height affects weight. Independence is both ways.

Independent variable: A variable on the right side of an equation, which is used as an explanation of the variable on the left side. Independent variables are mostly the antecedent factors that affect or suspected to affect the (dependent) outcome.

Index: A composite of two or more indicators, such BMI for obesity that combines height and weight, and Indrayan's smoking index for duration, quantity, type of smoking, and the time elapsed since quitting by exsmokers.

Index case: An affected person who might affect others also. In the case of infection, the infected person is an index case who can spread the disease. When a new person is infected, he can be an index case for other susceptibles.

Indicator: A single measurement that indicates the existence or magnitude of a condition. Signs-symptoms are indicators of a disease, smoking an indicator of MI risk, and IMR is an indicator of mortality: contrast it with an index, which is obtained by combining two or more indicators.

Indirectly standardized death rate: For age standardization, common age-specific death rates are used on the observed age-structure of two or more groups to recalculate the death rate. Common (called standard) age-specific death rates are chosen by the researcher. Age is the most frequent factor for standardization but similar standardization can be done for any factor. Indirect standardization is used when observed specific rates are unreliable due to small numbers, or are not available.

IndMed: The Indian counterpart of MedLine that includes abstracts from 75 Indian journals that are not covered by MedLine.

Induction: The method of reaching to a generalized conclusion after compiling the individual cases-from particular to general. This is the basic method used in medicine.

Infant mortality rate: The number of infant (a child of age less than one year) deaths in one year per thousand live births in the same year—perhaps the most sensitive single indicator of health for intercountry comparison.

Infectiousness: The property of a disease to be able to infect susceptibles on exposure: but generally used to measure how many can be infected. Measles is a highly infectious disease since an exposed susceptible is very likely to catch the infection.

Infectivity: The proportion actually got infected out of those exposed.

Interaction: A situation where simultaneous presence of two factors affects the outcome either negatively or positively so that the effect is not the same as the sum of their individual effects. It is called antagonism when the interaction effect is negative and called synergism when this is positive. But there could be other interactions that are not classifiable into any of these two groups.

International Classification of Diseases: See ICD.

Inter-observer variability: The variation between observers that occurs when the same measurement on the same subject is taken by different observers. A high inter-observer variability indicates poor reliability of the measurement.

Inter-quartile range: From first quartile value to the third quartile value: thus covering middle 50 percent values.

Interval estimation: The process of assigning a range of values to a parameter within which it is expected to lie.

Intervention study: A study of the impact of an intentionally introduced intervention. Experiments and trials are intervention studies.

Intra-observer variability: The variation that occurs when a measurement is taken repeatedly by the same observer. This indicates poor reliability of that observer.

Inverse probability: The conditional probability of P(B/A) opposed to P(A/B). This concept is often used to find the predictivity P(D+/T+) or P(D–/T–) when sensitivity P(T+/D+) and specificily P(T–/D–) are known.

Late expanding phase: The phase of demographic cycle when birth rate starts to decline and death rate is at a low level. The difference between birth rate and death rate is large and the population continues to expand.

Late neonatal mortality: Death of children of age 7 days to less than 28 days.

Left-skewed distribution: See skewed distribution.

Level of significance: The maximum tolerable probability of Type 1 error that is fixed in advance, such as 5 percent: denoted by α.

Life expectancy: The average number of years a person is expected to live in a given community on the basis of current pattern of mortality. It can be calculated 'at birth' or at any other age. A life expectancy of 36 years at age 40 means that the average life span after the age 40 years is 36 years in that community. Life expectancy is a mortality indicator measured in terms of survival duration.

Life table: A summary of the death and survival pattern of a group of people-generally for the entire population of an area, but can be used for patients of a particular disease also.

Limits of disagreement: A procedure for measuring extent of disagreement between quantitative measurements obtained by two methods, two laboratories, two sites, etc. on the same subjects. These limits are obtained as (mean of differences) ± 2(SD of differences). If these limits are far too wide that can change clinical management, the disagreement is considered beyond clinical tolerance.

Line diagram: A diagram showing the trend by a line.

Linear relationship: A relationship that moves in a line with either positive or negative slope. The essential feature of a linear relationship is that one variable changes exactly by same amount when the other changes by one unit. If systolic BP rises by ½ mm Hg per year of age over the entire adult age from 20 to 59, the relationship is linear in this age-interval. Linearity can include many variables. See multiple linear regression, also curvilinear relationship.

Literacy: Ability to read and write with understanding.

Literacy rate: Percentage of literates in population of age 7 years and above.

Logistic regression: The regression where the dependent variable is binary (or dichotomous). The independent variables may or may not be qualitative. This regression is based on a specific mathematical form, called logistic model, and straightaway gives the value of the odds ratio.

Longitudinal study: A study where the same set of individuals is periodically assessed for one or more defined outcomes.

Low stationary phase: The phase of demographic cycle when both birth rate and death rate are at low level. The difference between birth rate and death rate is nearly zero, and the population is stationary.

McNemar test: A statistical test for comparing differences in proportions when values are derived from paired (nonindependent) groups.

Mann-Whitney test: A nonparametric test for comparing central tendency in two groups: analogs to *t*-test for Gaussian data.

Masking: It is same as blinding.

Matching: Deleberately selecting control subjects that have the same characteristics as the cases except for the disease or the condition under study. In practice only a few characteristics can be matched. Mostly it is one-to-one matching, which is called pair-matching, but sometimes can be group-matching also. In the former, each control is matched with one case. In the latter, one group is matched with the other on average or for the pattern on the whole.

Maternal mortality ratio: Number of maternal deaths (i.e. due to puerperal causes) per thousand live births per year.

Mean: The average.

Measures of central tendency: It is same as central values.

Median: The most middle value obtained after arranging values in increasing or decreasing order: median seeks to divide the group in two halves, each with $n/2$ individuals. Sometimes in practice exactly equal halves are not possible, and they are divided into nearly equal halves.

Medical decision process: The process of taking decisions regarding diagnosis; treating or not treating a patient, what treatment to prescribe, when to stop, etc. after considering the chances of success of various alternatives, and their utility values in term of the likely outcome.

Medical ethics: The discipline that considers individual patient's welfare above every thing else—thus puts restrictions on how research involving human subjects should be done. Sometimes animal experimentation is also included in its domain.

Medical uncertainties: Uncertainties arising from various kinds of variations, lack of knowledge, partial compliance, errors, etc. in medical decision process.

Medically significant: A result that is capable of modifying the management of any aspect of health or disease.

MedLine: An electronic database of citations from more than 4500 medical journals published in different languages in different parts of the world. This is the most useful resource of medical research literature.

Memory lapse: See recall bias.

Meta-analysis: A procedure of combining evidence in different reports on the same aspect. If different trials on the same regimen report varying efficacy, they can be combined to come to a unified conclusion, which may command substantially more confidence than result of any one of the individual trials.

Metric scale: Measurement in terms of numerics such as blood glucose and cholesterol level: contrast it with measurement in terms of attributes such as gender and signs-symptoms. Metric scale gives rise to quantitative data.

Misclassification: Classifying diseased as healthy or nondiseased as diseased. The first could be called missed diagnosis and the second as misdiagnosis. In place of healthy/diseased there could be any other dichotomy.

Misdiagnosis: Diagnosing a person as suffering from a particular disease when he does not have that disease (the person can have any other disease).

Missed diagnosis: Not being able to detect a particular disease in a person when it is present.

Mode: The most commonly occurring value, i.e. a value seen in highest number of subjects.

Model: A simplified version of a complex process. A model could be mathematical, graphical, structural, etc.

Morbidity: Deviation from normal health.

Mortality rate: The number of deaths per thousand live births in one year: can be calculated for specific groups.

Multifactorial etiology: Occurrence of disease depending on multiple factors: hypertension is a univariate disease because the diagnosis depends entirely on BP level, but it has multifactorial etiology since its occurrence depends on hereditary factors, life stress, diet, obesity, etc. Malaria has single factor etiology.

Multiple controls: More than one control subject for each case. In a case-control setup, sometimes it is easier to enroll controls than cases. The reliability of the results can be increased in this situation by enrolling 2 or 3 or even 4 controls per case.

Multiple correlation coefficient: The degree of relationship of one quantitative variable with two or more simultaneously considered quantitative variables.

Multiple linear regression: A regression in which a dependent variable is sought to be explained by linear combination of more than one independent variables: such as regression of systolic BP on age, obesity, and socio-economic status. For one dependent and one independent variable, see simple linear regression.

Multiple regression: A regression that expresses the nature of relationship of one (dependent) variable on two or more of the other (independent) variables. This could be linear or nonlinear.

Multiplication rule (of probability): The probability of joint occurrence of two or more independents events can be obtained by multiplying the probabilities or their individual occurrence.

Multistage random sampling: The process of sampling where a subset is chosen at random from units at different stages. First stage units can be cities, second stage hospitals (within chosen cities), third stage wards (within chosen hospitals), and fourth stage patients (within chosen wards).

Multivariate analysis: A group of statistical procedures that considers several variables together for drawing a conclusion. If the variables are inter-related, as they would be in most situations, the results of multivariate analysis could be very different from separate univariate analyses.

Multivariate setup: A situation where several variables are considered simultaneously.

Mutually exclusive categories: Categories such that one person belongs to only one category, and cannot simultaneously belong to two or more categories.

Mutually exclusive events: The set of events wherein only one can occur at a point of time. Blood group of a patient would either be O, or A, or B or AB. These are mutually exclusive. Signs-symptoms such as pain, diarrhea and vomiting are not mutually exclusive—they can occur together in a patient.

Natural growth rate: The difference between birth rate and death rate in a particular year.

Necessary cause: A cause that must be present to change the outcome. Exposure to an infection is necessary for it to produce the disease such as measles but it is not sufficient since in some cases infection can remain subclinical and may not produce the disease. Hypertension is not a necessary cause of stroke (neither it is sufficient).

Negative association: When presence of one factor is associated with absence of the other, and vice-versa, in more subjects than expected by chance.

Negative correlation: When higher values of one variable are accompanied by lower values of the other, and vice-versa, i.e. the two variables tend to move in quantitatively reverse direction, such as body mass index and lung capacity.

Negative predictivity: Short for 'predictive value of a negative test.' This is the probability that a person with negative test really turns out to be free from the disease. Since a test is used only on suspected cases, the predictivity should be evaluated on the basis of suspected cases only.

Negative trial: A trial that reports that difference between the test and control regimen is not statistically significant.

Neonatal mortality rate: Deaths of neonates (children of age less than 28 days) in one year per thousand live births in the same year.

Net reproduction rate: Average number of female live births per woman during her entire reproductive span according to the existing age-specific fertility and adjusted for mortality of woman.

Nominal scale: Assessment of a characteristic in terms of names only. Blood group has a nominal scale since O, A, B and AS are just names with no order or no grading among them. The other type of scale for qualitative variable is ordinal where grading is present such as hypotensive, normotensive, probably hypertensive and definitely hypertensive.

Nonlinear relationship: A relationship which is characterized by a curve instead of a line. Estrogen level in a woman has a cyclic variation over menstrual periods, and thus the relationship is nonlinear. Many organisms multiply exponentially as the days after exposure pass, and not linearly.

Nonparametric test: A test of hypothesis that does not focus on any parameter such as mean. This does not require Gaussian or any other specific form of distribution of the variable. The usual tests such as *t* and *F* are based on means and require Gaussianity but chi-square is nonpararnetric. Other popular nonparametric tests are Mann-Whitney (or Wilcoxon), Kruskal-Wallis, and Friedman.

Nonresponse: Not being to able to collect full or partial information on subjects once they are included in a study. This can happen due to unrelated death, moving out of the area, left against medical advice, refusal to cooperate, etc.

Nonsampling errors: Opposed to sampling errors, these arise mostly due to lack of planning or due to lack of knowledge. The examples are presence of confounders, nonresponse, partial compliance, biased sample, inadequate measurement, etc.

Nonsense correlation: A correlation between two variables that incidentally occurs because each is related to a third irrelevant variable. Such correlation has no biological piausibility. For example, there is a correlation (negative) between cardiovascular mortality and birth rate in India over the past 30 years.

Normal deviate: The difference of a value from its mean when expressed in SD units, such as LDL cholesterol in a patient being more than 1.25 SD away from the mean in healthy subjects. Normal deviate is 1.25 in this example. Compared to the absolute difference, this deviate gives a more realistic assessment of how far the value is from mean. Generally, same as *z*-score.

Normal distribution: It is same as Gaussian distribution.

Normal level: A level generally seen in healthy individuals. This is not necessarily ideal or optimal: normal level may be different for children than for adults, or different for males than for females, etc.

Normal range: The range of values (of a quantitative medical measurement), which is generally seen in healthy individuals in a population or its specified segment.

Normalization (of variables): Subtracting mean from the value and dividing by the SD: thus making mean = 0 and SD = 1 for normalized values.

Notifiable diseases: Certain communicable diseases that are required to be notified for monitoring according to national and international regulations.

Nuclear family: Man, wife and children.

Null hypothesis: A hypothesis that says that there is no difference, or that asserts the existing knowledge, and is tested for refutation by the study.

Nurse-population ratio: Number of qualified nurses per 1000 population or the average population served by one qualified nurse.

Nurse-patient ratio: Number of patients are assigned to one qualified nurse for taking care in a stipulated hours according to their severity of illness (e.g. ICU 1:1).

Nursing research: Systematic inquiry designed to develop knowledge about issues of importance to the nursing profession.

Observational study: A study based on observation of the natural occurrences (no intervention).

Odds: The chance or frequency of occurrence or presence of a characteristic relative to its nonoccurrence or absence. If the chance of presence is 75 percent, the odds are 3:1.

Odds ratio: The ratio of odds in one group to the other (generally the control group).

Ogive: A line diagram showing cumulative frequencies.

One-sample *t*-test: The statistical criterion used to compare one sample mean with an externally determined mean. There is no second group for comparison.

One-sided alternative: A directional alternative hypothesis in the sense of asserting that the value can be only either more or less than the null value: contrast it with the two-sided alternative.

One-tailed test: While testing equality of two groups, it is sometimes not known before hand that which group could be better (or worse). For example, this happens when a test regimen is being compared with the existing regimen. This requires a two-tailed test. However, while comparing a test regimen with placebo, if there is an assurance that test regimen cannot be worse than placebo, one-tailed test is used.

One-to-one matching: See matching.

One-way classification: The division of subjects by only one characteristic, such as dividing cases of MI by their CPK level.

One-way design: A design for the study that investigates the effect of levels of only one factor. The levels could be two such as presence and absence, or more than two such as none, mild, moderate, and serious, but the factor is single in a one-way design.

Open-ended question: A question whose answer is allowed to be recorded in verbatim as given by the respondent: contrast it with a close-ended question that provides a list of possible answers.

Ordinal scale: A polytomous variable where the categories have defined order, such as severity of disease into mild, moderate, serious and critical. The 'distance' between mild and moderate is undefined. Division of blood group into O, A, B, and AB is polytomous but not ordinal since these blood groups do not have any order—none is better or worse than the other.

Outcome: A disease or a health condition of interest following exposure to antecedents. It may or may not be a result of the antecedents.

Outlier: A value that is far away from the other values. If duration of hospital stay after a cholecystectomy is 2, 3 or 4 days for most patients but happens to be 14 days for one patient because of complications, this value 14 days is an outlier.

Paired sample: The sample on which quantitative or qualitive measurements are made twice to evaluate the change in each subject such as before and after an intervention.

Paired *t*-test: The statistical criterion used to test whether the mean difference in pairs of values is significantly different.

Pair-matching: See matching.

Parallel tests: Using two or more test criteria in 'either/or' setup. A person is considered positive when either criterion is positive. This increases sensitivity but reduces specificity.

Parameter: A summary measure for any characteristic in the target population, such as percentage of cirrhosis patients with high AST, or rate of increase of systolic BP in healthy subjects per year of age. The parameter pertains to the entire population of interest and not to the sample.

Parity: The order of live birth.

Pathogenecity: The ability to produce the clinical manifestation of disease in an infected person. Measles is not only highly infectious but also highly pathogenic—the disease appears in most susceptibles when infected. Generally measured by the percentage of infected who develop the disease.

Pearsonian correlation coefficient: A measure of the degree of linear relationship between two quantitative variables. This ranges from –1 to +1 with zero in between indicating no linear relationship. A negative correlation means that increase in one is accompanied by decrease in the other or vice-versa, whereas a positive correlation means that both increase or decrease together at least to some extent.

Percentiles: Ninetynine cutpoints for the values of a measurement that divide a group of subjects into one hundred segments after arranging in ascending order such that each segment has the same number (n/100) of subjects.

Perinatal mortality rate: Still births (gestation 28 weeks or more) plus deaths within 7 days of life in one year per thousand (live births + still births).

Perinatal mortality ratio: Deaths from 28 weeks of gestation up to 7 days of life per 1000 live births in the same period.

Person-years: The sum total of years observed for different individuals. If one person is followed-up for 3 years, second for 1½ years and third for 2 years, then the person-years of follow-up is 3 + 1½ + 2 = 6½ years. Similarly, there could be person-weeks or person-months.

Phases of a trial: An RCT is generally the last phase of a trial when dosing and side-effects of the new regimen are fairly well determined. In phase I, the maximum tolerated dose and pharmacological properties are determined by a trial on a group of volunteers. The objectives of phase II are to establish clinical efficacy: incidence of side-effects, identify a dose schedule, and to collect further pharmacological data, Phase III is an RCT that is done on diverse patients after achieving success in the first two phases.

Physical quality of life index (PQLI): A combination of (i) infant mortality rate, (ii) expectation of life at one year, and (iii) literacy rate. This is supposed to adequately assess the physical aspects of quality of life at community level.

Pie diagram: A diagram showing the proportion of subjects in different groups or with different mutually exclusive characteristics by means of a segment of a circular pie.

Pilot study: A small-scale forerunner study to learn about the situation and the variables.

Placebo: An inert substance or a procedure that is neither harmful nor beneficial. The objective of placebo is that the subject gets the perception that he is receiving treatment-thus removing perception bias in trials.

Point estimate: Estimate of a parameter by a single value, opposed to an interval.

Polygon: It is same as frequency polygon.

Polytomous variable: A characteristic divided into three or more categories, such as severity of disease into mild, moderate, serious and critical, or site of injury as limbs, trunk, head, etc. A quantitative measurement such as cholesterol level can be made polytomous when divided into a small number of categories such as <100, 100–179, 180–249 and 250+ mg/dL.

Population: Statistically the totality of individuals or units of interest. There could be a 'Population' of blood samples collected in a year. If the interest is restricted to only suspected cases of liver diseases; the population comprises blood samples of such cases only. If the interest is further restricted to the cases attending OPD in a group of hospitals, the population is also accordingly restricted.

Population attributable risk: The risk in the total population minus the risk in unexposed subjects. This measures the impact on the population of eliminating that exposure.

Population dynamics: The changing scenario of the structure of population.

Population pyramid: A typical graphical presentation of the age-gender and structure of a population.

Positive association: When presence of one factor is associated with presence of the other, and absence with absence, in more subjects than expected by chance.

Positive correlation: When higher values of one variable are accompanied by higher values of the other and lower values with lower, i.e. they tend to move in the same direction.

Positive health: The ability to withstand the pressure of adverse situations.

Positive predictivity: Short for 'predictive value of a positive test'. This is the probability that a person with positive test really turns out to be suffering from the disease. Depends heavily on the prevalence of the disease. Since a test is used only on suspected cases, the predictivity should be evaluated on the basis of suspected cases only.

Posterior probability: See prior probability.

Post-marketing surveillance: Keeping a watch on outcome and side-effects of a formulation after it is introduced into the market.

Postneonatal mortality rate: Deaths from 28 days to less than 365 days of life per 1000 live births in the same period.

Post-test probability: The probability of occurrence of an event such as disease after the test results are available. See prior probability.

Poverty line: Minimum income required for essential food, clothing and housing.

Power: The probability that a study or a trial will be able to detect a specified difference. This is calculated as 1–Probability of Type II error—i.e. the probability of correctly concluding that a difference exists when it is indeed present. This measures the ability to demonstrate an association when one really exists.

Precision: Same as reliability but measured statistically as inverse of the variance.

Predictive validity (of a test): The average of the positive predictivity and negative predictivity of a test. This can be used as a combined measure of the two types of predictivities when both are equally important for the disease of interest.

Predictivity (of a test): See positive predictivity and negative predictivity.

Pregnancy wastage: Termination of pregnancy into abortion, miscarriage or still birth. Also called fetal loss.

Pretest probability: The probability of occurrence or presence of an event such as disease before the test results are available: generally the same as prevalence rate in the specified group: contrast it with post-test probability. See also prior probability.

Pretesting: Checking the workability, adequacy, reliability, etc. of a tool before using it for actual study. The tool could be an instrument, a laboratory procedure, a questionnaire, or any other.

Prevalence: The number of cases of interest present or existing at any specific time, usually at the time of the survey.

Prevalence rate: Prevalence per unit of population or per unit of susceptibles, such as percent, per thousand and per million. Note that prevalence rate is not a 'rate' as it does not signify frequency of occurrence—it is only a proportion. Conventionally, but wrongly, it is called a rate.

Prevalence ratio: Ratio of prevalence rate in one group to the other.

Prevalent cases: It is same as prevalence.

Primary data: Data that are directly collected from the respondents, opposed to secondary data that already exist in records, reports, articles, etc.

Prior probability: The chance of presence or occurrence of an event such as disease or death in a patient when nothing is known about the condition of the patient. Once something such as signs-symptoms-measurements are known, the diagnosis becomes substantially more focused and the probability changes. The latter is called the posterior probability. When further information becomes available, this posterior becomes prior probability and the new probability based on the fresh information becomes posterior.

Probability: A measure of belief in occurrence of an event or presence of a characteristic. This can be obtained either on the basis of theoretical considerations such as 1/6 for each of the 6 faces of a dice, on the basis of experience, or on the basis of frequency of occurrence out of total occurrences, but for latter the total occurrences must be very large. Probability is the degree of certainty of occurrence of an event on a 0 to 1 scale. Probability of death is 1 for all individuals but the probability of death of a pancreatic cancer case within 5 years of detection could be 0.6.

Proforma: A prototype or a sample of a format on which the observations are to be recorded.

Prophylactic trial: An experiment on a prophylactic measure such as prophylactic amnioinfusion for meconium-stained amniotic fluid at the lime of childbirth, or in the field such as iron supplementation to adolescent girls.

Proportion: The measure of how big is the part of a whole. The whole is considered as one. If 20 percent of a population have blood group A, the proportion is 0.20 or 1/5.

Proportional mortality: Deaths due to a cause or in any specific age-group as a fraction of the total deaths.

Prospective study: A study that investigates outcomes for known antecedents. The follow-up of subjects is inherent in this kind of study since the occurrence of outcome can take time.

Protocol: A comprehensive but concise statement regarding steps to be taken—the plan of a study.

Proximal measures: Measurements directly on outcome: contrast it with distal measures. Impact of vitamin A supplementation to children below three years can be measured proximally by rise in retinol level. In contrast, distally, the impact can be measured by growth pattern. Research results many times depend on appropriate choice of proximal measures for the outcome of interest around the world.

PubMed: An extension of MedLine database of articles published in selected journals around the world.

Purposive sampling: Nonrandom sampling to include subjects that serve the specific purpose, such as volunteers in phase I of clinical trials.

***P*-value:** The probability of Type I error, i.e. the chance that a difference or association is concluded when actually there is none.

Qualitative data: Set of observations on qualitative characteristics of individuals such as signs and symptoms. These can be nominal or ordinal. The only real summary measure for qualitative data, proportion of subjects with a specified characteristic, although for some ordinal data , scores can be assigned that can be treated as numerics.

Qualitative variable: A characteristic that is assessed in tenms of attributes such as gender and degree of severity of disease: a variable that yields qualitative data.

Quality of life: An assessment of the extent to which individual and social aspirations are met with regard to facilities and opportunities in life.

Quantitative data: Set of observations on characteristics that could be numerically expressed for an individual such as Hb level, BP and blood glucose level. Most common summary measures for quantitative data are mean and SD.

Quantitative variable: A characteristic that is measured in terms of numerics, such as creatinine level and parity of a woman: a variable that yields quantitative data.

Quartiles: Three cutpoints for values of a measurement that divide a group in four equal parts with regard to number of subjects, after the values are arranged in ascending order.

Questionnaire: A survey instrument that contains a predetermined series of questions that are supposed to put in verbatim to the respondents, or can be self-adrninistered. It contains space for recording responses also.

Random: Unpredictable, like lottery—generally when each unit has same chance of being picked up.

Random allocation: It is same as randomization.

Random error: An error that has no bias, and which is natural to occur in observations because biological or other variation beyond control. These errors are small, and some are positive, some negative so that the average is close to zero.

Random sampling: Sampling in a manner that the selection cannot be predicted. The chances of selection of various units can be equal or unequal. The popular methods of random sampling are simple systematic, stratified, cluster, and multistage.

Randomization: Allocation of subjects to different groups in a random manner. The objective is that unaccounted factors are almost equally distributed among groups, and there is no bias on this court.

Randomized controlled trial: A trial where there is a control group (in addition to the test group) and the allocation of subjects to the control and test groups is by random method. This is considered to be the ideal methodology to evaluate efficacy of a new regimen particularly when it is double-blind.

Range: From minimum value or a measurement to the maximum value.

Rate: The frequency with which events occur, such as deaths per year or new cases per month. Time is a ingredient of a rate. Generally measured per unit of population such as percent, per thousand and per million.

Ratio: Strength or magnitude or number of one quantity relative to the other, such as sex ratio and albumin globulin ratio.

RCT: Short for randomized controlled trial.

Recall bias: Not being able to recall events occurring far away in the past with the same frequency as those occurring recently. This introduces bias in favor of recent occurrences. Also occurs when disease cases are able to recall because of their current suffering but controls fail to recall as much.

Record linkage: A method to trace the same patient or subject appearing in various hospitals, clinics, registries, etc. so as to build up a more comprehensive record.

Reference population: Same as target population.

Reference values: Same as normal levels.

Regression coefficient: The quantity that delineates the average change in dependent variable for one unit change in independent variable. If regression coefficient of birth weight (in g) on maternal Hb level is +60, it means that birth weight increases on average by 60 g for each 1g/dL increase in maternal Hb level.

Regression equation: The nature of relationship of one characteristic with one or more of others, generally expressed as a mathematical equation that best fits the data.

Regression line: Graphical representation of linear regression.

Regressor: Same as independent variable.

Relationship: The phenomenon of change in one quantitative characteristic when the other changes. This change can be causal, incidental, or due to a third intervening variable.

Relative frequency: Frequency in a category divided by the total cases: the proportion of cases in a particular category.

Relative risk: Risk of occurrence of an outcome in the presence of one factor (exposure) relative to the risk in the presence of another (generally control, which means absence) factor.

Relative risk reduction: Reduction in absolute risk after an intervention as percentage of the risk in exposed group.

Reliability: Ability to repeat the performance. The performance could be poor but same performance every time means good reliability. Statistically, this means smaller variance in repeated measurements.

Repeatability: Same as reproducibility.

Repeated measures: When the same subject is observed repeatedly after specified time gaps, such as monitoring BP and heart rate at 1, 5, 10, 15 and 30 minutes after a surgical operation.

Replication: Trying the same regimen on more than one equivalent group so as to get an idea of the repeatability. Replications tend to increase the reliability of the results.

Reporting bias: Highlighting findings in a report that support a particular view at the cost of the other.

Reproducibility: The ability of a test or measurement to give same or nearly similar result when conducted in identical conditions.

Reproductive rate: The rate at which an index case infects others in the entire transmission phase. If the reproductive rate is one or more, the infection sustains itself and spreads in the population, like HIV is doing in some countries includinq India. If the reproductive rate is less than one, the infection will die down or will stabilize at a low level.

Research: Systematic inquiry that uses orderly, disciplined methods to answer questions or solve problems.

Research protocol: Statement on steps of research, including background information and rationale, objectives and hypotheses, review of literature, methodology, ethics, statistical evaluation, and references.

Retrospective cohort: Same as historical cohort.

Retrospective follow-up study: Same as historical cohort.

Retrospective study: A study that investigates antecedents for known outcomes.

Right-skewed distribution: See skewed distribution.

Risk: The chance of occurrence of an outcome of interest, generally calculate per year of exposure. It is not necessary that the outcome is adverse to health. Incidence is a measure of risk.

Risk difference: The difference in risk of occurrence of a condition in two setups, such as risk of glaucoma in vegetarians vs risk in nonvegetarians. Same as attributable risk.

Risk factor: A characteristic that is suspected to affect the outcome, such as obesity for hypertension.

Risk ratio: Same as relative risk.

Sample: A part of the target population, which is actually studied.

Sample registration system: A system of tracking all births and deaths occurring in selected sample areas across India. Ancillary information such as marriage, parity of birth, birth interval, age at death, etc. are also collected. Our information regarding various fertility and mortality rates in India and states is based on this system.

Sample size: The number of subjects or units in a sample.

Sampling: Choosing a part from the whole, such as choosing 300 childbirths out of 5000 in a hospital in one year for studying the intrauterine growth retardation.

Sampling bias: The bias due to (i) nonrandom sample such as volunteers that do not represent the target population, and (ii) small sample that fails to represent the entire spectrum of subjects.

Sampling error: Same as sampling fluctuation. This is not an error.

Sampling fluctuation: The tendency of different samples giving different results, even if drawn from the same target population. This happens because different samples contain individuals who are different from those in other samples.

Sampling fraction: The extent of sampling such as one out of eight, or one out of twenty.

Sampling frame: A list of units in the target population from which a sample is drawn.

Sampling method: Method of drawing sample—random or purposive.

Sampling unit: The unit used for sampling purposes. In a multistage sampling, the first stage sampling unit may be district, second stage PHC areas, third stage village, and fourth stage a family.

Sampling variation: Same as sampling fluctuation.

Scales of measurement: The system of differentiating one type of observation from the other. When names are used (opposed to grades) for differentiation, the scale is called nominal. Signs and symptoms are generally measured on nominal scale. Textual grades such as mild, moderate, serious, are measurements on ordinal scale. Numeric measurements such as body mass index are on metric scale.

Scatter diagram: A diagram displaying values of one variable for different values of the other variable by plotting points. This is also called the (x, y) plot.

Schedule: A form which contains a set of items on which information is to be obtained. It contains space also to record the responses.

Score: Quantification of a set of (mostly) qualitative or ordinal measurements such as APACHE score. Scores in medicine are used either to grade severity of a condition, or as an aid to diagnosis.

SD: Short for standard deviation.

Secondary attack rate: The number of new spells of sickness within the range of incubation period in exposed subjects as percentage of total subjects exposed to index cases.

Secondary data: The existing data in records, reports, or of previous surveys: contrast it with primary data that you generate.

Sensitivity: Ability to identify known positives as positive. If CPK ≥ 120 IU is present in 60 percent cases of known MI cases, then sensitivity of this cut-ott is 60 percent. Sensitivity is not a valid indicator of diagnostic value of the test. It only measures the intrinsic ability of a test to detect a disease when it is known to be present.

Sequential clinical trial: A clinical trial in which data are continuoulsy analysed and 'stop rules' are used to decide when the evidence about the interventions efficacy is sufficiently strong that experiment can be stopped.

Serial tests: Using two or more criteria in 'and' setup. That is, all the criteria should be positive to label the person as positive. This reduces sensitivity but increases specificity.

Sex outside marriage: Sexual activity among partners that are not married with one another.

Sex ratio: Number of females per 1000 males.

Sign test: A nonparametric test based on sign (negative or positive) of differences between two sets of observations. This test is used to compare two groups for their central tendency.

Significance: See statistical significance and medical significance.

Significance level: Same as level of significance.

Simple linear regression: A regression in which a dependent variable is sought to be explained by only one independent variable, such as regression of systolic BP on age. Other correlates are ignored in this setup and the relationship format is limited to linear.

Simple random sampling: Random sampling that gives equal chance of selection to every unit. This is like lottery.

Simple regression: Relationship between one independent and one dependent variable. This could be linear, curvilinear or nonlinear.

Single blind: When the subject alone is not informed that he is receiving test regimen or the control regimen in a trial. The doctor or assessor knows.

Skewed distribution: Opposed to symmetric such as Gaussian, a distribution is skewed when values on one side of mode vary much more than on the other side. It is called right-skewed when values more than mode have higher variability, and left-skewed when values less than mode have higher variability.

Smoking index: A measure of life-long burden of smoking with weightage for quantity of smoking, duration of smoking, type of smoking (filter/nonfilter/bidi/cigar), age at start, and duration elapsed since quitting by exsmokers.

Social class: Status in the society determined jointly by education, income and occupation.

Social classification: The division of individuals in classes on the basis of education, income and occupation.

Spearman's rank correlation: The correlation between ranks of two variables.

Specificity: Ability to identify known negatives as negative. If AFB is negative in 95 percent of the healthy subjects, its specificity is 95 percent. In practice, a test is rarely used on healthy subjects.

It is used on suspected cases. In them, the specificity may be very different.

Spectrum of disease: The percentage distribution of cases that get mild, moderate, serious and fatal form of disease; or infectivity, pathogenecity and virulence of a disease.

Spurious association: A false correlation that could arise due to presence of confounders, bias, or merely a chance.

Stable population: A population with same growth rate over a substantial period, say 5 years or more.

Standard deviation: Most common and generally most appropriate measure of dispersion obtained as positive square root of variance.

Standard error: Measure of variability of sample summaries. Just as the measurements such as Hb level differ from person-to-person, so do the sample statistics from sample-to-sample. Mean Hb level in one sample would be different from another sample even when both are drawn from the same target population. The extent, of variability in statistics such as mean and median is measured by their standard errors. Actually, this is the SD of mean or median or any other statistic as the case may be.

Standardization (of variables): Same as normalization of variables.

Standardization (of groups): The procedure that makes two different groups comparable by bringing them on to a common base or a common standard, such as age-standardization.

Standardized death rate (directly standardized): Recalculated death rate when one or more factors affecting deaths (such as age structure) are brought at par with the comparison group, or both brought to a common base. This substantially increases comparability that crude death rate lacks when one group is young and the other is old. Common base structure (called, standard) of population is chosen by the researcher.

Standardized mortality ratio: Ratio of actually observed deaths to expected deaths obtained after indirect standardization. If this ratio is more than one, the force of mortality is higher in the study group compared to the standard group.

Stationary population: A population with zero growth.

Statistic: A summary measure for any characteristic in the sample or the group actually studied, such as mean, median or SD of a sample, or proportion of subjects found affected in a sample.

Statistical analysis: Subjecting data to the rigors of statistical methods so that the uncertainty levels are either quantified and/or minimized.

Statistical power: Same as power.

Statistical significance: A result is statistically significant if the chance of wrongly rejecting null hypothesis is less than the prefixed level such as 5 percent. The implication is that chance differences in samples would produce that kind of result in less than 5 times out of 100—thus chance is not an explanation for that result, and it is most likely real.

Statistical test: A procedure to find *P*-value corresponding to a null hypothesis on the basis of the given data. Depending upon the type of data and the type of hypothesis, a large number of statistical tests are available. Most popular of these are student's *t*-test and chi-square test.

Statistical threshold (of normal range): Mean ± 2SD where mean and SD are obtained from measurements in a large number of healthy individuals. There is always a chance of nearly 5 percent of classifying healthy individuals with extreme values as sick when this range is used as normal.

Statistics: (i) As a singular, a science or discipline to manage uncertainties (ii) As a plural, data.

Still birth ratio: The number of still births per thousand live births in the same period of time.

Strata: The divisions obtained after stratification (the singular is stratum).

Stratification: Division of subjects into relevant groups.

Stratified random sampling: Separate simple random sampling from each group after stratification.

Structured questionnaire (or schedule): A questionnaire or a schedule that provides a list of possible responses and the respondent or the investigator is required only to mark response among the choices given. One of the choices couid be "Any other (specify)" to make them exhaustive.

Student's *t*-test: It is same as *t*-test.

Study design: It is same as design.

Sufficient cause: A cause that by itself is sufficient to change the outcome. Exposure to measles virus in a susceptible is sufficient to produce the disease. In fact this cause is both necessary and sufficient. Hanging by rope is sufficient to cause suicidal death but is not necessary as a cause for suicidal death.

Surrogate variable: A makeshift substitute variable when the measurements on actually required variable are not available. If the respondents are shy of revealing income, surrogates such as presence of own house, car, telephone and television can be used to assess the level of income. Since they are surrogate, they may or may not reveal the true status.

Survey: Same as descriptive study.

Susceptibility: 'Ability' to catch a disease. A person who is effectively immunized against tetanus is not susceptible to tetanus or a child is not susceptible to the usual STDs.

Systematic random sampling: Selection of individual at regular intervals depending on sampling fraction, after beginning with a random start.

Tabulation: Arrangement of data in rows and column of a table in a manner that makes them intelligible.

Target population: The larger group of person or patients of interest to which the sample results would finally apply. Sample is generally chosen from the target population. Also called reference population.

Tertiles: Two cutpoints for values of a measurement that divide a group into three equal parts—each part with same number ($n/3$) of subjects—after arranging in ascending order.

Test criterion: The formula used to calculate a value that determines statistical significance of a result.

Test group: The group of subjects that is receiving or has received a regimen under test.

Test of hypothesis: The statistical procedure used to test whether or not data provide sufficient evidence against a null hypothesis.

Test of significance: A statistical procedure to test whether or not the observations fall into a specified pattern, such as equal means of two or more groups, or following a linear trend. If they do not, the result is called statistically significant. This requires prior fixing of the level of significance that specifies the maximum tolerable probability of Type I error.

Total fertility rate: Expected number of live births per woman during her entire reproductive span according to the existing age-specific fertility rates. It is assumed that the women would remain alive during the entire reproductive span.

True score: A hypothetical score that would be obtained if a measure were infalliable.

Trial: An experiment on human subjects.

***t*-test:** A statistical criterion to test hypothesis on mean being a specified value, on equality or specified difference between two means, and for certain other parameters such as regression coefficient.

Two-sample *t*-test: The criterion used to compare means in two independent samples for finding statistical significance of their difference.

Two-sided alternative: An alternative hypothesis that stipulates that the parameter value can be higher or lower than the null value. Both directions are admissible. This type of alternative is setup when it is not known that the value is going to be higher or lower. Contrast it with one-side alternative.

Two-tailed test: See one-tailed test.

Two-way classification: Simultaneous division of subjects by two characteristics, such as dividing cases of MI by their CPK level and cholesterol level.

Two-way design: The design of a study that is planned to investigate the effect of levels of two antecedent factors, such as effect of obesity (BMI < 20.0, 20.0–24.9, 25.0–29.9 or 30.0+) and smoking (none, mild, moderate or severe) on blood glucose level. Their interaction can also be investigated in this kind of design.

Type I error: The error of rejecting a true null hypothesis, i.e. concluding that there is a difference when actually there is none. The sample or data might be such that this leads to such a wrong conclusion.

Type II error: The error of wrongly concluding that there is a difference when there is none because the data happen to indicate so.

Unit of analysis: The basic unit or focus of a researcher analysis; in nursing research, the unit of analysis is typically the individual study participant.

Unit of study: An entity such as individual, family or a hospital on which enquiries are made for collection of data. One study can have multiple units.

Unitary family: It is same as nuclear family.

Univariate analysis: The analysis regarding one variable at a time. The combined result of several univariate analyses may be very different from the result obtained by simultaneous consideration of these variables in a multivariate setup.

Universe: Statistically broader than target population. The broad group of subjects for which the findings could be generalized or implicated. For example, this could include future cases.

Validity (of a study): The ability of a study to provide correct conclusion, considering the representativeness and size of sample, validity of measurements, and the soundness of methods.

Validity (of measurement): Ability to hit the target (or around it): ability to assess what is really intended to be assessed. Weight by itself is not a valid indicator of obesity in adults but body mass index that uses height also is for a medical test, validity is measured by sensitivity, specificity and predictivities (positive and negative).

Variable: A characteristic that varies from person-to-person, or from situation-to-situation. Distance between various cities is a variable but distance between Delhi and Hong Kong is not a variable.

Variance: A measure of dispersion or scatteredness of data obtained as average of the squared deviations from mean.

Virulence: The ability to produce severe form of disease that can threaten life. Rabies is a highly virulent disease and cholera is not—measured as percentage of disease cases who go into severe form, including fatal cases.

Vital registration: The formal recording of the events of birth and deaths. This is done by a government functionary.

Volunteer studies: A study done on volunteers, opposed to randomly selected subjects. In a clinical trial setup, results from such studies can be used to identify tolerated dose and some side-effects of the test regimen but cannot be used to estimate efficacy.

Wedging a pie: Showing a segment of a pie diagram apart from the rest to highlight that segment.

Wilcoxon signed rank test: A nonparametric statistical test for paired sample situation based on sum of the ranks of differences with either positive or negative sign.

Wilcoxon sum rank test: A nonparametric statistical test for two-sample situation based on sum of the ranks of values in one sample when ranks are assigned jointly to the values in the two samples.

***z*-score:** Same as normal deviate, but some times measured from median instead of mean, particularly in assessing growth: difference of a value from group mean in terms of how many times of SD.

***z*-test:** A statistical test of hypothesis based on Gaussian distribution, generally used to compare two means or two proportions in large sample.

Appendix

Table	Description
A	Proportions of area under normal distribution curve
B	Critical valves of '*t*'
C	Conversion of '*r*' into '*z*'
D	Critical values of Pearson product moment correlation
E	Critical values of Spearman rank correlation.
F	Critical values of Chi-square.
G	Probabilities associated with values as small as observed values of *x* in the Binomial test
H	Significances of A_3 (Skewness)
I	Significances of A_4 (Kurtosis)
J	Critical values of K in the Kolmogrov-Smirnov two sample test when samples are small
K	F-Ratio
L	A Table to aid in the calculation of T scores
M	Standard scores (or Deviates) and ordinates corresponding to divisions of the area under the normal curve into a larger portion (B) A smaller portion, and (C) the value $\sqrt{BC}$
N	Values of R_t taken as the cosine of an angle
O	Table of squares and square roots of the numbers from 1-1000

Table A

Proportions of area under normal distribution curve

Fractional parts of the total area (taken as 0.1000) under the normal probability curve, corresponding to distances on the base-line between the mean and successive points laid off from the mean in units of standard deviation

Example: Between the mean and a point 1.38 σ $\left(\frac{x}{\sigma}=1.38\right)$ are found 41.62% of the entire area under the curve

$\frac{x}{\sigma}$	0.00	0.01	0.02	0.03	0.04	0.05	0.06	0.07	0.08	0.09
0.0	0000	0040	0080	0120	0160	0199	0239	0279	0319	0359
0.1	0398	0438	0478	0517	0557	0596	0636	0675	0714	0753
0.2	0793	0832	0871	0910	0948	0987	1026	1064	1103	1141
0.3	1179	1217	1255	1293	1331	1368	1406	1443	1480	1517
0.4	1554	1591	1628	1664	1700	1736	1772	1808	1844	1879
0.5	1915	1950	1985	2019	2054	2088	2133	2157	2190	2224
0.6	2257	2291	2324	2357	2389	2422	2454	2486	2517	2549
0.7	2580	2611	2642	2673	2704	2734	2764	2794	2823	2852
0.8	2881	2910	2939	2967	2995	3023	3051	3078	3106	3133
0.9	3159	3186	3212	3238	3264	3289	3315	3340	3365	3389
1.0	3413	3438	3461	3485	3508	3531	3554	3577	3599	3621
1.1	3643	3665	3686	3708	3729	3749	3770	3790	3810	3830
1.2	3849	3869	3888	3907	3925	3944	3962	3980	3997	4015
1.3	4032	4049	4066	4082	4099	4115	4131	4147	4162	4177

Contd...

Contd...

x/σ	0.00	0.01	0.02	0.03	0.04	0.05	0.06	0.07	0.08	0.09
1.4	4192	4207	4222	4236	4251	4265	4279	4292	4306	4319
1.5	4332	4345	4357	4370	4382	4394	4406	4418	4429	4441
1.6	4452	4463	4474	4484	4495	4505	4515	4525	4535	4545
1.7	4554	4564	4573	4582	4591	4599	4608	4616	4625	4633
1.8	4641	4649	4656	4664	4671	4678	4686	4693	4699	4706
1.9	4713	4719	4726	4732	4738	4744	4750	4756	4761	4767
2.0	4772	4778	4783	4788	4793	4798	4803	4808	4812	4817
2.1	4821	4826	4830	4834	4838	4842	4846	4850	4854	4857
2.2	4861	4864	4868	4871	4875	4878	4881	4884	4887	4890
2.3	4893	4896	4898	4901	4904	4906	4909	4911	4913	4916
2.4	4918	4920	4922	4925	4927	4929	4931	4932	4934	4936
2.5	4938	4940	4941	4943	4945	4946	4948	4949	4951	4952
2.6	4953	4955	4956	4957	4959	4960	4961	4962	4963	4964
2.7	4965	4966	4967	4968	4969	4970	4971	4972	4973	4974
2.8	4974	4975	4976	4977	4977	4978	4979	4979	4980	4981
2.9	4981	4982	4982	4983	4984	4984	4985	4985	4986	4986
3.0	4986.5	4986.9	4987.4	4987.8	4988.2	4988.6	4988.9	4989.3	4989.7	4990
3.1	4990.3	4990.6	4991.0	4991.3	4991.6	4991.8	4992.1	4992.4	4992.6	4992.9
3.2	4993.129									
3.3	4995.166									
3.4	4996.631									
3.5	4997.674									
3.6	4998.409									
3.7	4998.922									
3.8	4999.277									
3.9	4999.519									
4.0	4999.683									
4.5	4999.966									
5.0	4999.997133									

Table B

Critical value of '*t*'.

Table of *t*, for use in determining the significance of statistics

Example: When the *df* are 35 and $t = 2.03$, the 0.05 in column 3 means that 5 times in 100 trials a divergence as large as that obtained may be expected in the positive and negative directions under the null hypothesis

Degrees of freedom (1)	Probability (P) *0.10 (2)*	*0.05 (3)*	*0.01 (4)*	*0.01 (5)*
1	T = 6.34	T = 12.71	T = 31.82	T = 63.66
2	2.92	4.30	6.96	9.92
3	2.35	3.18	4.54	5.84
4	2.13	2.78	3.75	4.60
5	2.02	2.57	3.36	4.03

Contd...

Contd...

Degrees of freedom (1)	Probability (P) 0.10 (2)	0.05 (3)	0.01 (4)	0.01 (5)
6	1.94	2.45	3.14	3.71
7	1.90	2.36	3.00	3.50
8	1.86	2.31	2.90	3.36
9	1.83	2.26	2.82	3.25
10	1.81	2.23	2.76	3.17
11	1.80	2.20	2.72	3.11
12	1.78	2.18	2.68	3.06
13	1.77	2.16	2065	3.01
14	1.76	2.14	2.62	2.98
15	1.75	2.13	2.60	2.95
16	1.75	2.12	2.58	2.92
17	1.74	2.11	2.57	2.90
18	1.73	2.10	2.55	2.88
19	1.73	2.09	2.54	2.86
20	1.72	2.09	2.53	2.84
21	1.72	2.08	2.52	2.83
22	1.72	2.07	2.51	2.8223
23	1.71	2.07	2.50	2.81
24	1.71	2.06	2.49	2.80
25	1.71	2.06	2.48	2.79
26	1.71	2.06	2.48	2.78
27	1.70	2.05	2.47	2.77
28	1.70	2.05	2.47	2.76
29	1.70	2.04	2.46	2.76
30	1.70	2.04	2.46	2.75
35	1.69	2.03	2.44	2.72
40	1.68	2.02	2.42	2.71
45	1.68	2.02	2.41	2.69
50	1.68	2.01	2.40	2.68
60	1.67	2.00	2.39	2.66
70	1.67	2.00	2.38	2.65
80	1.66	1.99	2.38	2.64
90	1.66	1.99	2.37	2.63
100	1.66	1.98	2.36	2.63
125	1.66	1.98	2.36	2.62
150	1.66	1.98	2.35	2.61
200	1.65	1.97	2.35	2.60
300	1.65	1.97	2.34	2.59
400	1.65	1.97	2.34	2.59
500	1.65	1.96	2.33	2.59
1000	1.65	1.96	2.33	2.58
∞	1.65	1.96	2.33	2.58

Table C

Conversion of '*r*' into '*z*'

*Conversion of a person r into a corresponding Fisher's z coefficient**											
r	*z*	*r*	*z*	*r*	*z*	*r*	*z*	*r*	*z*	*r*	*z*
0.25	0.26	0.40	0.42	0.55	0.62	0.70	0.87	0.85	1.26	0.950	1.83
0.26	0.27	0.41	0.44	0.56	0.63	0.71	0.89	0.86	1.29	0.955	1.89
0.27	0.28	0.42	0.45	0.57	0.65	0.72	0.91	0.87	1.33	0.960	1.95
0.28	0.29	0.43	0.46	0.58	0.66	0.73	0.93	0.88	1.38	0.965	2.01
0.29	0.30	0.44	0.47	0.59	0.68	0.74	0.95	0.89	1.42	0.970	2.09
0.30	0.31	0.45	0.48	0.60	0.69	0.75	0.97	0.90	1.47	0.975	2.18
0.31	0.32	0.46	0.50	0.61	0.71	0.76	1.00	0.905	1.50	0.980	2.30
0.32	0.33	0.47	0.51	0.62	0.73	0.77	1.02	0.910	1.53	0.985	2.44
0.33	0.34	0.48	0.52	0.63	0.74	0.78	1.05	0.915	1.56	0.990	2.65
0.34	0.35	0.49	0.54	0.64	0.76	0.79	1.07	0.920	1.59	0.995	2.99
0.35	0.37	0.50	0.55	0.65	0.78	0.80	1.10	0.925	1.62		
0.36	0.38	0.51	0.56	0.66	0.79	0.81	1.13	0.930	1.66		
0.37	0.39	0.52	0.58	0.67	0.81	0.82	1.16	0.935	1.70		
0.38	0.40	0.53	0.59	0.68	0.83	0.83	1.19	0.940	1.74		
0.39	0.41	0.54	0.60	0.69	0.85	0.84	1.22	0.945	1.78		

**r*'s under 0.25 may be taken as equivalent to *z*'s

Table D

Critical value of Pearson product moment correlation

Correlation coefficients at the 5% and 1% levels of significance

Example: When N is 52 and *df* is 50, an *r* must be 0.273 to be significant at 0.05 level, and 0.354 to be significant at 0.01 level.

Degrees of freedom (N-2)	*0.05*	*0.01*	*Degrees of freedom (N-2)*	*0.05*	*0.01*
1	0.997	1.000	24	0.388	0.496
2	0.950	0.990	25	0.381	0.487
3	0.878	0.959	26	0.374	0.478
4	0.811	0.917	27	0.367	0.470
5	0.754	0.874	28	0.361	0.463
6	0.707	0.834	29	0.335	0.456
7	0.666	0.798	30	0.349	0.449
8	0.632	0.765	35	0.325	0.418
9	0.602	0.735	40	0.304	393
10	0.576	0.708	45	0.288	0.372
11	0.533	0.684	50	0.273	0.354
12	0.532	0.661	60	0.250	0.325
13	0.514	0.641	70	0.233	0.302
14	0.497	0.623	80	0.217	0.283
15	0.482	0.606	90	0.205	0.267
16	0.468	0.590	100	0.195	0.254
17	0.456	0.575	125	0.174	0.228

Contd...

Contd...

Degrees of freedom (N-2)	0.05	0.01	Degrees of freedom (N-2)	0.05	0.01
18	0.444	0.561	150	0.159	0.208
19	0.433	0.549	200	0.138	0.181
20	0.423	0537	300	0.113	0.148
21	0.413	0.526	400	0.098	0.128
22	0.404	0.515	500	0.088	0.115
23	0.396	0.505	1000	0.062	0.081

Table E

Critical value of Spearman Rank correlation

Values of rank—difference coefficients of correlation that are significant at the 0.05 and 0.01 levels (one-tail test)

N	0.05	0.01	N	0.05	0.01
5	0.900	1.000	16	0.425	0.601
6	0.829	0.943	18	0.399	0.564
7	0.714	0.893	20	0.377	0.534
8	0.643	0.833	22	0.359	0.508
9	0.600	0.783	24	0.343	0.485
10	0.564	0.746	26	0.329	0.465
12	0.506	0.712	28	0.317	0.448
14	0.456	0.645	30	0.306	0.432

Table F

Critical value of chi-square.

χ^2 Table. P gives the probability of exceeding the tabulated value of χ^2 for the specified number of degrees of freedom (*df*). The values of χ^2 are printed in the body of the table

df	0.95	0.90	0.80	0.70	0.50	0.30	0.20	0.10	0.05	0.02	0.01
1	0.00393	0.0158	0.0642	0.148	0.455	1.074	1.642	2.706	3.841	5.412	6.635
2	0.103	0.211	0.446	0.713	1.386	2.408	3.219	4.605	5.991	7.824	9.210
3	0.352	0.584	1.005	1.424	2.366	3.665	4.642	6.251	7.815	9.837	11.345
4	0.711	1.064	1.649	2.195	3.357	4.878	5.989	7.779	9.488	11.668	13.277
5	1.145	1.610	2.343	3.000	4.351	6.064	7.289	9.236	11.070	13.388	15.086
6	1.635	2.204	3.070	3.828	5.348	7.231	8.558	10.645	12.592	15.033	16.812
7	2.167	2.833	3.822	4.671	6.346	8.383	9.803	12.017	14.067	16.622	18.475
8	2.733	3.490	4.594	5.527	7.344	9.524	11.030	13.362	15.507	18.168	20.090
9	3.325	4.168	5.380	6.393	8.343	10.656	12.242	14.684	16.919	19.679	21.666
10	3.940	4.865	6.179	7.267	9.342	11.781	13.442	15.987	18.307	21.161	23.209
11	4.575	5.578	6.989	8.148	10.341	12.899	14.631	17.275	19.675	22.618	24.725
12	5.226	6.304	7.807	9.034	11.340	14.011	15.812	18.549	21.026	24.054	26.217
13	5.892	7.042	8.634	9.926	12.340	15.119	16.985	19.812	22.362	25.472	27.688
14	6.571	7.790	9.467	10.821	13.339	16.222	18.151	21.064	23.685	26.873	29.141
15	7.261	8.547	10.307	11.721	14.339	17.322	19.311	22.307	24.996	28.259	30.578

Contd...

Contd...

df	0.95	0.90	0.80	0.70	0.50	0.30	0.20	0.10	0.05	0.02	0.01
16	7.962	9.312	11.152	12.624	15.338	18.418	20.465	23.542	26.292	29.633	32.000
17	8.672	10.085	12.002	13.531	16.338	19.511	21.615	24.769	27.587	30.995	33.409
18	9.390	10.865	12.857	14.440	17.338	20.601	22.760	25.989	28.869	32.346	34.805
19	10.117	11.651	13.716	15.352	18.338	21.689	23.900	27.204	30.144	33.687	36.191
20	10.851	12.443	14.578	16.266	19.337	22.775	25.038	28.142	31.410	35.020	37.566
21	11.591	13.240	15.445	17.182	20.337	23.858	26.171	29.615	32.671	36.343	38.932
22	12.338	14.041	16.314	18.101	21.337	24.939	27.301	30.813	33.924	37.659	40.289
23	13.091	14.848	17.187	19.021	22.337	26.018	28.429	32.007	35.172	38.968	41.638
24	13.848	15.659	18.062	19.943	23.337	27.096	29.553	33.196	36.415	40.270	42.980
25	14.611	16.473	18.940	20.867	24.337	28.172	30.675	34.382	37.652	41.566	44.314
26	15.379	17.292	19.820	21.792	25.336	29.246	31.795	35.563	38.885	42.856	45.642
27	16.151	18.114	20.703	22.719	26.336	30.319	32.912	36.741	40.113	44.410	46.963
28	16.928	18.939	21.588	23.647	27.336	31.391	34.027	37.916	41.337	45.419	48.278
29	17.708	19.768	22.475	24.577	28.336	32.461	35.139	39.087	42.557	46.693	49.588
30	18.493	20.599	23.364	25.508	29.336	33.530	36.250	40.256	43.773	47.962	50.892

Table G

Probabilities associated with values as small as observed values of 'x' in Binomial test.

Cumulative proportions from the tail categories of Binomial distribution for $(\frac{1}{2} + \frac{1}{2})^N$, with N varying from 6 to 25 Categories C

C N	C 0 N	C 1 (N-1)	C 2 (N-2)	C 3 (N-3)	C 4 (N-4)	C 5 (N-5)	C 6 (N-6)	C 7 (N-7)	C 8 (N-8)	C 9 (N-9)
6	0.016	0.109								
7	0.008	0.062	0.227							
8	0.004	0.035	0.145							
9	0.002	0.020	0.090	0.254						
10	0.001	0.011	0.055	0.172						
11		0.006	0.033	0.113						
12		0.003	0.019	0.073	0.194					
13		0.002	0.011	0.046	0.133					
14		0.001	0.006	0.029	0.090					
15			0.004	0.018	0.059	0.151				
16			0.002	0.011	0.038	0.105				
17			0.001	0.006	0.025	0.072.	0.166			
18			0.001	0.004	0.015	0.048	0.119			
19				0.002	0.010	0.032	0.084	0.180		
20				0.001	0.006	0.021	0.058	0.132		
21				0.001	0.004	0.013	0.039	0.095	0.192	
22					0.002	0.008	0.026	0.067	0.143	
23					0.001	0.005	0.017	0.047	0.105	
24					0.001	0.003	0.011	0.032	0.076	0.154
25						0.002	0.007	0.022	0.054	0.115

Comment: Each entry is the probability of an outcome as extreme as the last category (0 head or N head, as in coin tossing), the next-to-the-last category (1 head or N-1 head), and so on (i.e. the probabilities are cumulative). Each probability is for one tail only. For a two-tail test, double the probability given.

Table H

Significance of A_3 (Skewness).

Upper 0.10 and 0.02 limits of A_3 (Skewness) when computed from random samples from a normal population

N	*0.10*	*0.02*
50	0.285	0.619
75	0.198	0.424
100	0.152	0.321
125	0.123	0.258
150	0.103	0.216
175	0.089	0.185
200	0.078	0.162
250	0.063	0.130
300	0.053	0.108
350	0.045	0.093
400	0.040	0.081
450	0.035	0.072
500	0.032	0.065
550	0.029	0.059
600	0.027	0.054
650	0.025	0.050
700	0.023	0.046
750	0.021	0.043
850	0.030	0.041
850	0.019	0.038
900	0.018	0.036
950	0.017	0.034
1000	0.016	0.032
1200	0.013	0.027
1400	0.012	0.023
1600	0.010	0.020
1800	0.009	0.018
2000	0.008	0.016
2500	0.006	0.013
3000	0.005	0.011
3500	0.005	0.009
4000	0.004	0.008
4500	0.004	0.007
5000	0.003	0.006

Table I

Significance of A_4 (Kurtosis).

Upper and lower 0.05 and 0.01 limits of A_4 (Kurtosis) when computed from random samples from a normal population

N	Lower limits		Upper limits	
	0.01	0.05	0.05	0.01
100	2.18	2.35	3.77	4.39
125	2.24	2.40	3.17	4.24
150	2.29	2.45	3.65	4.13
175	2.33	2.48	3.61	4.05
200	2.37	2.51	3.57	3.98
250	2.42	2.55	3.52	3.87
300	2.46	2.59	3.47	3.79
350	2.50	2.62	3.44	3.72
400	2.52	2.64	3.41	3.67
450	2.55	2.66	3.39	3.63
500	2.57	2.67	3.37	3.60
550	2.58	2.69	3.35	3.57
600	2.60	2.70	3.34	3.54
650	2.61	2.71	3.33	3.52
700	2.62	2.72	3.31	3.50
750	2.64	2.73	3.30	3.48
800	2.65	2.74	3.29	3.46
850	2.66	2.74	3.28	3.45
900	2.66	2.75	3.28	3.43
950	2.67	2.76	3.27	3.42
1000	2.68	2.76	3.36	3.41
1200	2.71	2.78	3.24	3.37
1400	2.72	2.80	3.22	3.34
1600	2.74	2.81	3.21	3.32
1800	2.76	2.82	3.20	3.30
2000	2.77	2.83	3.18	3.28
2500	2.79	2.85	3.16	3.25
3000	2.81	2.86	3.15	3.22
3500	2.82	2.87	3.14	3.21
4000	2.83	2.88	3.13	3.19
4500	2.84	2.88	3.12	3.18
5000	2.85	2.89	3.12	3.17

Table J

Critical values of K–S

Critical value of K-S. Critical values of K in the Kolmogorov-Smirnov two-sample test, when samples are small

N	*One-tail test*		*Two-tail test*		*N*	*One-tail test*		*Two-tail test*	
	α = 0.05	*= 0.01*	*α = 0.05*	*= 0.01*		*α = 0.05*	*= 0.01*	*α = 0.05*	*= 0.01*
3	3	–	–	–	18	8	10	9	10
4	4	–	4	–	19	8	10	9	10
5	4	5	5	5	20	8	10	9	11
6	5	6	5	6	21	8	10	9	11
7	5	6	6	6	22	9	11	9	11
8	5	6	6	7	23	9	11	10	11
9	6	7	6	7	24	9	11	10	12
10	6	7	7	8	25	9	11	10	12
11	6	8	7	8	26	9	11	10	12
12	6	8	7	8	27	9	12	10	12
13	7	8	7	9	28	10	12	11	13
14	7	8	8	9	29	10	12	11	13
15	7	9	8	9	30	10	12	11	13
16	7	9	8	10	35	11	13	12	
17	8	9	8	10	40	11	14	13	

Table K

'F'-ratio.

F-ratio for 0.05 (Roman) and 0.01 (Italics) levels of significance

	Degrees of freedom for greater mean square									
	1	*2*	*3*	*4*	*5*	*6*	*8*	*12*	*24*	*∞*
1	161.45	199.50	215.72	224.57	230.17	233.97	238.89	243.91	249.04	254.32
	4052.10	499.03	5403.49	5625.14	5764.08	5859.39	5981.34	6105.83	6203.16	6366.48
2	18.51	19.00	19.16	19.25	19.30	19.33	19.37	19.41	19.45	19.50
	98.49	99.01	99.17	99.25	99.30	99.33	99.36	99.42	99.46	99.50
3	10.13	9.55	9.28	9.12	9.01	8.94	8.84	8.74	8.64	8.53
	34.12	30.81	29.46	28.71	28.24	27.91	27.49	27.05	26.60	26.12
4	7.71	6.94	6.59	6.39	6.26	6.16	6.04	5.91	5.77	5.63
	21.20	18.00	16.69	15.98	15.52	15.21	14.80	14.37	13.93	13.46
5	6.61	5.79	5.41	5.19	5.05	4.95	4.82	4.68	4.53	4.36
	16.26	13.27	12.06	11.39	10.97	10.67	10.27	9.89	9.47	9.02
6	5.99	5.14	4.76	4.53	4.39	4.28	4.15	4.00	3.84	3.67
	13.74	10.92	9.78	9.15	8.75	8.47	8.10	7.72	7.31	6.88
7	5.59	4.74	4.35	4.12	3.97	3.87	3.73	3.57	3.41	3.23
	12.25	9.55	8.45	7.85	7.46	7.19	6.84	6.47	6.07	5.65
8	5.32	4.46	4.07	3.84	3.69	3.58	3.44	3.28	3.12	2.93
	11.26	8.65	7.59	7.01	6.63	6.37	6.03	5.67	5.28	4.86
9	5.12	4.26	3.86	3.63	3.48	3.37	3.23	3.07	2.90	2.71
	10.56	8.02	6.99	6.42	6.06	5.80	5.47	5.11	4.73	4.31

Contd...

Contd...

	Degrees of freedom for greater mean square									
	1	*2*	*3*	*4*	*5*	*6*	*8*	*12*	*24*	*∞*
10	4.96	4.10	3.71	3.48	3.33	3.22	3.07	2.91	2.74	2.54
	10.04	7.56	6.55	5.99	5.64	5.39	5.06	4.71	4.33	3.91
11	4.84	3.98	3.59	3.36	3.20	3.09	2.95	2.79	2.61	2.40
	9.65	7.20	6.22	5.67	5.32	5.07	4.74	4.40	4.02	3.60
12	4.75	3.88	3.49	3.26	3.11	3.00	2.85	2.69	2.50	2.30
	9.33	6.93	5.95	5.41	5.06	4.82	4.50	4.16	3.78	3.36
13	4.67	3.80	3.41	3.18	3.02	2.92	2.77	2.60	2.42	2.21
	9.07	6.70	5.74	5.20	4.86	4.62	4.30	3.96	3.59	3.16
14	4.60	3.74	3.34	3.11	2.96	2.85	2.70	2.53	2.35	2.16
	8.86	6.51	5.56	5.03	4.69	4.46	4.14	3.80	3.43	3.00
15	4.54	3.68	3.29	3.06	2.90	2.79	2.64	2.48	2.29	2.07
	8.68	6.36	5.42	4.89	4.56	4.32	4.00	3.67	3.29	2.87
16	4.49	3.63	3.24	3.01	2.85	2.74	2.59	2.42	2.24	2.01
	8.53	6.23	5.29	4.77	4.44	4.20	3.89	3.55	3.18	2.75
17	4.45	3.59	3.20	2.96	2.81	2.70	2.55	2.38	2.19	1.96
	8.40	6.11	5.18	4.67	4.34	4.10	3.79	3.45	3.08	2.65
18	4.41	3.55	3.16	2.93	2.77	2.66	2.51	2.34	2.15	1.92
	8.28	6.01	5.09	4.58	4.25	4.01	3.71	3.37	3.01	2.57
19	4.38	3.52	3.13	2.90	2.74	2.63	2.48	2.31	2.11	1.88
	8.18	5.93	5.01	4.50	4.17	3.94	3.63	3.30	2.92	2.49
20	4.35	3.49	3.10	2.87	2.71	2.60	2.45	2.28	2.08	1.84
	8.10	5.85	4.94	4.43	4.10	3.87	3.56	3.23	2.86	2.42
21	4.32	3.47	3.07	2.84	2.68	2.57	2.42	2.25	2.05	1.81
	8.02	5.78	4.87	4.37	4.04	3.81	3.51	3.17	2.80	2.36
22	4.30	3.44	3.05	2.82	2.66	2.55	2.40	2.23	2.03	1.78
	7.94	5.72	4.82	4.31	3.99	3.75	3.45	3.12	2.75	2.30
23	4.28	3.42	3.03	2.80	2.64	2.53	2.38	2.20	2.00	1.76
	7.88	5.66	4.76	4.26	3.94	3.71	3.41	3.07	2.70	2.26
24	4.26	3.40	3.01	2.78	2.62	2.51	2.36	2.18	1.98	1.73
	7.82	5.61	4.72	4.22	3.90	3.67	3.36	3.03	2.66	2.21
25	4.24	3.38	2.99	2.76	2.60	2.49	2.34	2.16	1.96	1.71
	7.77	5.57	4.68	4.18	3.86	3.63	3.32	2.99	2.62	2.17
26	4.22	3.37	2.98	2.74	2.59	2.47	2.32	2.15	1.95	1.69
	7.72	5.53	4.64	4.14	3.82	3.59	3.29	2.96	2.58	2.13
27	4.21	3.35	2.96	2.73	2.57	2.46	2.30	2.13	1.93	1.67
	7.68	5.49	4.60	4.11	3.78	3.56	3.26	2.93	2.55	2.10
28	4.20	3.34	2.95	2.71	2.56	2.44	2.29	2.12	1.91	1.65
	7.64	5.45	4.57	4.07	3.75	3.53	3.23	2.90	2.52	2.06
29	4.18	3.33	2.93	2.70	2.54	2.43	2.28	2.10	1.90	1.64
	7.60	5.42	4.34	4.04	3.73	3.50	3.20	2.87	2.49	2.03
30	4.17	3.32	2.92	2.69	2.53	2.42	2.27	2.09	1.89	1.62
	7.56	5.39	4.51	4.02	3.70	3.47	3.17	2.84	2.47	2.01
35	4.12	3.26	2.87	2.64	2.48	2.37	2.22	2.04	1.83	1.57
	7.42	5.27	4.40	3.91	3.59	3.37	3.07	2.74	2.37	1.90
40	4.08	3.23	2.84	2.61	2.45	2.34	2.18	2.00	1.79	1.52
	7.31	5.18	4.31	3.83	3.51	3.29	2.99	2.99	2.29	1.82

Contd...

Contd...

	Degrees of freedom for greater mean square									
	1	2	3	4	5	6	8	12	24	∞
45	4.06	3.21	2.81	2.58	2.42	2.31	2.15	1.97	1.76	1.48
	7.23	5.11	4.25	3.77	3.45	3.23	2.94	2.61	2.23	1.75
50	4.03	3.18	2.79	2.56	2.40	2.29	2.13	1.95	1.74	1.44
	7.17	5.06	4.20	3.72	3.41	3.19	2.89	2.56	2.18	1.68
60	4.00	3.15	2.76	2.52	2.37	2.25	2.10	1.92	1.70	1.39
	7.08	4.98	4.13	3.65	3.34	3.12	2.82	2.50	2.12	1.60
70	3.98	3.13	2.74	2.50	2.35	2.23	2.07	1.89	1.67	1.35
	7.01	4.92	4.07	3.60	3.29	3.07	2.78	2.45	2.07	1.53
80	3.96	3.11	2.72	2.49	2.33	2.21	2.06	1.88	1.65	1.31
	6.96	4.88	4.04	3.56	3.26	3.04	2.74	2.42	2.03	1.47
90		3.10	2.71	2.47	2.32	2.20	2.04	1.86	1.64	1.28
	6.92	4.85	4.01	3.53	3.23	3.01	2.72	2.39	2.00	1.43
100	3.94	3.09	2.70	2.46	2.30	2.19	2.03	1.85	1.63	1.26
	6.90	4.82	3.98	3.51	3.21	2.99	2.69	2.37	1.98	1.39
125	3.92	3.07	2.68	2.44	2.29	2.17	2.01	1.83	1.06	1.21
	6.84	4.78	3.94	3.47	3.17	2.95	2.66	2.33	1.94	1.32
150	3.90	3.06	2.66	2.43	2.27	2.16	2.00	1.82	1.59	1.18
	6.81	4.75	3.91	3.45	3.14	2.92	2.63	2.31	1.92	1.27
200	3.89	3.04	2.65	2.42	2.26	2.14	1.98	1.80	1.57	1.14
	6.76	4.71	3.88	3.41	3.11	2.89	2.60	2.28	1.88	1.21
300	3.87	3.03	2.64	2.41	2.25	2.13	1.97	1.79	1.55	1.10
	6.72	4.68	3.85	3.38	3.08	2.86	2.57	2.24	1.85	1.14
400	3.86	3.02	2.63	2.40	2.24	2.12	1.96	1.78	1.54	1.07
	6.70	4.66	3.83	3.37	3.06	2.85	2.56	2.23	1.84	1.11
500	3.86	3.01	2.62	2.39	2.23	2.11	1.96	1.77	1.54	1.06
	6.69	4.65	3.82	3.36	3.05	2.84	2.55	2.22	1.83	1.08
1000	3.85	3.00	2.61	2.38	2.22	2.10	1.95	1.76	1.53	1.03
	6.66	4.63	3.80	3.34	3.04	2.82	2.53	2.20	1.81	1.04
∞	3.84	2.99	2.60	2.37	2.21	2.09	1.94	1.75	1.52	
	6.64	4.60	3.78	3.32	3.02	2.80	2.51	2.18	1.79	

Table L

Calculation of T scores

Proportion below the point	T score	Proportion below the point	T score	Proportion below the point	T score
0.0005	17.1	0.100	37.2	0.900	62.8
0.0007	18.1	0.120	38.3	0.910	63.4
0.0010	19.1	0.140	39.2	0.920	64.1
0.0015	20.3	0.160	40.1	0.930	64.8
0.0020	21.2	0.180	40.8	0.940	65.5
0.0025	21.9	0.200	41.6	0.950	66.4
0.0030	22.5	0.220	42.3	0.960	67.5
0.0040	23.5	0.250	43.3	0.965	68.1
0.0050	24.2	0.300	44.8	0.970	68.8

Contd...

Contd...

Proportion below the point	T score	Proportion below the point	T score	Proportion below the point	T score
0.0070	25.4	0.350	46.1	0.975	69.6
0.010	26.7	0.400	47.5	0.980	70.5
0.015	28.3	0.450	48.7	0.985	71.7
0.020	29.5	0.500	50.5	0.990	73.3
0.025	30.4	0.550	51.3	0.993	74.6
0.030	31.2	0.600	52.5	0.995	75.8
0.035	31.9	0.650	53.9	0.9960	76.5
0.040	32.5	0.700	55.2	0.9970	77.5
0.050	33.6	0.750	56.7	0.9975	78.1
0.060	34.5	0.780	57.7	0.9980	78.7
0.070	35.2	0.800	58.4	0.9985	79.7
0.080	35.9	0.820	59.2	0.9990	80.9
0.090	36.6	0.840	59.9	0.9993	81.9
		0.860	60.8	0.9995	82.9
		0.880	61.7		

Table M

Standard scores (or deviates) and ordinates corresponding to divisions of the area under the normal curve into a larger proportion (B) and a smaller proportion (C); also the value $\sqrt{BC}$

B The larger area	Z Standard score	Y Ordinate	$\sqrt{BC}$	C The smaller area
1	2	3	4	5
0.500	0.0000	0.3989	0.5000	0.500
0.505	0.0125	0.3989	0.5000	0.495
0.510	0.0251	0.3988	0.4999	0.490
0.515	0.0376	0.3987	0.4998	0.485
0.520	0.0502	0.3984	0.4996	0.480
0.525	0.0627	0.3982	0.4994	0.475
0.530	0.0753	0.3978	0.4991	0.470
0.535	0.0878	0.3974	0.4988	0.465
0.540	0.1004	0.3969	0.4984	0.460
0.545	0.1130	0.3958	0.4980	0.455
0.550	0.1257	0.3951	0.4975	0.450
0.555	0.1383	0.3944	0.4970	0.445
0.560	0.1510	0.3944	0.4964	0.440
0.565	0.1637	0.3936	0.4958	0.435
0.570	0.1764	0.3928	0.4951	0.430
0.575	0.1891	0.3919	0.4943	0.425
0.580	0.2019	0.3909	0.4936	0.420
0.585	0.2147	0.3899	0.4927	0.415
0.590	0.2275	0.3887	0.4919	0.410

Contd...

Contd...

B *The larger area*	Z *Standard score*	Y *Ordinate*	$\sqrt{BC}$	C *The smaller area*
0.595	0.2404	0.3876	0.4909	0.405
0.600	0.2533	0.3863	0.4899	0.400
0.605	0.2663	0.3850	0.4889	0.395
0.610	0.2793	0.3837	0.4877	0.390
0.615	0.2924	0.3822	0.4867	0.385
0.620	0.3055	0.3808	0.4854	0.380
0.625	0.3186	0.3792	0.4841	0.375
0.630	0.3319	0.3776	0.4828	0.370
0.635	0.3451	0.3759	0.4814	0.365
0.640	0.3585	0.3741	0.4800	0.360
0.645	0.3719	0.3723	0.4785	0.355
0.650	0.3853	0.3704	0.4770	0.350
0.655	0.3989	0.3684	0.4754	0.345
0.660	0.4125	0.3664	0.4737	0.340
0.665	0.4261	0.3643	0.4720	0.335
0.670	0.4399	0.3621	0.4702	0.330
0.675	0.4538	0.3599	0.4684	0.325
0.680	0.4677	0.3576	0.4665	0.320
0.685	0.4817	0.3552	0.4645	0.315
0.690	0.4959	0.3528	0.4625	0.310
0.695	0.5101	0.3503	0.4604	0.305
0.700	0.5244	0.3477	0.4583	0.300
0.705	0.5388	0.3450	0.4560	0.295
0.710	0.5534	0.3423	0.4538	0.290
0.715	0.5681	0.3395	0.4514	0.285
0.720	0.2828	0.3366	0.4490	0.280
0.725	0.5978	0.3337	0.4465	0.275
0.730	0.6128	0.3306	0.4440	0.270
0.735	0.6280	0.3275	0.4413	0.265
0.740	0.6433	0.3244	0.4386	0.260
0.745	0.6588	0.3211	0.4359	0.255
0.750	0.6745	0.3178	0.4330	0.250
0.755	0.6903	0.3144	0.4301	0.245
0.760	0.7063	0.3109	0.4271	0.240
0.765	0.7225	0.3073	0.4240	0.235
0.770	0.7388	0.3036	0.4208	0.230
0.775	0.7554	0.2999	0.4176	0.225
0.780	0.7722	0.2961	0.4142	0.220
0.785	0.7892	0.2922	0.4108	0.215
0.790	0.8064	0.2882	0.4073	0.210
0.795	0.8239	0.2841	0.4037	0.205
0.800	0.8416	0.2800	0.4000	0.200
0.805	0.8596	0.2757	0.3962	0.195

Contd...

Contd...

B *The larger area*	Z *Standard score*	Y *Ordinate*	$\sqrt{BC}$	C *The smaller area*
0.810	0.8779	0.2714	0.3923	0.190
0.815	0.8965	0.2669	0.3883	0.185
0.820	0.9154	0.2624	0.3842	0.180
0.825	0.9346	0.2578	0.3800	0.175
0.830	0.9542	0.2531	0.3756	0.170
0.835	0.9741	0.2482	0.3712	0.165
0.840	0.9945	0.2433	0.3666	0.160
0.845	1.0152	0.2383	0.3619	0.155
0.850	1.0364	0.2332	0.3571	0.150
0.855	1.0581	0.2279	0.3521	0.145
0.860	1.0803	0.2226	0.3470	0.140
0.865	1.1031	0.2771	0.3417	0.135
0.870	1.1264	0.2115	0.3363	0.130
0.875	1.1503	0.2059	0.3307	0.125
0.880	1.1750	0.2000	0.3250	0.120
0.885	1.2004	0.1941	0.3190	0.115
0.890	1.2265	0.1880	0.3129	0.110
0.895	0.2536	0.1818	0.3066	0.105
0.900	1.2816	0.1755	0.3000	0.100
0.905	1.3106	0.1690	0.2932	0.095
0.910	1.3408	0.1624	0.2862	0.090
0.915	1.3722	0.1556	0.2789	0.085
0.920	1.4051	0.1487	0.2713	0.080
0.925	1.4395	0.1416	0.2634	0.075
0.930	1.4757	0.1343	0.2551	0.070
0.935	1.5141	0.1268	0.2465	0.065
0.940	1.5548	0.1191	0.2375	0.060
0.945	1.5982	0.1112	0.2280	0.055
0.950	1.6449	0.1031	0.2179	0.050
0.955	1.6954	0.0948	0.2073	0.045
0.960	1.7507	0.0862	0.1960	0.040
0.965	1.8119	0.0773	0.1838	0.035
0.970	1.8808	0.0680	0.1706	0.030
0.975	1.9600	0.0584	0.1561	0.025
0.980	2.0537	0.0484	0.1400	0.020
0.985	2.1701	0.0379	0.1226	0.015
0.990	2.3263	0.0267	0.0995	0.010
0.995	2.5758	0.0145	0.0705	0.005
0.996	2.6521	0.0118	0.0631	0.004
0.997	2.7478	0.0091	0.0547	0.003
0.998	2.8782	0.0063	0.0447	0.002
0.999	3.0902	0.0034	0.0316	0.001
0.9995	3.2905	0.0018	0.0224	0.0005

Table N

Values of r_t'

Values of r_t taken as the cosine of an angle

Example: Suppose that $r_t = \cos 45°$. Then $\cos 45° = 0.707$, and $r_t = 0.71$ (to two decimals)

Angle	*Cosine*	*Angle*	*Cosine*	*Angle*	*Cosine*
0	1.000	41	0.755	73	0.292
		42	0.743	74	0.276
5	0.996	43	0.731	75	0.259
		44	0.719	76	0.242
10	0.985	45	0.707	77	0.225
		46	0.695	78	0.208
		47	0.682	79	0.191
15	0.966	48	0.669	80	0.174
16	0.961	49	0.656		
17	0.956	50	0.643	81	0.156
18	0.951			82	0.139
19	0.946	51	0.629	83	0.122
20	0.940	52	0.616	84	0.105
		53	0.602	85	0.087
21	0.934	54	0.588		
22	0.927	55	0.574		
23	0.921	56	0.559	90	0.000
24	0.914	57	0.545		
25	0.906	58	0.530		
26	0.899	59	0.515		
27	0.891	60	0.500		
28	0.883				
29	0.875	61	0.485		
30	0.866	62	0.469		
		63	0.454		
31	0.857	64	0.438		
32	0.848	65	0.423		
33	0.839	66	0.407		
34	0.829	67	0.391		
35	0.819	68	0.375		
36	0.809	69	0.358		
37	0.799	70	0.342		
38	0.788				
39	0.777	71	0.326		
40	0.766	72	0.309		

Table O

Tables of square and square roots

Squares and square roots of the number from 1 to 1000

Number 1	*Square* 2	*Square root* 3	*Number* 4	*Square* 5	*Square root* 6
1	1	1.000	2	4	1.414
3	9	1.732	4	16	2.000
5	25	2.236	6	36	2.449
7	49	2.646	8	64	2.828
9	81	3.000	10	100	3.162
11	121	3.317	12	144	3.464
13	169	3.606	14	196	3.742
15	225	3.873	16	256	4.000
17	289	4.123	18	324	4.243
19	361	4.359	20	400	4.472
21	441	4.583	22	484	4.690
23	529	4.796	24	576	4.899
25	625	5.000	26	676	5.099
27	729	5.196	28	784	5.292
29	841	5.385	30	900	5.477
31	961	5.568	32	1024	5.657
33	1089	5.745	34	1156	5.831
35	1225	5.916	36	1296	6.000
37	1369	6.083	38	1444	6.164
39	1521	6.245	40	1600	6.325
41	1681	6.403	42	1764	6.481
43	1849	6.557	44	1936	6.633
45	2025	6.708	46	2116	6.782
47	2209	6.856	48	2304	6.928
49	2401	7.000	50	2500	7.071
51	2601	7.141	52	2704	7.211
53	2809	7.280	54	2916	7.348
55	3025	7.416	56	3136	7.483
57	3249	7.550	58	3364	7.616
59	3481	7.681	60	3600	7.746
61	3721	7.810	62	3844	7.874
63	3969	7.937	64	4096	8.000
65	4225	8.062	66	4356	8.124
67	4489	8.185	68	4624	8.246
69	4761	8.307	70	4900	8.367
71	5041	8.428	72	5184	8.485
73	5329	8.544			
75	5625	8.660			
77	5929	8.775			
79	6241	8.888			
81	6561	9.000			
83	6889	9.110			

Contd...

Contd...

Number 1	*Square* 2	*Square root* 3	*Number* 4	*Square* 5	*Square root* 6
85	7225	9.220			
87	7569	9.327			
89	7921	9.434			
91	8281	9.539			
93	8649	9.644			
95	9025	9.747			
97	9409	9.849			
99	9801	9.950			
101	10201	10.050			
103	10609	10.149			
105	11025	10.247			
107	11449	10.344			
109	11881	10.440			
111	12321	10.536			
113	12769	10.724			
115	13225				
117	13689				
119	14161				
121	14641				
123	15129				
125	15625				
127	16129				

Index

Page numbers followed by *f* refer to figure and *t* refer to table

D